Strength
of
Materials

in SI Units

Fourth Revised Edition

Foreword by

Dr JP Subrahmanyam

Strength of Materials

in SI Units

Fourth Revised Edition

for B Tech, BSc (Eng), BE, UPSC (IES), AMIE, GATE, and
Courses of Other Engineering Universities
(with Solved Papers)

SS Pathak

BSc, BSc (Engg) (Mechanical), M Tech
Assistant Professor
Department of Mechanical Engineering
Dr KN Modi Institute of Engineering and Technology, Modinagar
Utter Pradesh, India
E-mail: ss_pathak2000@yahoo.co.uk

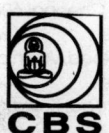

CBS Publishers & Distributors Pvt Ltd

New Delhi • Bengaluru • Chennai • Kochi • Kolkata • Mumbai
Bhopal • Bhubaneswar • Hyderabad • Jharkhand • Nagpur • Patna • Pune • Uttarakhand • Dhaka (Bangladesh)

Strength of
Materials

in SI Units

Fourth Revised Edition

ISBN: 978-93-86217-72-1

Copyright © Author and Publisher

Fourth Revised Edition: 2017

Reprint: 2019

First Edition: 2017
Second Revised Edition: 2011
Third Revised Edition: 2013
Reprints: 2008, 2009, 2010

Published by Satish Kumar Jain and produced by Varun Jain for

CBS Publishers & Distributors Pvt Ltd

4819/XI Prahlad Street, 24 Ansari Road, Daryaganj, New Delhi 110 002, India.
Ph: 23289259, 23266861, 23266867   Website: www.cbspd.com
Fax: 011-23243014   e-mail: delhi@cbspd.com; cbspubs@airtelmail.in.

Corporate Office: 204 FIE, Industrial Area, Patparganj, Delhi-110092
Ph: 4934 4934   Fax: 4934 4935   e-mail: publishing@cbspd.com; publicity@cbspd.com

Branches

- **Bengaluru:** Seema House 2975, 17th Cross, K.R. Road,
  Banasankari 2nd Stage, Bengaluru 560 070, Karnataka
  Ph: +91-80-26771678/79   Fax: +91-80-26771680   e-mail: bangalore@cbspd.com
- **Chennai:** 7, Subbaraya Street, Shenoy Nagar, Chennai 600 030, Tamil Nadu
  Ph: +91-44-26680620, 26681266   Fax: +91-44-42032115   e-mail: chennai@cbspd.com
- **Kochi:** Ashana House, No. 39/1904, AM Thomas Road, Valanjambalam, Ernakulam 682 016, Kochi, Kerala
  Ph: +91-484-4059061-65   Fax: +91-484-4059065   e-mail: kochi@cbspd.com
- **Kolkata:** 6/B, Ground Floor, Rameswar Shaw Road, Kolkata-700 014, West Bengal
  Ph: +91-33-22891126, 22891127, 22891128   e-mail: kolkata@cbspd.com
- **Mumbai:** 83-C, Dr E Moses Road, Worli, Mumbai-400018, Maharashtra
  Ph: +91-22-24902340/41   Fax: +91-22-24902342   e-mail: mumbai@cbspd.com

Representatives

• **Bhopal**	0-8319310552	• **Bhubaneswar**	0-9911037372	• **Hyderabad**	0-9885175004
• **Jharkhand**	0-9811541605	• **Nagpur**	0-9421945513	• **Patna**	0-9334159340
• **Pune**	0-9623451994	• **Uttarakhand**	0-9716462459	• **Dhaka (Bangladesh)**	01912-003485

Printed at: Glorious Printers, Daryaganj, New Delhi, India

Foreword

It gives me a great pleasure to write the Foreword to this book.

The subject of strength of materials is very important to all engineers, in particular students of mechanical, civil and material engineering.

I am sure this book will be a useful addition to the knowledge on the subject.

Dr JP Subrahmanyam
Ex-Professor and Head
Department of Mechanical Engineering
Indian Institute Technology, Delhi

Preface to
the Fourth Revised Edition

It gives me immense pleasure to present the fourth revised edition of the book *Strength of Materials* in the hands of the esteemed readers. The book has been written for second year engineering students as per the syllabi of all Indian universities. The colossal response to the third edition necessitated its thorough revision. I would like to thank the faculty and students of various universities for their suggestions to improve the book. The book is enlarged with addition of new text as well as numerical problems and their solutions along with previous years' questions and solutions. In this edition some calculation errors and misprints have been rectified.

In Chapters 7 to 10, additional material with examples and solutions has been added to enhance the elementary knowledge of the students. Theory and examples are supplemented with detailed explanations and illustrations. Topics, namely 2D and 3D stresses, Mohr's circle, deflection of beams, curved beam, column and strut, etc. have been profusely revised. SI units of measurement have been used.

I am thankful to Mr Satish Kumar Jain, MD, and Mr Y N Arjuna, Sr Vice President, Publishing, Editorial and Publicity, for bringing out the fourth revised edition in a very short period of time.

Although every effort has been taken to make this edition error free, suggestions and feedback are welcome on ss_pathak2000@yahoo.com.

SS Pathak

Contents in Brief

Contents

8. COMBINED STRESSES   8.1–8.12

9. SHEAR STRESSES IN BEAMS   9.1–9.24

10. DEFLECTION OF BEAMS   10.1 – 10.62

11. INDETERMINATE BEAM (Fixed and Continuous Beam)   11.1 – 11.17

12. TORSION   12.1 – 12.25

NOTATIONS

$a; a_1, a_2$ .... Distance; area
A, B, C .... Points; Constant
b .... Distance; width
d .... Distance; diameter; depth
e .... Eccentricity
E .... Modulus of elasticity; Young's Modulus
f .... Function
F .... Force
F_s .... Shear force
G .... Modulus of rigidity
$I; I_X, I_Y$ .... Moment of Inertia
I_{xy} .... Product of Inertia
$I_p; J$ .... Polar moment of Inertia
K .... Bulk Modulus; Stress concentration factor
k .... Radius of gyration; Stiffness of spring
l, L .... Span length
l_e .... Effective length
m .... Mass
M .... Bending moment
$M_x, M_y; M_z$ .... Resolved moment
p .... Pressure; Compressive stress
P .... Load; Power
r, R .... Radius
r_i .... Inner radius
r_o .... Outer radius
$\bar{r}$ .... Radius of Centroidal axis
R_N .... Radius of Neutral axis
T .... Torque; Temperature
u, v .... Rectangular coordinates
u .... Strain energy density; radial shift
V, v .... Volume
w .... Weight per unit length; distributed load intensity
W .... Weight; concentrated load
x, y, z .... Rectangular coordinates;
$\bar{x}, \bar{y}, \bar{z}$ .... Coordinate of centroid;
Z .... Section modulus
z .... Coordinate; intercept
$\alpha, \beta, \gamma, \theta; \phi$ .... Angle
α .... Coefficient of thermal expansion
γ .... Shearing strain; specific weight
$\delta; y$ .... Deflection
σ .... Stress; σ_1, σ_2 Principal stress
ε .... Strain
ε_l .... Longitudinal strain
ε_v .... Volumetric strain
τ .... Shear stress
ω .... Angular velocity
ρ .... Density
ν .... Poisson's Ratio
θ .... Slope of beam; twist of shaft.
NA .... Neutral Axis
CA .... Centroidal Axis

SIMPLE STRESSES AND STRAINS

1.1 INTRODUCTION

At the outset let us discuss what is strength of materials. We know that matter is made up of small particles called molecule. Molecules in solid are attached to each other by the force of cohesion. When we apply external force, the distance between the molecules tend to increase which is resisted by the force of cohesion.

As the force (applied) is increased, the resisting force (due to cohesion) also increases simultaneously till the maximum resistance is reached. **This maximum resistance offered by the material is called it's strength.** For example wall of gunbarrel must be able to resist pressure developed as a result of firing; piston cylinder must be able to resist pressure developed as a result of combustion; the wall of water pipe, steam pipe must be able to sustain pressure of fluid flowing through the pipe. **Strength of materials involves the analytical method of determining-strength, stiffness and stability of load carrying component of machine.**

In strength of material we consider that
— material is elastic
— deformation is small
— when machine member/structure is loaded these should neither break nor deform excessively

Many structural member/material like steel, Aluminium are perfectly elastic within limits *i.e.* if the load is not exceeding much.

The strength of materials depends on —
— the type of loading
— temperature
— internal structure of the material
  Let us start with the term load.

External force applied on the body is called load denoted by 'P'. It's SI unit is Newton.

Since Newton is small, force is expressed in Kilo-Newton and Mega Newton.

$$1 \text{ kN} = 10^3 \text{ N}$$

$$1 \text{ Mega Newton} = 10^6 \text{ N}$$
$$1 \text{ Giga Newton} = 10^9 \text{ N}$$

1.2 CLASSIFICATION OF LOAD

Load may be in the form of

— Axial load (P)

    (a) Tensile (P_t) (b) Compressive (P_c)

— Shear (τ)

— Torque (T)

— Moment (M)

Or Combination of these.

Load which is applied to most components in engineering is a combination (superposition) of these. For example, a rotating shaft which transmits power is subjected not only to torsion but also to bending and to direct shear. We will discuss these in details later.

Loads may also be classified on the basis of their variation with a respect to time as static, quasi-static and dynamic. Static loads are those which do not change their magnitude or direction or point of application with respect to time. Those loads which vary at a very small rate so that inertial effects may be neglected are called quasi-static. Loads of dynamic character change with time at a fast rate. The action of such loads set up vibration, fatigue etc. in the body.

As an engineer, we study the various types of load and its effect on the elastic bodies. We also analyze and design various machines and load bearing structure. Analysis and design of a given structure involve determination of stresses and deformations.
It has been observed that

    (i)   load may develop 'stress' and 'strain' in a body simultaneously.

    (ii) load may develop 'deflection' in a body i.e. in beam; cantilever etc.

    (iii) load may develop 'buckling' in the body i.e. the case of column.
We will discuss the effect of load on the elastic bodies in various chapters of this book.

1.3 STRESS OR ENGINEERING STRESS

When load is applied on an elastic body, internal resisting force is developed inside the material to counter the effect of the external force.

The internal resisting force per unit area of the body is called stress or enginneering stress and is denoted by the letter σ.

Difference between Stress and Pressure:

Stress is not same as pressure. Pressure is reserved for a specific stress state in which there is no shear components and all the normal components are equal.

Stress $(\sigma) = \dfrac{P}{A}$. It represents the **average value** of stress over the cross-section rather than the stress at a specific point of the cross-section.

So, if a body is loaded externally then internal forces are distributed throughout the region of the body and stresses will be caused. For the defination of stress, we intersect the body by a imaginary plane like shown in the Fig. 1.1 (a).

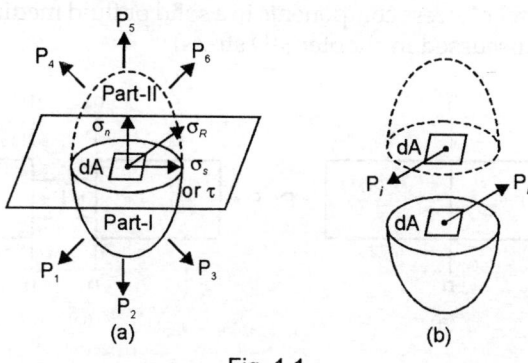

Fig. 1.1

Both parts of the body then interact through forces of equal magnitude and opposite in direction Fig. 1.1(b).

Let dP be the elementary load acting on an area dA of the cross-section then $\left(\dfrac{dP}{dA}\right)$ is the average stress on this element.

The limit $\sigma = \lim\limits_{\Delta A \to 0} \dfrac{\Delta P}{\Delta A} = \dfrac{dP}{dA}$ is called the stress* at a point of the cross-section.

The Standard Unit (SI unit) for stress is N/m^2 'or' Pascal. Typical level of stress are several million Pascals, so the most covenient unit for stress is the megapascal or MPa. The stress magnitude 1 MPa is equal to the pressure (p) at a depth (z) of about 100 m in water or 37 in rock using the relationship $p = \rho gz$, where

ρ = density of material

g = acceleration due to gravity

1 N/mm² = 1 MPa (mega pascal); 1 Pa = 1 N/m²

Mathematically, Stress** (σ) = $\dfrac{\text{Load}}{\text{Area}} = \dfrac{P}{A} \dfrac{N}{m^2}$

Stress is a tensor*** entity. The stress tensor characterizes the stress state at a point in the body. Stress is measured by photoelasticity technique (in this book we will compute the stress and check with the permissible stress or design stress for proper functioning of the machine member or structural member).

The stress at any point on a plane can be resolved into two components — one along normal and the other perpendicular to the normal *i.e.* tangent to the plane.

The component of stress along the normal is called the normal stress (σ_n) or direct stress (σ) and the component tangential to the plane is called the tangential stress (σ_s) or shear stress (τ).

---

*Six components are required to describe the state of stress at a point in a body under the most general loading condition which we will discuss in 3-D stress.

**Stress developed on the body due to application of load, should never exceed the ultimate tensile strength for brittle materials and yield strength for ductile materials.

***A physical quantity is said to be tensor if it is neither a scalar nor a vector.

(The complete set of stress components in a solid or fluid medium are written as τ_{ij} which will be discussed in chapter 3-D stress).

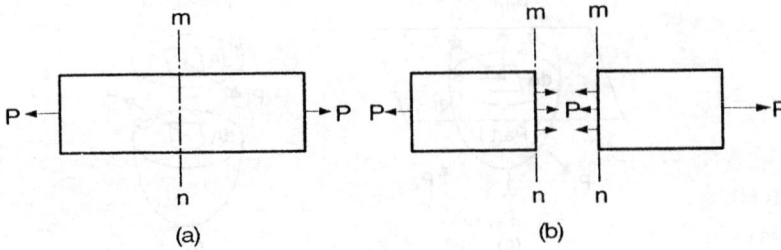

(a)   (b)

Fig. 1.2

Let us consider a prismatic bar having cross-sectional area A subjected to load P, then normal stress at any point of the bar $= \dfrac{P}{A}$.

The component of stress along x-axis and y-axis are written as σ_x and σ_y respectively. When an elastic body is subjected to stresses σ_x and σ_y along x and y-axes respectively then we call it biaxial stress system. Biaxial stress arises in the analysis of pressure vessel (thin); beams; shaft and many other structural parts.

When the normal stress acts outwards from the plane then it is called *tensile stress*.

Tensile stress is considered positive (+).

Similarly, normal stress acting towards the plane is called 'compressive stress' and it is considered negative (–).

A tensile stress tends to stretch the member (of machine part or structural part) apart, whereas, a compressive stress tends to compress the material of the load carrying member and shortens the member itself.

Shear Stress

When equal and opposite transverse loads P and P' of magnitude P are applied to a member AB, shearing stress τ are created over any section located between the points of application of two loads as shown in Fig. 1.3.

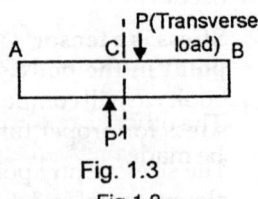

Fig. 1.3

Fig 1.3

In practice shearing stress act simultaneously with normal stress. However, there are cases where the shear stresses are considerably larger than the normal stresses and as such the normal streses are ignored in the analysis.

Riveted, bolted and welded joints are examples of simple shear.

Let us consider a rectangular block fixed at the lower surface and subjected to load P parallel to its surface as in Fig. 1.3(a).

By application of load P (which is tangenital), the plane gets distorted.

If A = Area of top or bottom of the block.

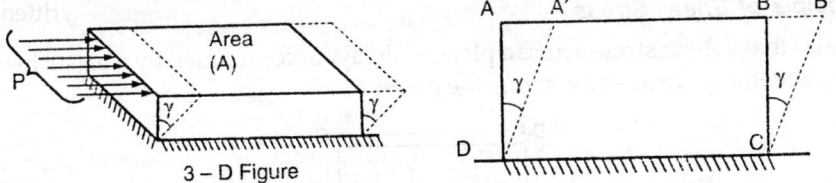

3 – D Figure

Fig 1.3(a)

Then shear stress $(\tau) = \dfrac{P}{A}$. The value obtained is an average value of shearing stress over the entire section.

Practical application shear stress are given below:

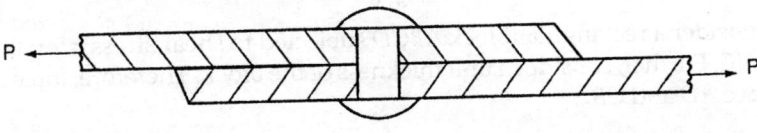

Fig 1.4

In this figure there is only one critical section of the rivet where the failure by shear can take place. This is called a case of single shear (Fig. 1.4).

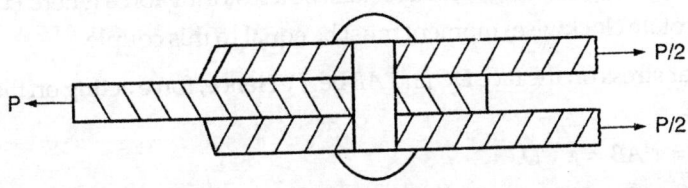

Fig 1.5

In the same manner, there is a case of double shear where the tendency of failure occurs at two sections as shown in Fig. 1.5.

Here, average shear stress $(\tau) = \left[\dfrac{P/2}{A}\right] = \left[\dfrac{P}{2A}\right]$

The other example of shear is punching operation by which small hole or slot can be made on the metal plates.

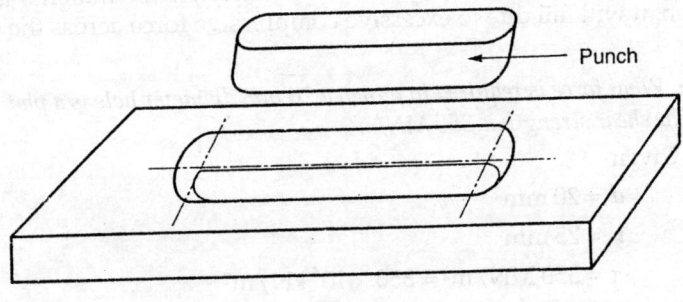

Fig. 1.6

Principle of Shear Stress

It states that a shear stress across a plane is always accompanied by a balancing or complementary shear stress across the plane.

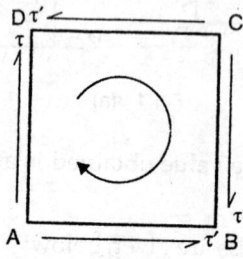

Fig. 1.7

Let us consider a rectangular block $ABCD$ subjected to shear stress τ on the face AD and BC. Further, consider a unit thickness of the block. Therefore, force acting on the face AD and CB,

$$P = \tau \cdot AD = \tau \cdot CB$$

Since these are equal and opposite forces so they will form a couple whose moment is equal to $\tau \times AD \times AB$.

If the block is in equilibrium then there must be a restoring force where ($\tau\uparrow$ and $\tau\downarrow$ will try to rotate clockwise) moment must be equal to this couple.

Let the shear stress on the face DC and AB be τ'. Hence, force acting on the face AB and CD are

$$P = \tau'AB = \tau'CD$$

These two forces ($\tau'AB$ and $\tau'CD$) will also form a couple (CCW).

Equating these two Moments

$$\tau \cdot AD \cdot AB = \tau'AB \cdot AD$$

$\therefore$
$$\tau = \tau'$$

As a result of shear forces which forms a couple, the diagonal BD will be subjected to tension whereas diagonal AC will be subjected to compression.

If the material of the machine under study is poor is tension, it will fail due to excessive tensile stress across diagonal BD. Similarly, if the material is poor in compression, it will fail due to excessive compressive force across the diagonal AC.

EXAMPLE 1: *What force is required to punch a 20 mm diameter hole is a plat that is 25 mm thick? The shear strength is 350 MN/m².*

SOLUTION Given

$$d = 20 \, mm$$
$$t = 25 \, mm$$
$$\tau = 350 \, MN/m^2 = 350 \times 10^3 \, kN/m^2$$

The resisting area is the shaded area along the perimeter and shearing force is equal to the punching force P.

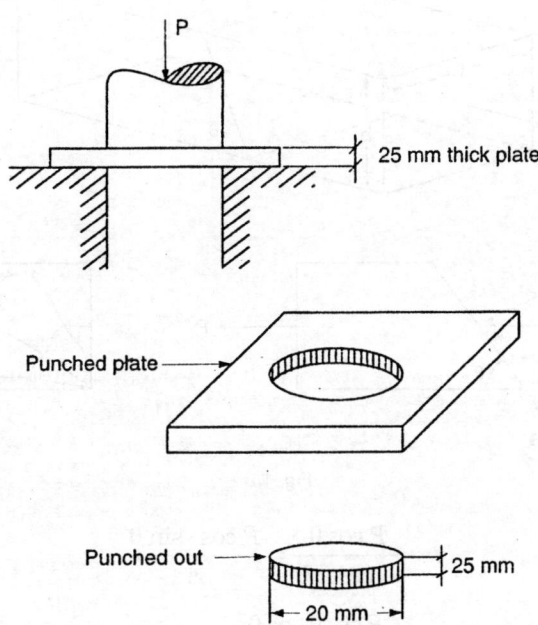

Fig. 1.8

Shearing force (P) = Shearing stress × Resisting area

$$= \tau \times \pi \times d \times t$$

$$= 350 \times 10^3 \times \left(\pi \times \frac{20}{10^3} \times \frac{25}{10^3} \right) \text{kN}$$

$$= 350 \times \frac{22}{7} \times 20 \times \frac{20}{10^3} \text{ kN}$$

$$= 550 \text{ kN} \qquad\qquad\qquad \textbf{Ans.}$$

EXAMPLE 2 *Two blocks of wood width 'b' and thickness 't' are glued together along the joint inclined at the angle θ as shown in the figure. Using the free body diagram show that*

the shearing stress on the glued joint is $\tau = \dfrac{P \sin 2\theta}{2A}$ *where A is the cross sectional area.*

SOLUTION Shear force (F_S) = τ · Area of oblique plane

$$= \tau \cdot A \operatorname{cosec} \theta \qquad\qquad \text{...(I)}$$

Further $\qquad\qquad F_S = P \cos \theta \qquad\qquad\qquad \text{...(II)}$

From I and II we have

$$\tau \cdot A \operatorname{cosec} \theta = P \cdot \cos \theta$$

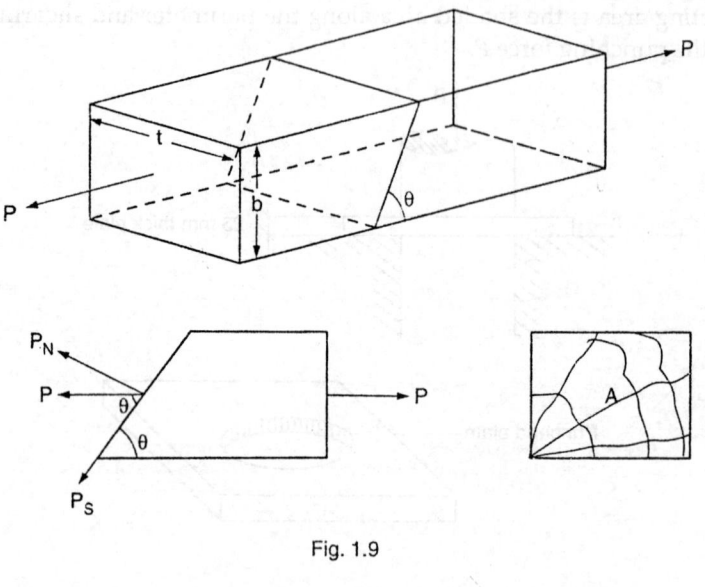

Fig. 1.9

$$\therefore \qquad \tau = \frac{P \cos \theta}{A \csc \theta} = \frac{P \cos \cdot \sin \theta}{A}$$

$$= \frac{2F \sin \theta \cos \theta}{2A}$$

$$= \frac{P}{2A} \sin 2\theta \qquad\qquad\qquad \textbf{Proved}$$

Bearing Stress (σ_{br})

When one body rests on another and transfers a load normal to it then such form of stress is called bearing stress.

Bearing stress is developed **at the surface in contact**.

$$\text{Bearing stress } (\sigma_{br}) = \frac{\text{Applied load}}{\text{Bearing Area}}$$

$$= \frac{P}{A_{br}}$$

where A_{br} = Bearing Area.

For flat surfaces in contact, the bearing area is the area over which the load is transferred from one member to other.

If two parts are having different area, then the smaller area is used.

Bearing stress is very important in design and in Building Construction.

EXAMPLE 1 *A rivet joint shown in figure has 110 mm wide plate and 20 mm rivet diameter. The allowable stresses are 120 MPa for bearing in the plate material and 60 MPa for shearing of the rivet. Determine*

(a) the minimum thickness of each plate and

(b) The largest average tensile stress in the plates.

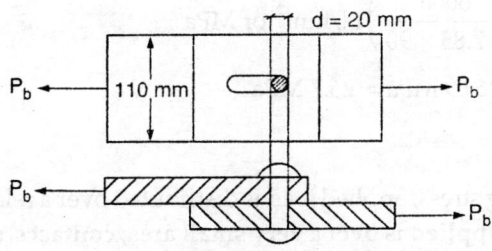

Fig. 1.10

SOLUTION Given

$$d = 20 \text{ mm}$$

$$\sigma_{bearing} = 120 \text{ MPa} = 120 \text{ N/mm}^2$$

$$\tau = 60 \text{ MPa} = 60 \text{ N/mm}^2$$

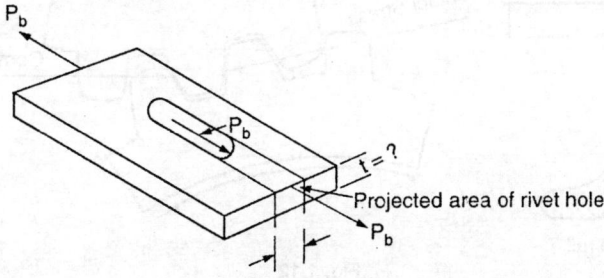

Fig. 1.11

(a) From shearing of rivet

$$P = \tau \cdot A_{rivet}$$

$$= 60 \times \frac{\pi}{4} (20)^2$$

$$= 6000 \, \pi \text{ Newton}$$

From bearing of plate material

$$P = \sigma_{bearing} \times A_{bearing}$$

$$6000 \, \pi = 120 \times (20t)$$

$$\therefore \qquad t = \left(\frac{6000 \, \pi}{120 \times 20} \right) \text{ mm} = 7.849 \simeq 7.85 \text{ mm} \qquad \textbf{Ans.}$$

(b) Largest average tensile stress in the plate

$$P = \sigma \cdot A$$

$$6000\,\pi = [7.85 \times (110 - 20)]$$

$$\sigma = \left(\frac{6000\,\pi}{7.85 \times 90}\right) \text{N/mm}^2 \text{ or MPa}$$

$$= 26.69\,\text{MPa} \simeq 26.7\,\text{MPa} \qquad \textbf{Ans.}$$

Contact Stress

In the case of bearing stress, applied load is distributed over a relatively large area. **But when the load applied is over a very small area, contact stress comes in the picture.**

Examples of contact stress are:

  (i) steel rail wheel on a rail

 (ii) two convex curved surfaces such as gear teeth in contact.

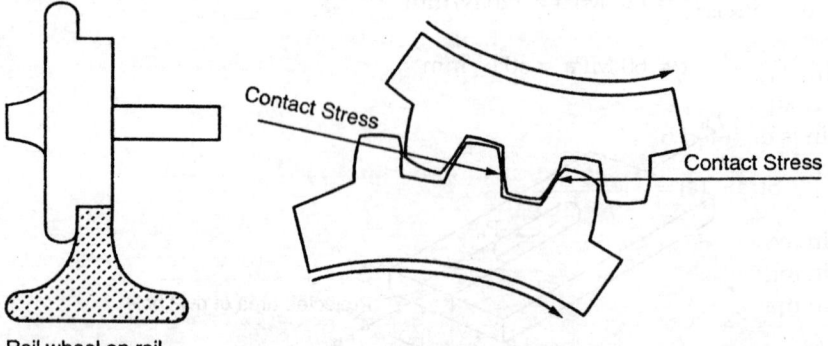

Rail wheel on rail

Fig. 1.12

Hydrostatic Stress*

This stress arises when body is subjected to equal external pressure at all points on the body *e.g.* when the body is immersed in a fluid at a large depth. Hydrostatic stress is compressive in nature and is equal to the pressure intensity to which the body is subjected. It is denoted by letter p.

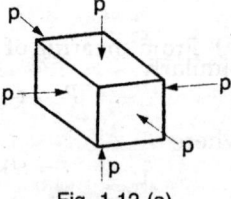

Fig. 1.12 (a)

True Stress

True stress is equal to the load divided by the instantaneous cross-sectional area through which it acts. True stress occurs due to the change in cross-section that occurs with changing load

$$\sigma = \frac{P}{A_i} \text{ where } A_i = \text{instantaneous Cross-sectional Area}$$

Besides these stresses discussed so far there are other types of stresses also. These are:

Residual Stress: Residual stresses are due to manufacturing process that leave a stress in a material. Welding leaves residual stresses in the metal welded.

---

*In metal forming process also hydrostatic stress arises.

Structural Stress: These stresses are produced in structural member because of the weights they support. These stresses are found in building foundation and framework as well as in machine parts.

Pressure Stress: Pressure stresses are induced in vessel containing pressurized fluid.

Flow Stress: Flow stress occurs when a mass of flowing fluid induce a dynamic pressure on a conduit wall.

Fatigue Stress: Fatigue stress arises due to cyclic loading. Rotation of shaft continuously develops a fatigue stress.

*These stresses are used in various engineering field.

1.4 STRAIN

The study of strain in a elastic body is the study of the displacement of points in the body relative to another when the body is deformed.

A load carrying member deforms under the influence of load applied.

Common forms of deformation or distortion** are —

(i) elongation   (ii) twisting
(iii) bending   (iv) shearing

Strain is also called unit deformation and is found by dividing the total deformation by the original length of bar.

Strain is denoted by letter epsilon (ε)

$$\text{Strain }(\varepsilon) = \frac{\text{Total deformation}}{\text{Original length}}$$

Strain may be longitudinal denoted by (ε_l)

Strain may be shear denoted by (γ or ϕ)

Strain may be volumetric denoted by (ε_v)

$\varepsilon_l = \dfrac{\Delta l}{l_i}$, where Δl = total elongation; l_i = original length, l_f = final length

∴ $\Delta l = (l_f - l_i)$

Similarly, $\varepsilon_v = \dfrac{\Delta V}{V}$, where ΔV = change in volume; V = original volume.

$\Delta V = (V_f - V_i)$

where V_f = final volume

V_i = initial volume

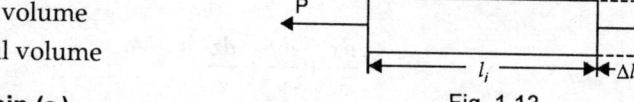

Longitudinal strain (ε_l)   Fig. 1.13

Longitudinal strain causes extension 'or' contraction in the body.

---

*Whether a machine member or structural member, stresses develop on these when loads are applied but as a designer or engineer, our aim should be to limit the stress by proper selection of material, factor of safety (FOS) and by suitable design in such a manner that machine member or structural member should not fail on application of loads. Unwanted stress leads to failure of the machine or structure.

**If the distortion disappears and the metal returns to its dimension upon removal of the load, the strain is called elastic strain. If the distortion disappears and metal remains distorted, the strain is called 'plastic strain'.

Shear strain (γ or ϕ)

Shear strain is the strain produced under shear stress.

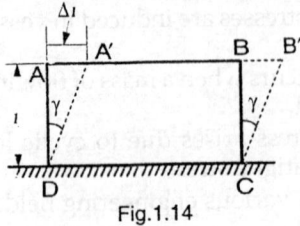

Fig.1.14

In the above figure

$$\text{Shear strain} = \tan \gamma = \frac{\Delta l}{l}$$

Shear strain causes angular distortion on the body.

Volumetric strain (ε_v) 'OR' Elastic dialation:

When a body is subjected to hydrostatic stress, it causes a change in the volume.

$$\varepsilon_v = \frac{\Delta V}{V}$$

Let a cuboid of sides x, y, and z are subjected to hydrostaic stress and as a result of stress its sides change by dx, dy and dz respectively.

$\therefore$ Change in volume $= (x + dx)(y + dy)(z + dz) - xyz$

$$= (xyz + xydz + yzdx + zxdy) - xyz$$

$$\left[\begin{matrix}\text{Neglecting smaller forms}\\ \text{viz } dx \cdot dy, dy \cdot dz \text{ etc.}\end{matrix}\right]$$

$$= yzdx + zxdy + xydz$$

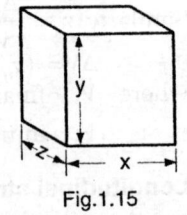

$\therefore$ Volumetric strain $(\varepsilon_v) = \dfrac{yzdx + zxdy + xydz}{xyz}$

$$= \frac{dx}{x} + \frac{dy}{y} + \frac{dz}{z}$$

Fig.1.15

$$= \varepsilon_x + \varepsilon_y + \varepsilon_z$$

This shows that volumetric strain is equal to the sum of linear strains in x, y and z direction.

1.5 MEASUREMENT OF STRAIN

The instrument by which strain is measured is called **extensiometer.** The most commonly used extensiometer are the resistance wire **electrical strain gauge** which is made of fine wire filament cemented on the surface of the body so that the wire of the strain gauge deforms as the surface of the body deforms. The operation of the strain gauge is based on the principle that as the wire elongates or shrinks, it's electrical resistance changes in proportion to the change of its length.

1.6 POISSON'S RATIO (v)

When a body is subjected to a load, strain occurs in the lateral direction also which is opposite in sign to that of the direction of load applied.

It has also been observed that lateral strain is always proportional to the longitudinal strain.

If you take a rubber piece having dia. 'd' and length l and if you apply a tensile load you will find that the length of rubber piece increases whereas the diameter decreases.

We define Poisson's ratio as the ratio of lateral strain to axial strain or longitudinal strain. Poisson's ratio is denoted by letter v (nu).

$$i.e. \quad \text{Poisson's ratio } (v) = \frac{\text{Lateral strain}}{\text{Axial strain}} = \frac{-\varepsilon_l}{\varepsilon_a}$$

$$= \frac{\text{Change in dia./original dia.}}{\text{Change in length/original length}} = -\frac{\Delta d/d}{\Delta l/l}$$

when the sample piece has circular section**.

The negative sign on the lateral strain is introduced to ensure that Poisson's Ratio (v) is a positive number.

Most commonly used metallic materials have a Poisson's ratio value between 0.25 and 0.35. Poisson's ratio is an elastic property of the material. For steel, it's value is approximately 0.3.

Elastomers and rubber may have Poisson's ratios approaching 0.50.

Approximate value of Poisson's Ratio (v) of various material are given below:

Material	Poisson's Ratio (v)
Aluminium	0.33
Brass	0.33
Cast Iron	0.27
*Concrete	0.10-0.25 (depending upon grade)
Copper	0.33
Phospher Bronze	0.35
Carbon and Alloy steel	0.29
Stainless steel (18-8)	0.30
Titanium	0.30

1.7 HOOK'S LAW

Hook's law states that within elastic limit stress is proportional to strain.

Mathematically $\sigma \propto \varepsilon$

or, $\sigma = E \cdot \varepsilon$ (when strain occurs in only one direction)

---

*Concrete is graded according to it's compressive strength which varies from 14 MPa to 48 MPa. Tensile strength of concrete is extremly low.

**Section may be rectangular square elliptical or any shape

In that case,

$$\text{Poisson's ratio } (v) = \frac{\text{Change in Cross Section Area/Original Cross Section Area}}{\text{Change in length/original length}}$$

This constant of proportionality (E) is called modulus of elasticity of the material. E is a measure of the stiffness of a material. E is determined by the slope of straight line portion of the stress–strain curve. A material having a steeper slope on the strain–strain curve will be stiffer and will deform less under load than a material having less steep slope (Fig. 1.16).

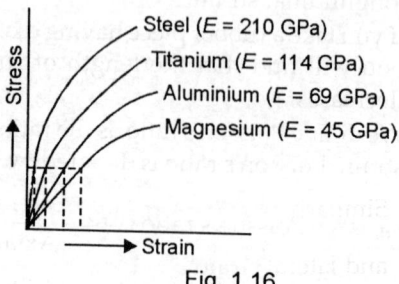

Fig. 1.16 illustrates the concept by showing the straight line portion of the stress-strain curve for steel, titanium, aluminium and magnesium.

Further, shear stress (τ) $\propto$ shear strain (γ)

or, $\tau = G \cdot \gamma$

$\therefore$ $G = \dfrac{\tau}{\gamma}$

Fig. 1.16

The constant of proportionality (G) is called the **'modulus of rigidity'**.

Hook's law is obeyed within certain limit by most ferrous alloys and other engineering materials such as concrete; timber and non-ferrous alloys with reasonable accuracy.

Poisson's ratio permits us to extend Hook's law of uniaxial stress to the biaxial and triaxial stresses also. Body subjected to σ_x and σ_y or σ_y and σ_z or σ_z and σ_x only are called biaxial stress and a body subjected to 3 stresses $i.e.$ σ_x; σ_y and σ_z are called 3-D stresses. Biaxial stresses and triaxial stresses arise in the analysis of pressure vessels, beams, shaft and any other structure parts.

If an element is subjected to tensile stresses in the x and y direction then the strain in the x direction due to tensile stress σ_x is $\dfrac{\sigma_x}{E}$.

Similtaneously, the tensile stress σ_y will produce lateral contraction in the x-direction of amout $(-)v \cdot \dfrac{\sigma_y}{E}$. So, the resultant strain in the x-direction will be

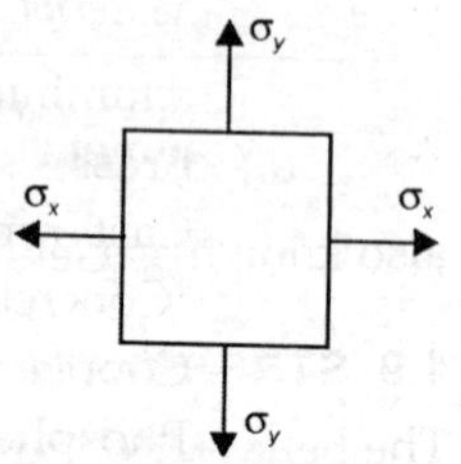

$$\varepsilon_x = \frac{\sigma_x}{E} - v \cdot \frac{\sigma_y}{E}$$

Similarly, total strain in the y-direction will be

$$\varepsilon_y = \frac{\sigma_y}{E} - v \cdot \frac{\sigma_x}{E}$$

Fig. 1.17

Poisson's ratio (v) are 0.25 to 0.30 for steel, approximately 0.33 for most other metals, 0.20 and 0.5 for concrete and rubber, respectively.

1.8 GENERALISED HOOK'S LAW (for Linear Elastic and Isotropic Materials)

Let an element of an elastic body is subjected to three dimensional stress σ_x, σ_y and σ_z along x, y and z axes, respectively.

Strain due to σ_x is $\varepsilon_x = \dfrac{\sigma_x}{E}$ (longitudinal)

and lateral strain $\varepsilon_y = \varepsilon_z = -v \cdot \dfrac{\sigma_x}{E}$ (lateral)

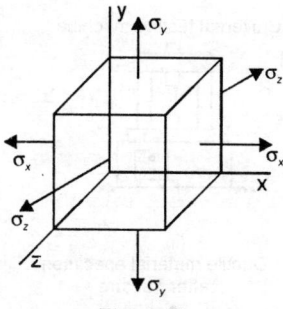

Fig. 1.18

Similarly, stress σ_y applied along y-axis produces longitudinal strain $\varepsilon_y = \dfrac{\sigma_y}{E}$

and lateral strain $\varepsilon_x = \varepsilon_z = -v \cdot \dfrac{\sigma_y}{E}$ and stress σ_z applied along z-axis produces

longitudinal strain $\varepsilon_z = \dfrac{\sigma_z}{E}$ and lateral strain $\varepsilon_x = \varepsilon_y = -v \cdot \dfrac{\sigma_z}{E}$

Therefore, total strain

along x-axis $\qquad \varepsilon_x = \dfrac{\sigma_x}{E} - v \cdot \dfrac{\sigma_y}{E} - v \cdot \dfrac{\sigma_z}{E}$

along y-axis $\qquad \varepsilon_y = \dfrac{\sigma_y}{E} - v \cdot \dfrac{\sigma_z}{E} - v \cdot \dfrac{\sigma_x}{E}$

along z-axis $\qquad \varepsilon_z = \dfrac{\sigma_z}{E} - v \cdot \dfrac{\sigma_x}{E} - v \cdot \dfrac{\sigma_y}{E}$

$\therefore \qquad \varepsilon_x + \varepsilon_y + \varepsilon_z = \dfrac{\sigma_x}{E}(1 - 2v) + \dfrac{\sigma_z}{E}(1 - 2v)$

$\therefore \qquad$ Volumetric strain $(\varepsilon_v) = (\varepsilon_x + \varepsilon_y + \varepsilon_z) = \left(\dfrac{\sigma_x + \sigma_y + \sigma_z}{E}\right)(1 - 2v)$

also known as Generalised Hook's law.

1.9 STRESS–STRAIN CURVE

The behaviour of ductile materials such as steel* which is subjected to tensile load is studied by a testing specimen in a tensile testing machine. Steel refers to alloy of iron and carbon and in many cases, other elements. Steels are classified as carbon steels, alloy steel and stainless steel.

The result of tensile test are expressed by means of stress–strain relationship and plotted in the form of a graph as shown in Fig. 1.18(a).

Stress–strain curve generated from tensile test result help engineers to know constitutive relationship between stress and strain for a particular material. The typical region in stress–strain curve are—

(a) elastic region (b) yielding (c) strain hardening (d) necking and failure

---

*According to American Iron and Steel Institute (AISI), a steel is considered to be carbon steel when carbon percentage is 0.16–0.29% (also called mild steel).

Density of mild steel = 7.85 g/cm³, $E = 210 \times 10^3$ MPa

Carbon steel is also called as plain carbon steel.

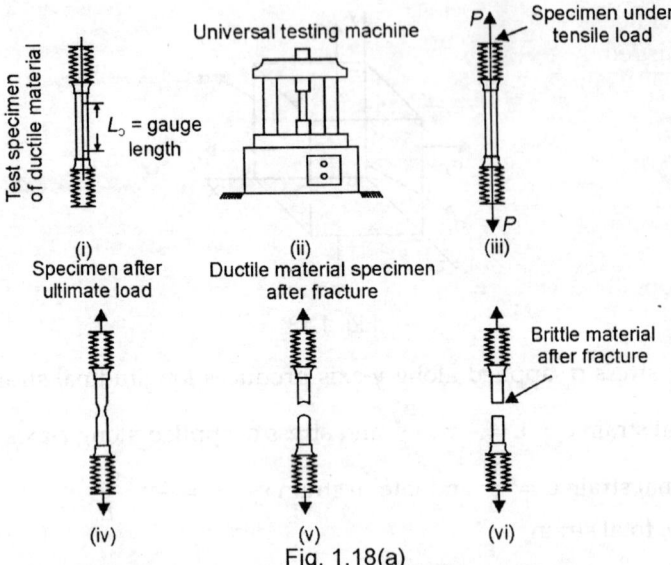

Fig. 1.18(a)

In the following graph:

      P denotes proportional limit E denotes elastic limit

      Y_1 denotes upper yield point Y_2 denotes lower yield point

      U denotes ultimate strength F denotes fracture point

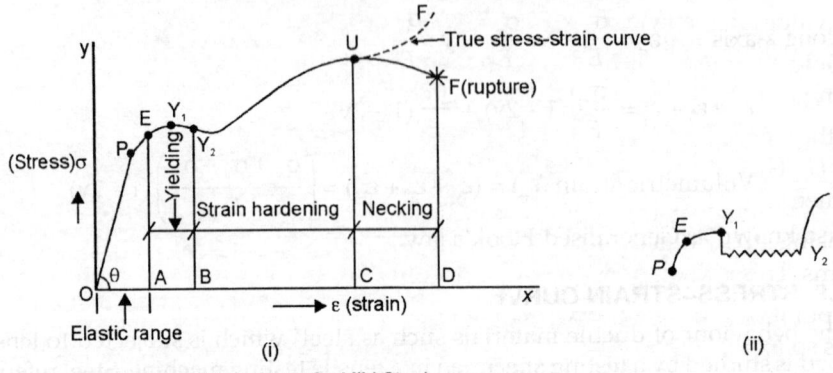

Stress–Strain Curve for Mild Steel

Fig. 1.18(b)

When the loads are increased gradually, the strain (ε) is proportional to load or stress up to point (P). So, P is called proportional limit. Hook's law is applicable in this region.

N.B.: Yield criterion often expressed as yield surface or yield locus, is an hypothesis concerning the limit of elasticity under any combination of stresses.

Lower carbon steels suffer from yield point runout where the material has two yield points. The first yield point (Y_1) is higher than second yield (Y_2) and yield drops dramatically (Y_2) after upper yield power (Y_1). If a low carbon steel is only stressed to some point between the upper and lower yield point then the surface may develop LUDER BANDS. A luder band is a localized band of plastic deformation which occurs in certain materials before fracture.

Even if the specimen is beyond P and up to E it will regain its initial size and shape when the load is removed. This indicates that the material is in elastic range upto point E. Therefore, E is called the elastic limit. **Elastic limit of the material is defined as the maximum stress without any permanent deformation.**

The proportional limit and elastic limit* are very close to each other and it is difficult to distinguish between points P and E on the stress-strain diagram.

Many a times these two are taken to be equal. When the specimen is stressed beyond E, plastic deformation occurs and material starts yielding. During this stage, it is not possible to recover the initial size and shape of the specimen on the removal of load.

Beyond E, the strain increases at a faster rate up to point Y_1 i.e., there is an appreciable increase in strain without much increase in stress.

In the case of mild stress (M.S.) there is small reduction in load and the curve drops down to point Y_2 immediately after yielding starts.

Y_1 is the upper yield point

and Y_2 is the lower yield point

upper and lower yield points can be obtained only in a carefully controlled test, otherwise the region from E and Y_1 to Y_2 merges in to one curve nearly horizontal apparently an increase of strain from 0.12% to 2% at a constant rate from Y_1 to Y_2, is an unstable region and the curve may show many peaks and valley as shown in Figure 1.18 (b). The onset of plastic deformation is called yielding of material. The lower value is called yield stress.

The yield strength is defined as the maximum stress at which a marked increase in elongation occurs without increases in the load.

After the yield point, if the load is increased further then the stress curve rises upto point U. The stress corresponding to point U is called ultimate stress of the specimen.

Increasing stress after yield point shows that material is becoming stronger as it deforms. This is known as ****work hardening or strain hardening.**

After point U, necking of specimen starts and at point F, fracture of test specimen occurs so F is called fracture point. The stress corresponding to point F is called 'Breaking stress'.

Dotted line in the curve shows the actual or true stress-strain diagram.

The structural steel that contains 0.2% carbon as an alloy is classified as low carbon steel. **With increase in carbon content, steel becomes less ductile but has higher yield stress and higher ultimate stress.**

For many ductile materials other than mild steel e.g., aluminium, copper etc. no **definite yield point is obtained. For such materials the shape of curve on stress-strain diagram is shown in Figure 1.18 (c).**

In this case, an arbitrary yield stress may be determined by offset method.

---

*Most of engineering structure are designed to function within their elastic range only.
**To remove strain hardening we use heat treatment process commonly known as annealing. After proper annealing the material returns to its original state.

In this method a line *MN* is drawn parallel to initial slope line *OA* on the stress-strain curve but is offset by some standard amount of strain such as 0.002 (or 0.2%). The intersection of line and the stress-strain curve defines the yield stress (*Y*). The yield stress determined in this way is called **Proof stress.**

High tensile steels, aluminium alloys, copper fall in this category.

The actual or true stress-strain curve is shown by dotted line in Fig. 1.18 (a) for mild steel and in Fig 1.18(c) for aluminium/copper.

Steel and aluminium alloy specimen exhibit ductile behaviour and a fracture occurs only after a considerable amount of deformation.

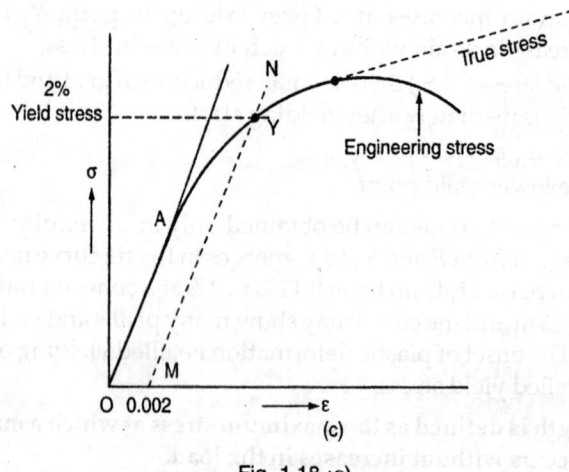

Fig. 1.18 (c)

The failure of steel and aluminium occur primarily due to shear strain along the plane forming 45° angle with the axis of the rod.

A typical 'cup and cone' fracture may be detected to steel and aluminium specimen. But the failure of cast iron occurs suddenly exhibiting a square fracture across the cross-section (See Figs. 1.18 (e) and (f)).

In the above discussion load was applied gradually. But under rapid or **impact loading*** two additional material parameters have relevance and these are—resilience and toughness.

Resilence defines the ability of material to absorb energy without suffering plastic strain.

Toughness defines the ability of material to absorb energy prior to fracture.

While using equation $\sigma = \varepsilon \cdot E$; it does not matter if we are loading or unloading the specimen, the stress-strain response is a straight line of slope *E*.

A material having proportional limit close to elastic limit such as steel is termed a linear, elastic material. For stress value below the elastic limit, the loading and unloading response follow the same path. All materials do not behave as that of steel.

_____

*We will discuss 'impact loading' in the chapter—strain energy and its application.

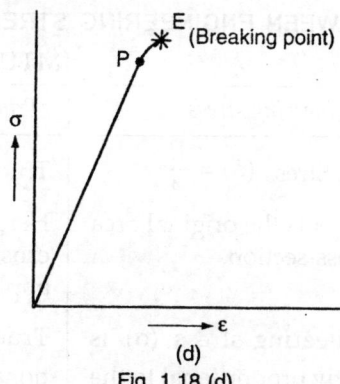

(d)

Fig. 1.18 (d)

Brittle materials do not exhibit the yield point. Materials that fail in tension at relatively low values of strains are classified as brittle materials. Examples are concrete, stone, cast iron, glass, ceramic material and many common alloys.

N.B. Stress-strain diagrams of various materials vary widely and different tensile tests conducted on the same material may yield different result depending upon the temperature of the specimen and the speed of the loading.

Stress-Strain Diagram for Concrete*

For a given steel, the **yield strength** is the same in both **tension** and **compression**.

For most 'brittle materials', ultimate strength in compression is much larger than the ultimate strength in tension. This is due to the presence of flaws such as microscopic cracks or Cavities which tend to weaken the material in tension. Properties in tension and compression of concrete is shown in Fig. 1.18(e).

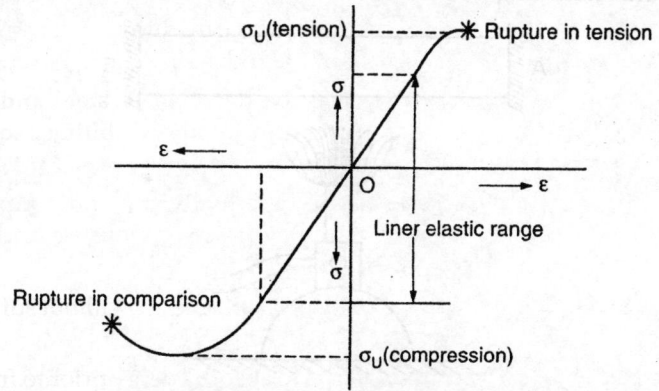

Fig. 1.18 (e) Stress-strain diagram for concrete

Value of E for common materials:

Material	E (GPa)
Steel	200-210
Copper	120
Aluminium	70
Bronze	83
Cast iron	100

*Concrete is an anisotropic material.

1.10 DIFFERENCE BETWEEN ENGINEERING STRESS AND TRUE STRESS

[MTU-2011-12 (2nd Semester)]

Particular	Engineering stress	True stress
1. Stress formula	Engg. Stress $(\sigma) = \dfrac{P}{A}$ Here, A is the original area of cross-section.	True stress $(\sigma_t) = \dfrac{P}{A}$ Here, A is the deformed area of cross-section after the load application.
2. Behaviour of material on application of load	Engineering stress (σ) is directly proportional to the load P, decreases with P during necking phase up to fracture point or breaking point of the specimen of ductile material.	True stress (σ_t) is proportional to P but also inversely proportional to A. True stress increases until rupture of the specimen occurs (See Fig. 1.18(a)).
3. Uses	Elastic behaviour of a deformable body is studied by Engineering stress.	Plastic behaviour of a material is studied by true stress.

1.11 THERMAL STRESS AND STRAIN

Owing to temperature variation in the material, stresses and strains are setup. Metal expand on heating and contract on cooling.

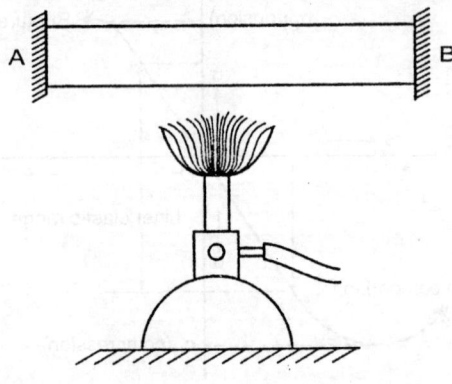

Fig. 1.19

If their expansion or contraction is prevented as shown in Fig. 1.19, then thermal stresses and strains are produced.

The increased length of the rod is given by

$$l_t = l_o\,(1 + \alpha\,\Delta T)$$

l_o = initial length of the rod

where l_t = final length of the rod at increased temperature

α = coefficient of thermal expansion

$$\Delta T = \text{rise in temperature}$$

$$= (T_f - T_i)$$

where T_f = final temperature and T_i = initial temperature

Thermal strain $(\varepsilon_l) = \dfrac{l_t - l_o}{l_o}$

$$= \dfrac{l_o(1 + \alpha\Delta T) - l_o}{l_o}$$

$$= \alpha\Delta T$$

and Thermal stress $(\sigma_{\text{thermal}}) = E \cdot \alpha \cdot \Delta T$.

1.12 THERMAL STRESSES IN COMPOSITE BAR (Fig. 1.20)

Let us consider a composite bar (rod-1 and tube 2) as shown in Fig. 1.20.

If the rod '1' and tube '2' were not connected with each other then their expansion would be $L \cdot \alpha_1 \Delta T$ and $L \cdot \alpha_2 \Delta T$ respectively.

However, as the two are connected at the ends so thermal stresses and strains will be produced.

Coefficient of expansion (α) is different for different materials. Here α_1 is more than α_2, so rod 1 will expand more than tube 2.

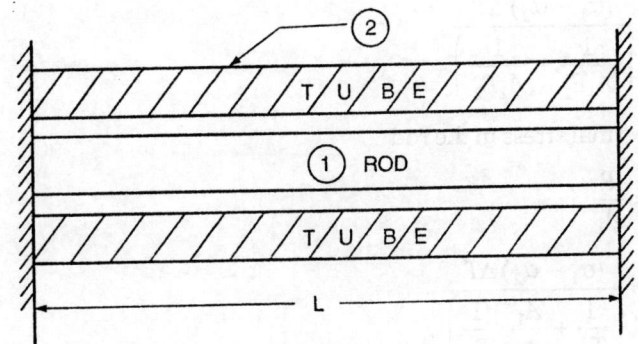

Fig. 1.20

Since there is no external force applied to the above composite bar, the sum of forces due to thermal stresses will be zero.

i.e. $\qquad P_2 - P_1 = 0$

or, $\qquad P_2 = P_1 = P$ (Assume)

Now, $\qquad \Delta L_1 + \Delta L_2 = L \cdot \alpha_1 \cdot \Delta T - L \cdot \alpha_2 \cdot \Delta T$

$$= L\Delta T(\alpha_1 - \alpha_2)$$

Also, $\qquad \Delta L_1 = \dfrac{PL}{A_1 E_1}$

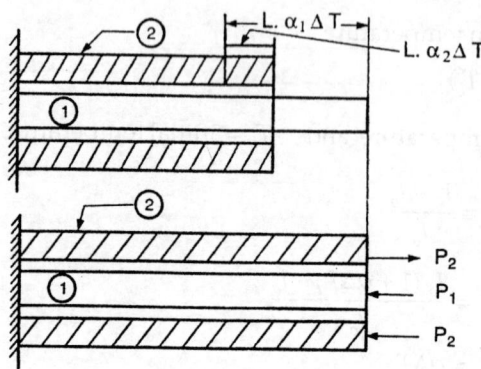

Fig. 1.21

and, $\Delta L_2 = \dfrac{PL}{A_2 E_2}$

$\therefore$ $\Delta L_1 + \Delta L_2 = PL\left(\dfrac{1}{A_1 E_1} + \dfrac{1}{A_2 E_2}\right)$

or, $L\Delta T (\alpha_1 - \alpha_2) = PL\left(\dfrac{1}{A_1 E_1} + \dfrac{1}{A_2 E_2}\right)$

$\therefore$ $P = \dfrac{(\alpha_1 - \alpha_2)\,\Delta T}{\left(\dfrac{1}{A_1 E_1} + \dfrac{1}{A_2 E_2}\right)}$

Therefore, thermal stress in the rod

$\sigma_1 = \dfrac{P}{A_1}$

$= \dfrac{(\alpha_1 - \alpha_2)\,\Delta T}{\left(\dfrac{1}{E_1} + \dfrac{A_1}{A_2}\cdot\dfrac{1}{E_2}\right)}$

and thermal stress in the tube

$\sigma_2 = \dfrac{P}{A_2} = \dfrac{(\alpha_1 - \alpha_2)\,\Delta T}{\left(\dfrac{A_2}{A_1}\cdot\dfrac{1}{E_1} + \dfrac{1}{E_2}\right)}$

EXAMPLE 1 *A steel rod is stretched between two rigid walls and carries a tensile load of 5000 N at 20°C. If the allowable stress is not to exceed 130 MPa at – 20°C, what is the minimum diameter of the rod? Assume $\alpha = 11.7\ \mu\ m/m\text{--}°C$ and $E = 200\ GPa$.*

SOLUTION   Actual expansing of steel rod = Free expansion of steel rod
                                                        + Expansion due to tensile load.

i.e. $\delta = \delta_{\text{thermal}} + \delta_{\text{tensile load}}$

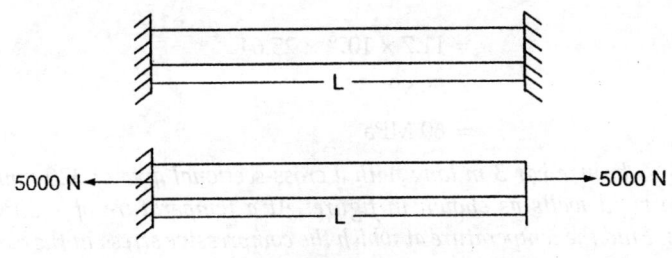

Fig. 1.22

$$\frac{\sigma \cdot L}{E} = L \cdot \alpha \cdot \Delta T + \frac{P \cdot L}{A \cdot E}$$

$$\sigma = L \alpha \, \Delta T \times \frac{E}{L} + \frac{PL}{AE} \times \frac{E}{L}$$

$$\sigma = \alpha E \Delta T + \frac{P}{A}$$

$$130 = 11.7 \times 10^{-6} \times 2 \times 10^{5} \times 40 + \frac{5000}{A}$$

$$\Rightarrow \qquad A = \left(\frac{5000}{36.4}\right)$$

or, $\qquad \dfrac{\pi}{4} d^2 = \dfrac{5000}{36.4}$

$$\therefore \qquad d = \sqrt{\frac{5000 \times 4}{36.4 \times \pi}}$$

$$= 13.22 \text{ mm} \qquad\qquad \textbf{Ans.}$$

EXAMPLE 2 *Steel railroad rails 10 m long are laid with a clearance of 3 mm at a temperature at 15°C. At what temperature will the rails just touch? What stress would be induced in the rails? At that temperature if there were no initial clearance? Assemed* $\alpha = 11.7 \; \mu m/m°C$ *and E = 200 GPa.*

SOLUTION $T_1 = ?$ and $T_2 = 15°C$

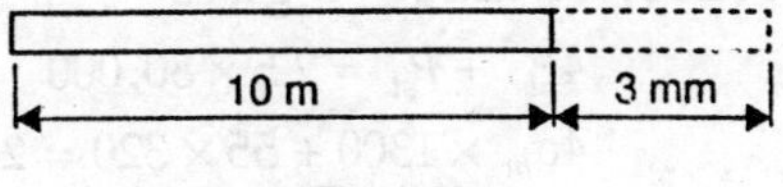

$$\delta_T = L \cdot \alpha \cdot \Delta T$$

$$= \alpha L \, (T_1 - T_2)$$

$$3 = 11.7 \times 10^{-6} \times 1000 \times (T_1 - 15)$$

$$\Rightarrow \qquad T_1 = 40.64°$$

Required stress $\sigma_{th} = \alpha \cdot E \cdot (T_1 - T_2)$

$$= 11.7 \times 10^{-6} \times 200 \times 10^{3} \, (40.64 - 15)$$

δ = 3mm

10 m   3 mm

Fig. 1.23

$$= 11.7 \times 10^{-6} \times 25.64$$

$$= 59.99$$

$$\simeq 60 \text{ MPa} \qquad \textbf{Ans.}$$

EXAMPLE 3 *A bronze bar 3 m long with a cross-sectional area of 320 mm² is placed between two rigid walls as shown in figure. At a temperature of – 20°C, the gap Δ = 2.5 mm. Find the temperature at which the compressive stress in the bar will be 35 MPa. (Use α = 18 × 10⁻⁶ m/m °C and E = 80 GPa)*

SOLUTION Here $\delta_{\text{thermal}} = \delta + \Delta$

$$\alpha \cdot L \cdot \Delta T = \frac{\sigma L}{E} + 2.5$$

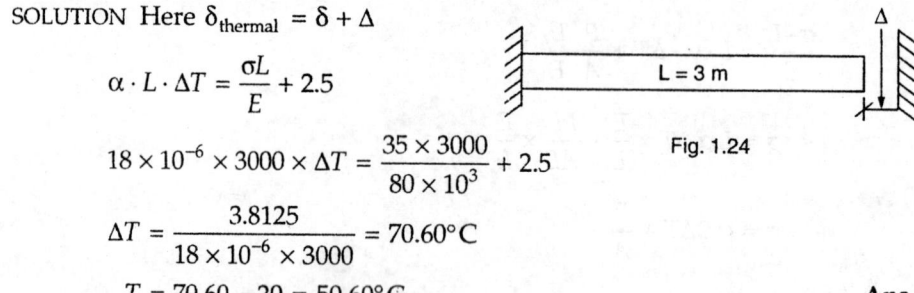

$$18 \times 10^{-6} \times 3000 \times \Delta T = \frac{35 \times 3000}{80 \times 10^3} + 2.5$$

Fig. 1.24

$$\Delta T = \frac{3.8125}{18 \times 10^{-6} \times 3000} = 70.60° \text{C}$$

$$T = 70.60 - 20 = 50.60° \text{C} \qquad \textbf{Ans.}$$

EXAMPLE 4 *A rigid bar of negligible weight is supported as shown in Fig. 1.25. If W = 80 kN. Compute the temperature change that will cause the stress in the steel rod to be 55 MPa.*

Assume the coefficient of linear expansion are 11.7 μm/m°C for steel and 18.9 μm/m°C for bronze.

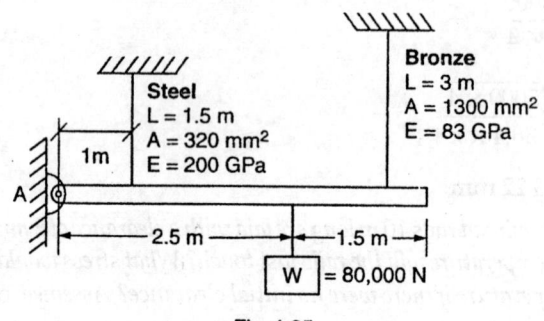

Fig. 1.25

SOLUTION $\Sigma M_A = 0$ gives

$$4P_{br} + P_{st} = 2.5 \times 80,000$$

$$4\sigma_{br} \times 1300 + 55 \times 320 = 2.5 \times 80,000$$

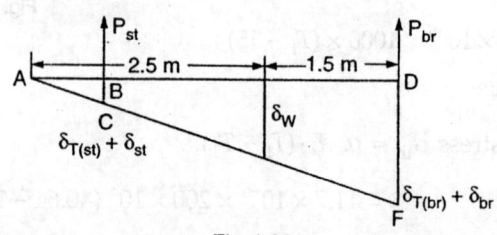

Fig. 1.26

$$\sigma_{br} = \frac{2.5 \times 80,000 - 55 \times 320}{4 \times 1300} = 35.08 \text{ MPa}$$

From similar triangles, ABC and ADF

$$\frac{\delta_T(st) + \delta_{ST}}{1} = \frac{\delta_T(br) + \delta_{br}}{4}$$

$$\delta_T(st) + \delta_{ST} = 0.25 \left[\delta_T(br) + \delta_{br} \right]$$

$$(\alpha \, L\Delta T)_{st} + \left(\frac{\sigma \cdot L}{E} \right)_{st} = 0.25 \left[(\alpha L\Delta T)_{br} \left(\frac{\sigma \cdot L}{E} \right)_{br} \right]$$

$$11.7 \times 10^{-6} \times 1500 \, \Delta T + \frac{55 \times 1500}{2000}$$

$$= 0.25 \left[18.9 \times 10^{-6} \times 3000 \, \Delta T + \frac{35.08 \times 3000}{83000} \right]$$

$$\Delta T = 28.3°\text{C}$$

A temperature drop of 28.3°C is needed to stress the steel to 55 MPa.

EXAMPLE 5 *At a temperature of 80°C, a steel tyre 12 mm thick and 90 mm wide that is to be shrunk on to a locomotive driving wheel 22 m in diameter just fits over the wheel, which is at a temperature of 25°C.*

Determine the contact pressure between the tyre and wheel after the assembly cools to 25°C. Neglect the deformation of the wheel caused by the pressure of the tyre.

Assume $\alpha = 11.7 \, \mu m/m°C$ and $E = 200 \, GPa$.

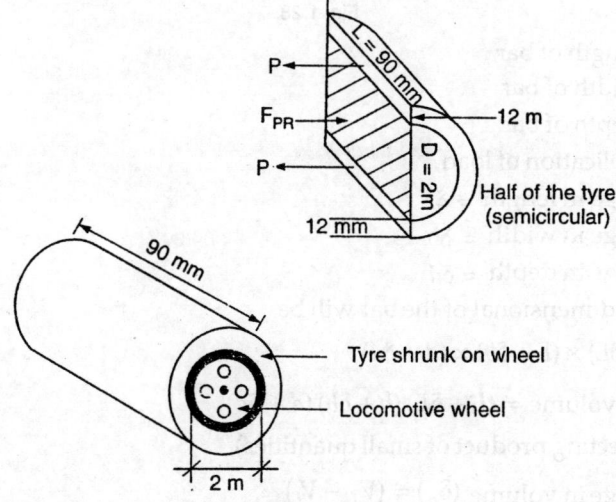

Fig. 1.27

SOLUTION We have

$$\delta = \delta_T$$

$$\frac{P \cdot L}{A \cdot E} = L \cdot \alpha \cdot \Delta T$$

$\Rightarrow \qquad\qquad P = AE\,\alpha\,\Delta T$

$$= (90 \times 12) \times 200 \times 10^3 \times 11.7 \times 10^{-6} \times (80 - 25)$$

$$= 1080 \times 200 \times 10^3 \times 11.7 \times 55$$

$$= 128996 \text{ Newton}$$

Now $\quad F_{\text{projected}} = 2P$

$\qquad p \cdot D \cdot L = 2P$

$\qquad p\,(2000)\,(90) = 2 \times 138996$

$\therefore \qquad\qquad p = 1.544 \text{ MPa}$ $\qquad\qquad\qquad\qquad\qquad$ **Ans.**

1.13 VOLUMETRIC STRAIN OF A RECTANGULAR BAR WHEN SUBJECTED TO UNIAXIAL LOAD *P*

Let a rectangular bar is subjected to load *P* along *x*-axis.

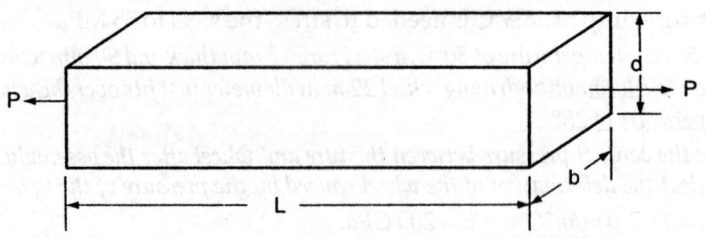

Fig. 1.28

Let $\quad L$ = length of bar
$\qquad\quad b$ = width of bar
and $\quad\;\; d$ = depth of bar.
Let due to application of load,
$\qquad\quad$ Change in length = δL
$\qquad\quad$ Change in width = δb
and $\quad$ Change in depth = δd
$\therefore \qquad$ Final dimensional of the bar will be

$\qquad (L \times \delta L) \times (b + \delta b) \times (d + \delta d)$

$\therefore \qquad$ Final volume $= (L + \delta L)(b + \delta b)(d + \delta d)$

$\qquad$ (neglecting product of small quantities)

$\therefore \qquad$ Change in volume $(\delta_v) = (V_f - V_i)$

$$= (Lbd + bd\delta L + Lb\delta d + Ld\delta d) - lbd$$

$$= bd\delta L + Lb\delta d + Ld\delta b$$

$\therefore \qquad$ Volumetric strain $(\varepsilon_v) = \dfrac{\delta V}{V}$

$$\varepsilon_v = \frac{\delta L}{L} + \frac{\delta d}{d} + \frac{\delta b}{b}$$

$\dfrac{\delta d}{d}$ and $\dfrac{\delta b}{b}$ are lateral strain.

$\therefore$ ε_v = longitudinal strain + 2 × lateral strain

= longitudinal strain − 2 × v longitudinal strain

$$= \frac{\delta L}{L} - 2 \times v \times \frac{\delta L}{L}$$

$\therefore$ Volumetric strain of rectangular bar subjected to uniaxial load P

$$= \frac{\delta L}{L}(1 - 2v)$$

1.14 VOLUMETRIC STRAIN OF A CYLINDERICAL ROD

Let the initial length of rod = L and dia. of rod = d

After uniaxial load P, let its length increases to $(L + \delta L)$ and diameter decrease to $(d - \delta d)$

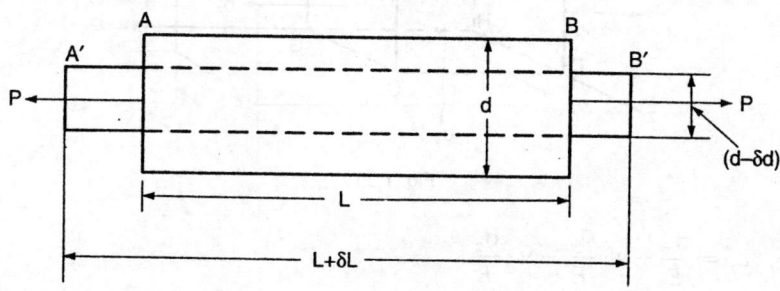

Fig. 1.29

$\therefore$ Change in volume $(\delta_v) = (V_f - V_i)$

$$= \frac{\pi}{4}\left\{(d - \delta d)^2 \cdot (L + \delta L)\right\} - \left\{\frac{\pi}{4}d^2 L\right\}$$

$$= \frac{\pi}{4}\left\{d^2 L - 2dL\delta d + d^2 \delta L - d^2 L\right\}$$

$$= \frac{\pi}{4}\left\{d^2 \delta L - 2dL\delta d\right\}$$

$\therefore$ Volumetric strain $(\varepsilon_v) = \dfrac{\delta_V}{V}$

$$= \frac{\dfrac{\pi}{4}(d^2 \delta L - 2dL \cdot \delta d)}{\dfrac{\pi}{4}d^2 L}$$

$$\therefore \qquad \varepsilon_v \text{ of cylinder rod} = \frac{\delta L}{L} - \frac{2\delta d}{d}$$

$$= \{ \text{longitudinal strain} - 2 \times \text{diametral strain} \}$$

1.15 VOLUMETRIC STRAIN OF A RECTANGULAR BLOCK SUBJECTED TO NORMAL STRESSES ON ALL ITS FACE

Let us consider a rectangular block having dimensions $x \times y \times z$ so that

$AB = x$

$BF = z$ and $BC = y$

Let the block is subjected to stress σ_x, σ_y and σ_z along x, y and z axes respectively. As a result of stresses the block will be strained along x, y and z axes. Let strain along x, y and z axes be $\varepsilon_x, \varepsilon_y$ and ε_z respectively.

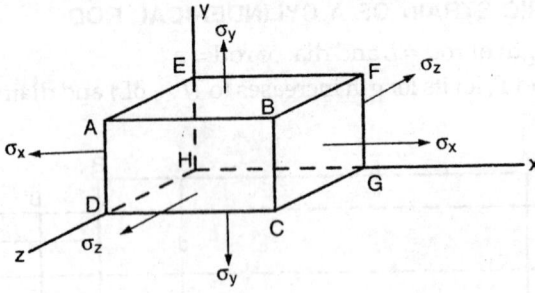

Fig. 1.30

Hence, $\varepsilon_x = \dfrac{\sigma_x}{E} - v \cdot \dfrac{\sigma_y}{E} - v \cdot \dfrac{\sigma_z}{E}$

$$\varepsilon_y = \frac{\sigma_y}{E} - v \cdot \frac{\sigma_x}{E} - v \cdot \frac{\sigma_z}{E}$$

$$\varepsilon_z = \frac{\sigma_z}{E} - v \cdot \frac{\sigma_x}{E} - v \cdot \frac{\sigma_y}{E}$$

Now, volumetric strain $(\varepsilon_v) = \varepsilon_x + \varepsilon_y + \varepsilon_z = \dfrac{\sigma_x}{E}(1-2v) + \dfrac{\sigma_y}{E}(1-2v) + \dfrac{\sigma_z}{E}(1-2v)$

$$= \left(\frac{\sigma_x}{E} + \frac{\sigma_y}{E} + \frac{\sigma_z}{E} \right) - \frac{2v}{E}(\sigma_x + \sigma_y + \sigma_z) = \frac{(\sigma_x + \sigma_y + \sigma_z)}{E} - \frac{2v}{E}(\sigma_x + \sigma_y + \sigma_z)$$

$$= \frac{(\sigma_x + \sigma_y + \sigma_z)}{E}[1 - 2v]$$

If a body is subjected to uniform hydrostatic pressure p, then each of the stress components is equal to $-p$, therefore volumetric strain

$$(\varepsilon_v) = \frac{-p-p-p}{E}(1-2v) = (-)\frac{3p}{E}(1-2v)$$

EXAMPLE 1 *A specimen of any given material is subjected to a uniform triaxial stress. Determine the theoretical maximum value of Poisson's ratio.*

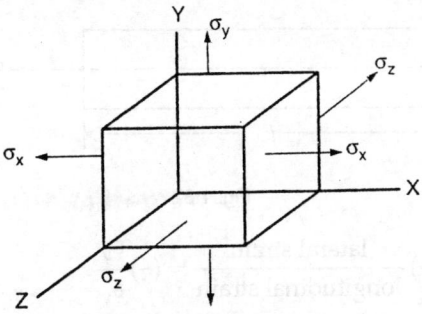

Fig. 1.31

SOLUTION Let the specimen (as shown in Figure) is subjected to σ_x, σ_y and σ_z along x, y and z axes respectively.

Then
$$\varepsilon_x = \frac{1}{E}[\sigma_x - v(\sigma_y + \sigma_z)] \qquad \text{...(I)}$$

$$\varepsilon_y = \frac{1}{E}[\sigma_y - v(\sigma_x + \sigma_z)] \qquad \text{...(II)}$$

$$\varepsilon_z = \frac{1}{E}[\sigma_z - v(\sigma_x + \sigma_y)] \qquad \text{...(III)}$$

Adding I, II, and III

$$\varepsilon_x + \varepsilon_y + \varepsilon_z = \frac{1}{E}(\sigma_x + \sigma_y + \sigma_z) - \frac{2v}{E}(\sigma_x + \sigma_y + \sigma_z)$$

$$= \frac{\sigma_x + \sigma_y + \sigma_z}{E}(1 - 2v) \qquad \text{...(IV)}$$

For uniform triaxial stress we have $\acute{\varepsilon}_x = \varepsilon_y = \varepsilon_z$ and $\sigma_x = \sigma_y = \sigma_z$

Hence, eq. (IV) reduces to

$$3\varepsilon = \frac{3\sigma}{E}\{1 - 2v\}$$

$$\varepsilon = \frac{\sigma}{E}\{1 - 2v\}$$

Since ε and σ must be of the same sign if follows that $(1 - 2v)$ must be positive *i.e.* $1 - 2v \geq 0$

$$\Rightarrow \qquad v \leq \left(\frac{1}{2}\right) \qquad \qquad \textbf{Ans.}$$

EXAMPLE 2 *A solid cylinder of diameter d has an axial load P. Show that it's change in diameter is* $\left(\dfrac{4Pv}{\pi Ed}\right)$.

SOLUTION The load can be considered tensile or compressive. Here, let us consider tensile load P.

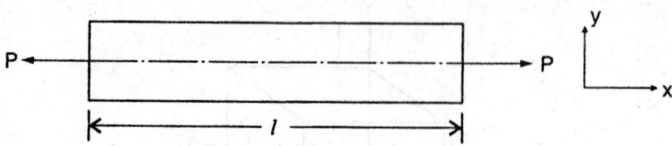

Fig. 1.32

Poisson ratio $(\nu) = (-) \dfrac{\text{lateral strain}}{\text{longitudinal strain}} = (-)\dfrac{\varepsilon_y}{\varepsilon_x}$

$\varepsilon_y = -\nu \cdot \varepsilon_x$

where ε_y = diametral strain along y-axis

ε_x = longitudinal strain along x-axis

$\left(\dfrac{\delta d}{d}\right) = -\nu \cdot \varepsilon_x$

$\delta d = -\nu \cdot d \cdot \varepsilon_x = -\nu \cdot d \cdot \dfrac{\Delta l}{l}$

$= -\nu \cdot d \cdot \dfrac{P}{AE}$

$= -\nu \cdot d \cdot \dfrac{P}{\dfrac{\pi}{4} d^2 E}$

$= (-) \dfrac{4P\nu}{\pi E d}$

(–) sign, since there is decrease in diameter when the cylinder is subjected to tensile load along x-axis.

EXAMPLE 3 *A rectantular block 1 m long, 0.4 m wide and 20 mm thick is subjected to biaxial stresses σ_x and σ_y acting along length and width respectively. If the increase in length is 0.6 mm and increases in width is 0.09 mm find*

   (a) σ_x and σ_y

   (b) change is thickness of the plate

   (c) change is volume of the plate

SOLUTION Given $\delta_l = 0.6$mm; $\delta_b = 0.09$mm; $\delta_z = 0$

$l = 1\text{m} = 1000\text{mm}$

$E = 200 \times 10^3\,\text{MPa or N/mm}^2$

$b = 0.4\text{m} = 400\,\text{mm}$

$t = 20\text{mm}$

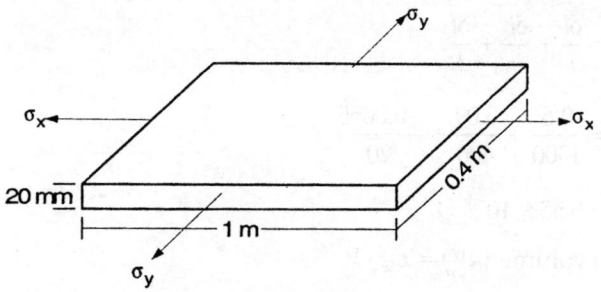

Fig. 1.33

(a) For biaxial system:

$$\varepsilon_x = \frac{1}{E}(\sigma_x - v \cdot \sigma_y)$$

$$\frac{\delta l}{l} = \frac{1}{E}(\sigma_x - v \cdot \sigma_y)$$

$$\frac{0.6}{1000} = \frac{1}{200 \times 10^3}(\sigma_x - 0.25\sigma_y)$$

$\therefore \qquad \sigma_x - 0.25\,\sigma_y = 120 \qquad\qquad\qquad\qquad \ldots\text{(I)}$

$$\varepsilon_y = \frac{1}{E}(\sigma_y - v \cdot \sigma_x)$$

$$\frac{\delta b}{b} = \frac{1}{E}(\sigma_y - v \cdot \sigma_x)$$

$$\frac{0.9}{400} = \frac{1}{200 \times 10^3}(\sigma_y - 0.25\sigma_x)$$

$\therefore \qquad -0.25\,\sigma_x + \sigma_y = 45 \qquad\qquad\qquad\qquad \ldots\text{(II)}$

Solving (I) and (II) $\sigma_x = 140$ MPa and $\sigma_y = 80$ MPa **Ans.**

(b) Change in thickness

$$\varepsilon_t = \frac{\delta t}{t} = \frac{1}{E}(\sigma_z - v \cdot \sigma_x - v\sigma_y)$$

$$\frac{\delta t}{20} = \frac{1}{200 \times 10^3}(0 - 0.25 \times 140 - 0.25 \times 80)$$

$\Rightarrow \qquad \delta t = -0.0055$ mm $\qquad\qquad\qquad\qquad\qquad$ **Ans.**

(c) Volumetric strain

$$\varepsilon_V = (\varepsilon_x + \varepsilon_y + \varepsilon_z)$$

$$= \frac{\delta l}{l} + \frac{\delta b}{b} + \frac{\delta t}{t}$$

$$= \frac{0.6}{1000} + \frac{0.09}{400} + \frac{-0.0055}{20}$$

$$= 0.55 \times 10^{-3}$$

So, change in volume $(dV) = \varepsilon_V \cdot V$

$$= 0.55 \times 10^{-3} \times (1000 \times 400 \times 20)$$

$$= 4400 \text{ mm}^3$$

Since value of dV is positive so there is increase in volume of the plate.   **Ans.**

EXAMPLE 4 *A circle of diameter d = 220 mm is made on a unstressed aluminium plate 400 mm × 400 mm and of thickness t = 20 mm. Forces acting on the plate cause normal stresses $\sigma_x = 80MPa$ and $\sigma_y = 140\,MPa$. For E = 70 GPa and $v = \frac{1}{3}$ determine:*

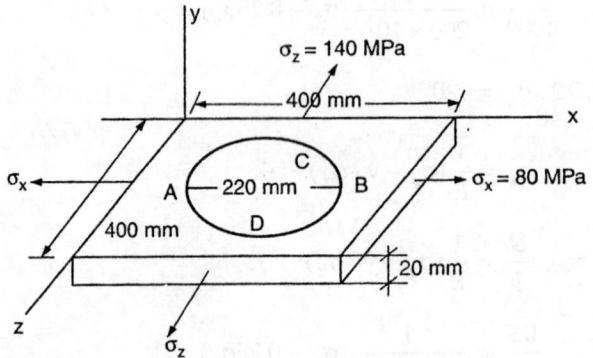

Fig. 1.34

(a) *change in length of diameter AB*   (b) *change in length of diameter CD*
(c) *change in thickness of the plate*   (d) *change in volume of the plate*

SOLUTION Given

$$\sigma_x = 80 \text{ MPa} = 80 \times 10^6 \text{ N/m}^2$$

$$\sigma_z = 140 \text{ MPa} = 140 \times 10^6 \text{ N/m}^2$$

$$E = 70 \times 10^9 \text{ N/m}^2$$

We know that by application of load stress and strain occurs in the material.

Let ε_x, ε_y and ε_z are the strain along x, y and z axes.

Then, $\varepsilon_x = \dfrac{\sigma_x}{E} - v \cdot \dfrac{\sigma_y}{E} - v \cdot \dfrac{\sigma_z}{E}$

$$= \frac{1}{E}[\sigma_x - v \cdot \sigma_y - v \cdot \sigma_z]$$

$$= \frac{10^6}{70 \times 10^9} = \left[80 - 0 - \frac{140}{3}\right]$$

$$= 0.476 \times 10^{-3}$$

$$\varepsilon_y = \frac{\sigma_y}{E} - v \cdot \frac{\sigma_x}{E} - v \cdot \frac{\sigma_z}{E}$$

$$= 0 - \frac{1}{3} \times \frac{80}{70 \times 10^3} - \frac{1}{3} \times \frac{140}{70 \times 10^3}$$

$$= -\frac{1}{3 \times 70 \times 10^3}[80 + 140]$$

$$= -1.047 \times 10^{-3}$$

$$\varepsilon_z = \frac{\sigma_z}{E} - v \cdot \frac{\sigma_x}{E} - v \cdot \frac{\sigma_y}{E}$$

$$= \frac{140}{70 \times 10^3} - \frac{1}{3} \times \frac{80}{70 \times 10^3} - 0$$

$$= \frac{1}{70 \times 10^3}\left[140 - \frac{80}{3}\right]$$

$$= 1.62 \times 10^{-3}$$

Now,

(a) Change in length in diameter AB i.e.

$$\delta_{AB} = \varepsilon_x \times d$$

$$= 0.476 \times 10^{-3} \times 220$$

$$= 0.1047 \text{ mm}$$

(b) Change in length in diameter CD i.e.

$$\delta_{CD} = \varepsilon_z \times d$$

$$= 1.62 \times 10^{-3} \times 220$$

$$= 0.356 \text{ mm}$$

(c) Change in thickness of plate i.e.

$$\delta_y = \varepsilon_y \times t$$

$$= -1.047 \times 10^{-3} \times 20 \text{ mm}$$

$$= -0.0209 \text{ mm (decreases in thickness)}$$

(d) Change in volume (δ_V)

$$= \varepsilon_V \times \text{original volume}$$

$$= \text{volumetric strain} \times \text{original volume}$$

Volumetric strain of aluminium plate is given by

$$\varepsilon_V = \frac{(\sigma_x + \sigma_y + \sigma_z)(1 - 2v)}{E}$$

$$= \frac{(80 + 0 + 140)\left(1 - 2 \times \dfrac{1}{3}\right)}{70 \times 10^9}$$

$$= 220 \times \frac{1}{3} \times \frac{1}{70 \times 10^9}$$

$$= \frac{220}{210} \times 10^{-9}$$

$\therefore$ Change in Volume (δ_V) $= \varepsilon_V \times V$

$$= \frac{22}{21} \times 10^{-9} \times (400 \times 400 \times 20)\,\text{mm}^3$$

$$= \frac{22}{21} \times 10^{-9} \times 32 \times 10^5\,\text{mm}^3$$

$$= \frac{22 \times 32}{21} \times 10^{-4}\,\text{mm}^3$$

$$= 33.523 \times 10^{-4}\,\text{mm}^3$$

$$= 3.352 \times 10^{-3}\,\text{mm}^3 \qquad \textbf{Ans.}$$

1.16 RELATION BETWEEN ELASTIC CONSTANTS (*E*, *K* AND *G*)

(a) *Relation between E and K:*

L = side of the cube

and dL = change in length of cube

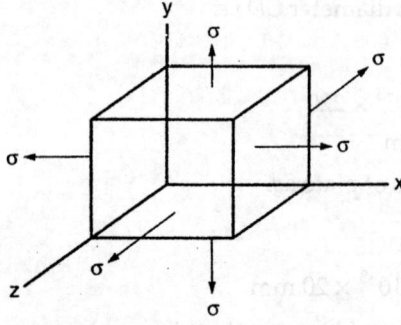

Fig. 1.36

Let the element of elastic body in the form of cube is subjected to equal tensile stress (σ) along x, y and z axes then total strain along x-axis.

$$\frac{dL}{L} = \frac{\sigma}{E} - v \cdot \frac{\sigma}{E} - v \cdot \frac{\sigma}{E}$$

$$= \frac{\sigma}{E}(1 - 2v) \qquad \qquad \qquad \text{...(i)}$$

Initial volume of the cube

$$(V) = L^3 \qquad \qquad \qquad \text{...(ii)}$$

Now, differentiating both sides, $dV = 3L^2 dL$

$$\therefore \qquad \left(\frac{dV}{V}\right) = \frac{3L^2 \times dL}{L^3} = \frac{3dL}{L}$$

$$\therefore \qquad \left(\frac{dL}{L}\right) = \left(\frac{dV}{3V}\right) \qquad \qquad \qquad \text{...(iii)}$$

From equation (i) and (iii)

$$\frac{dV}{3V} = \frac{\sigma}{E}(1 - 2v)$$

$$\frac{dV}{V} = \frac{3\sigma}{E}(1 - 2v)$$

$$\text{Bulk Modulus } (K) = \frac{\text{Stress}}{\text{Volumetric strain}}$$

$$= \frac{\sigma}{\dfrac{3\sigma}{E}(1 - 2v)}$$

$$K = \frac{E}{3(1 - 2v)}$$

$$\therefore \qquad \boldsymbol{E = 3K(1 - 2v)} \qquad \qquad \qquad \text{...(iv)}$$

(b) *Relation between E and G:* Let the block of side 'L' and thickness unity is subjected to shear stresses τ, at faces AB and CD, hence complementary shear stresses (τ) will be developed on faces AD and BC, as a result the cube is distorted to $ABC'D'$.

Now, strain in $AC = \dfrac{AC' - AC}{AC}$

$$= \frac{C'H}{AC}$$

$$= \frac{CC' \cos 45°}{AB\sqrt{2}}$$

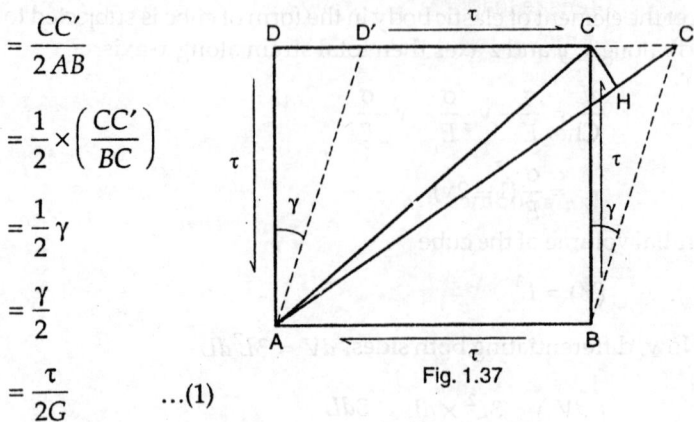

Fig. 1.37

$$= \frac{CC'}{2AB}$$

$$= \frac{1}{2} \times \left(\frac{CC'}{BC} \right)$$

$$= \frac{1}{2} \gamma$$

$$= \frac{\gamma}{2}$$

$$= \frac{\tau}{2G} \qquad ...(1)$$

Strair. along $AC = \dfrac{\tau}{E}$ and strain along $BD = (-) \, \text{v} \cdot \dfrac{\tau}{E}$ $\left[\text{Shear strain } (\gamma) = \dfrac{\tau}{G} \right]$

Further Strain along diagonal AC = strain due to tensile stress in AC

$$- \text{ strain due to compressive stress along } BD$$

$$= \left[\frac{\tau}{E} - \left(-\text{v} \frac{\tau}{E} \right) \right] = \left[\frac{\tau}{E} + \text{v} \cdot \frac{\tau}{E} \right]$$

So combined strain along $AC = \dfrac{\tau}{E}[1 + \text{v}]$ $\qquad ...(2)$

∴   From equation (1) and (2)

$$\frac{\tau}{2G} = \frac{\tau}{E}(1 + \text{v})$$

∴ $G = \dfrac{E}{2(1 + \text{v})}$ $\qquad ...(3)$

where G = modulus of rigidity

E = modulus of elasticity.

Eliminating v from equ. (3) we get the relation between three elastic constants

which is $E = \dfrac{9GK}{3K + G}$

EXAMPLE 1 *A bar of 30mm diameter is subjected to a axial pull of 60kN. The measured extension on a guauge length of 200mm is 0.09 mm and the change is diameter is 0.0039mm. Calculate the Poisson's ratio and the values of the three moduli.*

SOLUTION   Diameter of the bar = 30mm

$$\text{Area of the bar } (A) = \frac{\pi}{4} \times d^2 = \frac{\pi}{4} \times (30)^2 = 706.86 \text{ mm}^2$$

N.B.: If the direction of shear stress τ is reversed then also the same result will occur. In that case diagonal BD will be elongated and AC will be compressed simultaneously.

Tensile load = 60 kN = 6000 N

$\therefore$ Tensile stress $(\sigma) = \dfrac{6000}{706.86}$ N/mm^2 = 84.88 N/mm^2

Change in length $(\delta) = 0.09$ mm

Longitudinal strain $(\varepsilon_t) = \dfrac{\delta}{l} = \dfrac{0.09}{200} = 0.00045$

Young's Modulus $(E) = \dfrac{\sigma}{\varepsilon_l} = \left(\dfrac{84.88}{0.00045}\right) = 18862$ N/mm^2

Lateral strain $= \dfrac{\Delta d}{d} = \dfrac{0.0039}{30} = 0.00013$

Poisson's ratio $(\nu) = \dfrac{\text{lateral strain}}{\text{longitudinal strain}}$

$= \dfrac{0.00013}{0.00045} = \dfrac{13}{45}$

Let G be modulus of rigidity

We know that $\quad E = 2G(1 + \nu)$

$$188622 = 2G\left(1 + \dfrac{13}{45}\right)$$

$\therefore \qquad G = \dfrac{188622 \times 45}{2 \times 58}$

$$= 73172.327 \text{ N/mm}^2$$

Let K be the bulk modulus

We know that $\quad E = 3K(1 - 2\nu)$

$$188622 = 3K\left(1 - \dfrac{26}{45}\right)$$

$$K = \dfrac{188622 \times 45}{3 \times 19}$$

$$= 148912.1 \text{ N/mm}^2$$

Hence, $\qquad \nu = \dfrac{13}{45} = 0.28$

$\left.\begin{array}{l} E = 188622 \text{ N/mm}^2 \\[4pt] G = 73172.327 \text{ N/mm}^2 \\[4pt] K = 148912.1 \text{ N/mm}^2 \end{array}\right\}$ **Ans.**

1.17 EXPRESSION FOR THE ELONGATION *D* OF A VERTICAL BAR OF LENGTH *L*, UNIFORM CROSS-SECTIONAL AREA *A*, SUPPORTED AT ITS UPPER AND UNDER ITS OWN WEIGHT *W*

Let us consider an element of thickness dx at a distance x from the lower end of the bar. Let ρ is the mass density of bar material.

For length X, $W_x = \rho \cdot g \cdot A \cdot x$

As a result of this load portion of length dx will suffer small elongation $d\delta$ such that

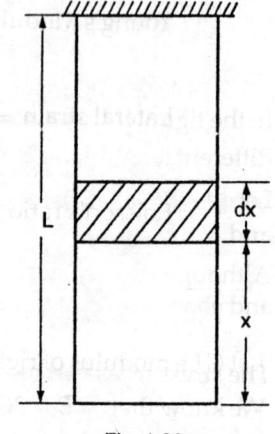

Fig. 1.38

$$d\delta = \frac{W \cdot dx}{A \cdot E}$$

$$= \frac{\rho \cdot g \cdot A \cdot x \cdot dx}{A \cdot E}$$

Total elongation $\delta = \int_0^L d\delta$

$$= \int_0^L \frac{\rho \cdot g \cdot A \cdot x \, dx}{A \cdot E}$$

$$= \frac{\rho g}{E} \int_0^L x \, dx$$

$$= \frac{\rho g L^2}{2E} \qquad \qquad ...(1)$$

Weight of bar $(W) = \rho \cdot g \cdot A \cdot L$

$\therefore \qquad \rho = \dfrac{W}{A \cdot L \cdot g}$

Substituting the value of P in the above equation we get,

$$\delta = \frac{W}{A \, L \, g} \times \frac{g \, L^2 \, L}{2E}$$

$\therefore \qquad \boxed{\delta = \dfrac{WL}{2AE}}^{*}$

1.18 PRINCIPLE OF SUPERPOSITION

When a number of loads are acting on a body then the resulting strain will be algebraic sum of the strain caused by individual loads.

While solving the problem by superposition principle, first the free body diagram is drawn, afterwards the deformation (increase or decrease) of the each section is obtained.

---

* δ and any computed value of dimensions viz d; l etc of the specimen should be expressed in **mm** while solving the numerical problem.

The total deformation (Increase or decrease) of the body will then be equal to the algebraic sum of the deformation of individual section.

Let us analyse bars of the varying sections:

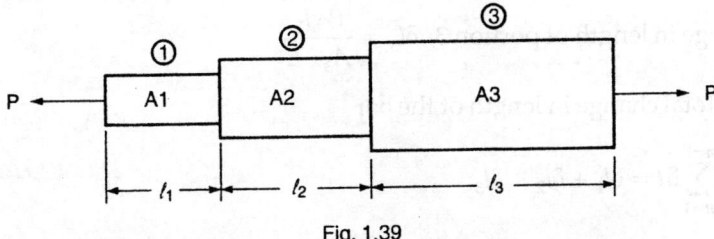

Fig. 1.39

In the figure there are three stepped bars of different cross-section A_1, A_2, A_3 and different length l_1, l_2 and l_3 respectively.

Let $\quad P$ = axial load acting on the bar

and $\quad E$ = Young's modulus of the bar.

Although each section is subjected to the same axial load P, yet the stresses, strain and change in lengths will be different.

The stress in section 1, $\quad \sigma_1 = \dfrac{P}{A_1}$

The stress in section 2, $\quad \sigma_2 = \dfrac{P}{A_2}$

The stress in section 3, $\quad \sigma_3 = \dfrac{P}{A_3}$

The strain in section 1, $\quad \varepsilon_1 = \dfrac{\sigma_1}{E} = \dfrac{P}{A_1 E}$

Similarly, strain in section 2, $\quad \varepsilon_2 = \dfrac{P}{A_2 E}$

and, $\qquad\qquad\qquad\qquad \varepsilon_3 = \dfrac{P}{A_3 E}$

Also, strain in portion 1 $= \dfrac{\text{Change in length of portion 1}}{\text{Original length of portion 1}}$

$$\varepsilon_1 = \dfrac{\delta l_1}{l_1}$$

$\therefore \quad$ Change in length of portion 1, $\delta l_1 = \varepsilon_1 \, l_1$

$$= \dfrac{P l_1}{A_1 E}$$

Similarly, change in length of portion 2, $\delta l_2 = \dfrac{P \cdot l_2}{A_2 \cdot E}$

and change in length of portion 3, $\delta l_3 = \dfrac{P \cdot l_3}{A_3 \cdot E}$

∴   Total change in length of the bar

$$\sum_{n=1}^{n=3} \delta l = \delta l_1 + \delta l_2 + \delta l_3$$

$$= \left[\frac{Pl_1}{A_1 E} + \frac{Pl_2}{A_2 E} + \frac{Pl_3}{A_3 E} \right]$$

$$= \frac{P}{E} \left[\frac{l_1}{A_1} + \frac{l_2}{A_2} + \frac{l_3}{A_3} \right]$$

This expression is used in solving the problem when a round bar/stepped bar/rectangular bar is subjected to axial load and the total change in length of the bar is needed.

In general total change in length of bar

$$\sum_{n=1}^{n=n} dl = \frac{P}{E} \left[\frac{l_1}{A_1} + \frac{l_2}{A_2} + \cdots + \frac{l_n}{A_n} \right]$$

EXAMPLE 1   *The loads acting on a 3 mm diameter has 6 meter total length divided into three segments as shown in figure. Find the total elongation of the bar (E = 210 GPa).*

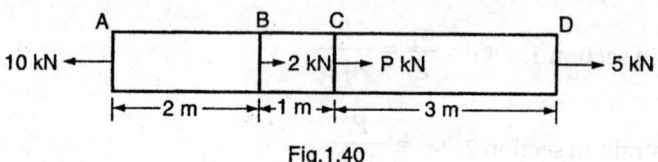

Fig.1.40

SOLUTION For static equilibrium $P + 2 + 5 = 10$

∴ $P = 3$ kN.

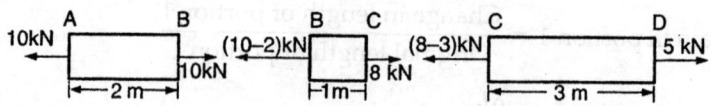

Fig. 1.41

Now, drawing *FBD*

$$A = \frac{\pi}{4} (d)^2 = 7.0714 \times 10^{-6} \text{ m}^2$$

∴   Total elongation of bar

$$= \frac{1}{EA} [P_{AB} \times L_{AB} + P_{BC} \times L_{BC} + P_{CD} \times L_{CD}]$$

$$= \frac{1}{210 \times 10^9 \times 7.0714 \times 10^{-6}}$$

$$\left[(10 \times 10^3 \times 2) + (8 \times 10^3 \times 1) + (5 \times 10^3 \times 3) \right] m$$

$$= \frac{10^3}{210 \times 7.0714 \times 10^3} [20 + 8 + 15]$$

$$= \frac{43}{210 \times 7.0714}$$

$$= 0.0289 \text{ m} = 28.95 \text{ mm}$$ **Ans.**

EXAMPLE 2 *A homogenous rod of constant cross-section is attached to unyielding supports. It carries an axial load P applied as shown in figure. Determine the reaction at A and B.*

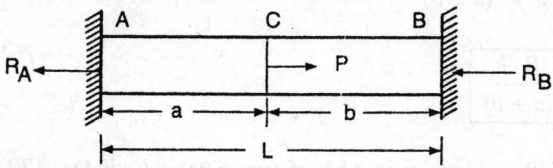

Fig. 1.42

SOLUTION Applying the condition of static equilibrium.

$$R_A + R_B = P$$ ...(1)

As the bar is fixed rigidly between supports.
Therefore, extension in portion AC = Contraction in portion CB.
Let us draw F.B.D. for portion AC and CB separately.

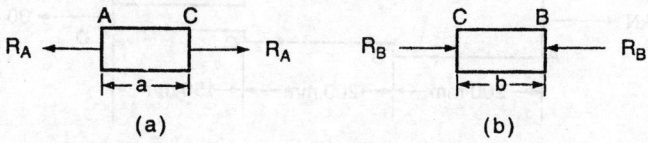

(a)   (b)

Fig. 1.43

$$\delta_{AC} = \frac{R_A \cdot a}{A \cdot E} \ ; \quad \delta_{CB} = \frac{R_B \cdot b}{A \cdot E}$$

Given $\delta_{AC} = \delta_{CB}$

∴ $$\frac{R_A \cdot a}{A \cdot E} = \frac{R_B \cdot b}{A \cdot E}$$

$$\frac{R_A}{R_B} = \frac{b}{a}$$

$$R_A = \left(\frac{b}{a}\right) \cdot R_B \qquad \qquad ...(2)$$

Substituting the value of R_A in eqn. (2)

$$\frac{b}{a} \cdot R_B + R_B = P$$

$$R_B \left(\frac{b}{a} + 1\right) = P$$

$$\boxed{R_B = \frac{P \cdot a}{a + b}} \qquad \qquad \textbf{Ans.}$$

and, $R_A = \left(\frac{b}{\not{a}}\right) \cdot \frac{P \cdot \not{a}}{(a + b)}$

$$\boxed{R_A = \frac{P \cdot b}{(a + b)}} \qquad \qquad \textbf{Ans.}$$

EXAMPLE 3 *A 550 mm long round bar of copper has a diameter of 30 mm over a length of 200 mm, diameter of 20 mm over a length of 200 mm and a diameter of 10 mm over its remaining length. Determine the stresses in each section and elongation of the rod when it is subjected to a pull of 30 kN. Assume E = 100 kN/mm².*

SOLUTION Axial pull $(P) = 30$ kN

$$= 30000 \text{ Newton}$$

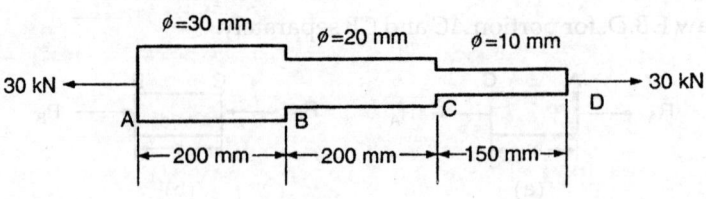

Fig. 1.44

Young's Modulus $(E) = 100$ kN/mm²

$$= 100 \times 10^3 \text{ N/mm}^2$$

$$= 10^5 \text{ N/mm}^2$$

Stress in portion AB, $\sigma_{AB} = \dfrac{P_{AB}}{A_{AB}}$

where, P_{AB} = load (Axial) in the portion AB

A_{AB} = cross-sectional area in the portion AB

$\therefore \qquad \sigma_{AB} = \dfrac{300 \times 10^3}{\dfrac{\pi}{4}(30)^2} = 42.463 \text{ N/mm}^2$

$A_{AB} = 706.5 \text{ mm}^2$

$A_{BC} = \dfrac{\pi}{4}(d)^2 = \dfrac{\pi}{4} \times (20)^2$

$A_{BC} = 314.28 \text{ mm}^2$

Similarly, $\sigma_{BC} = \dfrac{P_{BC}}{A_{BC}}$

$\qquad = \dfrac{30,0000}{\dfrac{\pi}{4} \times (20)^2} = 95.54 \text{ N/mm}^2$ **Ans.**

$A_{CD} = \dfrac{\pi}{4} \times (10)^2 \text{ mm}^2$

$\qquad = 78.57 \text{ m m}^2$

$\sigma_{CD} = \dfrac{30,000}{\dfrac{\pi}{4}(10)^2}$

$\qquad = 381.82 \text{ N/mm}^2$

$\therefore \qquad$ Total elongation of the rod

$(\delta) = \dfrac{P}{E} \cdot \left(\dfrac{L_1}{A_1} + \dfrac{L_2}{A_2} + \dfrac{L_3}{A_3} \right)$

$\qquad = \dfrac{30000}{(10)^5} \left(\dfrac{200}{706.85} + \dfrac{200}{314.28} + \dfrac{150}{78.57} \right)$

$\delta = 0.84 \text{ mm}$ **Ans.**

EXAMPLE 4 *A steel bar of 25 mm diameter is loaded as shown in Fig. 1.45. Calculate the stresses in each portion and the total elongation. Assume $E_{steel} = 200$ GPa.*

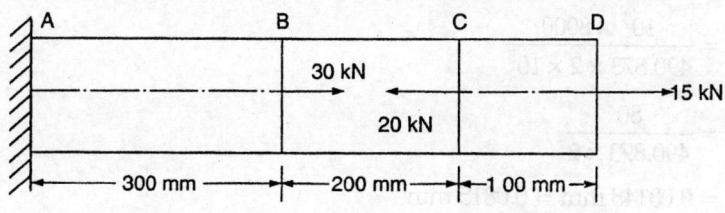

Fig. 1.45

SOLUTION Let us draw FBD of various portion of bar (starting from D for convenience).

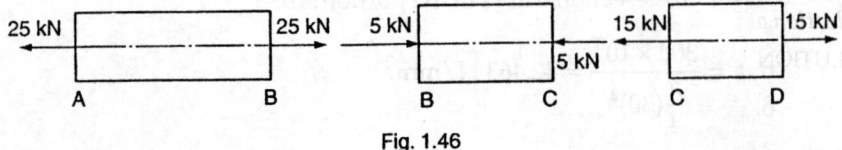

Fig. 1.46

C.S. area of the bar $= \dfrac{\pi}{4} \times d^2$

$$= \dfrac{\pi}{4} \times (25)^2$$

Hence, $A = 490.873 \text{ mm}^2$

$$\sigma_{AB} = \dfrac{P_{AB}}{A} = \dfrac{25 \times 10^3}{490.873}$$

$$= 50.93 \text{ MPa}$$

$$\sigma_{BC} = (-)\dfrac{P_{BC}}{A} \quad \text{(since load is compressive so negative sign used)}$$

$$= (-)\dfrac{5 \times 10^3}{490.873} = (-)10.186 \text{ MPa}$$

Total elongation

$$= \dfrac{1}{AE} \Sigma P_n \cdot L_n$$

$$= \dfrac{1}{AE} [P_{AB} \cdot L_{AB} - P_{BC} \cdot L_{BC} + P_{CD} \cdot L_{CD}]$$

$$= \dfrac{1}{490.873 \times 200 \times 10^3} [25 \times 10^3 \times 300 - 5 \times 10^3 \times 200 + 15 \times 10^3 \times 100]$$

$$= \dfrac{10^3}{490.873 \times 2 \times 10^5} [25 \times 300 - 5 \times 200 + 15 \times 100]$$

$$= \dfrac{10^3}{490.873 \times 2 \times 10^5} [7500 - 1000 + 1500]$$

$$= \dfrac{10^3 \times 8000}{490.873 \times 2 \times 10^5}$$

$$= \dfrac{80}{490.873 \times 2}$$

$$= 0.08148 \text{ mm} \simeq 0.0815 \text{ mm} \qquad\qquad\qquad \textbf{Ans.}$$

EXAMPLE 5 *A single axial load P = 50 kN is applied at end C of the brass road ABC. Knowing that E = 105 GPa, determine the diameter d of the portion BC for which the deflection at point C will be 3 mm.*

SOLUTION Applying formula

$$\delta_{total} = \delta_{AB} + \delta_{BC}$$

$$= \frac{P \cdot L_{AB}}{A_{AB} \cdot E_{AB}} + \frac{P \cdot L_{BC}}{A_{BC} \cdot E_{BC}}$$

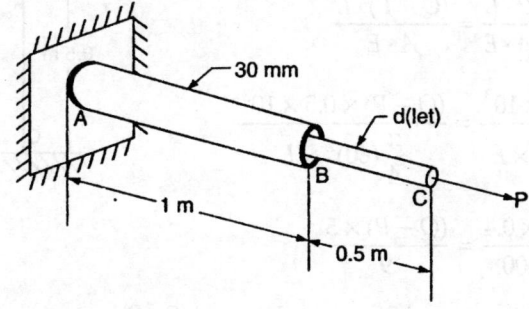

Fig. 1.47

$$E_{AB} = E_{BC} = E_{brass} = 105 \text{ GPa (given)}$$

$$= 105 \times 10^3 \text{ MPa}$$

$$3 = \frac{50 \times 10^3 \times 1 \times 10^3}{\frac{\pi}{4}(30)^2 \times 105 \times 10^3} + \frac{50 \times 10^3 \times 0.5 \times 10^3}{\frac{\pi}{4}(d)^2 \times 105 \times 10^3}$$

or

$$3 = \frac{50 \times 10^3 \times 10^3}{\frac{\pi}{4} \times 105 \times 10^3}\left[\frac{1}{(30)^2} + \frac{0.5}{(d)^2}\right]$$

or,

$$3 = \frac{4 \times 50 \times 10^3}{\pi \times 105}\left[\frac{1}{900} + \frac{0.5}{(d)^2}\right]$$

or,

$$\left(\frac{3 \times \pi \times 105}{4 \times 105 \times 10^3}\right) - \frac{1}{900} = \frac{0.5}{d^2}$$

or,

$$4.9455 \times 10^{-3} - 1.111 \times 10^{-3} = \frac{0.5}{d^2}$$

or,

$$\frac{3.8345}{10^3} = \frac{0.5}{d^2}$$

$$\Rightarrow \qquad d = 11.42 \text{ mm} \qquad \textbf{Ans.}$$

EXAMPLE 6 *In the given figure AB and BC are made of an aluminium for which E = 70 GPa. Knowing that the magnitude of P is 4 kN. Determine*

   (a) *the value of Q so that the deflection at A is zero*

   (b) *the corresponding deflection at B.*

SOLUTION   (a)   Given deflection at A = 0 and P = 4 kN

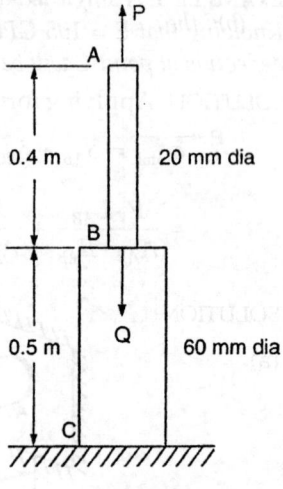

Fig. 1.48

$$\Rightarrow \qquad 0 = \frac{P \cdot L}{A \cdot E} - \frac{(Q - P) \cdot L}{A \cdot E}$$

$$\Rightarrow \qquad \frac{P \cdot L}{A \cdot E} = \frac{(Q - P) \cdot L}{A \cdot E}$$

$$\Rightarrow \qquad \frac{P \times 9.4 \times 10^3}{\frac{\pi}{4}(20)^2 \times E} = \frac{(Q - P) \times 0.5 \times 10^3}{\frac{\pi}{4}(60)^2 \times E}$$

$$\Rightarrow \qquad \frac{P \times 0.4}{400} = \frac{(Q - P) \times 5}{9}$$

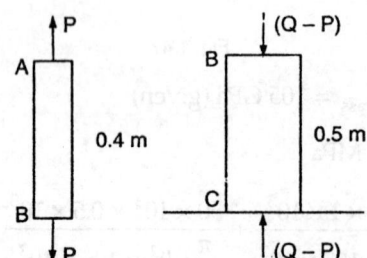

Fig. 1.49

$$\Rightarrow \qquad 36P = 5Q - 5P$$

$$\Rightarrow \qquad 41P = 5Q$$

$$\Rightarrow \qquad Q = \left(\frac{41}{5}\right)P = \frac{41}{5} \times 4 = \frac{164}{5}$$

$$\therefore \qquad \boxed{Q = 32.8 \text{ kN}} \qquad\qquad\qquad\qquad\qquad \textbf{Ans.}$$

(b) $$\qquad \delta_{BC} = \frac{(32.8 - 4) \times 10^3 \times 500 \times 28}{22 \times 3600 \times 70 \times 10^3}$$

$$= \frac{14.4}{198}$$

$$= 0.0727 \text{ mm}$$

EXAMPLE 7 *The specimen shown in Figure is made from a 25 mm diameter cylindrical steel rod with two 38 mm sleeves bonded to the rod as shown in figure. Knowing that E = 200 GPa, determine*

(a) the load P so that the total deformtion is 0.05 mm.

(b) the corresponding deformation of the central part BC.

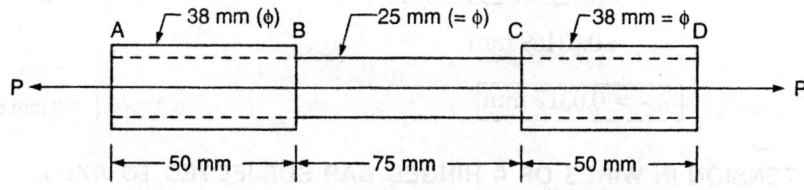

Fig. 1.50

SOLUTION Given δ_{total} = 0.05 mm; E = 200 GPa = 200 × 10³ MPa.

(a) $\delta_{\text{total}} = \delta_{AB} + \delta_{BC} + \delta_{CD}$, by superposition theorem

$$0.05 = \frac{P \cdot L_{AB}}{A_{AB} \cdot E} + \frac{P \cdot L_{BC}}{A_{BC} \cdot E} + \frac{P \cdot L_{CD}}{A_{CD} \cdot E}$$

$$0.05 = \frac{P}{E} \left[\frac{L_{AB}}{A_{AB}} + \frac{L_{BC}}{A_{BC}} + \frac{L_{CD}}{A_{CD}} \right]$$

$$0.05 = \frac{P}{200 \times 10^3} \left[\frac{50}{\frac{\pi}{4}(38)^2} + \frac{75}{\frac{\pi}{4}(25)^2} + \frac{50}{\frac{\pi}{4}(38)^2} \right]$$

$$\left(\frac{0.05}{1} \right) = \frac{P}{2 \times 10^5 \times \frac{\pi}{4}} \left[\frac{2 \times 50}{(38)^2} + \frac{75}{(25)^2} \right]$$

$$\frac{0.05}{1} = \frac{4P}{2\pi \times 10^5} \left[\frac{100}{(38)^2} + \frac{75}{(25)^2} \right]$$

$$\frac{0.05 \times 2\pi \times 10^5}{4} = P \times \left[\frac{100}{(38)^2} + \frac{75}{(25)^2} \right]$$

$$\frac{5 \times 2\pi \times 10^3}{4} = P \times (0.069252 + 0.12)$$

$$P = 41479 \text{ N}$$

$$= 41.479 \text{ kN}$$

$$\boxed{P = 41.5 \text{ kN}}$$ Ans.

(b) Corresponding to P = 41.5 kN, the central part BC

Deformation i.e. $\delta_{BC} = \dfrac{41.5 \times 10^3 \times 75}{\dfrac{\pi}{4}(25)^2 \times 200 \times 10^3}$

$$= \frac{41.5 \times 10^3 \times 75 \times 4 \times 7}{22 \times 625 \times 2 \times 10^5}$$

$$= 0.03169 \text{ mm}$$

$\therefore$ $\boxed{\delta_{BC} = 0.0317 \text{ mm}}$ **Ans.**

1.19 TENSION IN WIRES OF A HINGED BAR SUBJECTED TO AXIAL PULL (P)

EXAMPLE 1 *In the figure OABC is a rigid bar which is hinged at 0 and supported in a horizontal position by two identical steel wires. A vertical load P is applied at C. Find the tension T_1 and T_2 in the steel wires.*

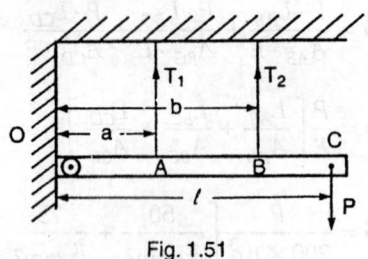

Fig. 1.51

SOLUTION The $T_1 + T_2 + F_y = P$

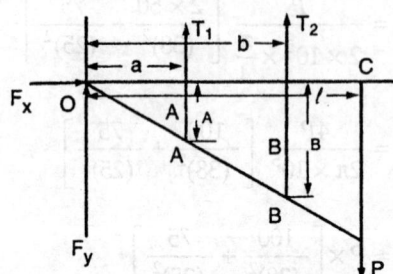

Fig. 1.52 Free body diagram

From Δs $OA'A$ and $OB'B$

$$\frac{\delta_A}{a} = \frac{\delta_B}{b} = \frac{T_1}{T_2} \qquad \qquad \ldots(1)$$

$$\frac{\delta_A}{\delta_B} = \frac{a}{b} = \frac{T_1}{T_2} \qquad \qquad \ldots(2)$$

Taking moment about O and equating it to zero

$$T_1 a + T_2 \cdot b = P \cdot l \qquad \qquad \ldots(3)$$

Given $\dfrac{a}{b} = \dfrac{T_1}{T_2}$

or $\qquad \dfrac{a^2}{b^2} = \dfrac{a\,T_1}{b\,T_2}$

or $\qquad \dfrac{a^2}{b^2} + 1 = \dfrac{a\,T_1 + b\,T_2}{b\,T_2}$ $\qquad\qquad$ (Adding 1 both sides)

or $\qquad \dfrac{a^2 + b^2}{b^2} = \dfrac{a\,T_1 + b\,T_2}{b\,T_2}$

$\therefore \qquad a\,T_1 + b\,T_2 = \dfrac{T_2\,(a^2 + b^2)}{b}$

Equation (3) reduces to

$$\dfrac{T_2(a^2 + b^2)}{b} = P \cdot l$$

$$\boxed{\begin{array}{l} \therefore \quad \dfrac{P \cdot b \cdot l}{(a^2 + b^2)} = T_2 \\[2mm] \text{Similarly } T_1 = \dfrac{P \cdot a \cdot l}{(a^2 + b^2)} \end{array}}$$

N.B: This can be used as a formula when P. a, b, l are given.

Let us confirm by the following example.

EXAMPLE 2 *A rigid bar OABC is hinged at A and supported in a horizontal position by two identical steel wires as shown in figure. A vertical load of 30 kN is applied at C. Find the tensile forces T_1 and T_2 induced in these wires by the vertical load.*

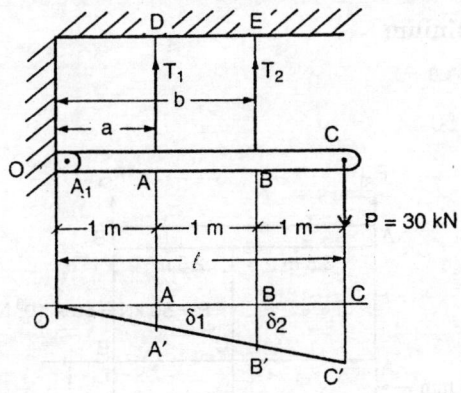

Fig. 1.53

SOLUTION By formula

$$T_1 = \dfrac{P \cdot a \cdot l}{(a^2 + b^2)}$$

$$= \frac{30 \times 10^3 \times 1 \times 3}{(1^2 + 2^2)}$$

$$= \frac{90,000}{5} = 18,000 \text{ Newton}$$

$$= 18 \text{ kN}$$

$$T_2 = \frac{P \cdot b \cdot l}{(a^2 + b^2)}$$

$$= \frac{6\overline{30} \times 10^3 \times 2 \times 3}{5_1}$$

$$= 36 \text{ kN} \qquad \textbf{Ans.}$$

EXAMPLE 3 *The rigid bar AB is attached to two vertical rods as shown in Fig. 1.54 is horizontal before the load P is apoplied. Determine the vertical movement of P if it's magnitude is 50 kN.*

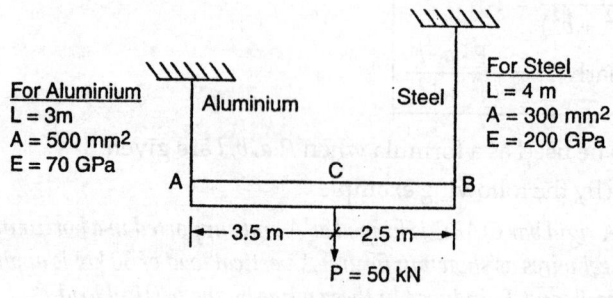

Fig. 1.54

SOLUTION **For Aluminium**

$$\Sigma M_B = 0 \text{ gives}$$

$$6P_{Al} = 2.5 \times 50$$

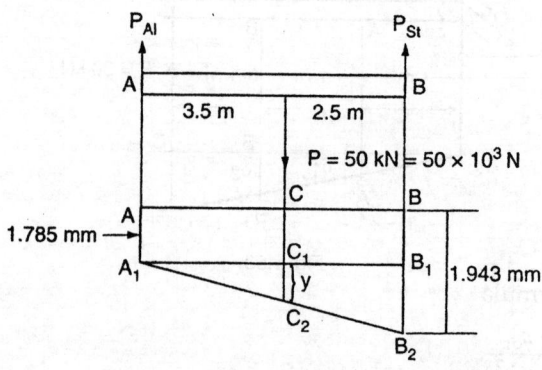

Fig. 1.55

$$\therefore \qquad P_{Al} = \frac{2.5 \times 50}{6}$$

$$= 20.83 \, kN = 20.83 \times 10^3 \, Newton$$

$$\delta_{Al} = \frac{P \cdot L}{A \cdot E} = \frac{20.83 \times 3 \times (1000)^2}{500 \times (70 \times 10^3)} mm$$

$$= \frac{20.83 \times 3000}{500 \times 70} mm = 1.785 \, mm$$

For Steel

$$\Sigma M_A = 0 \ \text{gives}$$

$$\sigma P_{st} = 3.5 \times 50$$

$$P_{st} = \frac{3.5 \times 50}{6} = 29.16 \, kN$$

$$= 19.16 \times 10^3 \, N$$

$$\sigma_{steel} = \frac{P \cdot L}{A \cdot E}$$

$$= \frac{29.16 \times 10^3 \times (4 \times 1000)}{300 \times 200 \times 10^3}$$

$$= \frac{29.16 \times 4000}{300 \times 200} = 1.943 \, mm$$

Now, from similar triangles $A_1C_1C_2$ and $A_1B_1B_2$

$$\frac{y}{A_1C_1} = \frac{B_1B_2}{A_1B_1}$$

$$\frac{y}{3.5} = \frac{1.943 - 1.785}{6}$$

$$\Rightarrow \qquad y = \frac{3.5 \times (1.943 - 1.785)}{6} = 0.092 \, mm$$

Now, vertical movement of P

$$= CC_2$$

$$= CC_1 + y$$

$$= 1.785 + 0.092$$

$$= 1.877 \, mm$$

Ans.

EXAMPLE 4 *The rigid bar AB and CD is shown in Fig. 1.56 are supported by pins A and C and the two rods. Determine the maximum force P that can be applied if its vertical movement is limited to 5 mm. Neglect the weights of all members.*

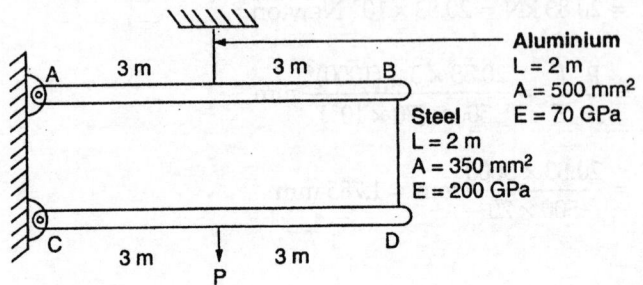

Fig. 1.56

SOLUTION Let us start from part AB.

$\Sigma M_A = 0$ gives

$$3P_{al} = 6P_{st}$$

$\therefore \qquad P_{al} = 2P_{st}$

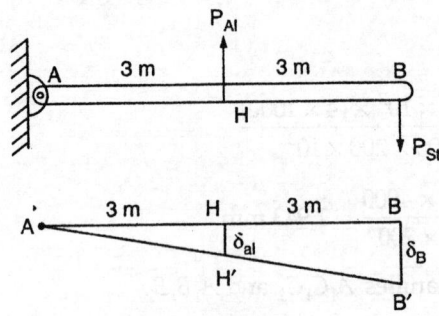

Fig. 1.57

Now, from similar triangles, ABB' and AHH' we get

$$\frac{BB'}{6} = \frac{HH'}{3}$$

$$\frac{\delta_B}{6} = \frac{\delta_{al}}{3}$$

$\therefore \qquad \delta_B = 2\delta_{al}$

$$= 2\left[\frac{P_{al} \cdot L}{A \cdot E}\right]$$

$$= 2\left[\frac{P_{al} \times 2000}{500 \times 70 \times 10^3}\right] = \frac{1}{8750}P_{al}$$

$$= \frac{1}{8750} \times 2P_{st}$$

$$= \frac{1}{4375} P_{st} \text{ is the movement of } B$$

Part CD

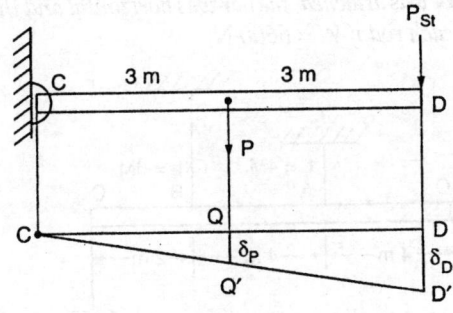

Fig. 1.58

Movement of D

$$\delta_D = \delta_{st} + \delta_B$$

$$= \frac{P \cdot L}{A \cdot E} + \frac{1}{4375} P_{st}$$

$$= \frac{P_{st} \times 2000}{300 \times 2 \times 10^5} + \frac{1}{4375} P_{st}$$

$$= 3.333 \times 10^{-5} P_{st} + 2.285 \times 10^{-4} P_{st}$$

$$= 2.618 \times 10^{-4} P_{st}$$

$\Sigma M_C = 0$ for static equilibrium

$$6P_{st} = 3P$$

$$P_{st} = \frac{1}{2}P$$

By similar triangles CQQ' and CDD'

$$\frac{\delta_P}{3} = \frac{\delta_D}{6}$$

$$\delta_P = \frac{1}{2}\delta_D$$

$$\left(\frac{5}{1000}\right) = \frac{1}{2} \times 2.618 \, P_{st} \times 10^{-4} \qquad [\because \delta_P = 5 \text{ mm}]$$

$$\therefore \qquad P_{st} = \left[\frac{0.005 \times 2}{2.618 \times 10^{-4}}\right]$$

or, $\dfrac{1}{2}P = 38.19$

$\therefore$ $P = 76.38$ kN   **Ans.**

EXAMPLE 5 *Two vertical rods attached to the light bar in Fig. 1.59 are identical except for length. Before the load W was attached, the bar was horizontal and the rods were stress free. Determine the load in each rod if W = 6600 N.*

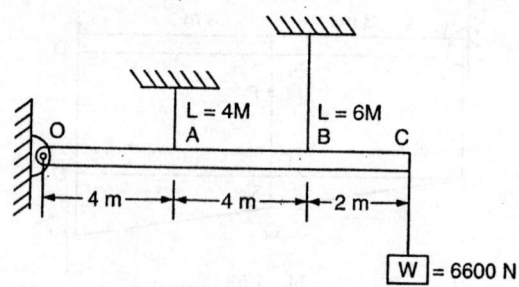

Fig. 1.59

SOLUTION $\Sigma M_O = 0$ gives

$4P_A + 8P_B = 10 \times 6600$

$P_A + 2P_B = 16500$ ...(I)

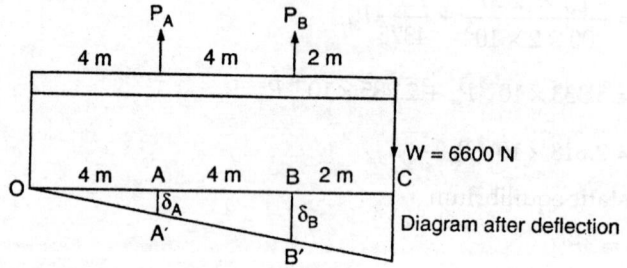

Fig. 1.60

Now, from similar triangle OAA' and OBB'

$\dfrac{\delta_A}{4} = \dfrac{\delta_B}{8}$

$\dfrac{P_A \cdot L_A}{A_A \cdot E_A} \times \dfrac{1}{4} = \dfrac{P_B \cdot L_B}{A_B \cdot E_B} \times \dfrac{1}{8}$

Since rods are identical except length

So $A_A = A_B = A$ (let)

$E_A = E_B = E$ (let)

$$\frac{P_A \cdot 4}{A \cdot E} \times \frac{1}{4} = \frac{P_B \cdot 6}{A \cdot E} \times \frac{1}{8}$$

$$P_A = \frac{3P_B}{4} \qquad \qquad \text{...(II)}$$

Substituting the value of P_A in equation (I)

$$\frac{3P_B}{4} + 2P_B = 16500$$

$$3P_B + 8P_B = 16500 \times 4$$

$$11P_B = 16500 \times 4$$

∴ $$P_B = \left(\frac{66000}{11}\right) = 6000 \text{ Newton}$$

$$P_A = 16500 - 2P_B$$

$$= 165000 - 12000$$

$$= 4500 \text{ Newton}$$

EXAMPLE 6 *The block of weight W hangs from the point at A. The bars AB and AC are pinned to the support at B and C. The C.S. area are 800 mm² for AB and 400 mm² for AC. Neglecting the weight of the bars, determine the maximum safe value of W if the stress in AB is limited to 110 MPa and in AC to 120 MPa.*

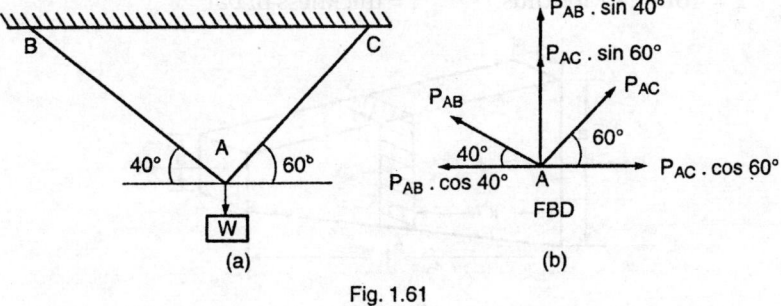

Fig. 1.61

SOLUTION Drawing F.B.D as in Fig. 1.50 (b) of joint A, we get

$\Sigma F_x = 0$ gives

$$P_{AC} \times 0.5 - P_{AB} \times 0.766 = 0 \qquad \qquad \text{...(1)}$$

$\Sigma F_y = 0$ gives

$$P_{AC} \times 0.866 + P_{AB} \times 0.642 - W = 0 \qquad \qquad \text{...(2)}$$

Solving (1) and (2) we get

$$P_{AB} = 0.508 \ W \qquad \qquad \left.\begin{array}{l} \sin 40 = 0.642 \\ \cos 40 = 0.766 \end{array}\right]$$

and, $$P_{AC} = 0.778 \ W$$

The value of W that will cause the stress in each bar to equal its maximum safe magnitude is determined as follows:

For AB:

$\because$ $P = \sigma \cdot A$

         $0.508\,W = 110 \times 10^6 \text{ N/m}^2 \times 800 \times 10^{-6} \text{ m}^2$

$\therefore$ $W = 173 \times 10^3 \text{ Newton}$

         $= 173 \text{ kN}$

For AC:

$\because$ $P = \sigma \cdot A$

         $0.778\,W = (120 \times 10^6 \text{ N/m}^2) \times (400 \times 10^{-6} \text{ m}^2)$

         $W = 61.7 \times 10^3 \text{ N}$

         $= 61.7 \text{ kN}$

The maximum safe value of W is the smaller one

$\therefore$ 61.7 kN   **Ans.**

1.20 EXPRESSION FOR THE TOTAL EXTENSION OF A UNIFORMLY TAPERING RECTANGULAR BAR WHEN SUBJECTED TO AXIAL LOAD *P*.

Let P = axial load on the bar L = length of the bar

            a = width of bigger end b = width of smaller end

            E = Young's Modulus t = thickness of bar

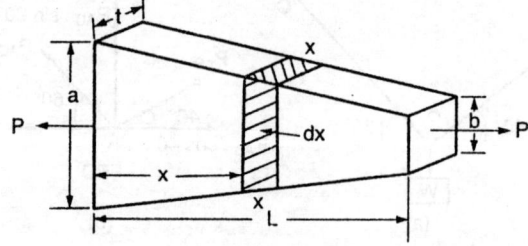

Fig. 1.52

Width of the bar of section $XX = a - \left(\dfrac{a-b}{L} \right) x$

$$= a - Kx \text{ where} \left(\frac{a-b}{L} \right) = K \text{ (Constant)}$$

Area at section XX = width × thickness

$$= (a - Kx)\,t$$

Stress at section XX,

$$\sigma_{XX} = \frac{P}{(a - Kx)\,t}$$

Extension of the small elemental length dx

$$= \text{Strain} \times \text{length } dx$$

$$= \frac{\text{Stress}}{E} \times dx$$

$$= \frac{\left[\dfrac{P}{(a - Kx)\,t}\right]}{E} \times dx$$

$$= \frac{P}{E\,(a - Kx)\,t} \times dx$$

Total extension of the bar $(dL) = \displaystyle\int_0^L \frac{P}{E\,(a - Kx)\,t}\,dx$

$$= \frac{P}{Et} \int_0^L \frac{dx}{(a - Kx)}$$

$$= \frac{P}{Et} \cdot \log_e\,[a - kx]_0^L \times \left(-\frac{1}{K}\right)$$

$$= -\frac{P}{Et}\,[\log_e\,(a - KL) - \log_e\,a]$$

$$= \frac{P}{Et}\left[\log_e\left(\frac{a}{a - KL}\right)\right]$$

$$= \frac{P}{Et\left(\dfrac{a - b}{L}\right)}\left[\log_e\left\{\frac{a}{a - \left(\dfrac{a - b}{L}\right) \cdot L}\right\}\right]$$

$$= \frac{PL}{Et\,(a - b)} \cdot \log_e\left(\frac{a}{b}\right) \quad \textbf{Ans.}$$

N.B. This may be treated as a formula.

EXAMPLE 1 *Find out the total elongation caused by an axial load of 100 kN applied to a flat bar 20 mm thick, tapering from a width of 120 mm to 40 mm in a length of 10 m as shown in Fig. 1.63. (Given E = 200 GPa.)*

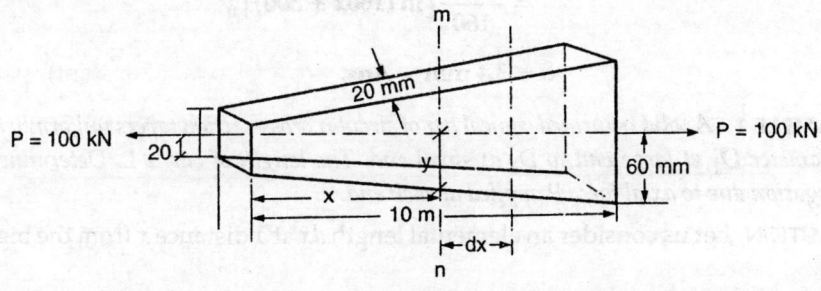

Fig. 1.63

SOLUTION From the question we find that cross-section is not constant so the equation $\sigma = \dfrac{P}{A}$ does not hold good in this problem.

However, it may be used to find the elongation on a differential length for which cross-section is constant.

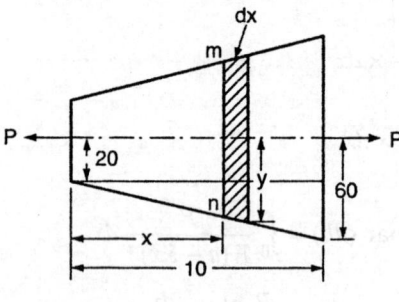

Fig. 1.64

At mn-section, $\dfrac{y - 20}{x} = \dfrac{60 - 20}{10}$

$\therefore$ $\quad y = (4x + 20)$ mm

Area of the section $(A) = 20 \times 2y = (160x + 800)$ mm^2

At mn, in a differential length dx, the elongation

$\because$ $\qquad \delta = \dfrac{P \cdot L}{AE}$

$\therefore$ $\qquad d\delta = \dfrac{(100 \times 10^3)\, dx}{(160x + 800)\,(10^{-6})\,(200 \times 10^9)}$

$\qquad\qquad = \left[\dfrac{0.500\, dx}{160x + 800} \right]$

$\therefore$ $\quad$ Total elongation $(\delta) = 0.500 \displaystyle\int_0^{10} \dfrac{dx}{160x + 800}$

$\qquad\qquad\qquad = \dfrac{0.500}{160} \left[\ln(160x + 800) \right]_0^{10}$

$\qquad\qquad\qquad \delta = 3.4$ mm   **Ans.**

EXAMPLE 2 *A solid truncated conical bar of circular cross-section tapers uniformly form a diameter D_1 at large end to D_2 at small end. The length of bar is L. Determine the elongation due to axial force P applied at each end.*

SOLUTION Let us consider an elemental length dx at a distance x from the bigger end.

∴ Diameter of the bar at x distance from bigger end

$$D_X = D_1 - (D_1 - D_2) \cdot \frac{x}{L}$$

$$= D_1 - mx, \text{ where } \left(\frac{D_1 - D_2}{L} \right) = m$$

∴ Sectional area at this section, $A_x = \frac{\pi}{4}(D_1 - mx)^2$

Axial strain at this section,

$$\varepsilon_x = \frac{\text{Axial stress}}{E}$$

$$= \frac{P/A_x}{E}$$

$$= \frac{P}{\frac{\pi}{4}(D_1 - mx)^2 \cdot E}$$

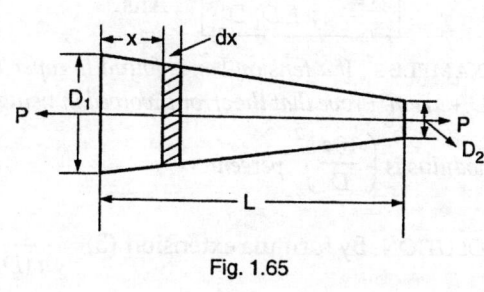

Fig. 1.65

Extension of the elemental length dx

$$= \varepsilon_x \times dx$$

$$= \frac{4P}{\pi(D_1 - mx)^2 E} dx$$

∴ Total extension of the bar

$$= \int_0^L \frac{4P\,dx}{\pi(D_1 - mx)^2 E}$$

$$= \frac{4P}{\pi E} \int_0^L (D_1 - mx)^{-2} dx$$

$$= \frac{4P}{\pi E} \left[\frac{1}{m(D_1 - mx)} \right]_0^L$$

$$= \frac{4P}{\pi Em} \left[\frac{1}{(D_1 - mL)} - \frac{1}{D_1 - m \times 0} \right]$$

$$= \frac{4P}{\pi Em} \left[\frac{1}{D_1(D_1 - D_2)} - \frac{1}{D_1} \right] \qquad \left[\because m = \frac{D_1 - D_2}{L} \right]$$

$$= \frac{4P}{\pi Em} \left[\frac{1}{D_2} - \frac{1}{D_1} \right]$$

$$= \frac{4P(D_1 - D_2)}{\pi E m\, D_1\, D_2}$$

$$= \frac{4P(D_1 - D_2)}{\pi E D_1 D_2 \left(\dfrac{D_1 - D_2}{L} \right)}$$

$$\boxed{\therefore \delta = \frac{4PL}{\pi E D_1 D_2}} \quad \textbf{Ans.}$$

EXAMPLE 3 *If a tension bar is found to taper uniformly from (D − a) cm to diameter (D + a) cm. Prove that the error involved in using the mean diameter to calculate Young's modulus is* $\left(\dfrac{10a}{D} \right)^2$ *percent.*

SOLUTION By formula extension $(\delta) = \dfrac{4PL}{\pi (D - a)(D + a) E}$

$$\therefore \qquad E = \frac{4PL}{\pi (D^2 - a^2)\,\delta}$$

In case we are to calculate E on the basis of mean diameter D, extension δ being the same

$$\therefore \qquad E = \frac{4PL}{\pi D^2 x}$$

$$\therefore \qquad \text{Error in calculating } E = \frac{4PL}{\pi (D^2 - a^2)\, x} - \frac{4PL}{\pi D^2 x}$$

and,   Error in calculating $E = \dfrac{\left[\dfrac{4PL}{\pi (D^2 - a^2)\, x} - \dfrac{4PL}{\pi D^2 x} \right] 100}{\dfrac{4PL}{\pi (D^2 - a^2)\, x}}$

$$= \frac{\left[\dfrac{1}{D^2 - a^2} - \dfrac{1}{D^2} \right] 100}{\dfrac{1}{D^2 - a^2}}$$

$$= 100 \left(\frac{a^2}{D^2} \right) = \left(\frac{10a}{D} \right)^2 \qquad \textbf{Proved.}$$

1.21 STRESSES IN COMPOSITE MEMBERS

A composite member is composed of two or more different materials joined together in such a way that the system is elongated or compressed as single unit.

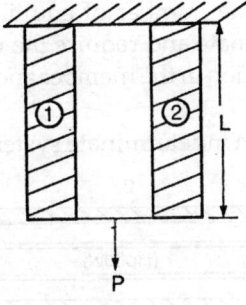

Fig. 1.66

In the figure composite bar of different materials have been shown.

Let P = total load on composite bar

L = length of each bar.

For   **Bar 1**   **Bar 2**

A_1 = Area of cross-section	A_2 = Area of cross-section
P_1 = load carried by it	P_2 = load carried by it
E_1 = Young's Modulus	E_2 = Young's Modulus
σ_1 = Stress induced	σ_2 = Stress induced

Total load on composite bar,

$$P = P_1 + P_2 \qquad \qquad \qquad ...(1)$$

The stress in bar 1, $\sigma_1 = \dfrac{P_1}{A_1}$

$$\therefore \qquad P_1 = \sigma_1 \cdot A_1 \qquad \qquad ...(2)$$

Similarly, $P_2 = \sigma_2 \cdot A_2 \qquad \qquad ...(3)$

Substituting the value of P_1 and P_2 in equation (1)

$$P = \sigma_1 A_1 + \sigma_2 A_2 \qquad \qquad ...(4)$$

Strain in bar (1), $\varepsilon_1 = \dfrac{\sigma_1}{E_1}$

Similarly, strain in bar (2), $\varepsilon_2 = \dfrac{\sigma_2}{E_2}$

We know, strain in bar 1 = Strain in bar 2

$$\boxed{\therefore \quad \dfrac{\sigma_1}{E_1} = \dfrac{\sigma_2}{E_2}} \qquad \textbf{Ans.}$$

1.22 STATICALLY INDETERMINATE MEMBERS

There are certain loaded members in which the equations of static equilibrium are not sufficient for a solution. This condition exists in structure where the number of unknown forces exceeds the number of equilibrium equations. Such cases are called statically indeterminate and require the use of addition relations that depend on the elastic deformation in the member and are known as **compatability equation.**

A compound bar is a case of an indeterminate system which is discussed below:

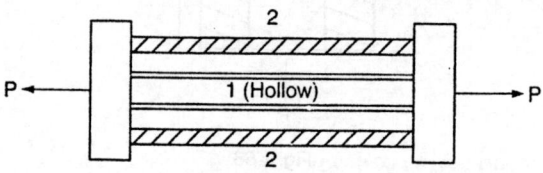

Fig. 1.67

Two bars of different materials (1 and 2) here make a composite bar or compound bar is subjected to load P.

Our objective is to find the load shared by hollow tube 1 and solid bar 2.

Applying condition of static equilibrium

$$P = P_1 + P_2 \qquad \qquad ...(I)$$

Applying compatibility equation

i.e. $\qquad \delta_1 = \delta_2 \qquad$ (i.e. deformation of bar is equal to tube)

$$\frac{P_1 L}{A_1 E_1} = \frac{P_2 L}{A_2 E_2} \quad (\text{As the length of 1 and 2 are equal } i.e. \ L_1 = L_2 = L)$$

or, $\qquad P_1 = \dfrac{P_2 A_1 E_1}{A_2 E_2} \qquad \qquad ...(II)$

Substituting P_1 in (I) we get

$$P = \frac{P_2 A_1 E_1}{A_2 E_2} + P_2$$

$$= \frac{P_2 A_1 E_1 + P_2 A_2 E_2}{A_2 E_2}$$

$$= \frac{P_2 (A_1 E_1 + A_2 E_2)}{A_2 E_2}$$

$\therefore \qquad P_2 = \dfrac{P \cdot A_2 E_2}{A_1 E_1 + A_2 E_2}$

Similarly, $\qquad P_1 = \dfrac{P \cdot A_1 E_1}{A_1 E_1 + A_2 E_2}$

EXAMPLE 1 *A compound tube is made by shrinking a thin sheet tube on a thin brass tube. A_s and A_b are the sectional areas of the steel and brass tubes and E_s and E_b are the corresponding values of Young's Modulus. Show that for any tensile load the extension of the compound tube is equal to that of a single tube of the same length and total cross sectional area but having a Young's modulus of* $\left(\dfrac{E_s A_s + E_b A_b}{A_s + A_b} \right)$.

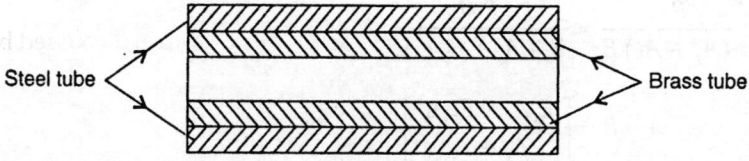

Fig. 1.68

SOLUTION Let the load on the compound tube be P.

Area of steel tube $= A_s$

Area of brass tube $= A_b$

Let the stresses in the steel tube and brass tube be σ_s and σ_b respectively therefore

$$\varepsilon_s = \varepsilon_b$$

or,

$$\left(\frac{\sigma_s}{E_s} \right) = \left(\frac{\sigma_b}{E_b} \right)$$

$\therefore$

$$\sigma_s = \frac{E_s}{E_b} \cdot \sigma_b$$

Load on steel + load on brass = total load on compound tube

$$\sigma_s \cdot A_s + \sigma_b \cdot A_b = P$$

$\therefore$

$$\frac{E_s}{E_b} \cdot \sigma_b \cdot A_s + \sigma_b \cdot A_b = P$$

$$\sigma_b \left[\frac{E_s}{E_b} \cdot A_s + A_b \right] = P$$

$\therefore$

$$\sigma_b = \left[\frac{E_b}{E_s A_s + E_b A_b} \right] \cdot P$$

$\therefore$ Extension of the compound tube $= dl =$ extension of steel or brass tube

$$dl = \frac{\sigma_b}{E_b} \cdot l$$

$$= \left[\frac{P}{E_s A_s + E_b A_b} \right] \cdot l \qquad \qquad \ldots(I)$$

Let E be the Young's Modulus of the tube of area (A_s) carrying the same load and undergoing the same extension.

$$dl = \left[\frac{P}{(A_s + A_b)\,E} \right] \qquad\qquad \text{...(II)}$$

From (I) and (II), we get

$$\frac{P \cdot l}{(A_s + A_b)\,E} = \frac{P \cdot l}{E_s \cdot A_s + E_b \cdot A_b}$$

$$\therefore \qquad E = \left[\frac{E_s A_s + E_b A_b}{A_s + A_b} \right]$$

EXAMPLE 2 *A load of 2 MN is applied on a short column of concrete 500 mm × 500 mm. The column is reinforced with four steel bars of 10 mm diameter, one in each corner. Find the stress in the concrete and steel bars. Take E for steel as $2.1 \times 10^5\,N/mm^2$ and for concrete $1.4 \times 10^5\,N/mm^2$* **(UPTU-2004)**

SOLUTION Given P = load applied = 2 MN

$$= 2 \times 10^6 \text{ Newton}$$

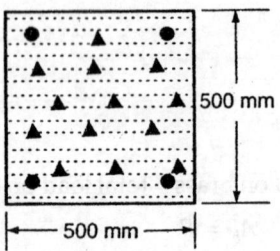

Fig.1.69

Area of column = (500×500) mm^2

$$= 250000 \text{ mm}^2$$

Area of 4 steel bars (As) = $\cancel{4} \times \dfrac{\pi}{\cancel{4}}\,(10)^2$

$$= 314.159 \text{ mm}^2$$

Area of concrete (Ac) = (Area of column – Area of steel bars)

$$= 250000 - 314.159$$

$$= 249685.841 \text{ mm}^2$$

Now, strain in steel = strain in concrete

$$\varepsilon_{\text{steel}} = \varepsilon_{\text{concrete}}$$

$$\frac{\sigma_s}{E_s} = \frac{\sigma_c}{E_c}$$

$$\therefore \qquad \sigma_s = \sigma_c \cdot \frac{E_s}{E_c}$$

$$= \sigma_c \times \frac{2.1 \times 10^5}{1.4 \times 10^4}$$

$$= 15\, \sigma_c \qquad \qquad \qquad \qquad \qquad ...(1)$$

Now, by figure we have,

Load on steel + load on concrete = Total load

$$\sigma_s\, A_s + \sigma_c\, A_c = P$$

$$15\, \sigma_c \times 314.159 + \sigma_c \times 249685.84 = 2000000$$

$$\boxed{\sigma_c = 7.86\, \text{N/mm}^2} \qquad \textbf{Ans.}$$

Putting the value of σ_c in the above equation (1).

$$\sigma_s = 15 \times 7.86\, \text{N/mm}^2$$

$$= 117.92\, \text{N/mm}^2 \qquad \textbf{Ans.}$$

EXAMPLE 3 *A reinforced concrete column 200 mm in diameter is designed to carry an axial compressive load of 300 kN. Determine the required area of the reinforcing steel if the allowable stresses are 6 MPa and 120 MPa for the concrete and steel respectively.*

$$E_{\text{concrete}} = 14\, \text{GPa}$$

$$E_{\text{steel}} = 200\, \text{GPa}$$

SOLUTION Given

$$\sigma_{co} = 6\, \text{MPa}$$

and $\qquad \sigma_{st} = 120\, \text{MPa}$

$$E_{co} = 14\, \text{GPa}$$

and $\qquad E_{st} = 200\, \text{GPa}$

Strain in column = Strain in steel

i.e. $\qquad \varepsilon_{co} = \varepsilon_{st}$

$$\frac{\sigma_{co}}{E_{con}} = \frac{\sigma_{st}}{E_{st}} \qquad \qquad \qquad [\because \sigma = \varepsilon \cdot E]$$

$$\frac{\sigma_{co}}{14 \times 10^3} = \frac{\sigma_{st}}{200 \times 10^3}$$

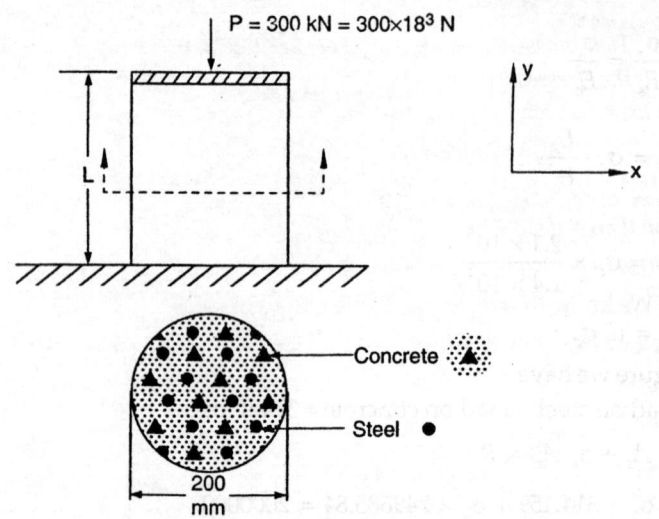

Fig. 1.70 Sectional Plan

$\therefore$ $\qquad$ $200\sigma_{co} = 14\sigma_{st}$

or, $\qquad$ $100\sigma_{co} = 7\sigma_{st}$

when $\qquad$ $\sigma_{st} = 120 \, \text{MPa}$

then $\qquad$ $100\sigma_{co} = 7 \times 120 \, \text{MPa}$

$\therefore$ $\qquad$ $\sigma_{co} = \dfrac{7 \times 120}{100} = 8.4 \, \text{MPa} > 6 \, \text{MPa}$

when $\qquad$ $\sigma_{co} = 6 \, \text{MPa}$

then $\qquad$ $100 \times 6 = 7 \times \sigma_{st}$

$\therefore$ $\qquad$ $\sigma_{st} = \dfrac{600}{7} = 85.71 < 120 \, \text{MPa}$

Using $\sigma_{co} = 6 \, \text{MPa}$ and $\sigma_{st} = 85.71 \, \text{MPa}$

Now $\Sigma F_y = 0$ gives $P_{\text{steel}} + P_{\text{concrete}} = 300$

$$\sigma_{st} \cdot A_{st} + \sigma_{co} \cdot A_{co} = 300 \times 10^3$$

$$85.71 \times A_{st} + 6 \times \left[\frac{\pi}{4}(200)^2 - A_{st} \right] = 3 \times 10^5$$

$$79.71 A_{st} + 6000\pi = 3 \times 10^5$$

$$A_{st} = \frac{3 \times 10^5 - 6000\pi}{79.71}$$

$$= 1397.92$$

$$= 1398 \, \text{mm}^2 \qquad \textbf{Ans.}$$

EXAMPLE 4 *Two brass rods and one steel rod together support a load as shown in figure 1.71. If the stresses in brass and steel are not to exceed 60 N/mm^2 and 120 N/mm^2, find the safe load that can be supported.*

Given, $E_{steel} = 2 \times 10^5 \, N/mm^2$

$E_{brass} = 1 \times 10^5 \, N/mm^2$

Cross-sectional area of steel rod = 1500 mm^2

Cross-section area of each brass rod = 1000 mm^2

SOLUTION We know that decrease in the length of steel rod, should be equal to the decrease in length of brass rod *i.e.* $\delta_{steel} = \delta_{brass}$.

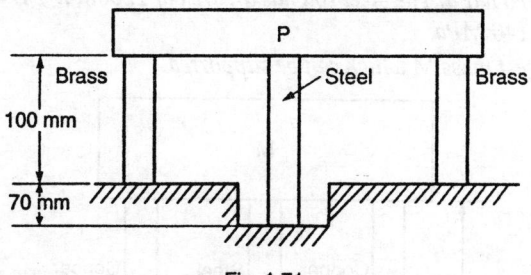

Fig. 1.71

Now, δ_{steel} = Strain in steel Rod × Length of steel rod

$$= \varepsilon_s \times L_s$$

Similarly, $\delta_{brass} = \varepsilon_b \times L_b$

where ε_s and ε_b are the strain in steel and brass rod respectively.

As $\delta_{steel} = \delta_{brass}$

∴ $\varepsilon_{steel} \cdot L_{steel} = \varepsilon_{brass} \cdot L_{brass}$

$$\frac{\varepsilon_{steel}}{\varepsilon_{brass}} = \frac{L_{brass}}{L_{steel}} = \frac{100}{170}$$

Now, $\sigma_{steel} = \varepsilon_{steel} \times E_{steel}$

and, $\sigma_{brass} = \varepsilon_{brass} \times E_{brass}$

∴ $\dfrac{\sigma_{steel}}{\sigma_{brass}} = \dfrac{\varepsilon_{steel} \times E_{steel}}{\varepsilon_{brass} \times E_{brass}}$

$$= \frac{100}{170} \times \frac{2 \times 10^5}{1 \times 10^5}$$

$$= 1.176$$

Total load (P) = load on steel rod + load on brass rods

$$\frac{\sigma_{steel}}{\sigma_{brass}} = 1.176$$

$$\therefore \quad \sigma_{\text{steel}} = 1.176 \times \sigma_{\text{brass}}$$

$$= 1.176 \times 60 \qquad \qquad (\text{As } \sigma_{brass} \neq 60 \text{ N/mm}^2 \text{ given})$$

$$= 70.56 \text{ N/mm}^2 < 120 \text{ N/mm}^2 \text{ of steel given hence accepted}$$

Therefore, safe load (P) = $\sigma_s \cdot As + \sigma_b \cdot A_b$

$$= 70.56 \times 1500 + 60 \times (2 \times 1000) = 105840 + 120000$$

$$= 225840 \text{ Newton} = 225.84 \text{ kN} \quad \textbf{Ans.}$$

EXAMPLE 5 *A rigid block of mass M is supported by three symmetrically spaced roads as shown in Fig. 1.72. Each copper rod has an area of 900 mm²; E = 120 GPa and the allowable stress is 70 MPa. The steel rod has an area of 1200mm², E = 200 GPa and the allowable stress is 140 MPa.*

Determine the largest mass M which can be supported.

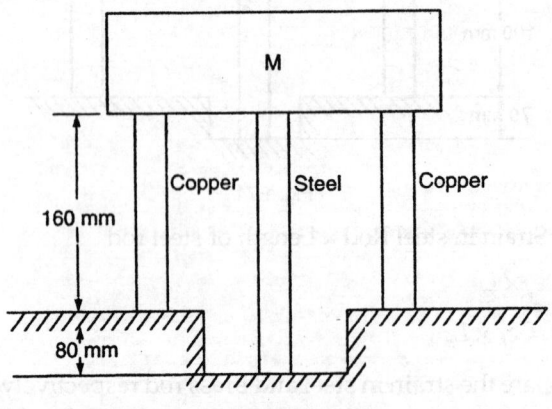

Fig. 1.72

SOLUTION It is evident that mass M causes the rods to deform equally

i.e. $$\delta_{co} = \delta_{st}$$

$$\left(\frac{\sigma \cdot L}{E} \right)_{co} = \left(\frac{\sigma \cdot L}{E} \right)_{st}$$

$$\frac{\sigma_{co} \times 160}{120 \times 10^3} = \frac{\sigma_{st} \times 240}{200 \times 10^3}$$

$$\sigma_{co} = \frac{240 \times 120 \times 10^3}{160 \times 200 \times 10^3} \sigma_{st} = 0.96_{st}$$

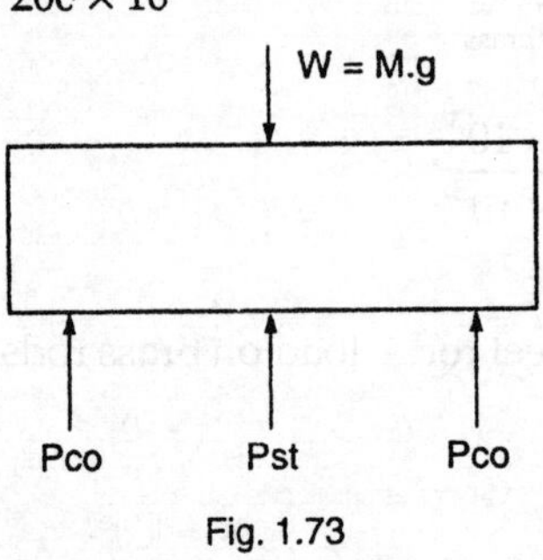

Fig. 1.73

when $\sigma_{st} = 140$ MPa, then $\sigma_{co} = 0.9 \times 140$ MPa

$\qquad = 126$ MPa > 70 MPa   Not OK

when $\quad \sigma_{co} = 70$ MPa

then $\quad \sigma_{st} = \dfrac{10}{9} \times \sigma_{co}$

$\qquad = \dfrac{10}{9} \times 70$ MPa

$\qquad = 77.78$ MPa < 140 MPa $\qquad$ Hence OK

Therefore using $\sigma_{co} = 70$ MPa

and $\qquad\qquad \sigma_{st} = 77.78$ MPa

Now, applying $\Sigma F_y = 0$ gives

$$2P_{co} + P_{st} = W$$

$$2\,(\sigma_{co} \times A_{co}) + \sigma_{st} \times A_{st} = M.g$$

$$2\,(70 \times 900) + 77.78 \times 1200 = M \times 9.81$$

$$M = \frac{2 \times 70 \times 900 + 77.78 \times 1200}{9.81}$$

$$= \frac{126000 + 93336}{9.81} = 22358.4 \text{ kg} \qquad\qquad \textbf{Ans.}$$

EXAMPLE 6 *A rigid plateform shown in figure has negligible mass and rests on two steel bars each 250 mm long. There centre bar is aluminium and 249.90 mm long. Compute the stress in the aluminium bar after the centre load P = 400 kN has been applied. For each steel bar the cross sectional area is 1200 mm² and G = 200 GPa and for the aluminium brass the area is 2400 mm² and E = 70 GPa.*

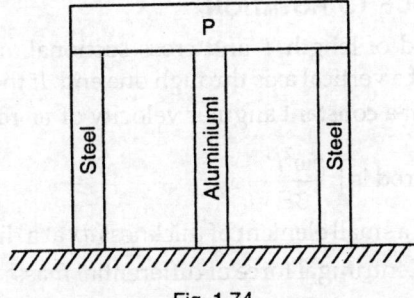

Fig. 1.74

SOLUTION Given $L_{steel} = 250$ mm

$\qquad\qquad L_{aluminium} = 249.90$ mm

Since applied load will deform rods equally so we have,

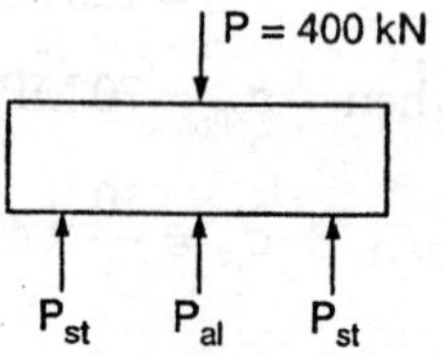

$$\sigma_{st} = \delta_{al} + 0.10$$

$$\left(\frac{\sigma \cdot L}{E}\right)_{co} = \left(\frac{\sigma \cdot L}{E}\right)_{al} + 0.10$$

$$\frac{\sigma_{st} \cdot L_{st}}{E_{st}} = \frac{\sigma_{al} \cdot L_{al}}{E_{al}} + 0.10$$

$$\frac{\sigma_{st} \times 250}{2 \times 10^5} = \frac{\sigma_{al} \times 249.90}{70 \times 10^3} \times 0.10$$

$$1.25 \times 10^{-3} \sigma_{st} = 3.57 \times 10^{-3} \sigma_{al} + 0.10$$

$$\sigma_{st} = 2.856\,\sigma_{al} + 80 \qquad\qquad\qquad \dots\text{(I)}$$

$\Sigma F_y = 0$ gives

$$P_{al} + 2P_{st} = 4 \times 10^5$$

$$\sigma_{al} \times A_{al} + 2\sigma_{st} \times A_{st} = 4 \times 10^5$$

$$\sigma_{al} \times 2400 + 2\,(2.856\,\sigma_{al} + 80) \times 1200 = 4 \times 10^5$$

$$2400\sigma_{al} + 6854.4\,\sigma_{al} + 192000 = 4 \times 10^5$$

$$9254.54\,\sigma_{al} + 192000 = 4 \times 10^5$$

$$9254.46\,\sigma_{al} = 208000$$

$$\therefore \qquad \sigma_{al} = \left(\frac{208000}{9254.46}\right)$$

$$= 22.475\ \text{MPa} \qquad\qquad \textbf{Ans.}$$

P = 400 kN

P_{st} P_{al} P_{st}

Fig. 1.75

1.23 ELONGATION DUE TO ROTATION

A uniform slender rod of length 'l' and cross sectional area A is rotating in a horizontal plane about a vertical axis through one end. If the unit mass of the rod is ρ and it is rotating at a constant angular velocity of ω rad/sec, show that the total elongation of the rod is $\left(\dfrac{\rho\omega^2 l^3}{3E}\right)$.

Proof: Let us consider a small element of thickness dx at a distance from origin O. Due to rotation, dP = Centrifugal force of differential mass

$$= dM \cdot \omega^2 x$$

$$= (\rho A dx)\,\omega^2 x$$

$$= \rho A\omega^2 x dx$$

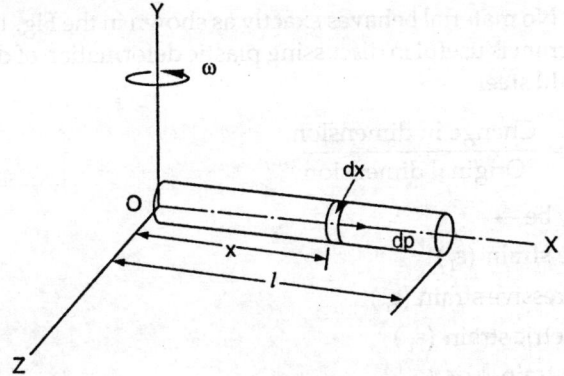

Fig. 1.76

Also, elemental deformation

$$d\delta = \frac{(\rho A\omega^2 x dx) \cdot x}{A \cdot E}$$

$$\int d\delta = \frac{\rho\omega^2}{E} \int_0^1 x^2 dx = \frac{\rho\omega^2}{E}\left[\frac{x^3}{3}\right]_0^1$$

$$\delta = \frac{\rho\omega^2}{E} \times \frac{l^3}{3}$$

$$= \frac{\rho\omega^2 l^3}{3E}$$

HIGHLIGHTS

1. Stress $(\sigma) = \dfrac{P}{A}$ assuming uniform distribution over the cross-section. Stress is a tensor. As long as the stress (σ) is less than the yield strength (σ_y) the material behaves elastically and obey's Hooke's law $\sigma = E\varepsilon$. When σ reaches the value σ_y, the material starts yielding and keeps deforming plastically under a constant load. If load is removed, unloading takes place along line *MN* parallel to the initial portion *OY* of the loading curve. The segment *ON* of the horizontal axis represents the strain corresponding to the permanent set or plastic deformation as a result from the loading and unloading of the

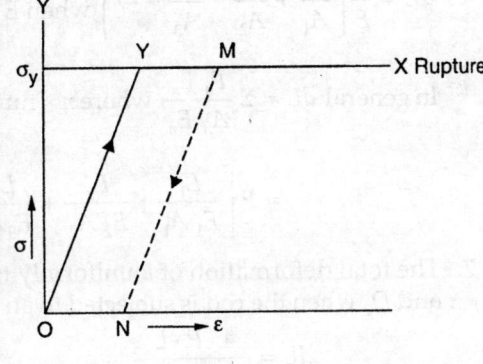

Fig. 1.77

specimen. No material behaves exactly as shown in the Fig. 1.77, this stress-strain diagram is useful in discussing plastic deformation of ductile material such as mild steel.

2. Strain $(\varepsilon) = \dfrac{\text{Change in dimension}}{\text{Original dimension}}$

Strain may be —

(a) Tensile strain (ε_t)

(b) Compressive strain (ε_c)

(c) Volumetric strain (ε_v)

(d) Shear strain ϕ or γ

3. Stress may be —

(a) Tensile stress (σ_t)

(b) Compressive stress (σ_c)

(c) Shear stress (τ)

4. Modulus of elasticity $(E) = \dfrac{\sigma}{\varepsilon}$ with the limit of Hook's law

$$= \frac{P/A}{\delta/l} = \frac{P}{A} \times \frac{l}{\delta}$$

$\therefore$ Change in dimension (linear) of uniform section *i.e.* prismatic bar

$$\delta = \left[\frac{P \cdot l}{A \cdot E} \right]$$

5. Factor of safety (f.o.s) $= \dfrac{\text{Ultimate stress}}{\text{Working stress}}$

6. *Principle of superposition*

Total change in length of a bar of different length and different diameter when subjected to an axial load P is given by

$$dL = \frac{P}{E} \left[\frac{L_1}{A_1} + \frac{L_2}{A_2} + \frac{L_3}{A_3} + \cdots \right] \quad \text{when } E \text{ is same}$$

In general $dL = \Sigma \dfrac{P_n L_n}{A_n E_n}$ where n = number of bar

$$= P \left[\frac{L_1}{E_1 A_1} + \frac{L_2}{E_2 A_2} + \frac{L_3}{E_3 A_3} + \cdots \right] \quad \text{where } E \text{ is different.}$$

7. The total deformation of a uniformly tapering circular rod of diameter D_1 and D_2 when the rod is subjected to an axial load P is given by

$$dL = \frac{4 \cdot P \cdot L}{\pi E D_1 D_2}$$

8. Total elongation (deformation) of a uniformly tapering rectangular bar when subjected to an axial load P is given by

$$dL = \frac{PL}{Et\,(a-b)} \cdot \log_e\left(\frac{a}{b}\right)$$

where L = total length of bar

t = thickness of bar

b = width at smaller end

a = width at bigger end

E = Young's modulus.

9. Elongation of a bar due to its own weight is given by

$$dL = \frac{WL}{2AE}$$

where W = weight of bar

L = length of bar

A = Area of cross-section of bar

E = modulus of elasticity of bar material.

10. In composite bar of equal length

(a) strain in each bar is equal

$$\varepsilon_1 = \varepsilon_2$$

i.e.
$$\frac{\sigma_1}{E_1} = \frac{\sigma_2}{E_2}$$

(b) Total load on the composite bar is equal to the sum of loads carried by each different material

i.e. $P = P_1 + P_2$

11. The stress induceed in the body due to change in temperature when the body is not allowed to expand or contract freely are known as thermal stress.

Thermal strain $(\varepsilon_{\text{temp}}) = \alpha \cdot T$

Thermal stress $(\sigma_{\text{th}}) = E \cdot \alpha \cdot \Delta T$

12. When a body is loaded axially it deforms longitudinally as well as transversely at right angle to the longitudinal direction.

The strain occurring in the longitudinal direction is known as longitudinal strain and that occurring in the transverse direction is known as lateral strain.

13. Within elastic limit, the ratio of lateral strain to the longitudinal strain is called Poisson's Ratio and is denoted by $\frac{1}{m}$ or μ or ν.

14. Longitudinal strain $(\varepsilon_l) = \dfrac{\delta l}{l}$

Lateral strain $(\varepsilon_b \text{ or } \varepsilon_d) = \dfrac{\delta_b}{b} \text{ or } \dfrac{\delta_d}{d}$

where δl = change in length

δb = change in width

δd = change in depth or diameter.

15. Volumetric strain $(\varepsilon_v) = \dfrac{\delta_V}{V}$

Volumetric strain (ε_v) for a rectangular bar subjected to an axial load P is given by

$$\varepsilon_v = \frac{\delta l}{l}(1 - 2v)$$

16. Volumetric strain for a rectangular bar subjected to three mutually perpendicular stresses is given by

$$\varepsilon_v = \frac{1}{E}(\sigma_x + \sigma_y + \sigma_z)(1 - 2v)$$

where σ_x, σ_y and σ_z are the stresses in x, y and z direction respectively.

17. Principle of complementary shear stress states that a set of shear stresses across a plane is always accompanied by a set of balancing shear stresses of the same magnitude across the plane and normal to it.

i.e. $\tau = \tau'$

18. When an element is subjected to simple shear stresses then :
    (i) The planes of maximum normal stresses are perpendicular to each other.
    (ii) The planes of maximum normal stresses are inclined at an angle of 45° to the plane of pure shear.
    (iii) One of the maximum normal stress is tensile while the other maximum normal stress is compressive.
    (iv) The maximum normal stress are of the same magnitude are equal to the shear stress on the plane of pure shear.

19. Volumetric strain of a cylindrical rod, subjected to an axial tensile load is given by

$$\varepsilon_v = \text{longitudinal strain} - 2 \times \text{strain of diameter}$$

$$= \frac{\delta l}{l} - 2 \cdot \frac{\delta d}{d}$$

20. The ratio of normal stress to the corresponding volumetric strain is called the Bulk Modulus and denoted by K.

21. The relation between Young's modulus and bulk modulus is given by

$$E = 3K(1 - 2v)$$

22. The relation between modulus of elasticity and modulus of rigidity is given by

$$E = 2G(1 + v)$$

modulus of rigidity is also denoted by G.

23. Relation between Young's modulus, Bulk modules and modulus of rigidity is following

$$E = \frac{9GK}{3K + G}$$

PROBLEMS FOR PRACTICE
(THEORETICAL)

1. Define the term — stress; strain; elasticity; elastic limit; Young's modulus and Modulus of rigidity.
2. State Hook's law.
3. Four section of a bar having different lengths and different diameter are subjected to axial pull P.
   Determine the total change in length of the bar. Assume Young's modulus of different sections same.
4. Define modular ratio; thermal stresses; thermal strain and Poisson's ratio.
5. What do you mean by a bar of uniform strength?
6. Find an expression for the rotal elongation of a bar due to its own weight when the bar is fixed at its upper end hanging freely at the lower end.

(NUMERICAL)

1. Find the maximum value of P in drawing if $P \not> 140$ MPa in steel and in Aluminium 90 MPa or in Bronze of 100 MPa.

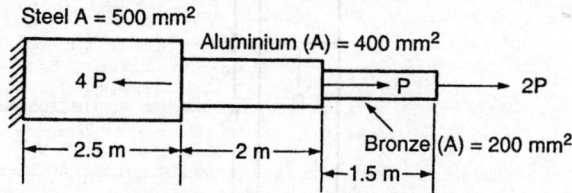

Fig. 1.78

2. Two blocks of wood width 'W' and thickness t are glued together along the joint inclined at an angle α as shown in Fig. 1.79. Using free body diagram show that the shearing stress on the glued joint is

$$\tau = \frac{P\alpha\sin^2\alpha}{2A}$$

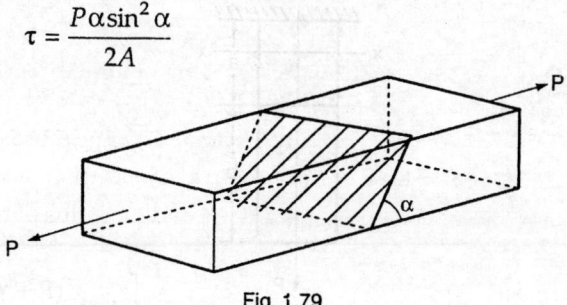

Fig. 1.79

3. A machine member is formed by connecting a steel bar to an aluminium bar as shown in Fig. 1.80. Assuming that the bars are prevented from buckling sideways, calculate the magnitude of force P, that will cause the total length of the member to decrease 0.30 mm. The values of elastic modulus for steel and aluminimum are 2×10^5 N/mm^2 and 6.5×10^4 N/mm^2 respectively.

[**Ans.** 406.22 kN]

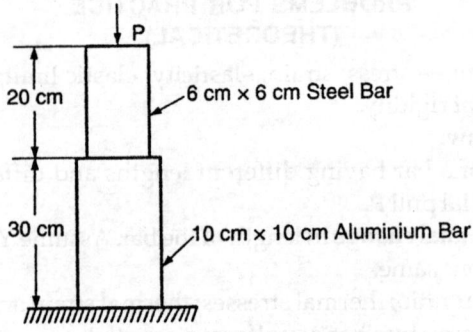

Fig. 1.80

4. Determine by taking into account the weight of bar, the displacement of the free end of bar shown in Fig.1.81. If its cross-sectional area is A the modulus of elasticity E and specific weight of material γ.

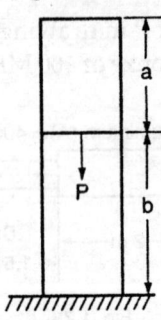

$$\left[\textbf{Ans.} \ \frac{Pb}{AE} + \frac{\gamma(a+b)^2}{2E} \right]$$

Fig. 1.81

5. Determine the displacement of section xx of the bar as shown in figure if its cross-section is A, modulus of elasticity E, and the specific weight of the material γ.

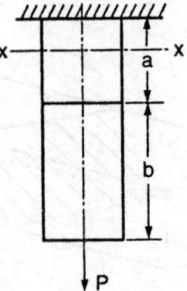

Fig. 1.82

$$\left[\textbf{Ans.} \ \frac{(P + \gamma Ab)a}{A \cdot E} + \frac{\gamma a^2}{2E} \right]$$

OBJECTIVE QUESTIONS

1. The factor of safety is the ratio of
   (a) working load or stress to ultimate load or stress
   (b) ultimate load or stress to yield load or stress
   (c) ultimate load or stress to working load or stress
   (d) yield load or stress to ultimate load or stress

2. Gauge length
   (a) is the total length of the specimen rod
   (b) is that part of the length over which measurement is made
   (c) there is no such length
   (d) none of the above

3. A prismatic bar is a bar of
   (a) maximum ultimate strength   (b) maximum yield strength
   (c) uniform cross-section   (d) varying cross-section

4. The gauge length is usually taken to be
   (a) 100 mm   (b) 75 mm
   (c) 50 mm   (d) 25 mm

5. The specimen rod under tension test has the following parameters
   (a) gauge length = 50 mm; diameter = 10 mm
   (b) gauge length = 50 mm; diameter = 12.5 mm
   (c) guage length = 25 mm; diameter = 25 mm
   (d) none of the above

6. The failure criteria for ductile materials is based on the following factor
   (a) ultimate strength   (b) shear strength
   (c) yield strength   (d) limit of proportionality

7. E and G are related by the equation
   (a) $E = 2G(1-v)$ (b) $E = 2G(1+v)$
   (c) $E = 3G(1-v)$ (d) $E = 3G(1+v)$

8. E and K are related by the equation
   (a) $E = 3K(1+2v)$ (b) $E = 3K(2-v)$
   (c) $E = 3K(1-2v)$ (d) $E = 3E(1-2v)$

9. The material becomes harder due to strain hardening. Strain hardening in case of structural steel occurs
   (a) between yield strength and ultimate strength
   (b) between limit of proportionality and yield strength
   (c) between ultimate strength and fracture point
   (d) none of the above

10. Structural steel forms neck before it breaks. Neck formation starts
    (a) before limit of proportionality   (b) after yield strength
    (c) before ultimate strength   (d) at ultiamte strength

11. Limiting values of Poission's ratio are
    (a) 0 to (+) 0.5   (b) 0 to (–) 0.5
    (c) 1 to (+) 0.5   (d) –1 to (+) 0.5

12. For mild steel, the ratio of modulus of elasticity in tension and compression (E_t/E_c) is equal to
    (a) 0.5   (b) 1   (c) 1.2   (d) 1.3

13. Ductile fracture generally takes place along planes on which the shear stress is
    (a) maximum   (b) minimum   (c) positive   (d) negative

14. The property of a material to undergo large uniform elongation before fracture (in tension) is known as
    (a) super elasticity   (b) super plasticity
    (c) visco elasticity   (d) visco plasticity

15. The percentage reduction in area during the tension test on a cast iron test specimen is
    (a) 5 – 10%   (b) 10 – 15%   (c) 0 – 3%   (d) 0 – 5%

16. The phenomenon under which the strain in a material varies under constant stress is called
    (a) strain hardening   (b) Bauschinger's effect
    (c) creep   (d) fatigue

17. The length, coefficient of thermal expansion and Young's Modulus of bar 'A' are twice that of bar 'B'. If the temperature of both bars is increased by the same amount while preventing any expansion, then the ratio of stress developed in bar A to that in bar B will be
    (a) 2   (b) 4   (c) 8   (d) 16

18. In the figure shear stress is 'τ' and shear strain $(\phi) = \left(\dfrac{\tau}{G}\right)$, then the diagonal strain will be
    (a) $\dfrac{\phi}{2}$ (b) $\dfrac{\phi}{4}$ (c) $\dfrac{\phi}{6}$ (d) $\dfrac{\phi}{8}$

19. If all the dimensions of a prismatic bar of cross-section suspended freely from the celing of a roof are doubled then the total elongation produced by its own weight will increase
    (a) eight times   (b) four times   (c) three times   (d) two times

20. A solid bar of uniform diameter D and length l is hung vertically from a ceiling. If the density of the material of the bar is ρ and the modulus of elasticity is E then the total elongation of the bar due to its own weight is
    (a) $\dfrac{\rho l}{2E}$ (b) $\dfrac{\rho l^2}{2E}$ (c) $\dfrac{\rho E}{2l}$ (d) $\dfrac{\rho E}{2l^2}$

21. In terms of bulk modulus (K) and modulus of rigidity (G), the Poisson's ratio can be expressed as
    (a) $\dfrac{3K - 2G}{6K + 4G}$ (b) $\dfrac{3K + 4G}{6K - 4G}$ (c) $\dfrac{3K - 2G}{6K + 2G}$ (d) $\dfrac{3K + 2G}{6K - 2G}$

22. A square section tapered bar of length l with sides l_1 and l_2 at its bigger and smaller end respectively is subjected to an axial pull. Taking E as the modulus of elasticity of the bar material, the elongation of the bar will be

(a) $\dfrac{2Pl}{El_1 l_2}$ (b) $\dfrac{P \cdot l}{2El_1 l_2}$ (c) $\dfrac{P \cdot l}{2E(l_1 + l_2)}$ (d) $\dfrac{P \cdot l}{E \cdot l_1 \cdot l_2}$

23. The elongation of conical bar of base diameter D hanging vertically, due to its own weight (when ρ = density of the material of the bar; l = length and E = (modulus of elasticity of the bar material) will be

(a) $\dfrac{\rho l^2}{2E}$ (b) $\dfrac{\rho l^2}{3E}$ (c) $\dfrac{\rho l^2}{4E}$ (d) $\dfrac{\rho \cdot l^2}{6E}$

24. A prismatic bar fixed at both ends is loaded by an axial load plating at a distance 'a' from one of the supports. The reaction at the supports will be

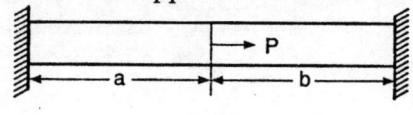

Fig. 1.83

(a) $\dfrac{Pb}{a+b} ; \dfrac{Pa}{a+b}$ (b) $\dfrac{P}{a(a+b)} ; \dfrac{P}{b(a+b)}$

(c) $\dfrac{2P}{a(a+b)} ; \dfrac{2P}{b(a+b)}$ (d) none of the above

25. For an isotropic elastic material, the number of independent elastic constant is
(a) 1 (b) 2 (c) 3 (d) 4

26. For most metals, Poisson's ratio is approximately
(a) 0.3 (b) 3 (c) 35
(d) none of the above

27. A material is called perfectly elastic if
(a) while loading or unloading, the deformation and recovery are instantaneous
(b) the recovery is complete and immediate
(c) the load-deformation curve has the same shape while loading or unloading
(d) All the above

ANSWERS

1. (c) 2. (b) 3. (c) 4. (c) 5. (b) 6. (a)
7. (b) 8. (c) 9. (a) 10. (d) 11. (d) 12. (b)
13. (a) 14. (b) 15. (c) 16. (a) 17. (b) 18. (a)
19. (b) 20. (a) 20. (a) 21. (c) 22. (d) 23. (d)
24. (a) 25. (b) 26. (a) 27. (d)

— ❖❖ —

2

COMPOUND STRESSES AND STRAINS

2.1 INTRODUCTION

Most machine members and structural parts are subjected to tensile stress/ compressive stress along with shear stress. Such a combination of stresses is called 'compound stress'.

Many real life stress situation are biaxial. When this occurs, it is very important to see as to how the stress combine to affect the structure. Any structure or portion of the structure will experience σ_x, σ_y and τ_{xy} as a function of x and y which vary in a continuous fashion throughout the region. In general, if a plane element is removed from a body, it will be subjected to the normal stresses σ_x and σ_y together with shearing stress τ_{xy}.

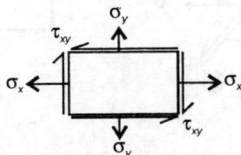

Some examples of regions where these kind of stress situation might occur are the surface of a pressure vessel, the skin of an aircraft or missile and the floor of a building.

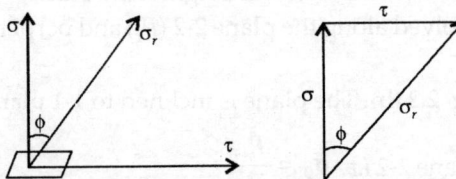

Let an element of any machine part is subjected to normal stress (σ) (tensile) along with shear stress (τ).

Then, the resultant stress $(\sigma_r) = \sqrt{\sigma^2 + \tau^2}$

and $\quad \tan \phi = \left(\dfrac{\tau}{\sigma}\right) \quad \therefore \quad \phi = \tan^{-1}\left(\dfrac{\tau}{\sigma}\right)$

where, ϕ is the angle which the resultant makes with the normal to the plane and is called 'obliquity'.

The study of compound stress is always associated with the plane on which its acts.

When the plane is normal to the axis of loading then it is called 'normal stress' or simply 'stress'.

2.2 STRESS AT A POINT ON INCLINED PLANE DUE TO UNIAXIAL LOAD

Let a prismatic bar is subjected to a tensile load P along the axis of the bar. Such a case is known as unidirectional loading.

Let us consider a point Q within the element where stress on an inclined plane is to be computed.

Through point Q three planes viz. 1-1, 2-2 and 3-3 are passed therefore 2-2, 3-3 are known as inclined plane.

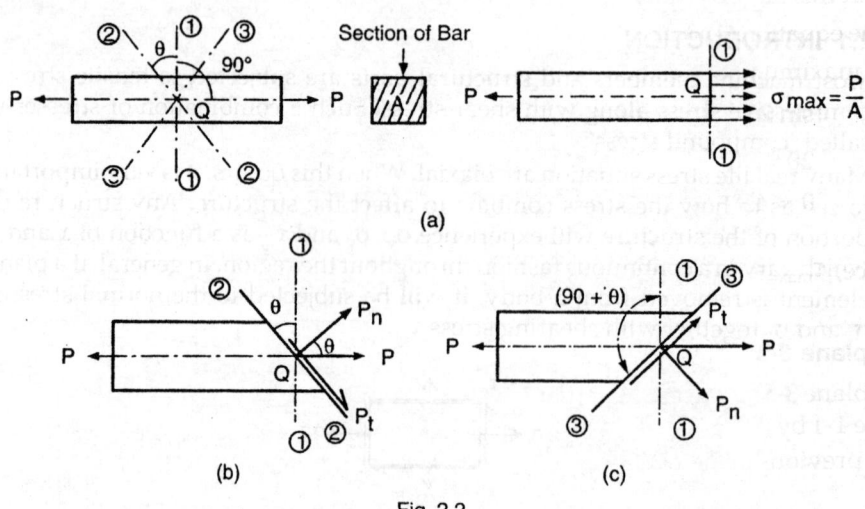

Fig. 2.2

For plane 2-2

For equilibrium, load P is drawn toward right hand side.

Load P has been resolved along the plane 2-2 (P_t) and perpendicular to the plane 2-2 as P_n.

This is shown in Fig. 2.2 (b). The plane is inclined to 1-1 plane by θ.

Normal stress on plane 2-2 *i.e.* $\sigma_\theta = \dfrac{P_n}{A}$

$$= \frac{P\cos\theta}{A\sec\theta}$$

$$= \frac{P}{A}\cdot\cos^2\theta \qquad\qquad …(1)$$

and Shear stress on plane 2-2 i.e. $\tau_\theta = \dfrac{P_t}{A}$

$$= \frac{P \sin \theta}{A \sec \theta} = \frac{P}{A} \cdot \sin \theta \cdot \cos \theta$$

$$= \frac{1}{2} \cdot \frac{P}{A} \cdot \sin 2\theta \qquad \qquad ...(2)$$

In equation (1), σ_θ is maximum when $\cos \theta$ is maximum. $\cos \theta$ will be maximum when $\theta = 0°$.

Hence, $\sigma_{max} = \left[\dfrac{P}{A} \right]$

When this happens, plane 2-2 coincides with plane 1-1.

In the equation (2).

τ_θ is maximum when $\sin 2\theta$ is maximum

or, $\quad \sin 2\theta = 1 = \sin 90°$

$\qquad 2\theta = 90°$

$\qquad \theta = 45°$

Hence, $\tau_{max} = \tau_{45°} = \dfrac{P}{2A}$

For plane 3-3

The plane 3-3 on the prismatic bar is shown in Fig. 2.2 (c). This plane is inclined to plane 1-1 by $(90° + \theta)$.

Like previous plane 2-2.

Normal stress on plane 3-3 i.e. $\sigma'_\theta = \dfrac{P_n}{A}$

$$= \frac{P \cos (90 + \theta)}{A \sec (90 + \theta)}$$

$$= \frac{P \sin \theta}{A \cdot \operatorname{cosec} \theta}$$

$$= \frac{P}{A} \cdot \sin^2 \theta \qquad \qquad ...(3)$$

and shear stress on plane 3-3 i.e. $\tau'_\theta = \dfrac{1}{2} \cdot \dfrac{P}{A} \cdot \sin 2 (90° + \theta)$

$$= -\frac{1}{2} \cdot \frac{P}{A} \cdot \sin 2\theta \qquad \qquad ...(4)$$

Adding equation (1) and (3)

$$\sigma_\theta + \sigma'_\theta = \frac{P}{A}$$

and adding (2) and (4)

$$\tau_\theta + \tau'_\theta = 0$$

or, $\tau_\theta = -\tau'_\theta$

So, we find that sum of normal stresses on two mutual perpendicular planes is constant and is equal to maximum normal stress. Shear stresses are equal and opposite in nature.

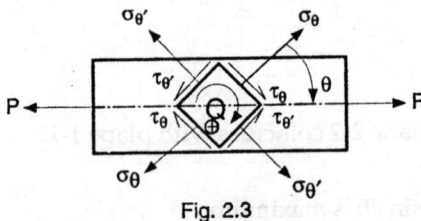

Fig. 2.3

Figure 2.3 shows that the point Q is stressed under uniaxial tensile load P.

The shear stresses on any surface of a body will be considered positive if it points in a direction corresponding to clockwise rotation about the centre inside the body otherwise negative sign. So we will refer shear stress τ_{xy} as clockwise (cw) or counter clockwise (ccw) according to how they tend to rotate the stress element. If cw then $\oplus$ ve if ccw then $\ominus$ ve.

Here, τ_θ is $\oplus$ ve as it is producing clockwise rotation at point Q.

If the load P is compressive in nature then at point Q, the stresses on mutually perpendicular planes will be as shown in Fig. 2.4.

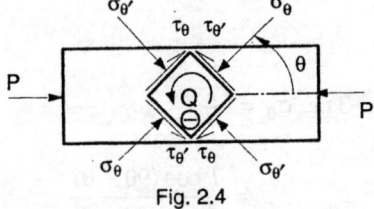

Fig. 2.4

Here, $\tau_{\theta'}$ is $\ominus$ ve as it is producing Anitclockwise rotation at point Q.

N.B.: Mohr suggested that the pair of shear stresses that give a clockwise couple must be taken as positive.

2.3 TWO DIMENSIONAL STRESS SYSTEM

In order to evaluate the normal stress (σ_θ) and shear stress (τ_θ) on the oblique plane a wedge shape like element ABC is taken and equilibrium condition is applied to get (σ_θ) and (τ_θ).

In the Fig. 2.5 ABC, wedge shape like element is taken. The given stresses σ_x and σ_y are then transformed parallel and perpendicular to σ_θ and τ_θ i.e. along x-axis and y-axis respectively. We shall assume $\sigma_x > \sigma_y$.

Let the thickness of wedge ABC be unity perpendicular to the plane of paper.

The resolved stresses are then multiplied with the area on which they are acting and ultimately by applying equation of equilibrium *i.e.*, $\Sigma F_x = 0$ and $\Sigma F_y = 0$ we get the expression for σ_θ and τ_θ.

$\Sigma F_y = 0$ gives

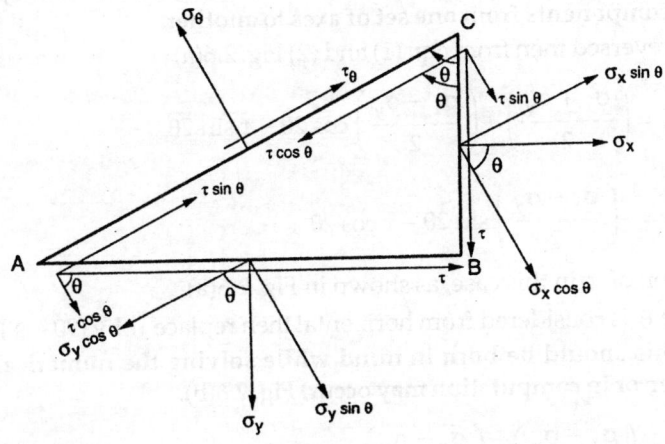

Fig. 2.5

$$\sigma_\theta \cdot AC \cdot 1 = \sigma_x \cdot \cos\theta \cdot BC + \tau \sin\theta \cdot BC + \sigma_y \sin\theta \cdot AB + \tau \cos\theta \, AB$$

$$\therefore \quad \sigma_\theta = \sigma_x \cdot \cos\theta \cdot \frac{BC}{AC} + \tau \sin\theta \cdot \frac{BC}{AC} + \sigma_y \sin\theta \cdot \frac{AB}{AC} + \tau \cos\theta \cdot \frac{AB}{AC}$$

$$= \sigma_x \cdot \cos\theta \cdot \cos\theta + \tau \sin\theta \cdot \cos\theta + \sigma_y \sin\theta \cdot \sin\theta + \tau \cos\theta \cdot \sin\theta$$

$$= \sigma_x \cdot \cos^2\theta + \sigma_y \sin^2\theta + 2\tau \sin\theta \cdot \cos\theta$$

$$= \sigma_x \left(\frac{1 + \cos\theta}{2} \right) + \sigma_y \left(\frac{1 - \cos 2\theta}{2} \right) + \tau \cdot \sin 2\theta$$

$$\boxed{\sigma_\theta = \left(\frac{\sigma_x + \sigma_y}{2} \right) + \left(\frac{\sigma_x - \sigma_y}{2} \right) \cos 2\theta + \tau \sin 2\theta} \qquad \qquad ...(1)$$

$\Sigma F_x = 0$ gives

$$\tau_\theta \cdot AC \cdot 1 = \tau \cos\theta \cdot BC - \tau \sin\theta \cdot AB + \sigma_y \cos\theta \cdot AB - \sigma_x \sin\theta \cdot BC$$

$$\therefore \quad \tau_\theta = \tau \cos\theta \cdot \frac{BC}{AC} - \tau \sin\theta \cdot \frac{AB}{AC} + \sigma_y \cos\theta \cdot \frac{AB}{AC} - \sigma_x \cdot \sin\theta \cdot \frac{BC}{AC}$$

$$= \tau \cos\theta \cdot \cos\theta - \tau \sin\theta \cdot \sin\theta + \sigma_y \cos\theta \cdot \sin\theta - \sigma_x \cdot \sin\theta \cdot \cos\theta$$

$$= -\frac{\sigma_x}{2} \cdot \sin 2\theta + \frac{\sigma_y}{2} \cdot \sin 2\theta + \tau \left(\cos^2\theta - \sin^2\theta \right)$$

$$\tau_\theta = -\left(\frac{\sigma_x - \sigma_y}{2}\right) \sin 2\theta + \tau \cos 2\theta \qquad \ldots(2)$$

Equation (1) and (2) are called transformation equation because they transform the stress components from one set of axes to another.

(a) If τ is reversed then from eqn (1) and (2) Fig. 2.6(a)

$$\sigma_\theta = \left(\frac{\sigma_x + \sigma_y}{2}\right) + \left(\frac{\sigma_x - \sigma_y}{2}\right) \cos 2\theta - \tau \sin 2\theta$$

and

$$\tau_\theta = -\left(\frac{\sigma_x - \sigma_y}{2}\right) \sin 2\theta - \tau \cos 2\theta$$

The direction of τ in this case, as shown in Fig. 2.6(a).

(b) If angle θ is considered from horizontal then replace θ by $(90 - \theta)$ in eqn. (1) and (2). **(This should be born in mind while solving the numerical problem otherwise error in computation may occur)** Fig. 2.6(b).

$$\sigma_\theta = \left(\frac{\sigma_x + \sigma_y}{2}\right) - \left(\frac{\sigma_x - \sigma_y}{2}\right) \cos 2\theta + \tau \sin 2\theta$$

and

$$\tau_\theta = -\left(\frac{\sigma_x - \sigma_y}{2}\right) \sin 2\theta - \tau \cos 2\theta$$

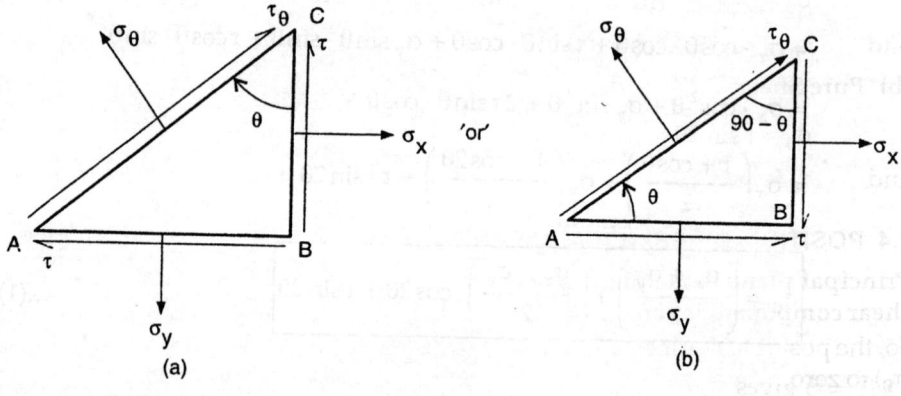

(a)   (b)

Fig. 2.6

The expression for the normal stress $\sigma_{\theta'}$ is obtained by replacing θ in eqn. (1) by the angle $(\theta + 90°)$.

Stresses on oblique plane is also represented by $\sigma_{x'}$, $\sigma_{y'}$ and $\tau_{x'y'}$ where $x'y'$ is the new set of axis when the element is rotated CCW by an angle θ with the earlier set of axes (x, y).

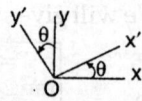

Since $\quad \cos(2\theta + 180) = -\cos 2\theta$

and $\quad \sin(2\theta + 180) = -\sin 2\theta$

So we have,

$$\sigma_{\theta'} = \frac{\sigma_x + \sigma_y}{2} - \frac{\sigma_x - \sigma_y}{2}\cos 2\theta - \tau \sin 2\theta \qquad ...(3)$$

Adding (1) and (3)

$$\sigma_\theta + \sigma_{\theta'} = \sigma_x + \sigma_y \qquad ...(4)$$

This shows that in the case of plane stress the sum of the normal stresses exerted on the cubic element of material is independent of the orientation of the element. If the body is subjected to normal stresses only *i.e.* σ_x and σ_y, then $\tau = 0$ and therefore, the equation (1) and (2) reduces to

$$\sigma_\theta = \left(\frac{\sigma_x + \sigma_y}{2}\right) + \left(\frac{\sigma_x - \sigma_y}{2}\right)\cos 2\theta \qquad ...(5)$$

and $\quad \tau_\theta = -\left(\frac{\sigma_x - \sigma_y}{2}\right)\sin 2\theta \qquad ...(6)$

Special Cases [Using equation (1) and (2)]

(a) Uniaxial:

$$\sigma_\theta = \sigma_x \cos^2 \theta \qquad\qquad \text{(As } \sigma_y = 0 \text{ and } \tau = 0)$$

and $\quad \tau_\theta = -\sigma_x \sin \theta \cdot \cos \theta$

(b) Pure Shear:

$$\sigma_\theta = \tau \sin 2\theta \qquad\qquad \text{(As } \sigma_x = 0 \text{ and } \sigma_y = 0)$$

and $\quad \tau_\theta = \tau \cos 2\theta$

2.4 POSITION OF PRINCIPAL PLANE

Principal plane is the plane on which there exist only normal stress and the shear component is zero.

So, the position of principal planes are obtained by equating the tangential stress (τ_θ) to zero.

i.e. $\quad -\left(\frac{\sigma_x - \sigma_y}{2}\right)\sin 2\theta + \tau \cos 2\theta = 0$

$\therefore \qquad \tan 2\theta = \left(\dfrac{2\tau}{\sigma_x - \sigma_y}\right)$

We will give suffix `p'

So $\quad \boxed{\tan 2\theta_p = \left(\dfrac{2\tau}{\sigma_x - \sigma_y}\right)} \qquad ...(7)$

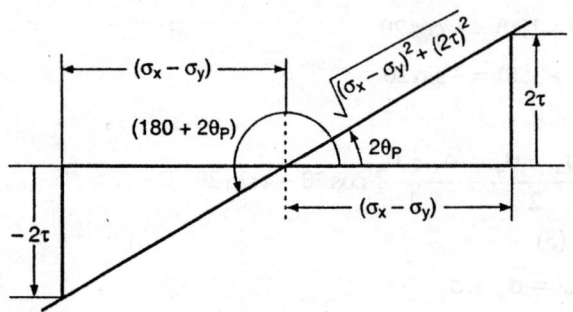

Fig. 2.7

Thus, there are two values of $2\theta_P$ differing by 180° and hence two values of θ_P differing by 90° is obtained.

Hence, principal planes are two planes at right angles.

$$\sin 2\theta_P = \frac{2\tau}{\sqrt{(\sigma_x - \sigma_y)^2 + (2\tau)^2}}$$

and

$$\cos 2\theta_P = \frac{\sigma_x - \sigma_y}{\sqrt{(\sigma_x - \sigma_y)^2 + (2\tau)^2}}$$

The value of major principal stress is obtained by substituting the values of $\sin 2\theta_P$ and $\cos 2\theta_P$ in equation (1).

Major principal stress

$$= \frac{1}{2}(\sigma_x + \sigma_y) + \frac{1}{2}(\sigma_x - \sigma_y) \times \frac{\sigma_x - \sigma_y}{\sqrt{(\sigma_x - \sigma_y)^2 + (2\tau)^2}} + \tau \times \frac{2\tau}{\sqrt{(\sigma_x - \sigma_y)^2 + (2\tau)^2}}$$

$$= \frac{(\sigma_x + \sigma_y)}{2} + \frac{1}{2} \cdot \frac{(\sigma_x - \sigma_y)^2}{\sqrt{(\sigma_x - \sigma_y)^2 + (2\tau)^2}} + \frac{2\tau^2}{\sqrt{(\sigma_x - \sigma_y)^2 + (2\tau)^2}}$$

$$= \frac{\sigma_x + \sigma_y}{2} + \frac{1}{2} \cdot \frac{(\sigma_x - \sigma_y)^2 + 4\tau^2}{\sqrt{(\sigma_x - \sigma_y)^2 + (2\tau)^2}}$$

$$= \frac{\sigma_x + \sigma_y}{2} + \frac{\sqrt{(\sigma_x - \sigma_y)^2 + 4\tau^2}}{2}$$

We denote major principal stress by σ_1

So, $\qquad \sigma_1 = \frac{1}{2}\left[(\sigma_x + \sigma_y) + \sqrt{(\sigma_x - \sigma_y)^2 + 4\tau^2} \right]$ ...(8)

Similarly, minor principal stress,

$$\sigma_2 = \frac{1}{2}\left[(\sigma_x + \sigma_y) - \sqrt{(\sigma_x - \sigma_y)^2 + 4\tau^2} \right] \qquad \qquad ...(9)$$

2.5 MAXIMUM SHEAR STRESS

The maximum value of shear stress on an inclined plane can be obtained by differentiating equation (2) w.r.t. θ and equating it to zero.

$$\frac{d\tau_\theta}{d\theta} = \frac{d}{d\theta}\left[-\left(\frac{\sigma_x - \sigma_y}{2}\right)\sin 2\theta + \tau\cos 2\theta \right] = 0$$

or, $\quad -\left(\dfrac{\sigma_x - \sigma_y}{2}\right) \times 2\cos 2\theta - 2\tau\sin 2\theta = 0$

or, $\quad \tan 2\theta = -\left(\dfrac{\sigma_x - \sigma_y}{2\tau}\right)$

Let us give suffix 's'

So, $\qquad \boxed{\tan 2\theta_S = -\left(\dfrac{\sigma_x - \sigma_y}{2\tau}\right)} \qquad \qquad ...(10)$

The equation (10) defines two values of $2\theta_S$ which are 180° apart and then the two values of θ_S are 90° apart.

Either of these values can be used to determine the orientation of the element corresponding to the maximum shear stress.

$$\tau_{max} = \left(\frac{\sigma_1 - \sigma_2}{2}\right)$$

Substituting the value of σ_1 and σ_2 from (8) and (9) we get

$$\boxed{\tau_{max} = \frac{1}{2}\sqrt{(\sigma_x - \sigma_y)^2 + 4\tau^2}} \qquad \qquad ...(11)$$

Normal stress corresponding to the condition of maximum shearing stress is

$$\sigma_{ave} = \frac{\sigma_x + \sigma_y}{2}$$

From eqn. (7) and (10) we observe that the angle $2\theta_S$ and $2\theta_P$ are 90° apart and therefore the angles θ_S and θ_P are 45° apart. We thus conclude, that the planes of maximum shearing stress are 45° to the principal planes.

EXAMPLES ON ANALYTICAL METHOD

EXAMPLE 1 *Two pieces of wood of section 50 mm × 40 mm are joined together along a plane at 60° with the x-axis. If the strength of the joint is 7.5 MPa in tension and 4 MPa in shear, determine the maximum force which the member can sustain.*

SOLUTION

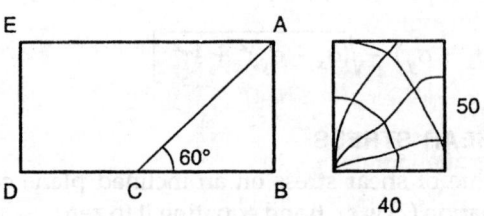

Fig. 2.8

In the figure two piece of wood are joined along plane AC making angle $60°$ with the x-axis. Redrawing the figure

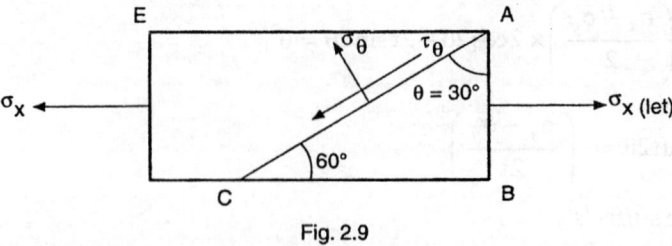

Fig. 2.9

Let the normal stress and shear stress on the plance AC be σ_θ and τ_θ respectively then by formula for uniaxial stress system

$$\sigma_\theta = \sigma_x \cos^2 \theta$$
$$7.5 = \sigma_x \cos^2 30°$$

$$\sigma_x = \left(\frac{7.5}{\cos^2 30°}\right) = 10 \text{ MPa} \qquad \qquad \dots(I)$$

and $\qquad \tau_\theta = -\dfrac{1}{2}\sigma_x \sin^2 \theta$

$$-4 = -\frac{1}{2}\sigma_x \sin 60° \qquad \qquad \text{(Assuming } \tau \text{ along } AC \text{ CCW)}$$

$$\therefore \qquad \sigma_x = \left(\frac{8}{\sin 60°}\right)$$

$$= 9.24 \text{ MPa} \qquad \qquad \dots(II)$$

For safety of the wooden joint, the maximum axial stress which should be taken is 9.24 MPa.

$\therefore \qquad$ Maximum force $= (50 \times 40) \times 9.245$ Newton
$$= 16480 \text{ N or } 16.48 \text{ kN}$$

EXAMPLE 2 *Show that in a material subjected to a biaxial stress system, the sum of normal components of stresses on any two planes at right angle to each other is constant.*

SOLUTION Let one plane is located at an angle θ then other plane will be at an angle $(\theta + 90°)$.

By Formula,

Normal stress at an angle θ,

$$\sigma_\theta = \frac{\sigma_x + \sigma_y}{2} + \frac{\sigma_x - \sigma_y}{2} \cos 2\theta + \tau \sin 2\theta \qquad \ldots(I)$$

and Normal stress at an angle $(\theta + 90°)$

$$\sigma_{\theta+90°} = \frac{\sigma_x + \sigma_y}{2} + \frac{\sigma_x - \sigma_y}{2} \cos 2(\theta + 90°) + \tau \sin 2(\theta + 90°)$$

$$= \frac{\sigma_x + \sigma_y}{2} - \frac{\sigma_x - \sigma_y}{2} \cos 2\theta - \tau \sin 2\theta \qquad \ldots(II)$$

Adding (I) and (II)

$\sigma_\theta + \sigma_{\theta+90°} = (\sigma_x + \sigma_y)$, which is independent of θ and hence constant for the given problem.

EXAMPLE 3 *At a point in a material sample $\sigma_x = 50$ MPa; $\sigma_y = 100$ MPa and $\tau_{xy} = -25$ MPa. Determine the normal and shear stresses on a plane at 45° to the y-axis.*

SOLUTION Normal stress $(\sigma_\theta) = \dfrac{\sigma_x + \sigma_y}{2} + \dfrac{\sigma_x - \sigma_y}{2} \cos 2\theta + \tau \sin 2\theta$

$$= \left(\frac{50 + 100}{2}\right) + \left(\frac{50 - 100}{2}\right) \cos 90° + (-25) \sin 90°$$

$$= 75 + 0 - 25$$

$$= 50 \text{ MPa (Tensile)} \quad \textbf{Ans.}$$

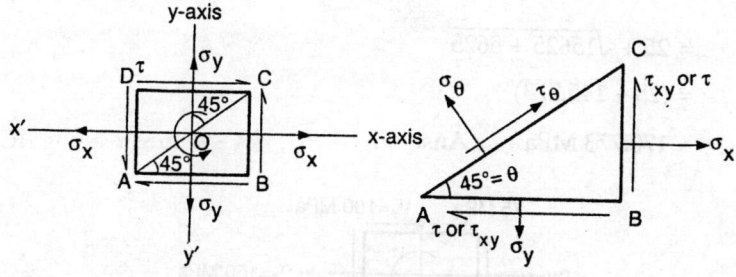

Fig 2.10

Shear stress $(\tau_\theta) = (-) \dfrac{\sigma_x - \sigma_y}{2} \sin 2\theta - \tau \cos 2\theta$

$$= (-1)\frac{50 - 100}{2} \times \sin 90° + (-25) \cos 90°$$

$$= + 25 - 0$$

$$= + 25 \text{ MPa} \quad \textbf{Ans.}$$

N.B. If in the problem $\tau_{xy} = +25$ MPa, then the figure would be like below

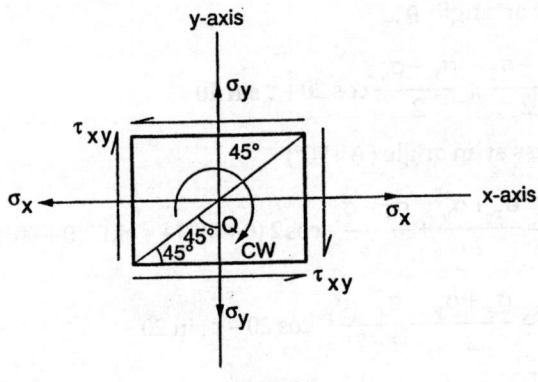

Fig. 2.11

Here, τ_{xy} is in the clockwise direction and so we will take $\tau \oplus$ ve.
For CCW direction ($\circlearrowleft$) we will take $\tau \ominus$ ve.

EXAMPLE 4 *The state of stress at a point in the material is*

$$\sigma_x = 150 \text{ MPa}; \sigma_y = -100 \text{ MPa}; \tau_{xy} = 75 \text{ MPa}$$

Determine maximum normal and shear stress.

SOLUTION Maximum normal stress *i.e.* maximum principal stress

$$\sigma_1 = \frac{\sigma_x + \sigma_y}{2} + \sqrt{\left(\frac{\sigma_x - \sigma_y}{2}\right)^2 + \tau^2 xy}$$

$$= \frac{150 - 100}{2} + \sqrt{\left(\frac{150 + 100}{2}\right)^2 + (75)^2}$$

$$= 25 + \sqrt{15625 + 5625}$$

$$= (25 + 145.773)$$

$$= 170.773 \text{ MPa} \qquad \textbf{Ans.}$$

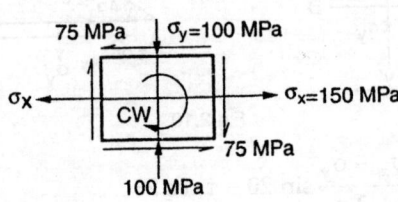

Fig. 2.12

Maximum shear stress

$$\tau_{max} = \sqrt{\left(\frac{\sigma_x - \sigma_y}{2}\right)^2 + \tau^2 xy}$$

$$= \sqrt{\left(\frac{150 + 100}{2}\right)^2 + (75)^2}$$

$$= 145.773 \text{ MPa} \qquad \textbf{Ans.}$$

∴   Maximum normal stress $= 170.773$ MPa

Maximum shear stress $= 145.773$ MPa

EXAMPLE 5 *A point in a strained material is subjected to a tensile stress of 65 N/mm² and compressive stress of 45 N/mm², acting on two mutually perpendicular planes and a shear stress of 10 N/mm² are acting on these plane.*

Find the normal stress, tangential stress and resultant stress on a plane inclined to 30° with the plane of the compressive stress. **(UPTU 3rd Sem. 2006-07; UPTU 3rd Sem. 2013-14)**

SOLUTION Since the plane is making 30° with the compressive stress, so it will make an angle 60° with tensile stress as shown in the figure. This was done in order to match the figure with theory 2.3 of this book and to apply the correct formula.

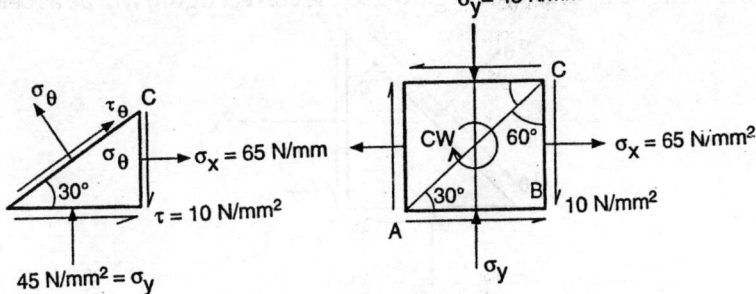

Fig. 2.13

Now, by formula,

$$\sigma_\theta = \frac{\sigma_x + \sigma_y}{2} + \frac{\sigma_x - \sigma_y}{2} \cos 2\theta + \tau \sin 2\theta$$

$$= \frac{65 - 45}{2} + \frac{65 + 45}{2} \cos 120° + 10 \sin 120°$$

$$= 10 + 55 \times \left(-\frac{1}{2}\right) + 10\left(\frac{\sqrt{3}}{2}\right)$$

$$= 10 - 27.5 + 5\sqrt{3}$$

$$= 10 - 27.5 + 8.65$$

$$= -8.84 \text{ N/mm}^2$$

$$\tau_\theta = -\left(\frac{\sigma_x - \sigma_y}{2}\right) \sin 2\theta + \tau \cos 2\theta$$

$$= -\left(\frac{65+45}{2}\right)\sin 120° + 10\cos 120°$$

$$= -55 \times \frac{\sqrt{3}}{2} - 10 \times \frac{1}{2}$$

$$= -27.5 \times 1.732 - 5$$

$$= -47.63 - 5$$

$$\therefore \qquad \tau_\theta = -52.63 \text{ N/mm}^2$$

(–)ve sign shows that direction of σ_θ and τ_θ will be opposite to that assumed.

Hence, resultant stress $(\sigma_r) = \sqrt{\sigma_\theta^2 + \tau_\theta^2}$

$$= \sqrt{(-8.84)^2 + (-52.63)^2} = 53.36 \text{ N/mm}^2$$

Since, the value of σ_θ and τ_θ is negative so the correct figure will be as below:

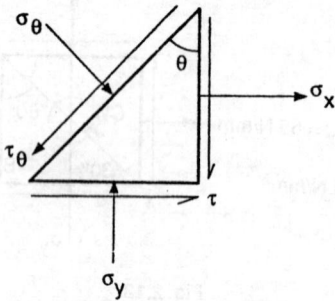

Fig. 2.14

EXAMPLE 6 *The state of stress at a given point in a machine component is as below:*

$$\sigma_x = 150 \text{ MPa}; \quad \sigma_y = -100 \text{ MPa}; \quad \tau_{xy} = 75 \text{ MPa}$$

The loading on the component is increased so that the stresses are increased 'k' times the the given values. Compute the maximum value of k if the material can withstand maximum normal and shear stresses of 500 MPa and 300 MPa respectively.   **(UPTU-2008)**

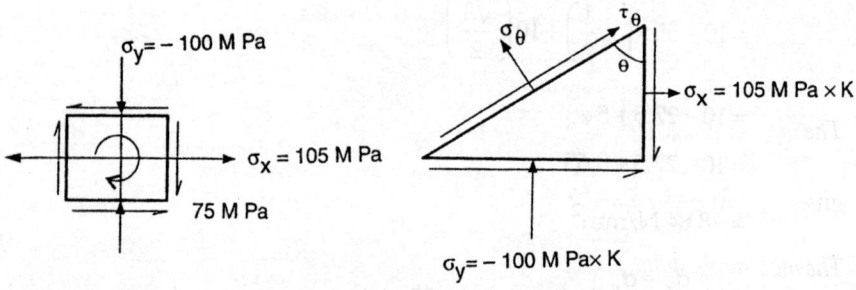

Fig. 2.15

SOLUTION   Given

$$\sigma_x = k \times 150 \text{ MPa}$$

$$\sigma_y = -k \times 100 \text{ MPa}$$

and $\tau_{xy} = k \times 75 \text{ MPa}$

Hence, Maximum normal stress i.e. the maximum principal stress

$$\sigma_1 = \frac{\sigma_x + \sigma_y}{2} + \sqrt{\left(\frac{\sigma_x - \sigma_y}{2}\right)^2 + \tau^2 xy}$$

$$= \frac{150k + (-100k)}{2} + \sqrt{\left\{\frac{150k - (-100k)}{2}\right\}^2 + (75k)^2}$$

$$= 25k + \sqrt{(125k)^2 + (75k)^2}$$

$$= 25k + 145.77k$$

$$= 170.77k$$

Given, 170.77 k = 500 MPa

$\therefore$ $k = 2.927$

Also, maximum shear stress

$$\tau_{max} = \sqrt{\left(\frac{\sigma_x - \sigma_y}{2}\right)^2 + \tau_{xy}^2}$$

$$= \sqrt{\left\{\frac{150k - (-100k)}{2}\right\}^2 + (75k)^2} = 145.77k$$

Given 145.77 k = 300

$\therefore$ $k = 2.05$

Hence, maximum value of $k = 2.05$.   **Ans.**

EXAMPLE 7 *In a Mohr's circle prove that*

(a) *On the plane of maximum shear stress, the normal and resultant strress components are given by*

$$\frac{\sigma_1 + \sigma_2}{2} \quad and \quad \sqrt{\frac{\sigma_1^2 + \sigma_2^2}{2}} \quad respectively$$

(b) *The maximum obliquity (ϕ_{max}) of the resultant stress with the normal to plane is given by* $\sin \phi = \left(\dfrac{\sigma_1 - \sigma_2}{\sigma_1 + \sigma_2}\right)$

(c) *The maximum obliquity (ϕ_{max}) occurs when $\theta = \sigma/2 + 45°$ where θ is the angle at which the plane is inclined to the σ_1-axis.*

SOLUTION

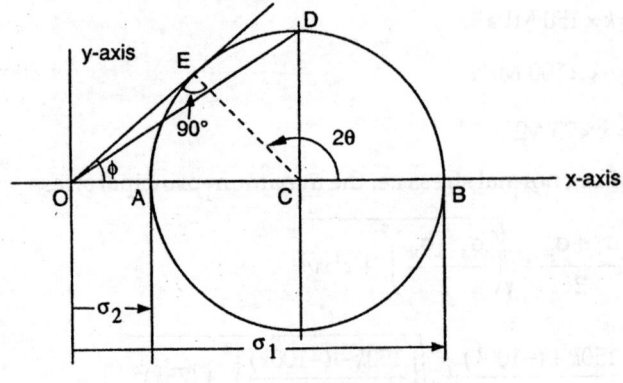

Fig. 2.16

(a) Normal stress on plane of maximum shear stress

$$= OC$$
$$= OA + AC$$
$$= \sigma_2 + \frac{\sigma_x - \sigma_y}{2}$$

∴   Normal stress $= \left(\dfrac{\sigma_x + \sigma_y}{2} \right)$ **Proved**

Resultant stress $(\sigma_r) = OD$

$$= \sqrt{OC^2 + CD^2}$$
$$= \sqrt{OC^2 + AC^2}$$
$$= \sqrt{\left(\frac{\sigma_x + \sigma_y}{2} \right)^2 + \left(\frac{\sigma_x - \sigma_y}{2} \right)^2}$$
$$= \sqrt{\frac{\sigma_1^2 + \sigma_2^2}{2}}$$ **Proved**

(b) The maximum obliquity (ϕ_{max}) occurs when OE is tangent to the circle i.e.

$$\angle CEO = 90°$$

∴ $\sin \phi = \dfrac{EC}{OC}$

$$= \frac{AC}{OC}$$

$$= \frac{\dfrac{\sigma_1 - \sigma_2}{2}}{\dfrac{\sigma_1 + \sigma_2}{2}} = \left(\frac{\sigma_1 - \sigma_2}{\sigma_1 + \sigma_2} \right)$$ **Proved**

(c) From geometry, $2\theta = \phi + 90°$

$\therefore \qquad \theta = \left(\dfrac{\phi}{2} + 45° \right)$ Proved

EXAMPLE 8 *The intensity of resultant stress on a plane AB shown in Figure 2.17 is 80 MPa (tensile) inclined at 30° to the normal to that plane. The normal component of stress on another plane BC at right angles to plane AB is 60 MPa. Determine*

(i) *the resultant stress on the plane BC*

(ii) *the principal stresses and the principal planes*

(iii) *the maximum shear stress and its plane.*

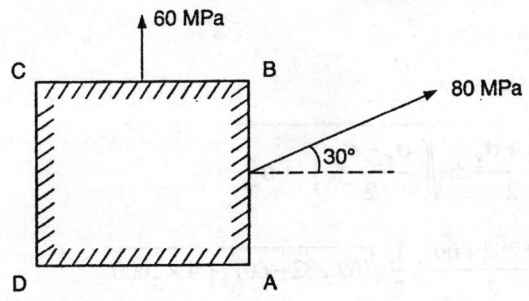

Fig. 2.17

SOLUTION

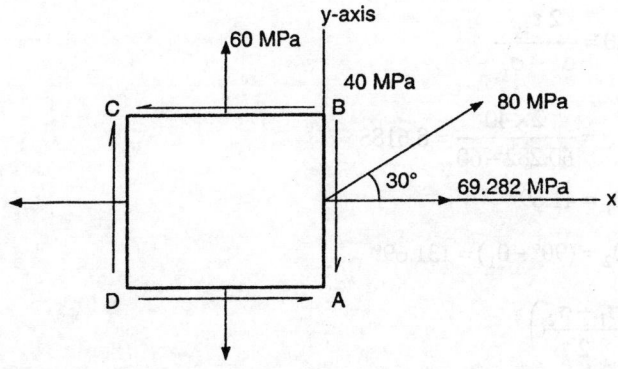

Fig. 2.18

After resolving 80 MPa along x-axis and y-axis respectively we get σ_x and τ_{xy}

$\sigma_x = 80 \cos 30°$

$= \cancel{80}^{40} \times \dfrac{\sqrt{3}}{\cancel{2}}$

$= 40 \times 1.732 = 69.282$ MPa

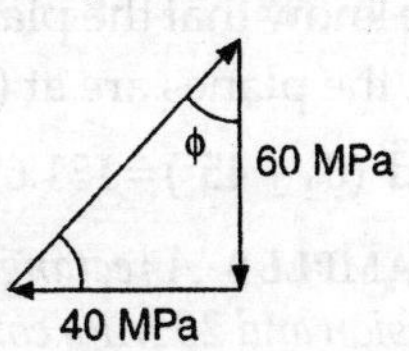

Fig. 2.19

$$\tau_{xy} = 80 \sin 30°$$

$$= 80 \times \frac{1}{2} = 40 \text{ MPa}$$

(*i*) Resultant stress on plane *BC*,

$$\sigma_r = \sqrt{60^2 + 40^2} = \sqrt{3600 + 1600}$$

$$= \sqrt{5200} = 72.111 \text{ MPa} \qquad \qquad \textbf{Ans.}$$

$$\tan \phi = \left(\frac{\tau}{\sigma_n}\right) = \left(\frac{40}{60}\right) = 0.66$$

∴ $\phi = 33.42°$

(*ii*) the principal stresses,

$$\sigma_{1,2} = \frac{\sigma_x + \sigma_y}{2} \pm \sqrt{\left(\frac{\sigma_x - \sigma_y}{2}\right)^2 + \sigma_{xy}^2}$$

$$= \frac{69.282 + 60}{2} \pm \frac{1}{2}\sqrt{(69.282 - 60)^2 + 4 \times 1600}$$

$$= 64.641 \pm 40.268$$

$$= 104.909 \text{ MPa}; \ 24.373 \text{ MPa}$$

$$\tan 2\theta = \frac{2\tau_{xy}}{\sigma_x - \sigma_y}$$

$$= \frac{2 \times 40}{60.282 - 60} = 8.6188$$

$$\theta_1 = 41.69°$$

$$\theta_2 = (90° - \theta_1) = 131.69°$$

(iii) $\tau_{max} = \left(\frac{\sigma_1 - \sigma_2}{2}\right)$

$$= \frac{104.909 - 24.373}{3} = 40.268 \text{ MPa}$$

We know that the planes of maximum shear stress are 45° to the principal planes. So, the planes are at ($\theta_1 + 45°$) = 41.69 + 45 = 86.69°.

and ($\theta_2 + 45°$) = 131.69 × 45° = 176.69° **Ans.**

EXAMPLE 9 *A rectangular block is subjected to a two perpendicular stresses of 20 MPa tension and 20 MPa compression. Dtermine the stresses on planes inclined at (a) 30°, (b) 45°, (c) 60° with the x-axis.*

SOLUTION

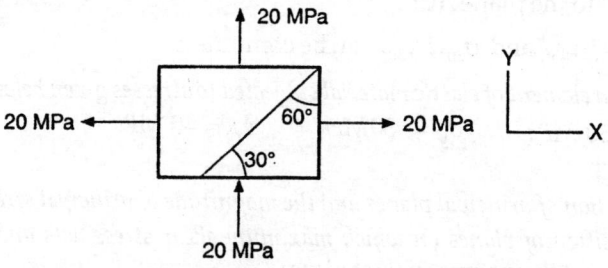

(a)   Fig. 2.20

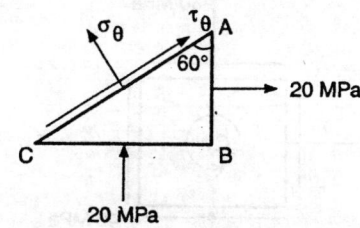

(b)   Fig. 2.21

First, we will convert the angle making with y-axis as per theory given in this book in section 2.3.

Here, $\theta = 60°$ with the y-axis.

$\therefore \qquad \sigma_\theta \text{ or } \sigma_{60°} = \sigma_x \cos^2 \theta + \sigma_y \sin^2 \theta$

$$= 20 (\cos^2 60° - \sin^2 60°)$$

$$= 20 \left(\frac{1}{4} - \frac{3}{4} \right)$$

$$= -20 \times \frac{2}{4} = -10 \text{ MPa (Compression)} \qquad \textbf{Ans.}$$

$\tau_{60°} = -\frac{1}{2} (\sigma_x - \sigma_y) \sin 2\theta$

$$= -\frac{1}{2} (20 + 20) \times \sin 120°$$

$$= -20 \times \sin 60°$$

$$= -20 \times \frac{\sqrt{3}}{2} = -10\sqrt{3}$$

$$= -17.320 \text{ MPa (CCW)}$$

$$= -17.32 \text{ MPa (CCW)} \qquad \qquad \textbf{Ans.}$$

i.e. downward to the plane AC.

Similarly, $\sigma_{45°}$; $\tau_{45°}$ and $\sigma_{30°}$; $\tau_{30°}$ can be computed.

EXAMPLE 8 *An element of elastic material subjected to stresses given below:*

$$\sigma_x = 50 \text{ MPa} \qquad \sigma_y = -30 MPa \qquad \tau_{xy} = 40 \text{ MPa}$$

Find

(a) *the position of principal planes and the magnitude of principal stresses*

(b) *The position of planes on which maximum shear stress acts and calculate the normal and shear stress on these planes.*

SOLUTION (a)

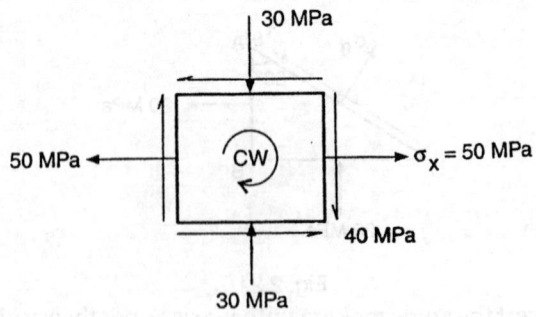

30 MPa

50 MPa ← CW → σ_x = 50 MPa

40 MPa

30 MPa

Fig. 2.22

By the formula, the principal stresses are given by

$$\sigma_{1,2} = \frac{\sigma_x + \sigma_y}{2} \pm \sqrt{\left(\frac{\sigma_x - \sigma_y}{2}\right)^2 + \tau_{xy}^2}$$

$$= \frac{50 - 30}{2} \pm \sqrt{\left(\frac{50 - 30}{2}\right)^2 + (40)^2}$$

$$= 10 \pm \sqrt{3200}$$

$$= (10 \pm 56.56) \text{ MPa}$$

Therefore, the major principal stress is

$$\sigma_1 = 10 + 56.56 = 66.56 \text{ MPa (Tensile)} \qquad \textbf{Ans.}$$

And the miner principal stress is

$$\sigma_2 = 10 - 56.56 = -46.56 \text{ MPa (Compressive)} \qquad \textbf{Ans.}$$

Position of principal planes:

$$\tan 2\theta_p = \left(\frac{2\tau_{xy}}{\sigma_x - \sigma_y}\right)$$

$$= \frac{2 \times 40}{50 - (-30)} = \frac{80}{80} = 1$$

$$= \tan 45° \text{ and } \tan (180 + 45°)$$

$$= \tan 45° \text{ and } \tan 225°$$

$$\theta_p = 22.5° \text{ and } 112.2°$$

$$\therefore \qquad \theta_{p_1} = 22.5° \text{ and } \theta_{p_2} = 112.2° \qquad\qquad \textbf{Ans.}$$

(b) Let θ_S be the angle made by the planes of maximum shear stress.

We know that θ_S and θ_P are 45° apart

So $\qquad \theta_S = (45 + 22.5°) \text{ and } (45 + 112.5°)$

$$= 67.5° \text{ and } 157.5°$$

$$\therefore \qquad \theta_{S_1} = 67.5° \text{ and } \theta_{S_2} = 157.5°$$

The Normal Stresses on the planes of maximum shear stress are:

For $\theta = 67.5°$

$$\sigma_\theta = \frac{\sigma_x + \sigma_y}{2} + \frac{\sigma_x - \sigma_y}{2} \cos 2\theta + \tau_{xy} \sin 2\theta$$

$$= \frac{50 - 30}{2} + \frac{50 + 30}{2} \cos 135° + 40 \times \sin 135°$$

$$= 10 - 28.28 + 28.28$$

$$= 10 \text{ MPa} \qquad\qquad \textbf{Ans.}$$

For $\theta = 157.5°$

$$\sigma_\theta = \frac{50 - 30}{2} + \frac{50 + 30}{2} \cos 315° + 40 \times \sin 315°$$

$$= 10 - 28.28 + 28.28$$

$$= 10 \text{ MPa} \qquad\qquad \textbf{Ans.}$$

The shear stresses on the planes of maximum shear stress are:

For $\theta = 67.5°$

$$\tau_\theta = -\frac{\sigma_x - \sigma_y}{2} \sin 2\theta + \tau_{xy} \cos 2\theta$$

$$= -\frac{50 + 30}{2} \sin 135° + 40 \cos 135°$$

$$= -28.28 - 28.28$$

$$= -56.56 \text{ MPa} \qquad\qquad \textbf{Ans.}$$

For $\theta = 157.5°$

$$\tau_\theta = -\frac{50 + 30}{2} \sin 315° + 40 \cos 315°$$

$$= 28.28 + 28.28$$

$$= 56.56 \text{ MPa} \qquad\qquad \textbf{Ans.}$$

EXAMPLE 11 *In a biaxial stress system, the stresses at a point are:* $\sigma_x = 25$ *MPa;* $\sigma_y = -40$ *MPa and* $\tau_{xy} = 30$ *MPa. Find the principal stresses, position of the principal planes and* τ_{max} . *Also compute the stresses on a plane inclined at 30° to the vertical.*

(UPSC Engg. Services 2001)

SOLUTION   By Formula, the principal stresses are

$$\sigma_{1,2} = \frac{\sigma_x + \sigma_y}{2} \pm \sqrt{\left(\frac{\sigma_x - \sigma_y}{2}\right)^2 + \tau_{xy}^2}$$

$$= \frac{25 - 40}{2} \pm \sqrt{\left(\frac{25 - 40}{2}\right)^2 + (30)^2}$$

$$= -7.5 \pm \sqrt{1056.25 + 900}$$

$$= (-7.5 \pm 44.23) \text{ MPa}$$

∴   Major principal stress (σ_1)

$$= -7.5 + 44.23 = 36.73 \text{ MPa (Tensile)}$$ **Ans.**

And the minor principal stress is (σ_2)

$$= -7.5 - 44.23 = -51.73 \text{ MPa (Compressive)}$$ **Ans.**

$$\tau_{max} = \left(\frac{\sigma_1 - \sigma_2}{2}\right) = \frac{36.73 + 51.73}{2}$$

$$= \frac{88.46}{2} \text{ MPa} = 44.23 \text{ MPa}$$ **Ans.**

The principal planes are given by,

$$\tan 2\theta_p = \left(\frac{2\tau_{xy}}{\sigma_x - \sigma_y}\right)$$

$$= \frac{2 \times 30}{25 - (-40)} = \frac{\overset{12}{\cancel{60}}}{\underset{13}{\cancel{65}}} = 0.923$$

or $2\theta_p = 42.70°$ and $222.70°$ **Ans.**

∴ $\theta_p = 21.35°$ and $111.35°$ **Ans.**

The normal stress on the inclined plane is given by

$$\sigma_\theta = \frac{\sigma_x + \sigma_y}{2} + \frac{\sigma_x - \sigma_y}{2} \cos 2\theta + \tau_{xy} \sin 2\theta$$

$$= \frac{25 - 40}{2} + \frac{25 - (-40)}{2} \cos 60° + 30 \sin 60°$$

$$= -7.5 + 32.5 \times 0.5 + 30 \times 0.866$$

$$= -7.5 + 16.25 + 25.98$$
$$= 34.73 \text{ MPa} \hspace{4cm} \textbf{Ans.}$$

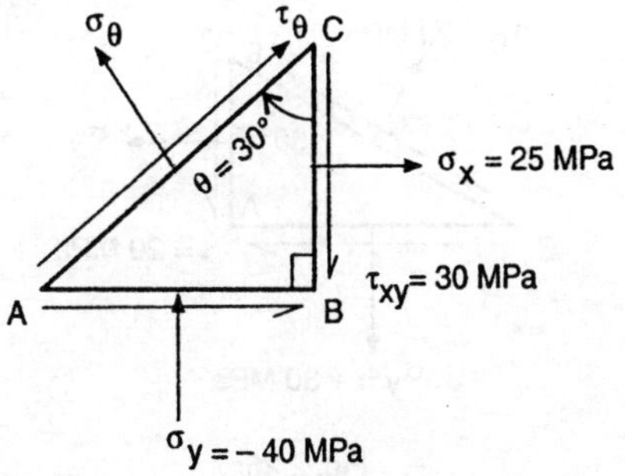

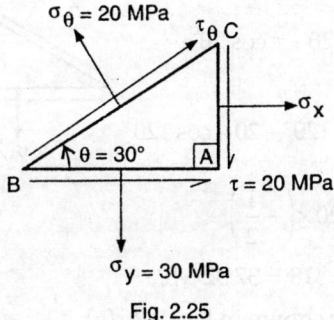

Fig. 2.23

The shear stress on the inclined plane is given by

$$\tau_\theta = -\frac{\sigma_x - \sigma_y}{2} \sin 2\theta + \tau_{xy} \cos 2\theta$$

$$= \frac{\sigma_y - \sigma_x}{2} \sin 2\theta + \tau_{xy} \cos 2\theta$$

$$= \frac{-40 - 25}{2} \sin 60° + 30 \cos 60°$$

$$= -32.5 \times 0.866 + 30 \times 0.5$$

$$= -28.145 + 15$$

$$= -13.145 \text{ MPa} \hspace{3cm} \textbf{Ans.}$$

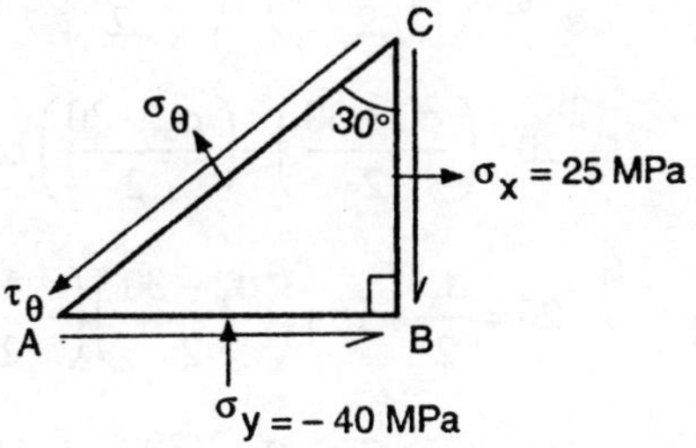

Fig. 2.24

So, the direction of τ will be downward the plane AC. The final figure is shown in Fig. 2.24.

EXAMPLE 12 *In a biaxial stress system, certain material under load on plane AB carries a tensile direct stress of 30 MPa and shear stress of 20 MPa while another plane BC carries a tensile direct stress of 20 MPa and a shear stress.*

If the planes are inclined to one another at 30° and plane AC at right angles to plane AB carries a direct stress unknown in magnitude and nature then find

(a) *The magnitude and nature of the direct stress on AC*

(b) *The value of the shear stress on BC*

(c) *The principal stress.* (**UPSC Engg. Services**)

SOLUTION

Fig. 2.25

Since, we have derived formula for σ_θ and τ_θ when the inclined plane is making angle with the vertical so first of all redraw the figure as below:

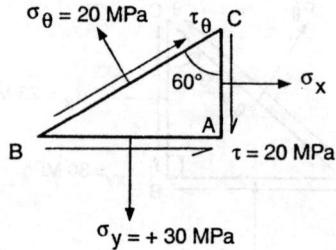

Fig. 2.26

We know from formula that

$$\sigma_\theta = \left(\frac{\sigma_x + \sigma_y}{2}\right) + \left(\frac{\sigma_x - \sigma_y}{2}\right) \cos 2\theta + \tau \sin 2\theta$$

$$20 = \left(\frac{\sigma_x + 30}{2}\right) + \left(\frac{\sigma_x - 30}{2}\right) \cos 120° + 20 \sin 120°$$

or, $$20 = \frac{\sigma_x}{2} + 15 + \left(\frac{\sigma_x - 30}{2}\right)\left(-\frac{1}{2}\right) + \overset{10}{\cancel{20}} \times \frac{\sqrt{3}}{\cancel{2}}$$

or, $$20 - 15 = \frac{\sigma_x}{2} - \frac{\sigma_x}{4} + \frac{30}{4} + 10\sqrt{3}$$

or, $$5 - \frac{30}{4} - 10\sqrt{3} = \frac{\sigma_x}{4}$$

or, $$\frac{20 - 30 - 40\sqrt{3}}{4} = \frac{\sigma_x}{4}$$

$\therefore$ $$\sigma_x = -10 - 40\sqrt{3} = -10 - 40 \times 1.732$$

$$= -10 - 69.28 = -79.28 \text{ MPa (Compressive in nature)}$$

(*b*) Now, applying formula for shear stress
We have,

$$\tau_\theta = \left(\frac{\sigma_y - \sigma_x}{2}\right) \sin 2\theta + \tau \cos 2\theta$$

$$= \frac{30 + 78.28}{2} \times \sin 120° + 20 \times \cos 120°$$

$$= 54.64 \times 0.866 + 20 \times \left(-\frac{1}{2}\right)$$

Fig. 2.26 (a)

$$= 47.318 - 10 = 37.318 = 37.32 \text{ MPa}$$

So, the revised diagram is shown in Fig. 2.26 (a).

(c) The principal stresses are given by

$$\sigma_1, \sigma_2 = \left(\frac{\sigma_x + \sigma_y}{2}\right) \pm \sqrt{\left(\frac{\sigma_x - \sigma_y}{2}\right)^2 + \tau_{xy}^2}$$

$$= \frac{-79.28 + 30}{2} \pm \sqrt{\left(\frac{-79.28 - 30}{2}\right)^2 + (20)^2}$$

$$= -24.64 \pm 58.18$$

$$= 33.54 \text{ MPa}; \ (-) 82.82 \text{ MPa}$$

∴ $\sigma_1 = 33.54$ MPa and $\sigma_2 = (-)82.82$ MPa **Ans.**

Alternative Method (from First Principle)

In this method all the forces acting on the face AC and AB of the wedge will be resolved parallel to BC and perpendicular to BC and then equation of equilibrium $\Sigma F_x = 0, \Sigma F_y = 0$ will be applied to get the value of σ_θ and τ_θ (as is done in the derivation of σ_θ and τ_θ in section 2.3 but this method is not advisable since it takes much time to solve the problem and time management is very essential. **However, if you are asked to solve the problem in examination from first principle then the same should be adopted.**

EXAMPLE 13 *In a unstressed steel plate, a circle of 100 mm diameter is cut. The plate is loaded as shown in figure. As a result of loading the circle changes into the ellipse. Determine the major and minor axes.*

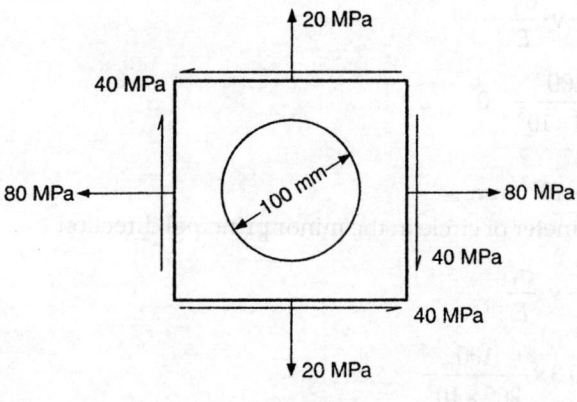

Fig. 2.27

SOLUTION

Principal stresses $\sigma_{1,2} = \dfrac{80 + 20}{2} \pm \sqrt{\left(\dfrac{80 - 20}{2}\right)^2 + (40)^2}$

$$= 50 \pm \sqrt{900 + 1600}$$

$$= 50 \pm 50$$

$$= 100 \text{ MPa} \text{ and } 0$$

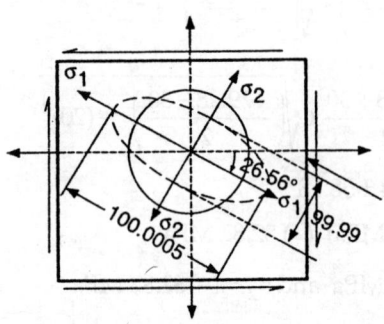

Fig. 2.28

Direction of Principal plane,

$$\tan 2\theta_P = \frac{2\tau}{\sigma_x - \sigma_y}$$

$$= \frac{2 \times 40}{80 - 20} = \left(\frac{4}{3}\right)$$

$$\therefore \qquad \theta_P = 26.56°$$

Change in diameter of circle in the major principal direction

$$= \frac{\sigma_1}{E} - v \cdot \frac{\sigma_2}{E}$$

$$= \frac{\cancel{100}^{2}}{\cancel{200} \times 10^3} - 0$$

$$= 0.5 \times 10^{-3} \text{ mm}$$

Change in diameter of circle in the minor principal direction

$$= \frac{\sigma_2}{E} - v \cdot \frac{\sigma_1}{E}$$

$$= 0 - 0.3 \times \frac{\cancel{100}^{2}}{\cancel{200} \times 10^3}$$

$$= -0.15 \times 10^{-3} \text{ mm}$$

Hence, major axis of ellipse $= 100 + 0.5 \times 10^{-3} = 100.0005$ mm

And minor axis of ellipse $= 100 - 0.15 \times 10^{-3} = 99.99$ mm $\simeq 100$ mm   **Ans.**

EXAMPLE 14 (a) A bar of cross sectional area 800 mm^2 is acted upon by axial tensile force of 50 kN applied at each end of the bar. Determine the normal and shear stress on a plane inclined at 30° to the direction of loading.

(b) *For what inclination of the plane, maximum shear stress does occur?*

Find out the normal and shear stress for the plane of maximum shear stress.

SOLUTION (a)

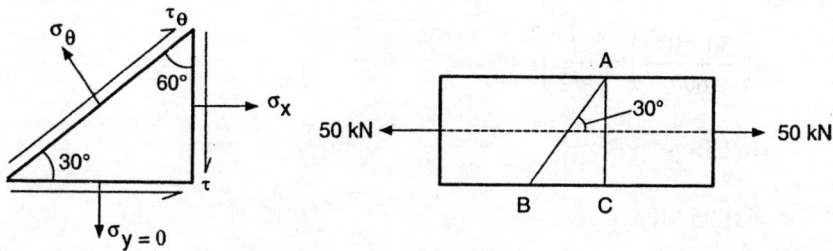

Fig. 2.29

Normal stress $\quad(\sigma_\theta \text{ or } \sigma_{60°}) = \sigma_x \cos^2\theta + \sigma_y^2 \sin^2\theta$

$$= \left(\frac{P}{A}\right).\cos^2\theta + 0 \qquad\qquad \left[\because \sigma_y = 0\right]$$

$$= \left(\frac{50\times10^3}{800}\right).\cos^2(60)^2$$

$$= 62.5 \text{ N/mm}^2 \times \left(\frac{1}{2}\right)^2$$

$$= 62.5 \text{ MPa} \times \frac{1}{4}$$

$$= 15.625 \text{ MPa}$$

Shear stress $(\sigma_\theta) = \dfrac{1}{2}\sigma_x \sin 2\theta$

$\therefore \qquad\qquad \tau_\theta = \dfrac{1}{2}\sigma_x \sin(60°\times2)$

$$= \frac{1}{2}\times\left(\frac{50\times10^3}{800}\right)\times\frac{\sqrt{3}}{2}$$

$$= 27.06 \text{ N/mm}^2$$

$$= 27.06 \text{ MPa}$$

(b) The shear stress $\tau_\theta = \dfrac{1}{2}\sigma_x \sin 2\theta$ will be maximum when $\sin 2\theta = 1 = \sin 90°$

i.e. when $\theta = 45°$

In that case

Normal stress $(\sigma_{45°}) = \sigma_x \cos^2 \theta$

At $\theta = 45°$

$$= \left(\frac{50 \times 10^3}{800} \right) \times \left(\frac{1}{\sqrt{2}} \right)^2$$

$$= 62.5 \times \frac{1}{2}$$

$$= 31.25 \text{ MPa}$$

Shear stress $(\tau_{45°}) = \frac{1}{2} \sigma_x \sin 2\theta$

At $\theta = 45°$

$$= \frac{1}{2} \times 62.5 \times \sin 90°$$

$$= \frac{1}{2} \times 62.5 \times 1 = 31.25 \text{ MPa}$$ **Ans.**

EXAMPLE 15 *A steel bolt 25 mm diameter is subjected to a direct tension of 15 kN and a shearing force of 10 kN. Determine the resultant stress across a plane inclined at an angle of 60° to the longitudinal axis of the bolt.*

SOLUTION

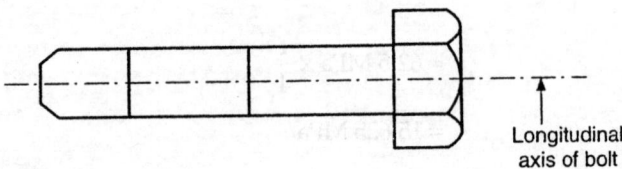

Fig. 2.30

Let us take a small portion of the bolt for the analysis.

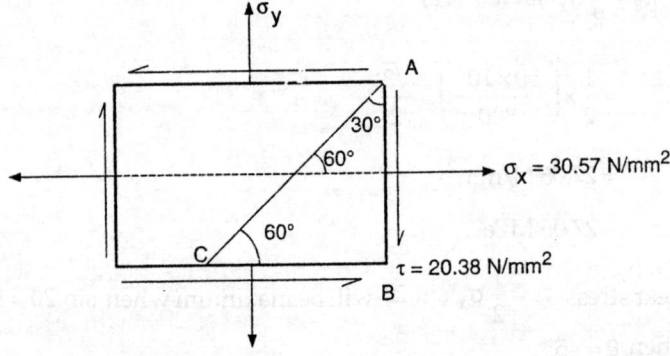

Fig. 2.31

It is given that the plane AC is inclined $60°$ to the longitudinal axis of the bolt. Therefore, angle with the y-axis willbe $(90 - 60) = 30° = \theta$. This was done to use the formula as given in this book.

Therefore, applying the formula for normal stress (σ_θ) on the oblique plane AC and shear stress (τ_θ). Let us redraw the figure

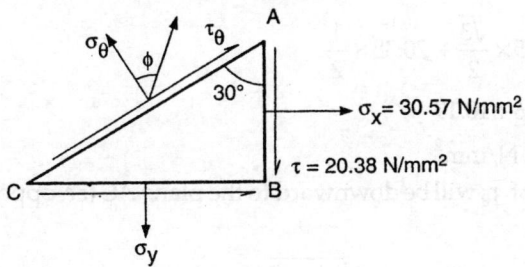

Fig. 2.32

Area of bolt $= \dfrac{\pi}{4} \times (25)^2 = 490.625 \text{ mm}^2$

Longitudinal stress (σ_x) on the bolt $= \dfrac{15 \times 10^3}{490.625}$

$\therefore \qquad \sigma_x = 30.57 \text{ N/mm}^2 \text{ (Tensile)}$

Shear stress (τ) on the bolt $= \dfrac{10 \times 10^3}{490.625}$

$\qquad \tau = 20.38 \text{ N/mm}^2$

Now, we have, $\sigma_x = 30.57 \text{ N/mm}^2$

$\qquad \sigma_y = 0$

and $\qquad \tau = 20.38 \text{ N/mm}^2$

Normal stress (σ_θ) on the oblique plane AC

$= \left(\dfrac{\sigma_x + \sigma_y}{2} \right) + \left(\dfrac{\sigma_x - \sigma_y}{2} \right) . \cos 2\theta + \tau . \sin 2\theta$

$= \dfrac{30.57 + 0}{2} + \dfrac{30.57 - 0}{2} . \cos 60° + 20.38 . \sin 60°$

$= 15.285 + 15.285 \times \dfrac{1}{2} + 20.38 \times \dfrac{\sqrt{3}}{2}$

$= 15.285 + 7.6425 + 17.64$

$= 40.56 \text{ Newton/mm}^2$

Shear stress (τ_θ) on the oblique plane AC

$$= -\left(\frac{\sigma_x - \sigma_y}{2}\right).\sin 2\theta + \tau.\cos 2\theta$$

$$= -\frac{30.57}{2} \times \sin 60° + 20.38 \times \cos 60°$$

$$= -7.6425 \times \frac{\sqrt{3}}{2} + \overset{10.19}{\cancel{20.38}} \times \frac{1}{\cancel{2}}$$

$$= -13.236 + 10.19$$

$$= -3.046 \text{ N/mm}^2$$

So, the direction of τ_θ will be downward to the plane AC (*i.e.* opposite to the shown in figure).

Now, the resultant stress $(\sigma_r) = \sqrt{\sigma_\theta^2 + \tau_\theta^2}$

$$= \sqrt{(40.56)^2 + (-3.046)^2}$$

$$= 40.67 \text{ N/mm}^2$$

Angle of obliquity (ϕ) *i.e.* the angle which the resultant stress (σ_r) makes with normal stress (σ_θ) is

$$\phi = \tan^{-1}\left(\frac{\tau_\theta}{\sigma_\theta}\right)$$

$$= \tan^{-1}\left(\frac{3.046}{40.56}\right) = 4.29° \hspace{3cm} \textbf{Ans.}$$

EXAMPLE 16 *A rectangular element of a structure is subjected to direct stresses of 75 N/mm² (tensile) and 40 N/mm² (compressive) acting on two mutually perpendicular planes. These stresses are accompanied by shear stress of intensity 20 N/mm². Determine the principal stresses, location of principal planes.*

Also determine the maximum shear stress and the planes on which it acts.

SOLUTION Given

$$\sigma_x = 75 \text{ N/mm}^2, \hspace{1cm} \sigma_y = -40 \text{ N/mm}^2, \hspace{1cm} \tau_{xy} = +20 \text{ N/mm}^2$$

By formula, principal stresses are given by

$$\sigma_{1,2} = \frac{\sigma_x + \sigma_y}{2} \pm \sqrt{\left(\frac{\sigma_x - \sigma_y}{2}\right)^2 + \tau_{xy}^2}$$

$$= \frac{75 - 40}{2} \pm \sqrt{\left(\frac{75 - 40}{2}\right)^2 + (20)^2}$$

$$= 17.5 \pm \sqrt{3306.25 + 400}$$

$$= 17.5 \pm 60.88 \text{ N/mm}^2$$

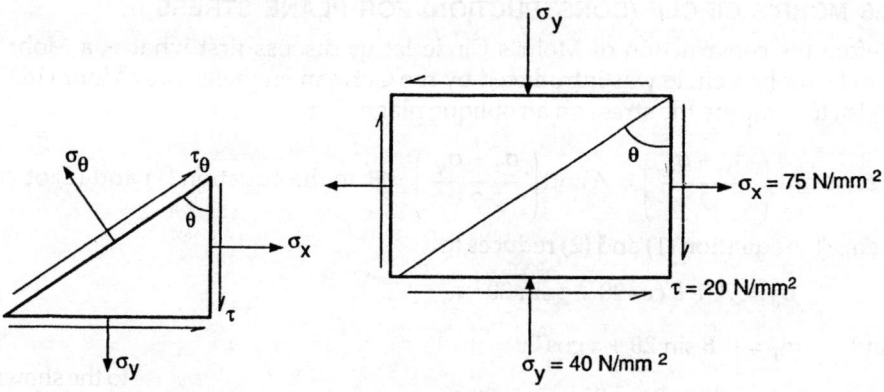

Fig. 2.33

$\therefore$ Major principal stress $(\sigma_1) = 78.38\,\text{N/mm}^2$ (Tensile)

And   Minor principal stress $(\sigma_2) = 17.5 - 60.88 = -43.38\,\text{N/mm}^2$

(compressive)

Position of principal planes can be known by applying formula as given below:

$$\tan 2\theta_P = \frac{2\tau}{\sigma_x - \sigma_y}$$

$$= \frac{2 \times 20}{75 + 40} = \frac{40}{115}$$

$2\theta_P = 19.17°$ and 199.17

$\therefore$ $\theta_P = 9.58°$ and $99.58°$

$= 9°\,35'$ and $99°\,35'$

$\therefore$ $\theta_{P_1} = 9°\,35'$ and $\theta_{P_2} = 99°\,35'$

$$\tau_{max} = \frac{\sigma_1 - \sigma_2}{2}$$

$$= \frac{78.38 + 43.38}{2} = 60.88\,\text{N/mm}^2$$

Angular position of the plane carrying maximum shear stress are

$$\theta_{s_1} = (\theta_{P_1} + 45°)$$

$$= 9°\,35' + 45° = 54°\,35'$$

$$\theta_{s_2} = \theta_{P_2} + 45°$$

$$= 99°\,35' + 45° = 144°\,35'$$

2.6 MOHR'S CIRCLE (CONSTRUCTION) FOR PLANE STRESS

Before the construction of Mohr's Circle let us discuss first what is a Mohr's Circle. Mohr's circle was introduced by the German engineer Otto Mohr (1835–1918) to compute the stress on an oblique plane.

Let us put $\left(\dfrac{\sigma_x + \sigma_y}{2}\right) = A$ and $\left(\dfrac{\sigma_x - \sigma_y}{2}\right) = B$ in the equation (1) and (2) of 2.3

hence the equation (1) and (2) reduces to

$$\sigma_\theta = A + B\cos 2\theta + \tau \sin 2\theta$$

and $\qquad \tau_\theta = -B \sin 2\theta + \tau \cos 2\theta$

$\therefore \qquad (\sigma_\theta - A) = B \cos 2\theta + \tau \sin 2\theta$

and $\qquad \tau_\theta = -B \sin 2\theta + \tau \cos 2\theta$

Now, squarring and adding these two we get

$$(\sigma_\theta - A)^2 + \tau_\theta^2 = B^2 + \tau^2$$

Now, substituting the value of A and B

$$\left(\sigma_\theta - \frac{\sigma_x + \sigma_y}{2}\right)^2 + (\tau_\theta - 0)^2 = \left(\frac{\sigma_x - \sigma_y}{2}\right)^2 + \tau^2$$

or, $\qquad \left(\sigma_\theta - \dfrac{\sigma_x + \sigma_y}{2}\right)^2 + (\tau_\theta - 0)^2 = \dfrac{(\sigma_x - \sigma_y)^2 + 4\tau^2}{4}$

or, $\qquad \left(\sigma_\theta - \dfrac{\sigma_x + \sigma_y}{2}\right)^2 + (\tau_\theta - 0)^2 = \left(\dfrac{\sqrt{(\sigma_x - \sigma_y)^2 + 4\tau^2}}{(2)^2}\right)^2$

or, $\qquad \left(\sigma_\theta - \dfrac{\sigma_x + \sigma_y}{2}\right)^2 + (\tau_\theta - 0)^2 = \left(\dfrac{1}{2}\sqrt{(\sigma_x - \sigma_y)^2 + 4\tau^2}\right)^2$

Now, let us recall the equation of circle which is $(x - a)^2 + (y - b)^2 = R^2$, where a and b are the co-ordinate of centre and R is the radius of the circle.

Therefore, Mohr's Circle is a circle having the co-ordinate of centre $\left(\dfrac{\sigma_x + \sigma_y}{2}; 0\right)$

and radius $(R) = \dfrac{1}{2}\sqrt{(\sigma_x - \sigma_y)^2 + 4\tau^2}$

Now, let us see as to how the Mohr's Circle is constructed under various condition of loading. The various stresses have been levelled in the Fig. 2.33.

N.B. A complete graphical representation of any symmetric 2D tensor (stress, strain, inertia etc.) in all orientation is given by Mohr's circle.

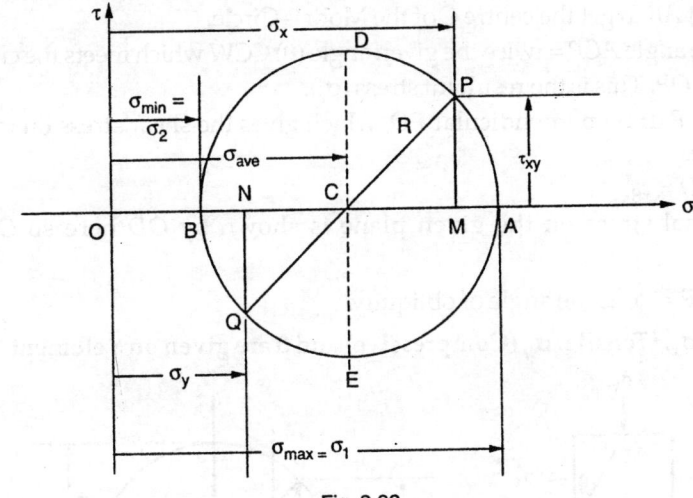

Fig. 2.33

Sign Convention:

For constructing Mohr circle, following sign convention should be adopted:

1. Positive normal stresses (tensile) are to the right.
2. Negative normal stresses (compressive) are to the left.
3. Shear stresses that tend to rotate the stress element clockwise (CW) are plotted upward on the τ-axis.
4. Shear stresses that tend to rotate the stress element counter clockwise (CCW) are plotted downward.

(a) When σ_x, σ_y and θ are given on a element also given ($\sigma_x > \sigma_y$).

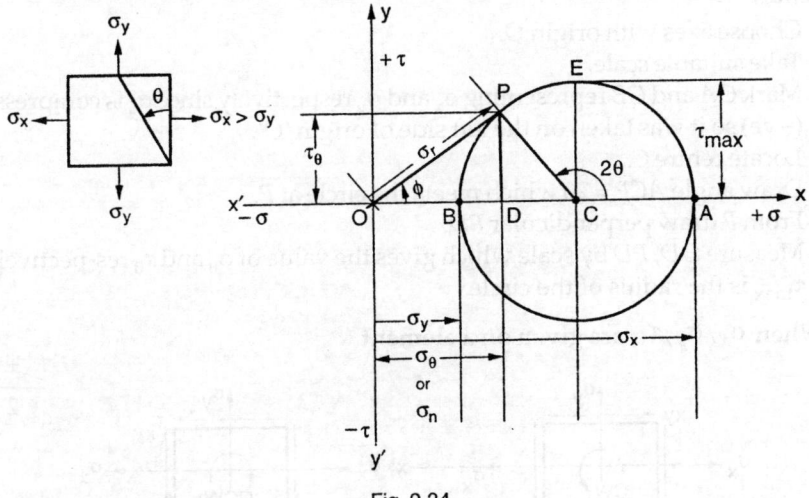

Fig. 2.34

Procedure:

(i) Draw axes with origin O.

(ii) Take suitable scale *i.e.* neither big nor small.

(iii) Make OA and OB representing σ_x and σ_y respectively.

(iv) Bisect AB to get the centre C of the Mohr's Circle.

(v) Make angle ACP = twice the given angle (θ) CCW which meets the circle at P.

(vi) Meet OP. This is the resultant stress (σ_r).

(vii) From P draw perpendicular PD, which gives the shear stress on the given plane.

So, $PD = \tau_\theta$.

Normal stress on the given plane is shown by OD here so $OD = \sigma_\theta$ or σ_n.

(viii) $\angle COP = \phi$, is the angle of obliquity.

(b) When σ_x, (Tensile) σ_y (Compressive) and θ are given on a element

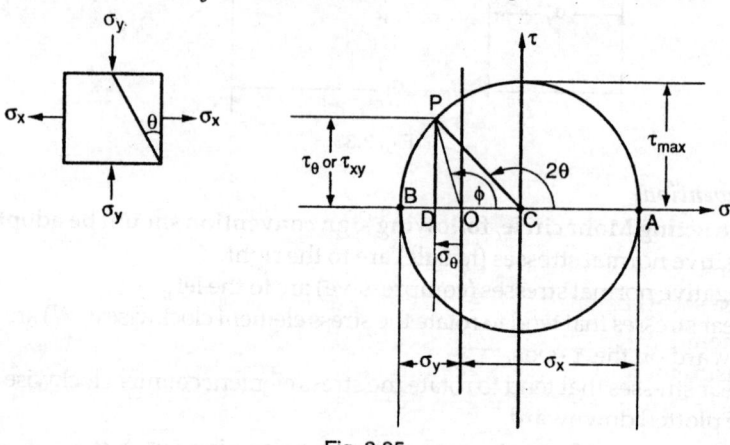

Fig. 2.35

Procedure:

(i) Choose axes with origin O.

(ii) Take suitable scale.

(iii) Mark OA and OB representing σ_x and σ_y respectively since σ_y is compressive (– ve) so it was taken on the left side of origin 'O'.

(iv) Locate centre C.

(v) Draw angle $ACP = 2\theta$ which meets the circle at P.

(vi) From P draw perpendicular PD.

(vii) Measure OD, PD by scale which gives the value of σ_θ and τ_θ res-pectively.

(viii) τ_{max} is the radius of the circle.

(c) When σ_x, σ_y, τ_{xy} are given on a element

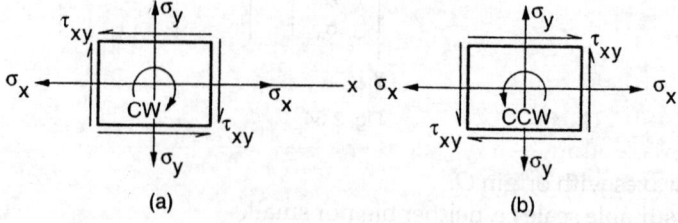

(a)   (b)

Fig. 2.36

Procedure:

(i) Draw xx' and yy' axes representing the σ_x and σ_y respectively as shown in Fig. 2.37.

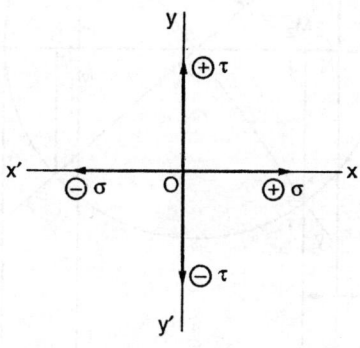

Fig. 2.37

(ii) Choose suitable scale so that the given problem can be accomodated in the given sheet/page.

Remember that scale should be such that one can draw circle and take the measurement of the desired thing e.g. σ_1, σ_2, τ, τ_{max}, ϕ etc.

(iii) Take $\oplus$ normal stress on the R.H.S of O and $\ominus$ stress on the LHS of O

$\oplus$ shear stress τ is taken above xx'

$\ominus$ shear stress τ is taken below xx'

Further, clockwise rotation of τ is considered $\oplus$ and counter clockwise rotation of τ is considered $\ominus$.

In the given Fig. 2.36 (a) τ_{xy} is CW so $\oplus$ve, hence will be plotted above xx' as shown in Fig. 2.37. In Fig. 2.36 (b) τ_{xy} is counter clock wise so $\ominus$, hence will be plotted below xx' as shown in Fig. 2.37.

(d) When σ_x, σ_y, τ_{xy} and θ are given on a element

Procedure:

(i) Choose axes with origin O.

(ii) Take suitable scale.

(iii) Mark σ_x and σ_y by OM_1 and OM_2.

(iv) Draw perpendicular on M_1 and M_2.

(v) Mark $M_1Q = M_2T = \tau_{xy}$ or τ (τ_{xy} or τ both are same)

(vi) Meet QT which meets the σ-axis at C. This is the centre of circle.

(vii) With C draw a circle which meets σ-axis at A and B.

(viii) *At CQ, Make an angle of $2\theta^*$ (i.e., twice the given angle θ) CCW and draw line $x'y'$ which meets the circle at P_1 and P_2.*

---

* Angle 2θ is always made CCW regardless of where point Q is located.

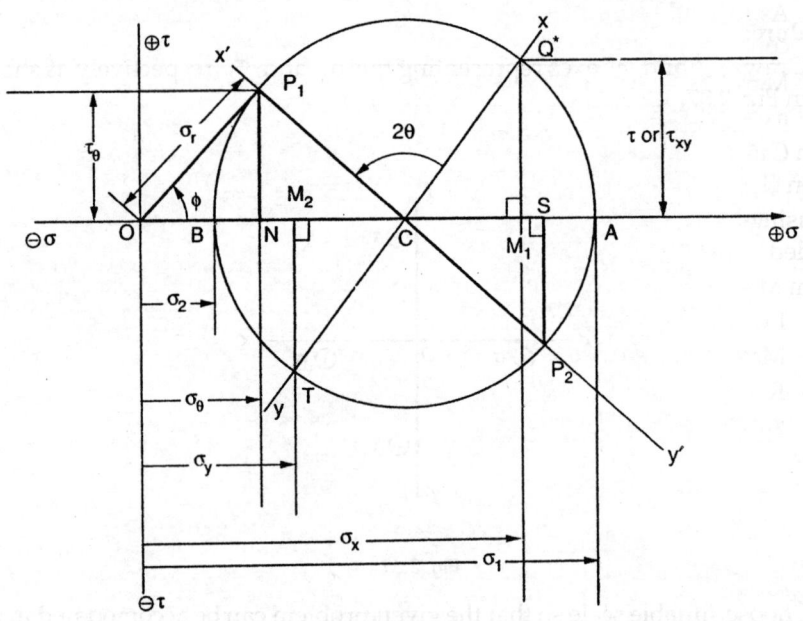

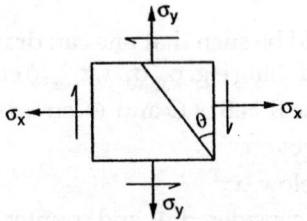

Fig. 2.38

(ix) Meet P_1O, measure this on scale and convert the same into the stress unit. This gives the resultant stress (σ_r).

(x) Measure $\angle COP_1$, this is known as angle of obliquity (ϕ).

From the drawn Mohr's circle we get

    Normal stress (σ_θ) = ON

    Shear stress (τ_θ) = P_1N

    Resultant stress (σ_r) = P_1O

    Angle of obliquity (ϕ) = $\angle COP_1$

    Maximum Principal stress (σ_1) = OA

    Minimum Principal stress (σ_2) = OB

Summary of Procedure for section 2.6 (c) with detailed Construction of Mohr's Circle

1. Take $OA = \sigma_x$ on suitable scale. Similarly, mark $OB = \sigma_y$ on suitable scale.

2. As in Fig. 2.36 (a) CW shear stress has been given so it will be +ve and constructed above xx'.

3. Mark $AP \oplus$ ve τ_{xy} on suitable scale. Make $BQ = AP$. Meet PQ which meets x-axis at C (Fig. 2.39).

With C as centre and radius CP draw a circle, which is the required circle for the given element shown in Fig. 2.36 (a). Construction is shown in Fig. 2.39.

By using Mohr's circle, one can save time and besides no formula cramming is needed.

From Mohr's circle one can find:

(i) Principal stresses (σ_1 and σ_2)

(ii) Maximum shear stress (τ_{max})

(iii) Resultant stress (σ_r)

(iv) Angle of obliquity (ϕ) etc.

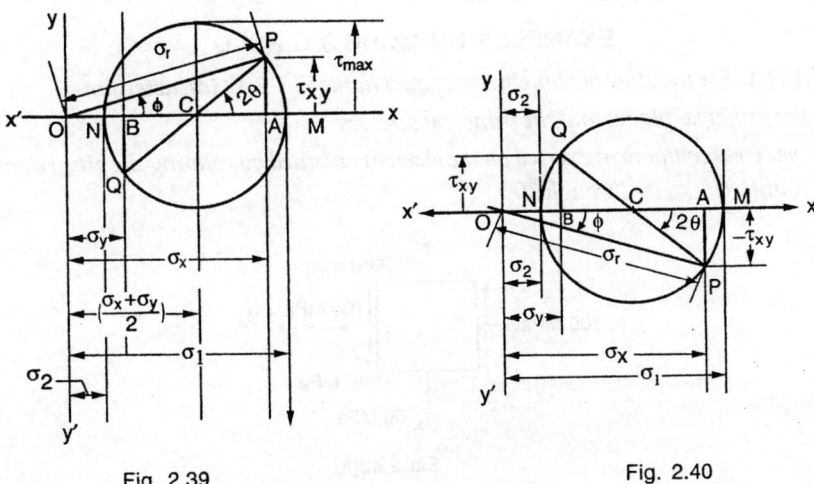

| Fig. 2.39 | Fig. 2.40 |

N.B: Angle of obliquity (ϕ) is the angle which the resultant stress (σ_r) makes with the normal stress. If τ_{xy} is $\oplus$ ve, ϕ is positive and if τ_{xy} in $\ominus$ ve, ϕ is negative. In Fig. 2.39, ϕ is $\oplus$ ve and in Fig. 2.40, ϕ is $\ominus$ ve.

For the element shown in Fig. 2.36 (b) where, τ_{xy} is CCW so $\ominus$ will be plotted below xx' as shown in Fig. 2.40. Mohr's Circle is shown in Fig. 2.40 for the element shown in Fig. 2.36 (b).

If we compare Fig. 2.39 and Fig. 2.40, everything remains the same except the plane to which orientation changes from CCW to CW. When τ_{xy} changes from $\oplus$ to $\ominus$.

(e) Mohr's Circle for torsional loading:

X and Y are located τ-axis

Radius of Mohr's circle $R = \dfrac{T \cdot C}{J}$ or $\dfrac{T \cdot C}{I_p}$

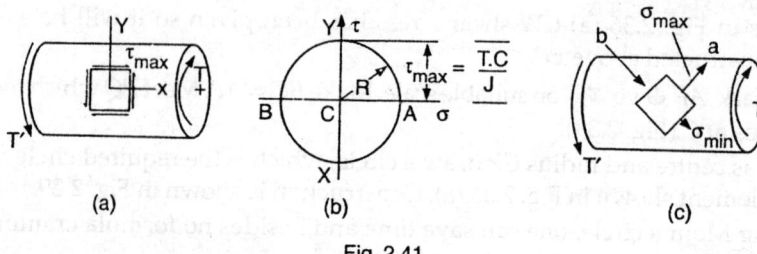

Fig. 2.41

Point A and B defines the principal plane

and the principal stresses, $\sigma_{max, min} = \pm R = \pm \dfrac{T \cdot C}{J}$

Mohr's circle is also applicable to transformation involving two dimensional strains and moment of inertia of plane areas because these quantities follow the same transformation law as do stresses.

EXAMPLES ON MOHR'S CIRCLE

EXAMPLE 1 *For the state of plane stress shown in the Fig. 2.42 (a), determine:*

(a) *the principal planes and the principal stresses.*

(b) *the stress component exerted on the element obtained by rotating the given element counterclockwise through 30°.*

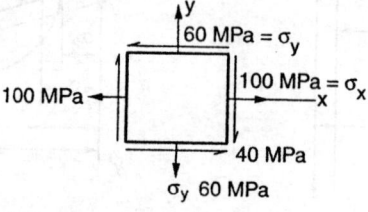

Fig. 2.42(a)

SOLUTION The abscissa of C, which represents $\sigma_{average}$ and radius of the circle can be measured directly or calculated as follows.

$$\sigma_{ave} = OC = \left(\frac{\sigma_x + \sigma_y}{2} \right) = \frac{1}{2} (100 + 60) = 80 \text{ MPa}$$

$$R = \sqrt{CM^2 + MP^2}$$

$$CM = OM - OC = 100 - 80 = 20 \text{ MPa}$$

$\therefore \qquad R = \sqrt{20^2 + 40^2}$

$\qquad = \sqrt{400 + 1600}$

$\qquad = \sqrt{2,000}$

$\qquad = 44.72 \text{ MPa}.$

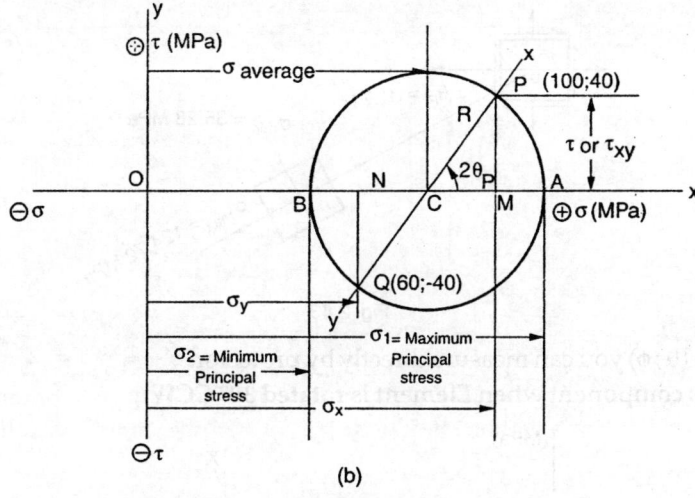

(b)

Fig. 2.42

(a) Principal plane and principal stresses

We rotate the diameter PQ clockwise through $2\theta_P$ until it coincides with the diameter AB then, we have,

$$\tan 2\theta_P = \frac{PM}{CM}$$

$$= \frac{40}{20}$$

$$= 2$$

$$2\theta_P = 63.43°$$

$$\theta_P = 31.71° \, CW \, \text{⤸} \quad \textbf{Ans.}$$

The principal (σ_1 and σ_2) stresses are represented by the abscissas of point A and B.

$$\sigma_{max} = \sigma_1 = OA = OC + CA$$

$$= \sigma_{av} + \text{Radius of circle}$$

$$= 80 + 44.72$$

$$= 124.72 \, \text{MPa} \quad \textbf{Ans.}$$

$$\sigma_{min} = \sigma_2 = OB = OC - CB$$

$$= 80 - 44.72$$

$$= 35.28 \, \text{MPa} \quad \textbf{Ans.}$$

Now, we obtain the orientation for the principal plane as shown below in Fig. 2.43.

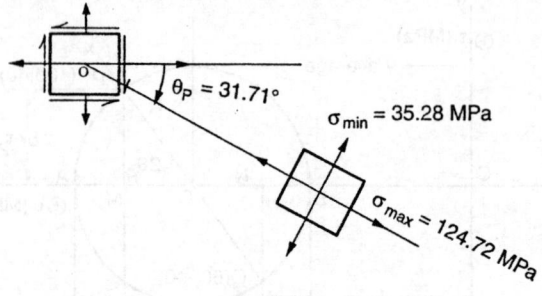

Fig. 2.43

The angle $(\theta ; \phi)$ you can measure directly by protector.

(b) Stress component when Element is rotated 30° CCW

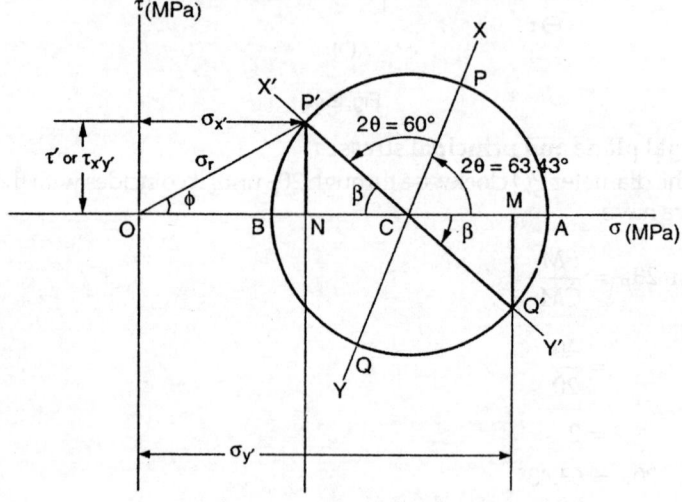

Fig. 2.44

Point P' and Q' on Mohr's circle that correspond to the stress components on the rotated element are obtained by rotating PQ counter clockwise through $2\theta = 60°$.
Now, we get

$$(\beta) = 180° - 60° - 63.43°$$

$$= 56.57° \quad \textbf{Ans.}$$

Normal stress $(\sigma_{x'})$ after rotating the stress element by $30° = ON$

$$= OC - NC = OC - P'C \cos \beta$$

$$= 80 - 44.72 \cos 56.57°$$

$$= 80 - 44.72 \times 0.5508$$

$$= 80 - 24.63$$

$$= 55.36 \text{ MPa} \qquad \textbf{Ans.}$$

Normal stress $(\sigma_{y'}) = OM = OC + CM = OC + CQ' \cos \beta$

$$= OC + CQ' \cos 56.57°$$

$$= 80 + 42.72 \cos 56.57°$$

$$= 80 + 23.53 = 103.53 \text{ MPa}$$

Shear stress $\tau_{x'y'}$ or $\tau' = P'N$

$$= P'C \sin 56.57°$$

$$= 44.72 \sin 56.57°$$

$$= 44.72 \times 0.8345$$

$$= 37.32 \text{ MPa} \quad \textbf{Ans.}$$

Resultant stress $= OP' = \sigma_r$

$$= \sqrt{ON^2 + NP'^2}$$

$$= \sqrt{(55.36)^2 + (37.32)^2}$$

$$= 66.76 \text{ MPa}$$

Angle of obliquity $(\phi) = \tan^{-1}\left(\dfrac{P'N}{ON}\right)$

$$= \tan^{-1}\left(\dfrac{37.32}{55.36}\right)$$

$$= 33.98° \quad \textbf{Ans.}$$

N.B: You can evaluate these measuring by scale and then converting it into the stress scale you have chosen the desired stresses can be computed.

The angle $(\theta; \phi)$ you can measure directly by protector.

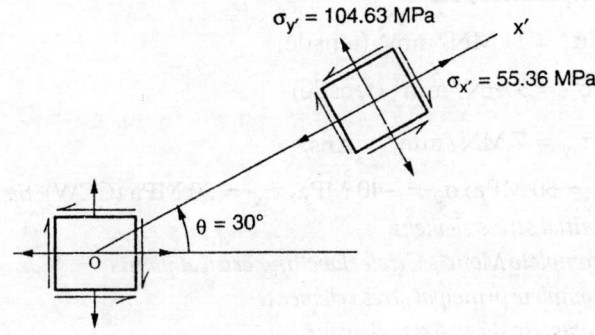

Fig. 2.45

EXAMPLE 2 *At a point in the cross-section of a loaded member, the maximum principal stress is 15 MN/mm² tensile and maximum shear stress of 8 MN/mm².*

Using Mohr's Circle, Find the state of stress on a plane making 30° with the plane of maximum principal stress.

SOLUTION Let us choose scale first, Mohr's circle has been drawn as per procedure discussed earlier.

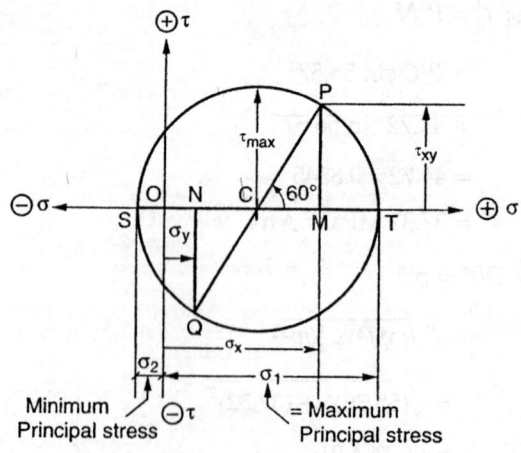

Fig. 2.46

Let 1 cm = 3 MN/mm²

$\therefore$ $\quad$ $15\,\text{MN/mm}^2 \Rightarrow 5\,\text{cm}$

and $\quad$ $8\,\text{MN/mm}^2 \Rightarrow 2.6\,\text{cm}$

(Since τ_{max} will be radius of Mohr circle

$\therefore$ $\quad$ $\tau_{max} = R = 2.6$ cm on scale after measuring = 8 MN/mm² (after converting the scale)

On measurement by scale the stresses on a plane making 30° with the plane of maximum principal stress are —

$$OM = \sigma_x = 11\,\text{MN/mm}^2 \text{ (tensile)}$$

$$ON = \sigma_y = 3\,\text{MN/mm}^2 \text{ (tensile)}$$

$$PM = \tau_{xy} = 7\,\text{MN/mm}^2 \quad \textbf{Ans.}$$

EXAMPLE 3 $\sigma_x = 60$ MPa; $\sigma_y = -40$ MPa; $\tau_{xy} = 30$ MPa (CCW) *then*

(a) *Draw the initial stress element.*

(b) *Draw the complete Mohr's Circle, labelling critical points*

(c) *Draw the complete principal stress element.*

(d) *Draw the complete shear stress element.*

SOLUTION Let 10 MPa = 1 cm on scale

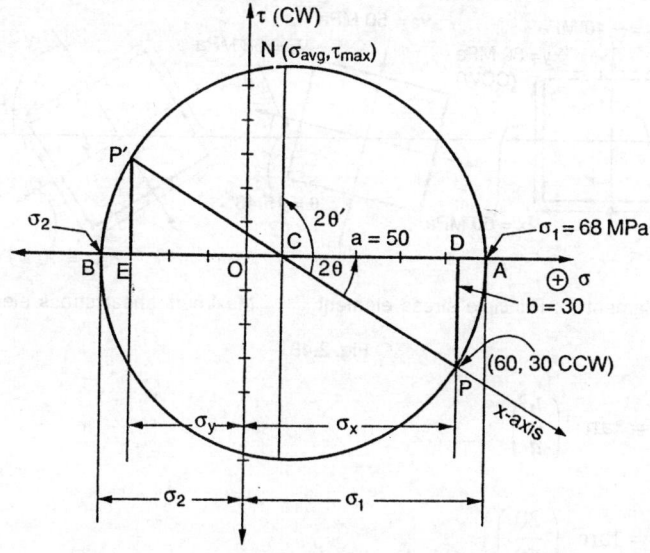

Fig. 2.47

$$\sigma_{avg} = \frac{1}{2}(\sigma_x + \sigma_y)$$

$$= \frac{1}{2}(60 - 40)$$

$$= 10 \text{ MPa}$$

On Measuring $\sigma_1 = 6.8 \text{ cm}$

$$= OA = 68 \text{ MPa}$$

$$\sigma_2 = OB$$

$$= 5 \text{ cm} = 50 \text{ MPa}$$

τ_{max} = radius of the circle

$$= CP$$

$$= CN$$

$$= 6 \text{ cm}$$

$$= 60 \text{ MPa}$$

$$a = \frac{1}{2}(\sigma_x - \sigma_y)$$

$$= \frac{1}{2}(60 + 40)$$

$$= 50 \text{ MPa}$$

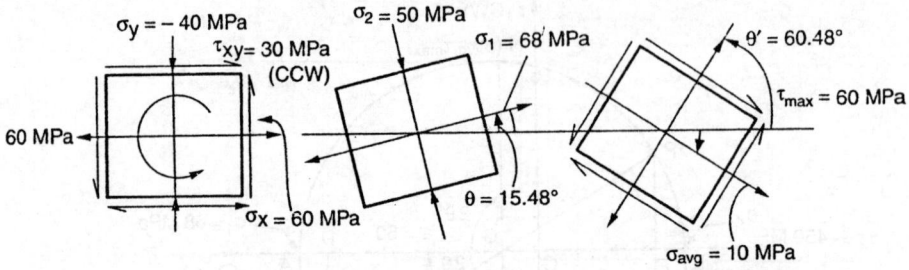

Initial stress element   Principle stress element   Maximum shear stress element

Fig. 2.48

$$2\theta = \tan^{-1}\left(\frac{b}{a}\right)$$

$$= \tan^{-1}\left(\frac{30}{50}\right)$$

$$= \tan^{-1}(0.6)$$

$$= 30.96$$

$$\theta = 15.48°$$

From Mohr's circle, $2\theta' = 90° + 2\theta$

$$= 90° + 30.96°$$

$$= 120.96°$$

$$\theta' = 60.48°$$

EXAMPLE 4 *A point in a load carrying member is subjected to the following stress condition:*

$$\sigma_x = 500 \text{ MPa; } \sigma_y = -400 \text{ MPa; } \tau_{xy} = 200 \text{ MPa (CW)}$$

Then,
   (a) Draw the initial stress element.
   (b) Draw the complete Mohr's Circle, labelling critical points.
   (c) Draw the complete principal stress element.
   (d) Draw the maximum shear stress element.

SOLUTION Let 100 MPa = 1 cm on scale

∴   500 MPa = 5 cm

and   400 MPa = 4 cm

        200 MPa = 2 cm

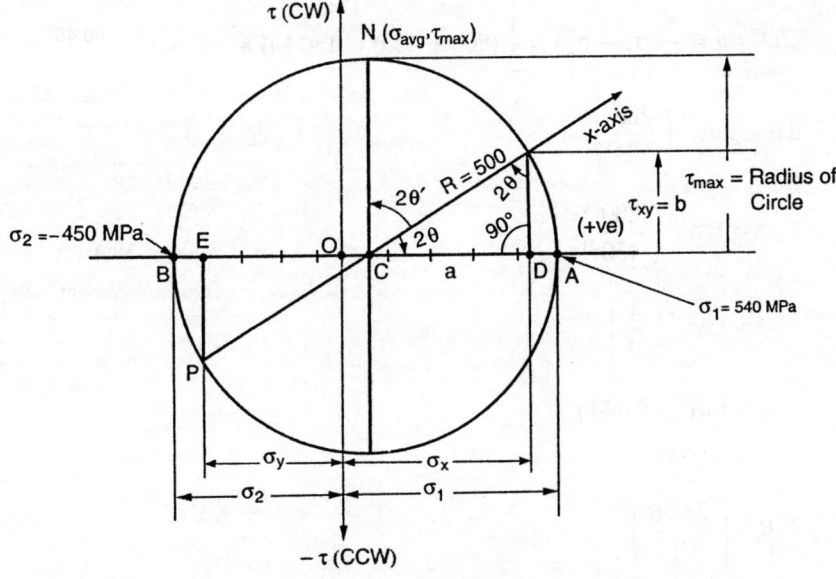

Fig. 2.49

Given $\sigma_x = 500$ MPa

$\sigma_y = -400$ MPa

and $\tau_{xy} = 200$ MPa

On measuring OA,

$\sigma_1 = 5.4$ cm

$= 5.4 \times 100$ MPa

$= 540$ MPa

and $\sigma_2 = OB$

$= 4.5$ cm

$= 4.5 \times 100$ MPa

$= -450$ MPa (As point 'B' is on the left side of O)

$\tau_{max} = CN =$ radius of the circle

$= CP$

$= 5$ cm

$= 5 \times 100$ MPa

$= 500$ MPa

$\sigma_{avg} = \dfrac{1}{2}(\sigma_x + \sigma_y)$

$= \dfrac{1}{2}(500 - 400)$

$= 50$ MPa

$$CD = a = \frac{1}{2}(\sigma_x - \sigma_y) = \frac{1}{2}(500 + 400) = 450 \text{ MPa}$$

$$2\theta = \tan^{-1}\left(\frac{200}{CD}\right)$$

$$= \tan^{-1}\left(\frac{200}{450}\right)$$

$$= \tan^{-1}\left(\frac{4}{9}\right)$$

$$= \tan^{-1}(0.444)$$

$$= 23.96°$$

$$\therefore \quad \theta = \left(\frac{23.96}{2}\right)°$$

$$= 11.98° \text{ CW from } x\text{-axis}$$

$$2\theta' = \tan^{-1}\left(\frac{a}{b}\right)$$

$$= \tan^{-1}\left(\frac{450}{200}\right)$$

$$= \tan^{-1}\left(\frac{9}{4}\right)$$

$$= \tan^{-1}(2.25)$$

$$= 66.03°$$

$$\therefore \quad \theta' = 33.01° \text{ CCW from } x\text{-axis.}$$

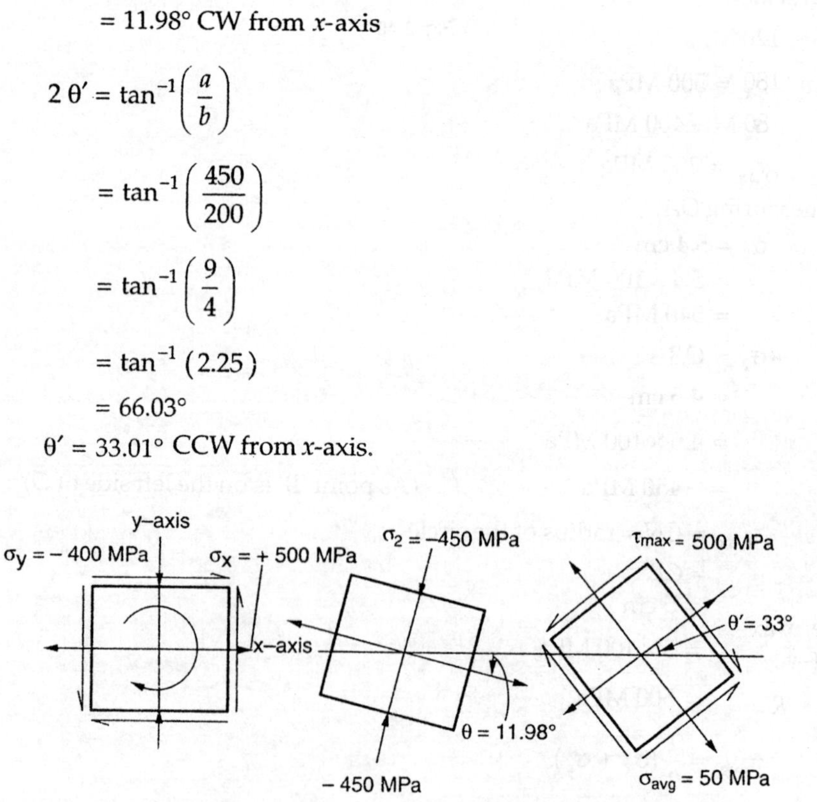

Initial Stress element   Principle stress element   Maximum shear stress element

Fig. 2.50

EXAMPLE 5 *A point in a load carrying member is subjected to the following stress condition*

$$\sigma_x = -120 \text{ MPa} ; \ \sigma_y = 180 \text{ MPa}; \ \tau_{xy} = 80 \text{ MPa (CCW)}$$

Then

(a) *Draw the initial stress element.*

(b) *Draw complete Mohr's circle.*

(c) *Draw the complete principal stress element.*

(d) *Draw the complete shear stress element.*

SOLUTION

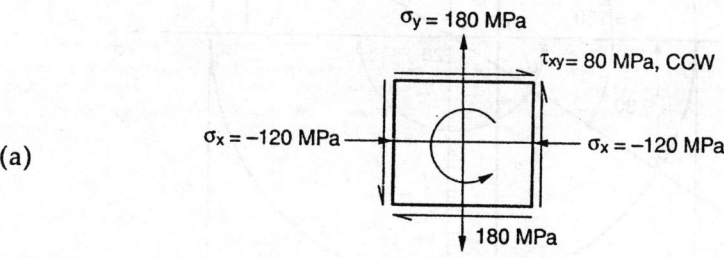

(a)

Fig. 2.51

Let on scale 1 cm = 20 MPa

∴   120 MPa = 6 cm

180 MPa = 9 cm

80 MPa = 4 cm.

(b) $\sigma_{avg} = \dfrac{1}{2}(\sigma_x + \sigma_y)$

$= \dfrac{1}{2}(-120 + 180)$

$= 30 \text{ MPa}$

$a = \dfrac{1}{2}(\sigma_x - \sigma_y)$

$= \dfrac{1}{2}(-120 - 180)$

$= \dfrac{1}{2} \times (-300)$

$= -150 \text{ MPa}$

$\tau = 80 \ (CCW) = b$

Hence, x-axis is in the third quadrant (Fig. 2.52) since σ_x is negative and τ_{xy} is CCW (–v.

$R = \sqrt{a^2 + b^2}$

$= \sqrt{(-150)^2 + (80)^2}$

$= \sqrt{22500 + 6400}$

$= 170 \text{ MPa}$

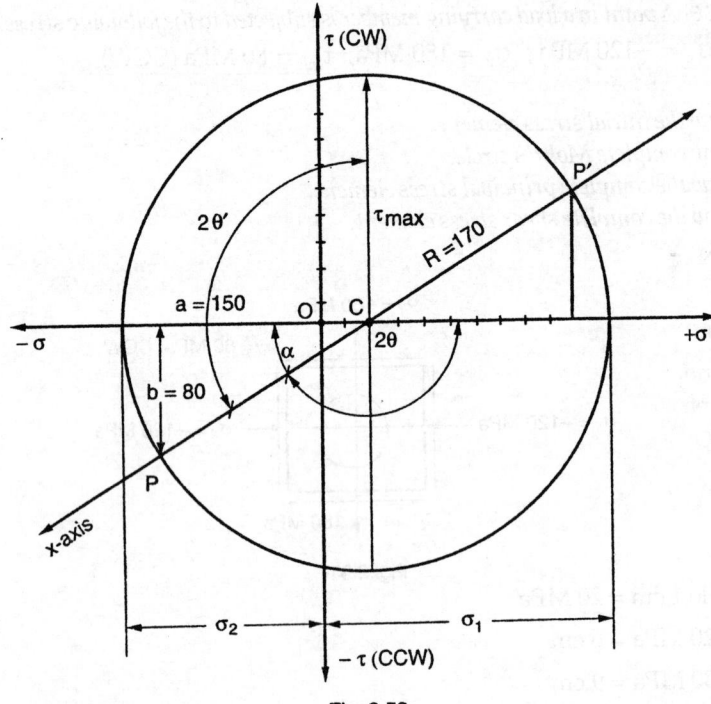

Fig. 2.52

$$\alpha = 28.07°$$
$$2\theta = 180 - \alpha$$
$$= 151.93°$$
$$\theta = 75.96° \text{ CCW}$$
$$2\theta' = (90° + \alpha)$$
$$= 90 + 28.07°$$
$$= 118.07°$$
$$\theta' = 59.04° \text{ CW}$$

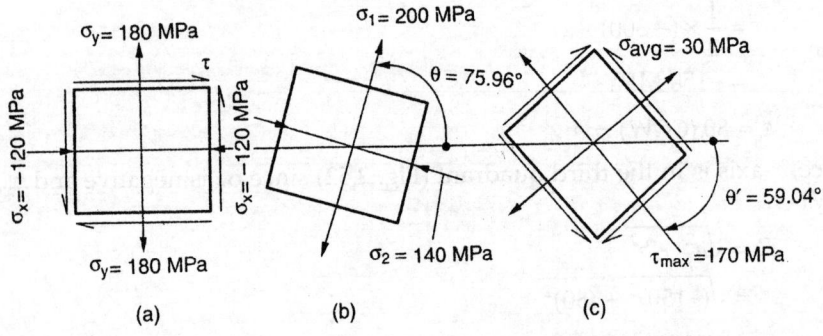

(a)	(b)	(c)
Initial stress element	Principal stress element	Maximum shear stress element

Fig. 2.53

On measuring, maximum principal stress $(\sigma_1) = 10$ cm

$$= 10 \times 20 \text{ MPa}$$

$$= 200 \text{ MPa}$$

Minimum Principal stress $(\sigma_2) = 7$ cm

$$= 7 \times 20 \text{ MPa}$$

$$= 140 \text{ MPa}$$

EXAMPLE 6 *Given* $\sigma_x = -30$ MPa, $\sigma_y = 20$ MPa, $\tau_{xy} = 40$ MPa (CW)

(a) *Draw initial stress element*

(b) *Draw the complete Mohr's Circle*

SOLUTION

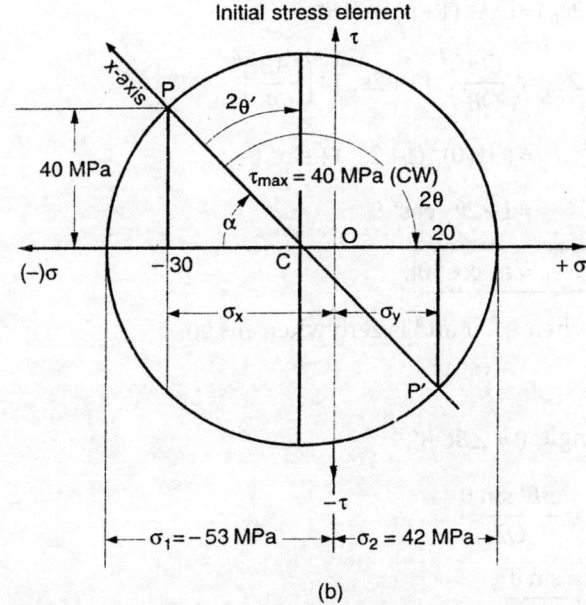

(a)

(a)
Initial stress element

(b)

(b)

Fig. 2.54

Here, x-axis is in the 2nd quadrant since σ_x is negative and τ_{xy} is CW (+).

2.7 STRAIN ANALYSIS

Strains on an oblique plane due to **Uniaxial strain.**

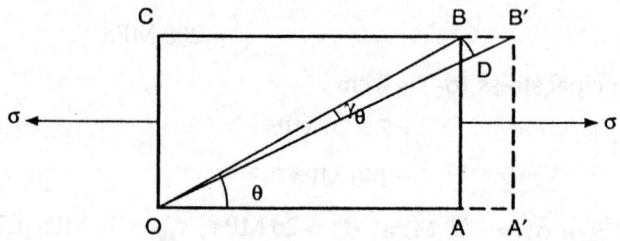

Fig. 2.55

Let us consider a small element $OABC$ of a elastic body of length dx is subjected to uniaxial stress σ as such body is strained to ε_x i.e. AA'.

Let ε_θ and γ_θ be the normal and shear strain on the oblique plane OB.
The length OA is increased to OA' and AB becomes $A'B'$.

Thus, $OB' = OB(1+\varepsilon_\theta)^*$

$\because$ $(OB')^2 = (OA')^2 + (A'B')^2$

$\therefore$ $OB^2(1+\varepsilon_\theta)^2 = OA^2(1+\varepsilon_x)^2 + AB^2$

If strains are small than ε_θ^2 and ε_x^2 can be neglected

$\therefore$ $OB^2(1+2\varepsilon_\theta) = OA^2(1+\varepsilon_x) + AB^2$

or, $1 + 2\varepsilon_\theta = \left(\dfrac{OA}{OB}\right)^2 (1+2\varepsilon_x) + \left(\dfrac{AB}{OB}\right)^2$

$= (\cos\theta)^2 (1+2\varepsilon_x) + \sin^2\theta$

$= 1 + 2\varepsilon_x \cos^2\theta$

$\boxed{\therefore \ \varepsilon_\theta = \varepsilon_x \cos^2\theta}$

ε_θ is maximum when $\theta = 0$ and is zero when $\theta = 90°$

$\therefore$ $\varepsilon_{max} = \varepsilon_x$

γ_θ = change in angle $\theta = \angle BOB'$

$= \left(\dfrac{BD}{OB}\right) = \dfrac{BB' \sin\theta}{OB}$

$= (OA\,\varepsilon_x) \cdot \dfrac{\sin\theta}{OB}$

$^*\varepsilon_\theta = \dfrac{OB' - OB}{OB} \Rightarrow OB' = OB(1+\varepsilon_\theta)$

$$= \cos\theta \cdot \varepsilon_x \cdot \sin\theta$$

$$= \frac{\varepsilon_x}{2} \cdot \sin 2\theta$$

$\gamma_\theta = $ is maximum when $\theta = 45°$

$$\therefore \qquad \gamma_\theta \max = \left(\frac{\varepsilon_x}{2}\right)$$

2.8 SHEAR STRAIN

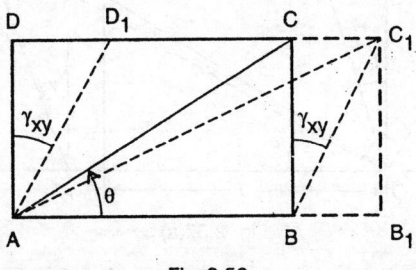

Fig. 2.56

Let the rectangular body $ABCD$ be deformed to ABC_1D_1 under the action of shearing force so that shear strain is τ_{xy}. Let the normal strain is ε_n.

$$CC_1 = BC \cdot \gamma_{xy}$$

$$AC_1 = (1 + \varepsilon_n) \cdot AC$$

Squaring both sides

$$(AC_1)^2 = (1 + \varepsilon_n)^2 \cdot (AC)^2$$

$$(AB_1)^2 + (B_1C_1)^2 = (1 + 2\varepsilon_n + \varepsilon_n^2) \cdot AC^2$$

or, $\qquad (AB + BB_1)^2 + (B_1C_1)^2 = (1 + 2\varepsilon_n + \varepsilon_n^2) \cdot AC^2$

or, $\qquad (AB + CC_1)^2 + (BC)^2 = (1 + 2\varepsilon_n) \cdot AC^2 \qquad$ [Neglecting ε_n^2 being small]

or, $\qquad (AB + BC \cdot \gamma_{xy})^2 + (BC)^2 = (1 + 2\varepsilon_n) \cdot AC^2$

or, $\qquad (1 + 2\varepsilon_n) = \left(\frac{AB}{AC}\right)^2 + 2 \cdot \frac{AB}{AC} \cdot \frac{BC}{AC} \cdot \gamma_{xy} + \left(\frac{BC}{AC}\right)^2$

or, $\qquad 1 + 2\varepsilon_n = \cos^2\theta + 2\cos\theta \cdot \sin\theta \cdot \gamma_{xy} + \sin 2\theta$

or, $\qquad 1 + 2\varepsilon_n = 1 + \gamma_{xy} \sin 2\theta$

$$\therefore \qquad \varepsilon_n = \left(\frac{\gamma_{xy}}{2}\right) \cdot \sin 2\theta$$

ε_n is maximum when $\theta = 45°$

$$\therefore \qquad (\varepsilon_n)_{max} = \frac{\gamma_{xy}}{2}$$

2.9 BIAXIAL STRAINS

Let us consider a small rectangular element $OABC$ of an elastic body. Let the normal strains along the X and Y axes be ε_x and ε_y respectively and let the shearing strain in the XY plane be γ_{xy}. Let ε_θ be the normal strain on diagonal OB. Further, let us select X' axis along the diagonal OB and Y' axis perpendicular to it

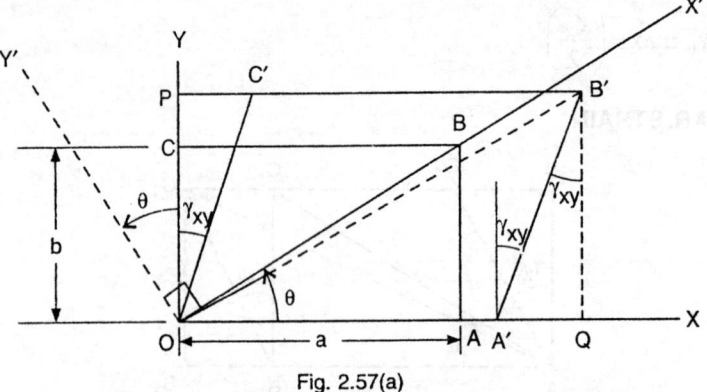

Fig. 2.57(a)

The axis $X'Y'$ is oriented at an angle θ CCW to the X-Y set of axis.
The deformed shape of the element is shown by $OA'B'C'$.

Let $OB = l$

Then
$$\varepsilon_\theta = \frac{OB' - OB}{OB} = \left(\frac{OB'}{OB} - 1\right)$$

$$OB' = OB \cdot (1 + \varepsilon_\theta)$$

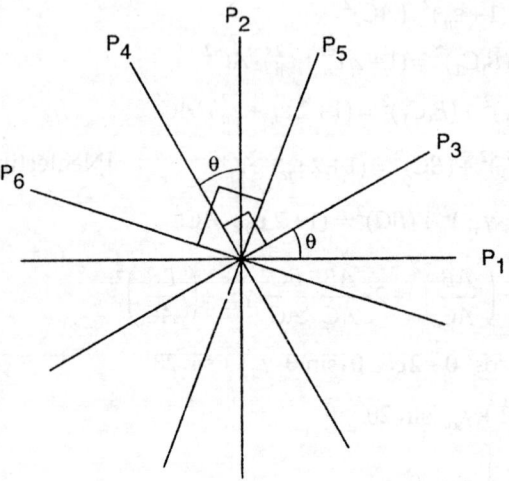

Fig. 2.57(b)

In Fig. 2.57(a) a number of planes are marked as points on the circumference of the circle and the actual orientation of plane is shown in Fig. 2.57(b).

The various planes are described as follow:

P_1, P_2 are general planes at right angles to each other.

P_3, P_4 are planes with major and minor principal strains

P_5, P_6 are the plane with maximum shear strains.

EXAMPLE 1 *The normal strains at a point in a material are* $\varepsilon_x = 15 \times 10^{-3}$, $\varepsilon_y = 10 \times 10^{-3}$. *Determine the normal and shearing strains on a plane inclined 30° with* ε_x *by drawing Mohr's circle.*

SOLUTION   Let $10 \times 10^{-3} = 5$ cm on scale

Plane $15 \times 10^{-3} = 7.5$ cm on scale

The Mohr's circle has been constructed as discussed earlier.

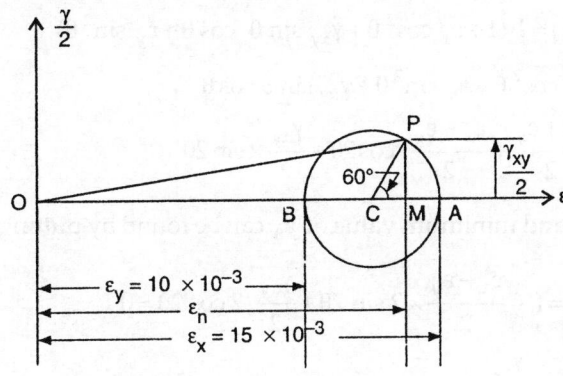

Fig. 2.58

On measuring normal strain $OM = \varepsilon_n = 14 \times 10^{-3}$

Shearing Strain $(\gamma_{xy}) = 2 \times PM$

$$= 2 \times (2 \times 10^{-3}) \text{ radian}$$

$$= 4 \times 10^{-3} \text{ radian} \qquad \textbf{Ans.}$$

EXAMPLE 2 *The state of strain at a point is defined by* $\varepsilon_x = 20 \times 10^{-3}$; $\varepsilon_y = 10 \times 10^{-3}$; $\gamma_{xy} = \pm 20 \times 10^{-3}$.

Determine the normal and shearing strains on a plane inclined at 30° with ε_x.

Also, determine the principal strains, principal planes and maximum shear strain verify the result by analytical method. [Refer to Fig. 2.57(a)]

SOLUTION   Let $OB = l$

$\therefore \qquad a = l \cos \theta, \qquad b = l \sin \theta \qquad$ and $OB' = l(1 + \varepsilon_\theta)$

Further, $AA' = \varepsilon_x a = l \varepsilon_x \cos \theta$

$PC = \varepsilon_b b = l \varepsilon_y \sin \theta$

and $\qquad A'Q = b \cdot \gamma_{xy} = l \cdot \gamma_{xy} \sin \theta \qquad\qquad$ (Strains are small)

Now, $OB' = \sqrt{(OQ)^2 + (QB')^2}$

$$= \sqrt{(OA + AA' + A'Q)^2 + (QB')^2}$$

$$= \sqrt{(l\cos + l\,\varepsilon_x\cos\theta + l\,\gamma_{xy}\sin\theta)^2 + \{l\sin\theta\,(1+\varepsilon_y)\}^2}$$

Neglecting infinitesimals of the second order

$$OB' = l\cdot\sqrt{1 + 2\,\varepsilon_x\cos^2\theta + 2\gamma_{xy}\sin\theta\cos\theta + 2\varepsilon_y\sin^2\theta}$$

Expanding by binomial theorem and neglecting infinitesimals of order 2 and higher

$$OB' = l\,(1 + \varepsilon_x\cos^2\theta + \gamma_{xy}\sin\theta\cos\theta + \varepsilon_y\sin^2\theta)$$

$$l\,(1+\varepsilon_\theta) = l\cdot(1 + \varepsilon_x\cos^2\theta + \gamma_{xy}\sin\theta\cdot\cos\theta + \varepsilon_y\sin^2\theta)$$

∴ $\varepsilon_\theta = \varepsilon_x\cos^2\theta + \varepsilon_y\sin^2\theta + \gamma_{xy}\sin\theta\cos\theta$

$$= \frac{\varepsilon_x + \varepsilon_y}{2} + \frac{\varepsilon_x - \varepsilon_y}{2}\cdot\cos 2\theta + \frac{\gamma_{xy}}{2}\times\sin 2\theta \qquad\qquad \ldots\text{(I)}$$

The maximum and minimum value of ε_θ can be found by putting $\dfrac{d\varepsilon_\theta}{d\theta} = 0$

∴ $\left(\dfrac{d\varepsilon_\theta}{d\theta}\right) = (-)\dfrac{\varepsilon_x - \varepsilon_y}{2}\times 2\sin 2\theta + \dfrac{\gamma_{xy}}{2}\cdot 2\cos 2\theta = 0$

∴ $\tan 2\theta = \dfrac{\gamma_{xy}}{\varepsilon_x - \varepsilon_y}$

$\sin 2\theta = \dfrac{1}{\sqrt{\operatorname{cosec}^2 2\theta}}$

$$= \frac{1}{\pm\sqrt{1 + \cot^2 2\theta}}$$

$$= \frac{1}{\pm\sqrt{1 + \dfrac{1}{\tan^2 2\theta}}}$$

$$= \frac{\tan 2\theta}{\pm\sqrt{1 + \tan^2 2\theta}}$$

$$= \frac{\dfrac{\gamma_{xy}}{\varepsilon_x - \varepsilon_y}}{\pm\sqrt{1 + \dfrac{\gamma_{xy}^2}{(\varepsilon_x - \varepsilon_y)^2}}}$$

$$= \frac{\gamma_{xy}}{\sqrt{(\varepsilon_x - \varepsilon_y)^2 + \gamma_{xy}^2}}$$

$$\cos 2\theta = \pm\sqrt{1 - \sin^2 2\theta}$$

$$= \sqrt{1 - \frac{\gamma_{xy}^2}{(\varepsilon_x - \varepsilon_y)^2 + \gamma_{xy}^2}}$$

$$= \frac{(\varepsilon_x - \varepsilon_y)}{\pm\sqrt{(\varepsilon_x - \varepsilon_y)^2 + \gamma_{xy}^2}}$$

Substituting the values of $\sin 2\theta$ and $\cos 2\theta$ in each (I).

We get,

$$\varepsilon_{\theta_{max, min}} = \frac{\varepsilon_x + \varepsilon_y}{2} + \frac{\varepsilon_x - \varepsilon_y}{2} \times \frac{\varepsilon_x - \varepsilon_y}{\pm\sqrt{(\varepsilon_x - \varepsilon_y)^2 + \gamma_{xy}^2}}$$

$$+ \frac{\gamma_{xy}}{2} \times \frac{\gamma_{xy}}{\pm\sqrt{(\varepsilon_x - \varepsilon_y)^2 + \gamma_{xy}^2}}$$

$$= \frac{\varepsilon_x + \varepsilon_y}{2} + \frac{(\varepsilon_x - \varepsilon_y)^2 + \gamma_{xy} \cdot \gamma_{xy}}{\pm\sqrt{(\varepsilon_x - \varepsilon_y)^2 + \gamma_{xy}^2}}$$

$$= \frac{\varepsilon_x + \varepsilon_y}{2} + \frac{(\varepsilon_x - \varepsilon_y)^2 + \gamma_{xy} \cdot \gamma_{xy}}{\pm 2\sqrt{(\varepsilon_x - \varepsilon_y)^2 + \gamma_{xy}^2}}$$

$$= \frac{\varepsilon_x + \varepsilon_y}{2} \pm \frac{(\varepsilon_x - \varepsilon_y)^2 + \gamma_{xy}^2}{2\sqrt{(\varepsilon_x - \varepsilon_y)^2 + \gamma_{xy}^2}}$$

$$\therefore \quad \varepsilon_{\theta_{max, min}} = \frac{\varepsilon_x + \varepsilon_y}{2} \pm \sqrt{\frac{(\varepsilon_x - \varepsilon_y)^2 + \gamma_{xy}^2}{2}}$$

Let us denote max value of θ by θ_1
and min value of θ by θ_2
then

$$\varepsilon_{\theta_1, \theta_2} = \frac{\varepsilon_x + \varepsilon_y}{2} \pm \sqrt{\frac{(\varepsilon_x - \varepsilon_y)^2 + \gamma_{xy}^2}{2}}$$

$$= \frac{1}{2}\left[(\varepsilon_x + \varepsilon_y) \pm \sqrt{(\varepsilon_x - \varepsilon_y)^2 + \gamma_{xy}^2} \right]$$

ε_{θ_1} and ε_{θ_2} are called the 'principal strains'. We can write simply ε_1 and ε_2 only.

Like stress analogy we can say that

$$\text{Shearing strain } (\varepsilon_s) = (-)\frac{\varepsilon_x - \varepsilon_y}{2}\sin 2\theta + \frac{\gamma_{xy}}{2}\cos 2\theta$$

We can, therefore, construct a 'Mohr's circle of strain' for obtaining normal and shear strain on different planes at a point in a stressed body.

The sign convention for 'Mohr's circle of strain' will be similar to that for the stress circle which can be stated as below:

1. Positive normal strain or tensile strain will be plotted to the right of origin 'O' on the horizontal axis and negative strain to the left of origin 'O'.

2. Shear strain $\left(\varepsilon_s - \dfrac{\gamma}{2}\right)$ is to be plotted along the vertical axis.

   The shearing strain associated with a C.W. shearing stress is to be plotted vertically upward (↑).

   The shearing strain associated with a CCW shearing stress is to be with a CCW shearing stress is to be plotted vertically downward (↓)

3. A rotation of θ in the actual plane in any sense (say CW) corresponds to a rotation of 2θ in the Mohr's circle in the same sense (i.e. CW in this case). A typical Mohr's circle of strain is shown in figure below:

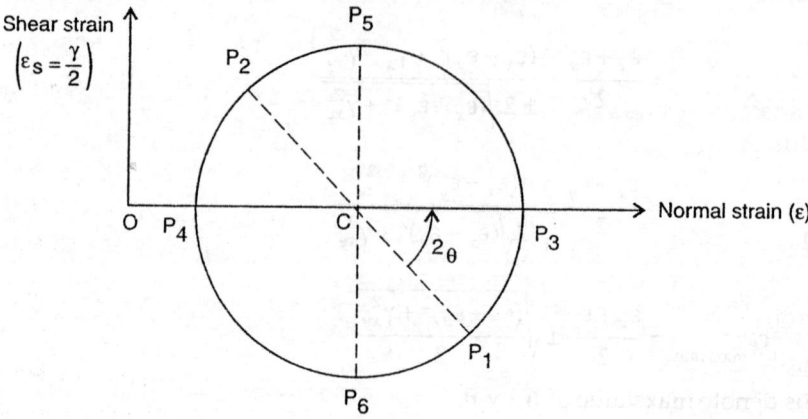

Fig. 2.59

Let $\quad 1\times 10^{-3} = 0.5$ cm on scale

Hence, $\quad 10\times 10^{-3} = 5$ cm

And $\quad 20\times 10^{-3} = 10$ cm

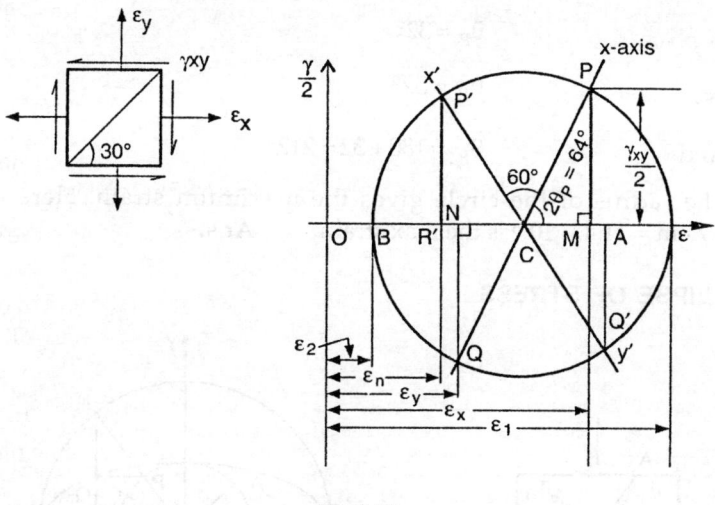

Fig. 2.60

Procedure

(i) Firstly suitable scale was chosen so that the given problem can be constructed in the space provided.

(ii) OM and ON was marked corresponding to ε_x and ε_y.

(iii) On M and N perpendiculars were drawn and $\dfrac{\gamma_{xy}}{2} = \pm 10 \times 10^{-3} = 5$ cm was

made by P and Q respectively.

(iv) P and Q was connected by line which meets the normal strain axis at C. This is the centre of Mohr's circle. The circle meets the strain axis at A and B which corresponds to principal strains ε_1 and ε_2 respectively.

(v) Make angle $60°$ CCW on PQ and $P'Q'$ is now the plane for the given condition after rotation of the original plane PQ by $60°$

(vi) Drop perpendicular from P' to strain (ε) axis meeting at R'.

(vii) Measure OR' and $P'R'$. This gives the value of normal strain (ε_n) and shear

strain $\left(\dfrac{\gamma_{xy}}{2}\right)$ respectively.

(viii) For principal plane (θ_P) either measure the angle PCM or compute $\left(\dfrac{PM}{CM}\right)$.

This will give the value of $2\theta_P$ or $\tan 2\theta_P$. Find θ_P which is half of $2\theta_P$.

This is first principal plane (θ_{P_1}).

For the other plane (θ_{P_2}) add $180°$ to θ_1. Hence, $\theta_{P_2} = (180° + \theta_{P_1})$.

In this case indirect measurement of angle by protector we see

$$2\theta_P = 64°$$

$$\therefore \qquad \theta_P = 32°$$

i.e., $\qquad \theta_{P_1} = 32°$

And $\qquad \theta_{P_2} = 180 + 32 = 212°$

(ix) The radius of the circle gives the maximum strain. Here radius is 5.7 cm $= 11.4 \times 10^{-3}$ is the max strain. **Ans.**

2.10 ELLIPSE OF STRESS

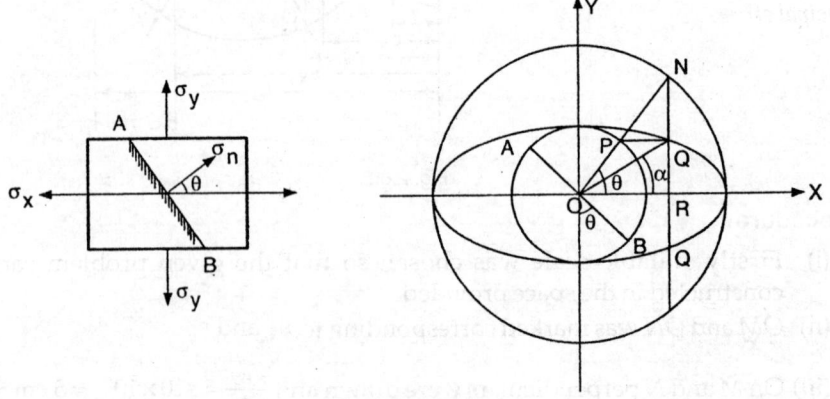

Fig. 2.61

Procedure for Construction

1. Take O as centre and draw two circles with radii proportional to σ_x and σ_y respectively.
2. Through O draw ON perpendicular to the interface AB as shown, to cut the inner circle at P and outer circle at N.
3. Through N draw a line NR perpendicular to OX and through P, draw line PQ perpendicular to OY to cut the line NR at Q. Join OQ.

From the diagram:

$$OR = \sigma_x \cos \theta$$

$$QR = \sigma_y \sin \theta$$

$$OQ = \sqrt{OR^2 + QR^2}$$

$$= \sqrt{\sigma_x^2 \cos^2 \theta + \sigma_y^2 \sin^2 \theta}$$

$$= \sigma_r$$

Therefore, OQ gives the resultant σ_r for the plane.

and $\quad \tan \alpha = \dfrac{\sigma_y \sin \theta}{\sigma_x \cos \theta}$

$\qquad\quad = \dfrac{\sigma_y}{\sigma_x} \cdot \tan \theta$

Point Q may be established for diffrerent values of θ. The locus of Q will give an ellipse.

EXAMPLE *At a point, the principal stresses are 100 MN/m² and 60 MN/m² both tensile. Find by the ellipse of stress the resultant stress on a plane inclined at 35° to the major principal stress.*

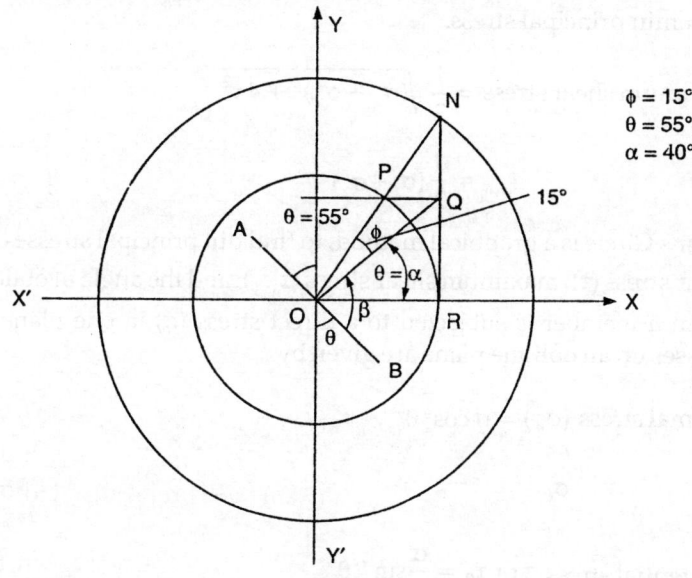

Fig. 2.62

SOLUTION The given plane is at 35° to the major principal stress or at 55° to the major principal plane.

Steps:
1. With O as centre draw two circle with radii proportional to 100 MN/m² and 60 MN/m² respectively.
2. Through O, draw ON perpendicular to the interface AB as shown to cut the inner circle in P and outer circle in N.
3. Through N, drawn NR perpendicular to OX.
4. Through P, draw line PQ perpendicular to OY to cut the line NR in Q.
5. Join OQ.

Now, the resultant stress $(\sigma_r) = OQ = 75.5 \text{ MN/m}^2$ (on measuring)

$$\alpha = \angle ROQ = 40°$$

and, $\qquad\qquad$ Obliquity $(\phi) = \angle PCQ = 15°$ $\qquad\qquad\qquad$ **Ans.**

HIGHLIGHTS

1. Resultant stress $(\sigma_R) = \sqrt{\sigma^2 + \tau^2}$ at angle to normal $\phi = \tan^{-1}\left(\dfrac{\tau}{\sigma}\right)$.

2. Pure shear equivalent to equal tension and compression on planes at $45°$.

3. Principal plane is the plane of zero shear.

4. Principal stresses $\sigma_1 \, \sigma_2 = \dfrac{1}{2}(\sigma_x + \sigma_y) \pm \dfrac{1}{2}\sqrt{(\sigma_x - \sigma_y)^2 + 4\tau^2}$

   σ_1 = max principal stress

   σ_2 = min principal stress.

5. Maximum shear stress $= \dfrac{1}{2}\sqrt{(\sigma_x - \sigma_y)^2 + 4\tau^2}$

   $\therefore \qquad\qquad \tau_{max} = \dfrac{1}{2}(\sigma_1 - \sigma_2)$

6. Mohr's Circle is a graphical method, to find out principal stresses (σ_1, σ_2); Shear stress (τ); maximum shear stress (τ_{max}); and the angle of obliquity (ϕ).

7. When a member is subjected to a direct stress (σ) in one plane then the stresses on an oblique plane are given by

   Normal stress $(\sigma_n) = \sigma \cos^2 \theta$

   or

   σ_θ

   Tangential stress τ or $\tau_\theta = \dfrac{\sigma}{2}\sin 2\theta$

   Maximum normal stress $= \sigma$

   Maximum shear stress $= \dfrac{\sigma}{2}$

8. The normal stresses acting on principal planes are called principal stresses. The maximum normal stress is called major (σ_1) principal stress and the minimum principal stress is called minor principal stress (σ_2).

9. There are two methods to determine the stresses on oblique plane
   (i) Analytical Method
   (ii) Graphical Method (Mohr's Circle)

10. The angle made by the resultant stress with the normal of the oblique plane is known as obliquity. It is denoted by ϕ.

    Mathematically $\tan \phi = \left(\dfrac{\sigma_t}{\sigma_n}\right)$

11. When a member is subjected to two direct stresses σ_x, σ_y in two mutually perpendicular directions accompanied by a simple shear stress (τ) then the stresses on an oblique plane inclined at angle θ are given by

Normal stress $(\sigma_n) = \dfrac{\sigma_x + \sigma_y}{2} + \dfrac{\sigma_x - \sigma_y}{2} \cos 2\theta + \tau \sin 2\theta$

Tangential stress $(\sigma_t) = -\left(\dfrac{\sigma_x - \sigma_y}{2}\right) \sin 2\theta + \tau \cos 2\theta$

Position of principal planes are given by

$$\tan 2\theta_p = \left[\dfrac{2\tau}{\sigma_x - \sigma_y}\right]$$

12. The planes of maximum and minimum normal stresses are at an angle 90° to each other.

13. Uniaxial strain (i.e. ε_θ and γ_θ)

    (a) Normal strain $(\varepsilon_\theta) = \varepsilon_x \cdot \cos^2 \theta$

    ε_θ is maximum when $\theta = 0$; ε_θ is zero when $\theta = 90°$ $\therefore \varepsilon_{\theta(min)} = 0$.

    $\therefore \quad \varepsilon_{\theta(max)} = \varepsilon_x$

    (b) Shear strain $(\gamma_\theta) = \dfrac{\varepsilon_x}{2} \sin 2\theta$

    γ_θ is maximum when $\theta = 45°$

    $\therefore \quad \gamma_{\theta(maximum)} = \dfrac{\varepsilon_x}{2}$

    $\gamma_{\theta(minimum)} = 0$

14. Biaxial strain

    (a) When a body is subjected to Biaxial strain ε_x, ε_y and γ_{xy} then

    Normal strain $(\varepsilon_\theta) = \dfrac{\varepsilon_x + \varepsilon_y}{2} + \dfrac{\varepsilon_x - \varepsilon_y}{2} \cos 2\theta + \dfrac{\gamma_{xy}}{2} \sin 2\theta$

    $\varepsilon_{\theta\,max,min} = \dfrac{\varepsilon_x + \varepsilon_y}{2} \pm \sqrt{\dfrac{(\varepsilon_x - \varepsilon_y)^2 + \gamma_{xy}^2}{2}}$

    If max value is θ_1 and min value is θ_2 then

    $$\varepsilon_{\theta_1,\theta_2} = \dfrac{\varepsilon_x + \varepsilon_y}{2} \pm \sqrt{\dfrac{(\varepsilon_x - \varepsilon_y)^2 + \gamma_{xy}^2}{2}} = \dfrac{1}{2}\left[(\varepsilon_x + \varepsilon_y) \pm \sqrt{(\varepsilon_x - \varepsilon_y)^2 + \gamma_{xy}^2}\right]$$

ε_{θ_1} and ε_{θ_2} are called maximum principal strain and minimum principal strain respectively.

(b) Shearing strain $(\varepsilon_s) = (-)\dfrac{\varepsilon_x - \varepsilon_y}{2} \sin 2\theta + \dfrac{\gamma_{xy}}{2} \cos 2\theta$

15. There are two methods of computing strain on oblique plane.
    (a) Analytical Method i.e. by formula
    (b) Graphical Method (Mohr's Circle)

PROBLEMS FOR PRACTICE
(THEORETICAL)

1. Define principal plane; principal stress; angle of obliquity.

2. A rectangular bar subjected to σ_x (Tensile) and σ_y (Tensile) along x and y-axis respectively. Prove that the normal stress (σ_n or σ_θ) and shear stress (τ_θ) on an oblique plane which is inclined at an angle of θ with the y-axis are given by

$$\sigma_\theta = \frac{\sigma_x + \sigma_y}{2} + \frac{\sigma_x - \sigma_y}{2} \cos 2\theta$$

and $\tau_\theta = -\left(\dfrac{\sigma_x - \sigma_y}{2}\right) \sin 2\theta$

3. Derive an expression for the major and minor principal stresses on an oblique plane, when the elastic body is subjected to direct stresses in two mutually perpendicular directions accompained by a shear stress.

4. Write a note on Mohr's circle of stresses for the following conditions:
   (a) when σ_x, σ_y, τ_{xy} are given
   (b) when σ_x, σ_y, τ_{xy} and θ are given
   (c) when σ_x and σ_y are given
   (d) when τ_{xy} is given.

(NUMERICAL)

1. The stresses at a point in a bar are 200 N/mm² (tensile) and 100 N/mm² (compressive). Determine the resultant stress in magnitude and directions on a plane inclined at 60° to the axis of the major stress. Determine τ_{max} in the material at that point.

2. At a section in a beam, the tensile stress due to bending is 50 N/mm² and shear stress is 20 N/mm². Determine the magnitude and direction of the principal stresses and calculate the maximum shear stress.

3. A piece of elastic material is subjected to stresses as follows:
   Tensile stress 50 N/mm² and Shear stress 40 N/mm² on one plane, compressive stress 35 N/mm² and complementary shear stress 40 N/mm² on the second plane, no stress on the third plane.

Find (a) the principal stresses and positions of the planes on which they act.

(b) the position of planes on which there is no normal stress.

4. Show that the sum of two normal components of the stresses on any two planes at right angles is constant in a material subjected to a two dimensional stress system.

5. A elastic body is subjected to normal stresses of 30 N/mm^2 and 60 N/mm^2 tensile, alongwith a shearing stress of 22.5 N/mm^2. Find the value of the principal stresses and the inclination of the principal planes to the direction of the 60 N/mm^2 stress.

ANSWERS

1. $\sigma_r = 180\ \text{N/mm}^2$; $\phi = 46.12°$; $\tau_{max} = 150\ \text{N/mm}^2$

2. $\sigma_1 = 57\ \text{N/mm}^2$ (Tensile); $\sigma_2 = 7\ \text{N/mm}^2$ (Compressive);
   $\sigma_3 = 0$; $\theta_{P_1} = 70°40'$; $\theta_{P_2} = 160°40'$; $\tau_{max} = 32\ \text{N/mm}^2$

3. (a) Principal stress $\sigma_1 = 65.9\ \text{N/mm}^2$ (Tensile);
   $\sigma_2 = 50.9\ \text{N/mm}^2$ (Compressive)
   $\theta_{P_1} = 21°40'$ (CCW); $\theta_{P_2} = 68°21'$ (CW)

   (b) $\theta = 48°21'$ to the principal plane.

5. $72\ \text{N/mm}^2$; $18\ \text{N/mm}^2$ $61°48'$; $151°48'$.

OBJECTIVE QUESTIONS

1. A plane stress condition is one in which
   (a) the body is subjected to stresses acting in one direction only
   (b) the body is subjected to stresses acting in two directions
   (c) the body is subjected to stresses acting in three directions
   (d) none of the above

2. A principal plane is a plane of
   (a) minimum tensile stress   (b) maximum tensile stress
   (c) maximum shear stress   (d) zero shear stress

3. Maximum shear stress acts on a plane which is
   (a) inclined at 45° to the principal planes
   (b) inclined at 30° to the principal planes
   (c) inclined at 60° to the principal planes
   (d) none of the above

4. The radius of Mohr's circle is equal to
   (a) shear stress
   (b) sum of the two principal stresses
   (c) difference of the two principal stresses
   (d) one half of the difference of two principal stresses

5. If a rectangular element is subjected to like principal stresses σ_1 and σ_2 in two mutually perpendicular direction along x and y, the maximum shear stress would occur along
   - (a) plane normal to x-axis
   - (b) plane normal to y-axis
   - (c) plane at 45° to y-direction
   - (d) plane at 45° and 135° to y-direction

6. Stress can be measured directly by
   - (a) extension meter
   - (b) strain gauge
   - (c) photoelasticity
   - (d) dial gauges

7. A material whose shear strength is more than half of its tensile strength when subjected to uniaxial tension will fail by
   - (a) tensile stress
   - (b) compressive stress
   - (c) shear stress
   - (d) bending stress

8. The plane of maximum shear stress at any point are inclined to the principal planes through that point at an angle of
   - (a) 0°
   - (b) 45°
   - (c) 90°
   - (d) 180°

9. In Mohr's circle of strain, y-axis represents
   - (a) normal strain
   - (b) shear strain
   - (c) half of normal strain
   - (d) half of shear strain

10. In a plane stress problem, there are normal tensile stresses σ_x and σ_y accompanied by shear stress τ_{xy} at a point along orthogonal Cartesian coordinate x and y respectively. It is observed that the minimum principal stress on a certain plane is zero then
    - (a) $\tau_{xy} = \sqrt{\sigma_x + \sigma_y}$
    - (b) $\tau_{xy} = \sqrt{\sigma_x - \sigma_y}$
    - (c) $\tau_{xy} = \sqrt{\dfrac{\sigma_x}{\sigma_y}}$
    - (d) $\tau_{xy} = \sqrt{\sigma_x \cdot \sigma_y}$

ANSWERS

1. (b)   2. (d)   3. (a)   4. (d)   5. (d)   6. (c)
7. (a)   8. (b)   9. (d)   10. (d)

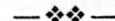

3

3-D STRESS

3.1 INTRODUCTION

The concept of stress was introduced by 'Cauchy'. According to Cauchy, stress is a measure of average amount of force exerted per unit area of the surface within a deformable body. In otherwords, it is a measure of intensity of the total internal force within a deformable body across the imaginary surface. These internal forces are produced between the particles in the body as a result of external force applied to the body.

As the loaded deformable body is assumed to be Continuum, these internal forces are distributed continuously within the volume of the material body.

From the definition of stress, we find that the average normal stress $(\sigma) = \dfrac{P}{A}$. Here, we assumed that stress is uniformly distributed. But in general stress is not uniformly distributed over a section of a material body and consequently the stress at a point on a given area is different from the average stress over the entire area. According to Cauchy, the stress at a point in a object is completely defined by tensor τ_{ij} of second order known as **Cauchy Stress Tensor**. It has nine components and written in the matrix form as below:

$$\tau_{ij} = \begin{bmatrix} \tau_{xx} & \tau_{xy} & \tau_{xz} \\ \tau_{yx} & \tau_{yy} & \tau_{yz} \\ \tau_{zx} & \tau_{zy} & \tau_{zz} \end{bmatrix}$$

But,
$$\tau_{xx} = \sigma_x$$
$$\tau_{yy} = \sigma_y$$
$$\tau_{zz} = \sigma_z$$

Hence,
$$\tau_{ij} = \begin{bmatrix} \sigma_x & \tau_{xy} & \tau_{xz} \\ \tau_{yx} & \sigma_y & \tau_{yz} \\ \tau_{zx} & \tau_{zy} & \sigma_z \end{bmatrix}$$ General stress tensor

This is a matrix representation of the 3-D stress or stress tensor. The diagonal elements of a matrix are normal stresses and the off diagonal elements are shear stresses.

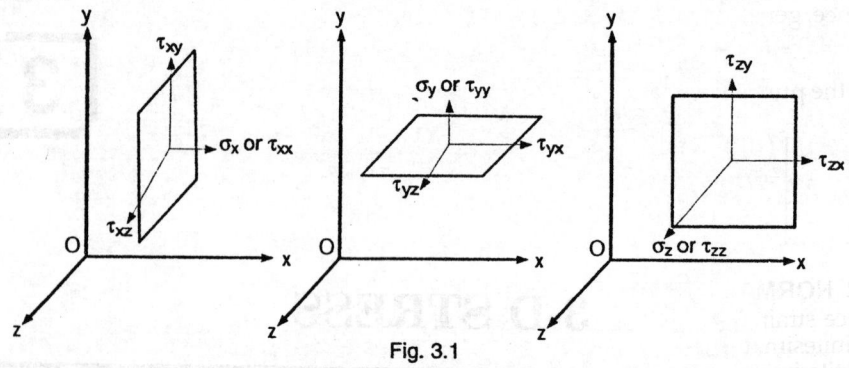

Fig. 3.1

The term 'Stress Tensor' is used to specify the state of stress at a point.

τ_{xy} represents the shear stress acting perpendicular to x-axis and parallel to the y- axis.

Conversely, τ_{yx} acts perpendicular to the y-axis and parallel to x-axis. It can be shown that in the absence of unbalance body moments, these tensor are symmetric *i.e.,* $\tau_{xy} = \tau_{yx}$; $\tau_{xz} = \tau_{zx}$; and $\tau_{yz} = \tau_{zy}$. So **only six stress components are required to describe the stress state at a point instead of nine. The six components are** $\sigma_x, \sigma_y, \sigma_z, \tau_{xy}, \tau_{yz}$ **and** τ_{zx}.

For a principal stress system, *i.e.* no shear, the matrix reduces to

$$\begin{bmatrix} \sigma_1 & 0 & 0 \\ 0 & \sigma_2 & 0 \\ 0 & 0 & \sigma_3 \end{bmatrix}$$ called principal stress tensor

and when $\sigma_1 = \sigma_2 = \sigma_3 = \bar{\sigma}$ then it is called hydrostatic stress tensor represented as below:

$$\begin{bmatrix} \bar{\sigma} & 0 & 0 \\ 0 & \bar{\sigma} & 0 \\ 0 & 0 & \bar{\sigma} \end{bmatrix}$$ hydrostatic stress tensor

a general stress is divided into two parts, one due to a hydrostatic stress $\bar{\sigma} = \left(\dfrac{\sigma_1 + \sigma_2 + \sigma_3}{3} \right)$ and the other due to shearing deformations.

Tensor notation for pure shear *i.e.* when $\sigma_x = \sigma_y = \sigma_z = 0$, the tensor becomes

$$\begin{bmatrix} 0 & \tau_{xy} & \tau_{xz} \\ \tau_{yx} & 0 & \tau_{yz} \\ \tau_{zx} & \tau_{zy} & 0 \end{bmatrix}$$ pure shear tensor

Therefore, we observe that general stress tensor is the combination of hydrostatic stress tensor and the pure shear tensor.

Hence, general three dimensional stress state
= hydrostatic stress state + pure shear state.

So, the pure shear state of stress in tensor form can be presented as below:

$$\begin{bmatrix} (\sigma_1 - \bar{\sigma}) & 0 & 0 \\ 0 & (\sigma_2 - \bar{\sigma}) & 0 \\ 0 & 0 & (\sigma_3 - \bar{\sigma}) \end{bmatrix}$$

3.2 NORMAL STRAIN

Since strain vary from point to point, the definition of strain must relate to an infinitesimal element. Normal strain indicates how much line segments in the infinitesimal element in the x, y, z direction change. These strains are labelled as $\varepsilon_x, \varepsilon_y, \varepsilon_z$.

If an elastic body is loaded provided material does not rupture, then displacement at any point can be completely given by three single valued components u, v and w along x, y and z-axes respectively.

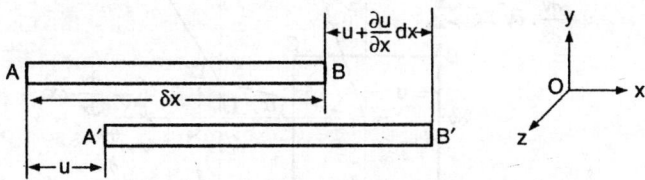

Fig. 3.2

The normal strain can be derived in terms of these displacement.
If the displacement of A is u

then displacement of B is $\left(u + \dfrac{\partial u}{\partial x} \cdot \delta x \right)$

So, increase in length $= \left(u + \dfrac{\partial u}{\partial x} \cdot \delta x - u \right) = \dfrac{\partial u}{\partial x} \cdot \delta x$

Strain along x-axis $= \varepsilon_x$

$$= \frac{\text{Change in length}}{\text{Original length}}$$

$$= \frac{\left(\dfrac{\partial u}{\partial x} \right) \cdot \delta x}{\delta x}$$

$$= \left(\frac{\partial u}{\partial x} \right)$$

Hence, $\varepsilon_x = \dfrac{\partial u}{\partial x}$

Similarly, $\varepsilon_y = \dfrac{\partial u}{\partial y}$

and $\varepsilon_z = \dfrac{\partial u}{\partial z}$

Normal strain produce dialations.

3.3 SHEAR STRAIN

Engineering Shear Strain is defined as the change in angle between two originally orthogonal material lines. Shear strain indicates the change in angle of right angle in the x-y, y-z and z-x plane. These angles are measured in radians and strains are labelled as γ_{xy}, γ_{yz}, and γ_{zx}.

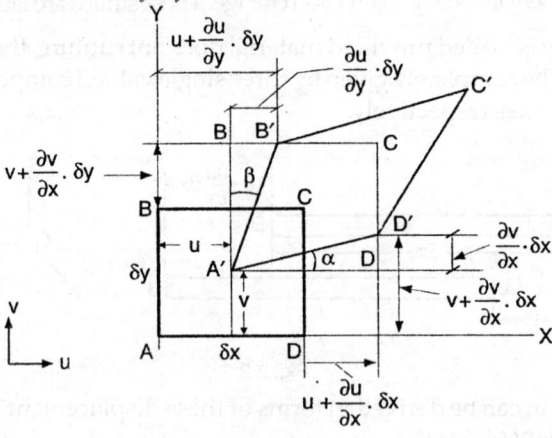

Fig. 3.3

We can derive shear strain in terms of displacements.

Consider a two dimensional infinitesimal material element with dimensions $\delta x \times \delta y$ which after deformation takes the form of a rhombus $A'B'C'D'$.

Let u, v, and w be the displacements along x, y and z-axes.

In the figure engineering shear strain γ_{xy} is the change in angle between lines AB and AD.

For Plane XY, total shear strain $\gamma_{xy} = (\alpha + \beta)$ (Since α and β are small)

$$= \tan \alpha + \tan \beta$$

$$= \left(\frac{DD'}{A'D} + \frac{BB'}{A'B} \right)$$

$$= \frac{\left(\dfrac{\partial v}{\partial x}\right) \cdot \delta x}{\delta x} + \frac{\left(\dfrac{\partial u}{\partial y}\right) \cdot \delta y}{\delta y}$$

$$= \left\{ \frac{\partial v}{\partial x} + \frac{\partial u}{\partial y} \right\}$$

Similarly, for plane YZ, $\gamma_{yz} = \left\{ \dfrac{\partial w}{\partial y} + \dfrac{\partial v}{\partial z} \right\}$

and for plane ZX, $\gamma_{zx} = \left\{ \dfrac{\partial u}{\partial z} + \dfrac{\partial w}{\partial x} \right\}$

Thus,

$$\varepsilon_x = \frac{\partial u}{\partial x} \qquad \gamma_{xy} = \frac{\partial v}{\partial x} + \frac{\partial u}{\partial y}$$

$$\varepsilon_y = \frac{\partial v}{\partial y} \quad \text{and} \quad \gamma_{yz} = \frac{\partial w}{\partial y} + \frac{\partial v}{\partial z}$$

$$\varepsilon_z = \frac{\partial w}{\partial z} \qquad \gamma_{zx} = \frac{\partial u}{\partial z} + \frac{\partial w}{\partial x}$$

are known as Cauchy's infinitesimal strain tensor. **The kinematics of a deformable body usually described in terms of the displacement vector and strain tensor.** Let us concentrate for XY plane only

We have three strains, $\varepsilon_x = \dfrac{\partial u}{\partial x}$

$$\varepsilon_y = \frac{\partial v}{\partial y}$$

$$\gamma_{xy} = \frac{\partial u}{\partial y} + \frac{\partial v}{\partial x}$$

The normal and shear strain together express the strain tensor which is analogous to stress tensor.

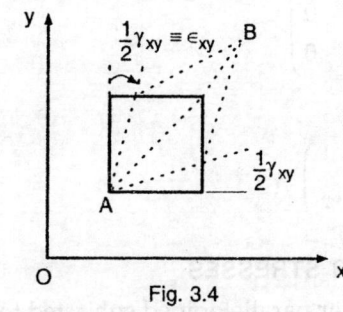

Fig. 3.4

$$\varepsilon_{xy} = \varepsilon_{yx} = \frac{\gamma_{xy}}{2} = \frac{\gamma_{yx}}{2}$$

$$\varepsilon_{yz} = \varepsilon_{zy} = \frac{\gamma_{yz}}{2} = \frac{\gamma_{zy}}{2}$$

$$\varepsilon_{zx} = \varepsilon_{xz} = \frac{\gamma_{zx}}{2} = \frac{\gamma_{xz}}{2}$$

(Since linear strain of diagonal is equal to half the shearing strain).

'Strain Tensor' in Matrix form can be expressed as

$$\varepsilon_{ij} \equiv \begin{pmatrix} \varepsilon_x & \dfrac{\gamma_{xy}}{2} & \dfrac{\gamma_{xz}}{2} \\ \dfrac{\gamma_{yx}}{2} & \varepsilon_y & \dfrac{\gamma_{yz}}{2} \\ \dfrac{\gamma_{zx}}{2} & \dfrac{\gamma_{zy}}{2} & \varepsilon_z \end{pmatrix} \equiv \begin{pmatrix} \varepsilon_{xx} & \varepsilon_{xy} & \varepsilon_{xz} \\ \varepsilon_{yx} & \varepsilon_{yy} & \varepsilon_{yz} \\ \varepsilon_{zx} & \varepsilon_{zy} & \varepsilon_{zz} \end{pmatrix}$$

The strain tensor is symmetric

i.e. $\varepsilon_{xy} = \varepsilon_{yx}$

$$\varepsilon_{xz} = \varepsilon_{zx}$$

$$\varepsilon_{yz} = \varepsilon_{zy}$$

We can write ε_{ij} for the 'strain tensor'.

For two dimensional problem $\varepsilon_3 = 0$ and we have plain strain.

The tensor for this situation is

$$\begin{pmatrix} \varepsilon_{xx} & \varepsilon_{xy} & 0 \\ \varepsilon_{yx} & \varepsilon_{yy} & 0 \\ 0 & 0 & 0 \end{pmatrix}$$

or

$$\begin{pmatrix} \varepsilon_1 & 0 & 0 \\ 0 & \varepsilon_2 & 0 \\ 0 & 0 & 0 \end{pmatrix}$$

or

$$\begin{pmatrix} \varepsilon_1 & 0 \\ 0 & \varepsilon_2 \end{pmatrix}$$

3.4 NORMAL AND SHEAR STRESSES

Let us consider a rectangular parallelopiped subjected to the three dimensional stress system.

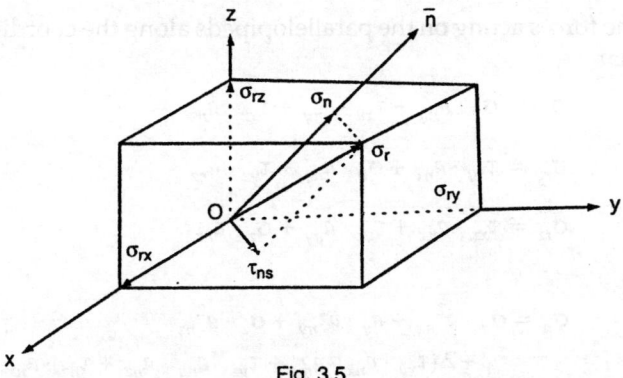

Fig. 3.5

Let σ_r be resultant stress on a plane passing through the point O.

Let σ_{rx}, σ_{ry} and σ_{rz} be its components along the three axes of reference.

The direction* cosines of the resultant stress are

$$a_{rx} = \frac{\sigma_{rx}}{\sigma_r}; a_{ry} = \frac{\sigma_{ry}}{\sigma_r}; a_{rz} = \frac{\sigma_{rz}}{\sigma_r}$$

Let σ_n and τ_{ns} be the normal and shear stress on the plane whose normal $\bar{n}$ has direction cosines $a_{nx}; a_{ny}; a_{nz}$.

$$\sigma_n = \sigma_r \cdot a_{nr}$$

where

$$a_{nr} = a_{nx} \cdot a_{rx} + a_{ny} \cdot a_{ry} + a_{nz} \cdot a_{rz}$$

$\therefore$

$$\sigma_n = \sigma_r (a_{nx} \cdot a_{rx} + a_{ny} \cdot a_{ry} + a_{nz} \cdot a_{rz})$$

$$= \sigma_{rx} \cdot a_{nx} + \sigma_{ry} \cdot a_{ny} + \sigma_{rz} \cdot a_{nz}$$

---

*We define a plane in space by direction cosine. Any direction cosine is termed as a_{ij} which is equal to the cosine of the angle between any two lines i and j. According to this system, l, m, n are a_{nx}, a_{ny} and a_{nz} respectively.

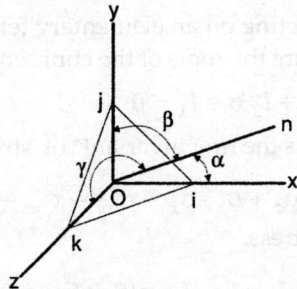

Fig. 3.6 Direction cosine

In the Fig. 3.6, there is a plane ABC, the normal to the plane is ON. ON is making α, β, γ with x, y and z axes respectively. The cosines of these angles are known as direction cosine. The three direction cosines are $\cos\alpha = l$, $\cos\beta = m$ and $\cos\gamma = n$ determines the inclination of plane ABC in space.

Resolving the forces acting on the parallelopipeds along the coordinate axes, we can show that

$$\sigma_{rx} = \sigma_x \cdot a_{nn} + \tau_{xy} \cdot a_{ny} + \tau_{xz} \cdot a_{nz}$$

$$\sigma_{ry} = \tau_{xy} \cdot a_{nx} + \sigma_y \cdot a_{ny} + \tau_{yz} \cdot a_{nz}$$

$$\sigma_{rz} = \tau_{xz} \cdot a_{nx} + \tau_{yz} \cdot a_{ny} + \sigma_z \cdot a_{nz}$$

Therefore,

$$\sigma_n = \sigma_x \cdot a^2_{nx} + a_y \cdot a^2_{ny} + \sigma_z \cdot a^2_{nz}$$
$$+ 2 \left(\tau_{xy} \cdot a_{nx} \cdot a_{ny} + \tau_{yz} \cdot a_{ny} \cdot a_{nz} + \tau_{nz} \cdot a_{nx} \cdot a_{nz} \right)$$

Now, $$\sigma_r^2 = \sigma_n^2 + \tau_{ns}^2$$

$\therefore$ $$\tau_{ns} = \sqrt{\sigma_r^2 - \sigma_n^2}$$

where, $$\sigma_r^2 = \left(\sigma_{rx}^2 + \sigma_{ry}^2 + \sigma_{rz}^2 \right)$$

The direction cosines of the shear stress may be determined as follows:

Let a_{sx}; a_{sy}; a_{sz} be the direction cosines of τ_{ns}.

Now, $$\sigma_{rx} = \sigma_n \cdot a_{nx} + \tau_{ns} \cdot a_{sx}$$

Similarly, $$a_{sx} = \frac{1}{\tau_{ns}} \left[\sigma_{rx} - \sigma_n \cdot a_{nx} \right]$$

$$a_{sy} = \frac{1}{\tau_{ns}} \left[\sigma_{ry} - \sigma_n \cdot a_{ny} \right]$$

and $$a_{sz} = \frac{1}{\tau_{ns}} \left[\sigma_{rz} - \sigma_n \cdot a_{nz} \right]$$

3.5 PRINCIPAL STRESSES

By considering the forces acting on an elementary tetrahedron, it can be shown that the principal stresses are the roots of the cubic equations,

$$\sigma^3 - I_1 \sigma^2 + I_2 \sigma - I_3 = 0$$

where $I_1 = \sigma_x + \sigma_y + \sigma_z$ is the first invariant* of stress.

$I_2 = \sigma_x \cdot \sigma_y + \sigma_y \cdot \sigma_z + \sigma_z \cdot \sigma_x - \tau^2_{xy} - \tau^2_{yz} - \tau^2_{xz}$ is the second invariant of stress.

$I_3 = \sigma_x \cdot \sigma_y \cdot \sigma_z + 2\,\tau_{xy} \cdot \tau_{yz} \cdot \tau_{zx} - (\sigma_x \cdot \tau^2_{yz} + \sigma_y \cdot \tau^2_{zx} + \sigma_{zx} \cdot \tau^2_{xy})$ is the third invariant of stress.

---

*In the context of stress tensor, invariants are such quantities that do not change with rotation of axes.

The cubic equation has 3 roots. These roots $(\sigma_1; \sigma_2; \sigma_3)$ **are called the principal normal stress at a given point.** The cubic equation can be solved by a **hit and trial procedure** or by **Newton-Rapson method****.

3.6 PRINCIPAL DIRECTION

For the three principal stresses σ_1, σ_2 and σ_3 the principal directions may be determined as follows:

For σ_1 stress, let

$$A_1 = \begin{vmatrix} (\sigma_y - \sigma_1) & \tau_{yz} \\ \tau_{yz} & (\sigma_z - \sigma_1) \end{vmatrix}$$

$$B_1 = -\begin{vmatrix} \tau_{xy} & \tau_{yz} \\ \tau_{yz} & (\sigma_z - \sigma_1) \end{vmatrix}$$

$$C_1 = -\begin{vmatrix} \tau_{xy} & (\sigma_z - \sigma_1) \\ \tau_{yz} & \tau_{yz} \end{vmatrix}$$

Then,

$$\sigma_{nx_1} = \frac{A_1}{\sqrt{A_1^2 + B_1^2 + C_1^2}}$$

$$\sigma_{ny_1} = \frac{B_1}{\sqrt{A_1^2 + B_1^2 + C_1^2}}$$

$$\sigma_{nz_1} = \frac{C_1}{\sqrt{A_1^2 + B_1^2 + C_1^2}}$$

Similarly, direction cosines of other stresses can be determined.

SOLVED PROBLEMS

EXAMPLE 1 *At a point in a stressed material the Cartesian Stress Components are:*

$$\sigma_x = -40; \sigma_y = 80; \sigma_z = 120 \; MPa$$

and,

$$\tau_{xy} = 72; \tau_{yz} = 46; \tau_{xz} = 32 \; MPa$$

Calculate the normal, shear and resultant stresses on a plane whose normal makes an angle of 48° with the x-axis and 61° with the y-axis. **(UPTU 2003-2004)**

SOLUTION

$$a_{nx} = \cos 48°$$

$$= 0.66913$$

$$a_{ny} = \cos 61°$$

$$= 0.48481$$

$$a_{nz} = \sqrt{1 - a_{nx}^2 - a_{ny}^2}$$

**See any book on 'Numerical Methods' for Newton Rapson Method.

$$= \sqrt{1 - 0.44773 - 0.23504}$$

$$= 0.56323$$

$$\sigma_{rx} = \sigma_x \cdot a_{nx} + \tau_{xy} \cdot a_{ny} + \tau_{xz} \cdot a_{nz}$$

$$= -40 \times 0.66913 + 72 \times 0.48481 + 32 \times 0.56323$$

$$= -26.76 + 34.91 + 18.02$$

$$= 26.17 \text{ MPa}$$

$$\sigma_{ry} = \tau_{xy} \cdot a_{nx} + \sigma_y \cdot a_{ny} + \tau_{yz} \cdot a_{nz}$$

$$= 72 \times 0.66913 + 80 \times 0.48481 + 46 \times 0.56323$$

$$= 48.18 + 38.78 + 25.91$$

$$= 112.87 \text{ MPa}$$

$$\sigma_{rz} = \tau_{xz} \cdot a_{nx} + \tau_{yz} \cdot a_{ny} + \sigma_z \cdot a_{nz}$$

$$= 32 \times 0.66913 + 46 \times 0.48981 + 120 \times 0.56323$$

$$= 21.41 + 22.30 + 67.58$$

$$= 111.29 \text{ MPa}$$

Resultant stress $\quad (\sigma_r) = \sqrt{\sigma_{rx}^2 + \sigma_{ry}^2 + \sigma_{rz}^2}$

$$= \sqrt{(26.17)^2 + (112.87)^2 + (111.29)^2}$$

$$= \sqrt{685 + 12739 + 12385}$$

$$= \sqrt{25809}$$

$$= 160.85 \text{ MPa}$$

Normal stress $(\sigma_n) = \sigma_{rx} \cdot a_{nx} + \sigma_{ry} \cdot a_{ny} + \sigma_{rz} \cdot a_{nz}$

$$= 26.17 \times 0.66913 + 112.87 \times 0.48481 + 111.29 \times 0.56323$$

$$= 17.51 + 54.72 + 62.68$$

$$= 134.91 \text{ MPa}$$

Shear stress, $\tau_{ns} = \sqrt{\sigma_r^2 - \sigma_n^2}$

$$= \sqrt{25809 - 18200}$$

$$= \sqrt{7609}$$

$$= 87.23 \text{ MPa}$$

EXAMPLE 2 *In a triaxial stress system, the six components of the stress at a point are given below:*

$$\sigma_x = 6 \text{ MN/m}^2 \quad \tau_{xy} = \tau_{yx} = 1 \text{ MN/m}^2$$

$$\sigma_y = 5 \text{ MN/m}^2 \quad \tau_{yz} = \tau_{zy} = 3 \text{ MN/m}^2$$

$$\sigma_z = 4 \text{ MN/m}^2 \quad \tau_{zx} = \tau_{xz} = 2 \text{ MN/m}^2$$

Find the magnitude of three principal stresses. **(UPTU 2002-2003)**

SOLUTION Principal stresses can be found by

Solving the equation $\sigma^3 - I_1 \sigma^2 + I_2 \sigma - I_3 = 0$

where $I_1, I_2\ I_3$ are the first invariant, second invariant and third invariant of stress.

$$I_1 = \sigma_x + \sigma_y + \sigma_z$$

$$I_2 = \sigma_x\sigma_y + \sigma_y\sigma_z + \sigma_z\sigma_x - \tau^2_{xy} - \tau^2_{yz} - \tau^2_{zx}$$

and, $I_3 = \sigma_x\sigma_y\sigma_z + 2\,\tau_{xy} \cdot \tau_{yz} \cdot \tau_{zx} - (\sigma_x \cdot \tau^2_{yz} + \sigma_y \cdot \tau^2_{zx} + \sigma_z \cdot \tau^2_{xy})$

Substituting the value of $\sigma_x, \sigma_y, \sigma_z, \tau_{xy}, \tau_{yz}$ and τ_{zx} we get

$$I_1 = \sigma_x + \sigma_y + \sigma_z$$

$$= 6 + 5 + 4$$

$$= 15\ \text{MN/m}^2$$

$$I_2 = \sigma_x\sigma_y + \sigma_y\sigma_z + \sigma_z \cdot \sigma_x - \tau^2_{xy} - \tau^2_{yz} - \tau^2_{zx}$$

$$= 6 \times 5 + 5 \times 4 + 4 \times 6 - 1^2 - 3^2 - 2^2$$

$$= 60$$

$$I_3 = \sigma_x\sigma_y\sigma_z + 2\,\tau_{xy} \cdot \tau_{yz} \cdot \tau_{zx} - (\sigma_x \cdot \tau^2_{yz} + \sigma_y \cdot \tau^2_{zx} + \sigma_z \cdot \tau^2_{xy})$$

$$= 6 \times 5 \times 4 + 2 \times 1 \times 3 \times 2 - (6 \times 3^2 + 5 \times 2^2 + 4 \times 1^2)$$

$$= 120 + 12 - (54 + 20 + 4)$$

$$= 132 - 78$$

$$= 54$$

Now, substituting the values of I_1, I_2 and I_3 in the eqn.

$\sigma^3 - I_1 \sigma^2 + I_2 \sigma - I_3 = 0$ we get

$\sigma^3 - 15\sigma^2 + 60\,\sigma - 54 = 0$

This is cubic equation in σ so we will get three roots σ_1, σ_2 and σ_3 after solving the above equation.

Solving by hit and trial method, we get,

$$\sigma_1 = 9\ \text{MN/m}^2$$

$$\sigma_2 = 4.732\ \text{MN/m}^2$$

$$\sigma_3 = 1.248\ \text{MN/m}^2 \qquad \textbf{Ans.}$$

EXAMPLE 3 *At a point P in a body* $\sigma_x = 30\ kN/cm^2$; $\sigma_y = -10\ kN/cm^2$ *and* $\sigma_z = 10\ kN/cm^2$ *and* $\tau_{xy} = \tau_{yz} = \tau_{zx} = 10\ kN/cm^2$. *Determine the normal and shearing stress on a plane that is equally inclined to all the three axes.*   **(UPTU 2001-02)**

SOLUTION A plane that is equally inclined to all the three axes will have

$$a_{nx} = a_{ny} = a_{nz} = \frac{1}{\sqrt{3}}$$

Normal stress $\sigma_n = \sigma_x \cdot a^2_{nx} + \sigma_y \cdot a^2_{ny} + \sigma_z \cdot a^2_{nz}$

$$+ 2(\tau_{xy} \cdot a_{nx} \cdot a_{ny} + \tau_{yz} \cdot a_{ny} \cdot a_{nz} + \tau_{zx} \cdot a_{nz} \cdot a_{nx})$$

$$= \frac{1}{3}(30 - 10 + 10 + 20 + 20 + 20)$$

$$= 30 \text{ kN/cm}^2 \qquad \textbf{Ans.}$$

$$\sigma_{rx} = \sigma_x \cdot a_{nx} + \tau_{xy} \cdot a_{ny} + \tau_{xz} \cdot a_{nz}$$

$$= \frac{1}{\sqrt{3}}(30 + 10 + 10)$$

$$= \frac{50}{\sqrt{3}}$$

$$\sigma_{ry} = \tau_{xy} \cdot a_{nx} + \sigma_y \cdot a_{ny} + \tau_{yz} \cdot a_{nz}$$

$$= \frac{1}{\sqrt{3}}(10 - 10 + 10)$$

$$= \frac{10}{\sqrt{3}}$$

$$\sigma_{rz} = \tau_{xz} \cdot a_{nx} + \sigma_{yz} \cdot a_{ny} + \tau_z \cdot a_{nz}$$

$$= \frac{1}{\sqrt{3}}(10 + 10 + 10)$$

$$= \frac{30}{\sqrt{3}}$$

Hence, $\sigma_r = \sqrt{\sigma^2_{rx} + \sigma^2_{ry} + \sigma^2_{rz}}$

$$= \sqrt{\left(\frac{50}{\sqrt{3}}\right)^2 + \left(\frac{10}{\sqrt{3}}\right)^2 + \left(\frac{30}{\sqrt{3}}\right)^2}$$

$$= \sqrt{\frac{2500}{3} + \frac{100}{3} + \frac{900}{3}}$$

$$= \sqrt{\frac{3500}{3}}$$

$$\tau_{ns} = \text{Shear Stress}$$

$$= \sqrt{\sigma_r^2 - \sigma_n^2}$$

$$= \sqrt{\frac{3500}{3} - 900}$$

$$= \sqrt{\frac{3500 - 2700}{3}}$$

$$= \sqrt{\frac{800}{3}}$$

$$= \sqrt{\frac{400 \times 2}{3}}$$

$$= 20 \times \sqrt{\frac{2}{3}}$$

$$= 20 \times \sqrt{0.6666}$$

$$= 16.32 \, \text{kN} / \text{cm}^2 \qquad \textbf{Ans.}$$

3.7 DIFFERENTIAL EQUATIONS OF EQUILIBRIUM   (UPTU 2007-08)

The equation of equilibrium describes how stress can vary within a body. The equation apply to viscous fluids, plastics and elastic solids.

State of stress in a body varies from point to point in all the directions. The variation of stress can be observed in the Fig. 3.7.

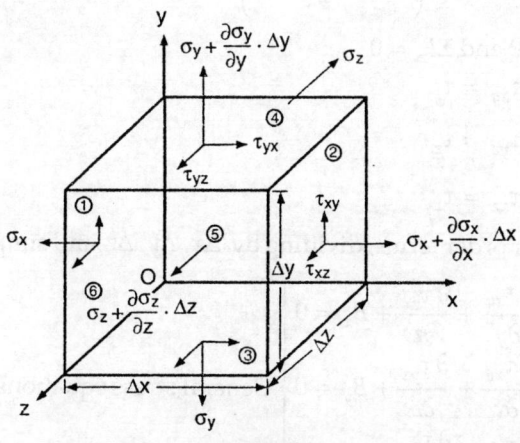

Fig. 3.7

Consider a small rectangular element with sides Δx, Δy and Δz isolated from it's parent body.

We shall deal with average values of the stress components on each face.

On the left side *i.e.* on face 1, the average stress components are σ_x, τ_{xy} and τ_{xz}.

On the right hand face *i.e.* face 2, the average stress components are

$$\sigma_x + \frac{\partial \sigma_x}{\partial x} \Delta x; \ \tau_{xy} + \frac{\partial \tau_{xy}}{\partial x} \Delta x; \ \tau_{xz} + \frac{\partial \tau_{xz}}{\partial x} \Delta x$$

Similarly, the stress components on the six faces of the element are as follows:

Face 1, $\sigma_x ; \tau_{xy} ; \tau_{xz}$

Face 2, $\sigma_x + \dfrac{\partial \sigma_y}{\partial x} \Delta x; \ \tau_{yx} + \dfrac{\partial \tau_{xy}}{\partial x} \Delta x; \ \tau_{xz} + \dfrac{\partial \tau_{xz}}{\partial x} \cdot \Delta x$

Face 3, $\sigma_y ; \tau_{yx} ; \tau_{yz}$

Face 4, $\sigma_y + \dfrac{\partial \sigma_y}{\partial y} \Delta y; \ \tau_{yx} + \dfrac{\partial \tau_{yx}}{\partial y} \Delta x; \ \tau_{yz} + \dfrac{\partial \tau_{yz}}{\partial y} \Delta y$

Face 5, $\sigma_z ; \tau_{zx} ; \tau_{zy}$

Face 6, $\sigma_z + \dfrac{\partial \sigma_z}{\partial z} \Delta z ; \ \tau_{zx} + \dfrac{\partial \tau_{zx}}{\partial zx} \Delta z; \ \tau_{zx} + \dfrac{\partial \tau_{zy}}{\partial z} \Delta z$

Let the body force components per unit volume in the x, y and z directions are B_x, B_y and B_z.

For equilibrium in x-direction $\Sigma F_x = 0$

$$\Rightarrow \quad \left(\sigma_x + \frac{\partial \sigma_x}{\partial x} \Delta x \right) \Delta y \, \Delta z - \sigma_x \, \Delta y \, \Delta z + \left(\tau_{yx} + \frac{\partial \tau_{yx}}{\partial y} \Delta y \right) \Delta z \, \Delta x - \tau_{yx} \, \Delta z \, \Delta x$$

$$+ \left(\tau_{zx} + \frac{\partial \tau_{yx}}{\partial z} \Delta z \right) \Delta x \, \Delta y - \tau_{zx} \, \Delta x \, \Delta y + F_x \cdot \Delta x \, \Delta y \, \Delta z = 0$$

Similarly, $\Sigma F_y = 0$ and $\Sigma F_z = 0$

Moreover, $\qquad \tau_{xy} = \tau_{yx}$

$$\tau_{yz} = \tau_{zy}$$

$$\tau_{xz} = \tau_{zx}$$

Cancelling higher order terms, dividing by $\Delta x, \Delta y, \Delta z$ and simplifying, we get

$$\left.\begin{array}{l} \dfrac{\partial \sigma_x}{\partial x} + \dfrac{\partial \tau_{xy}}{\partial y} + \dfrac{\partial \tau_{zx}}{\partial z} + B_x = 0 \\[3mm] \dfrac{\partial \sigma_y}{\partial y} + \dfrac{\partial \tau_{xy}}{\partial x} + \dfrac{\partial \tau_{yz}}{\partial z} + B_y = 0 \\[3mm] \dfrac{\partial \sigma_z}{\partial z} + \dfrac{\partial \tau_{xz}}{\partial x} + \dfrac{\partial \tau_{yz}}{\partial y} + B_z = 0 \end{array}\right\} \text{General stress equations of equilibrium}$$

where, B_x, B_y and B_z are the components of body force in x, y and z direction.

The above three equations must be satisfied at all points throughout the volume of the body.

The conditions of equilibrium expressed in the form of partial differential equations give us an idea as to how the stresses are distributed inside the body.

3.8 COMPATIBILITY*

A body that deforms without developing any gap/overlap is called compatible body. Comatibility conditions are mathematical conditions that determine whether a particular deformation will leave a body in compatible state.

Compatibility have both mathematical and physical significance. From mathematicsl viewpoint, they establish that the displacement field, as expressed by u, v, w is a single valued and continuous. Physically this means that body must be connected together.

The smooth deformation describes the continuity property of the element and commonly called the continuum expression or compatibility expression.

Let there be a solid plane that undergoes deformation due to application of load.

Then $$\varepsilon_{xx} = \frac{\partial u_x}{\partial x} \text{ and } \varepsilon_{yy} = \frac{\partial u_y}{dy}$$

where, u_x and u_y are the component of displacement vector.

Taking its second derivatives, we have $\dfrac{\partial^2 \varepsilon_{xx}}{\partial y^2} = \dfrac{\partial^3 u_x}{\partial y^2 \cdot \partial x}$ and $\dfrac{\partial^2 \varepsilon_{yy}}{\partial x^2} = \dfrac{\partial^3 u_y}{\partial x^2 \cdot \partial y}$

Now, substituting the value of ε_{xx} and ε_{yy}

$$\frac{\partial^2 \varepsilon_{xx}}{\partial y^2} = \frac{\partial^2}{\partial x \cdot \partial y}\left(\frac{\partial u_x}{\partial y}\right) \quad \text{...(I)} \quad \text{and} \quad \frac{\partial^2 \varepsilon_{yy}}{\partial x^2} = \frac{\partial^2}{\partial x \cdot \partial y}\left(\frac{\partial u_y}{\partial x}\right) \quad \text{...(II)}$$

---

*Let us discuss the meaning of compatibility.

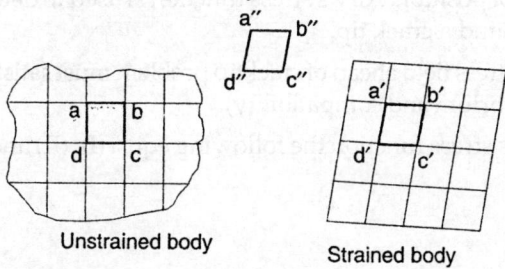

Unstrained body   Strained body

Fig. 3.8

Let us consider an element *abcd* of 2 D-body which deforms to parallelogram $a'\,b'\,c'\,d'$ then each element of the deformed body should have a similar shape. Hence, if we isolate an element $a''b''c''d''$ from the deformed body leaving a gap $a'\,b'\,c'\,d'$, the shape and size of the isolated element and the gap should be identical for compatibility.

Adding (I) and (II), we get

$$\left(\frac{\partial^2 \varepsilon_{xx}}{\partial y^2} + \frac{\partial^2 \varepsilon_{yy}}{\partial x^2}\right) = \frac{\partial^2}{\partial x\,\partial y}\left(\frac{\partial u_x}{\partial y}\right) + \frac{\partial^2}{\partial x\,\partial y}\left(\frac{\partial u_y}{\partial x}\right)$$

$$= \frac{\partial^2}{\partial x\,\partial y}\left(\frac{\partial u_x}{\partial y} + \frac{\partial u_y}{\partial x}\right)$$

$$\therefore \qquad \left(\frac{\partial^2 \varepsilon_{xx}}{\partial y^2} + \frac{\partial^2 \varepsilon_{yy}}{\partial x^2}\right) = \frac{\partial^2 \gamma_{xy}}{\partial x\cdot\partial y} \qquad\qquad\text{(III)}$$

This is called compatibility Expression in terms of strain.

Compatibility equation can be written in terms of stress also.

We know that

$$\varepsilon_{xx} = \frac{1}{E}\cdot(\sigma_{xx} - \nu\sigma_{yy})$$

$$\varepsilon_{yy} = \frac{1}{E}\cdot(\sigma_{yy} - \nu\sigma_{xx})$$

$$\gamma_{xy} = \frac{2(1+\nu)}{E}\cdot\tau_{xy}$$

Substituting these in equation (III)

$$\frac{\partial^2}{\partial y^2}\left\{\frac{1}{E}(\sigma_{xx} - \nu\sigma_{yy})\right\} + \frac{\partial^2}{\partial x^2}\left\{\frac{1}{E}(\sigma_{yy} - \nu\sigma_{xx})\right\} - \frac{\partial^2}{\partial x\cdot\partial y}\left\{\frac{(2+2\nu)}{E}\cdot\tau_{xy}\right\} = 0$$

is the compatibility equation in term of stress.

3.9 AIRY'S STRESS FUNCTION

Airy's stress function is a function that uniquely defines the stress in an elastic body as a function of position. Airy's stress function is used to determine the stress and strain field around a crack tip.

The solution to the stress field ahead of cracktip problem must satisfy all equilibrium requirement (equilibrium and compatibility).

According to Airy's stress function the following eqns. (I), (II) and (III) hold true.

$$\sigma_{xx} = \frac{\delta^2\psi}{\delta y^2} \qquad\qquad\qquad\qquad \ldots\text{(I)}$$

$$\sigma_{yy} = \frac{\delta^2\psi}{\delta x^2} \qquad\qquad\qquad\qquad \ldots\text{(II)}$$

and $\qquad \tau_{xy} = \frac{-\delta^2\psi}{\delta x\cdot\delta y} \qquad\qquad\qquad\qquad \ldots\text{(III)}$

Equilibrium condition is given below:

$$\frac{\delta\sigma_{xx}}{\delta x} + \frac{\delta\tau_{xy}}{\delta y} = 0 \qquad \dots \text{(IV)}$$

or,

$$\frac{\delta}{\delta x}\left(\frac{\delta^2 y}{\delta y^2}\right) + \frac{\delta}{\delta y}\left(-\frac{\delta^2\psi}{\delta x \cdot \delta y}\right) = 0$$

or,

$$\frac{\delta^3\psi}{\delta x \cdot \delta y^2} - \frac{\delta^3\psi}{\delta x \cdot \delta y^2} = 0 \qquad \dots \text{(V)}$$

Compatibility condition from Section 3.8 of equation (III) is

$$\frac{\delta^2\varepsilon_{xx}}{\delta y^2} + \frac{\delta^2\varepsilon_{yy}}{\delta x^2} - \frac{\delta^2\gamma_{xy}}{\delta x \cdot \delta y} = 0$$

$$\frac{\delta^2}{\delta y^2}\left\{\frac{1}{E}(\sigma_{xx} - v \cdot \sigma_{yy})\right\} + \frac{\delta^2}{\delta x^2}\left\{\frac{1}{E}(\sigma_{yy} - v \cdot \sigma_{xx})\right\}$$

$$-\frac{\delta^2}{\delta x \cdot \delta y}\left\{\frac{(2+2v)}{E} \cdot \tau_{xy}\right\} = 0$$

$$\frac{\delta^2}{\delta y^2}\left[\frac{1}{E}\left\{\frac{\delta^2\psi}{\delta y^2} - v \cdot \frac{\delta^2\psi}{\delta x^2}\right\}\right] + \frac{\delta^2}{\delta x^2}\left[\frac{1}{E}\left\{\frac{\delta^2\psi}{\delta x^2} - v \cdot \frac{\delta^2\psi}{\delta y^2}\right\}\right]$$

$$-\frac{\delta^2}{\delta x \cdot \delta y}\left\{\frac{2+2v}{E}\left(-\frac{\delta^2\psi}{\delta x \cdot \delta y}\right)\right\}$$

This simplifies to

$$\frac{1}{E}\left\{\frac{\delta^4\psi}{\delta y^4} - v \cdot \frac{\delta^4\psi}{\delta y^2 \cdot \delta x^2} + \frac{\delta^4\psi}{\delta x^4} - v \cdot \frac{\delta^4\psi}{\delta x^2 \cdot \delta y^2}\right\}$$

$$+\frac{2}{E}\cdot\left\{\frac{\delta^4\psi}{\delta x^2 \cdot \delta y^2} + v \cdot \frac{\delta^4\psi}{\delta x^2 \cdot \delta y^2}\right\} = 0$$

$$\frac{\delta^4\psi}{\delta x^4} + 2\cdot\frac{\delta^4\psi}{\delta x^2 \delta y^2} + \frac{\delta^4\psi}{\delta y^4} = 0$$

This equation is also known as biharmonic equation and can be expressed as $\nabla^2 \cdot (\nabla^2\psi) = 0$.

where, $\nabla^2 \cdot \psi$ is the Laplacian Operator.

EXAMPLE 1 *At a point inside a body, the displacement field is linear and is given as below. Calculate various components of strain.*

$$\begin{bmatrix} u \\ v \\ w \end{bmatrix} = \begin{bmatrix} 0.10 & 0.05 & 0.04 \\ 0.03 & -0.02 & 0.03 \\ -0.04 & +0.04 & -0.02 \end{bmatrix}\begin{bmatrix} x \\ y \\ z \end{bmatrix}$$

SOLUTION   The various strain components are:

$$\varepsilon_{xx} = \frac{\partial u}{\partial x} \qquad\qquad \gamma_{xy} = \frac{\partial v}{\partial x} + \frac{\partial u}{\partial y}$$

$$\varepsilon_{yy} = \frac{\partial v}{\partial y} \qquad\qquad \gamma_{yz} = \frac{\partial w}{\partial y} + \frac{\partial v}{\partial z}$$

$$\varepsilon_{zz} = \frac{\partial w}{\partial z} \qquad\qquad \gamma_{zx} = \frac{\partial u}{\partial z} + \frac{\partial w}{\partial x}$$

$$\varepsilon_{xx} = \frac{\partial}{\partial x}(0.10x + 0.05y + 0.04z) = 0.10$$

$$\varepsilon_{yy} = \frac{\partial}{\partial y}(0.03x - 0.02y + 0.03z) = -0.02$$

$$\varepsilon_{zz} = \frac{\partial}{\partial z}(-0.04 + 0.04y - 0.02z) = -0.02$$

and $$\gamma_{xy} = \frac{\partial}{\partial x}(0.03x - 0.02y + 0.03z) + \frac{\partial}{\partial y}(0.10x + 0.05y + 0.04z)$$

$$= 0.03 + 0.05 = 0.08$$

$$\gamma_{yz} = \frac{\partial}{\partial y}(-0.04x + 0.04y - 0.02z) + \frac{\partial}{\partial z}(-0.03x - 0.02y + 0.03z)$$

$$= 0.04 + 0.03 = 0.07$$

$$\gamma_{zx} = \frac{\partial}{\partial z}(0.10x + 0.05y + 0.04z) + \frac{\partial}{\partial x}(-0.04x + 0.04y - 0.02z)$$

$$= 0.04 - 0.04 = 0$$

Thus, we have

$$\varepsilon_{ij} = \begin{bmatrix} \varepsilon_{xx} & \gamma_{xy} & \gamma_{xz} \\ \gamma_{xy} & \varepsilon_{yy} & \gamma_{yz} \\ \gamma_{xz} & \gamma_{yz} & \varepsilon_{zz} \end{bmatrix} = \begin{bmatrix} 0.10 & 0.08 & 0 \\ 0.08 & -0.02 & 0.07 \\ 0 & 0.07 & -0.02 \end{bmatrix} \qquad \textbf{Ans.}$$

EXAMPLE 2 *The stresses in the three principal direction are* $+ 65\ MN/m^2$; $+ 20MN/m^2$; *and* $- 85\ MN/m^2$. *Find the principal strain. Take* $\mu = 0.3$ *and* $E = 200GN/m^2$.

(UPTU-2006-07)

SOLUTION   Given $\sigma_x = 65\ MN/m^2$

$$\sigma_y = 20\ MN/m^2 \text{ and } \sigma_z = (-)85\ MN/m^2$$

$$\mu = 0.3$$

$$E = 200 \times 10^3\ MN/m^2$$

Strain along x-axis $(\varepsilon_x) = \dfrac{\sigma_x}{E} - \mu \cdot \dfrac{\sigma_y}{E} - \mu \cdot \dfrac{\sigma_z}{E}$

$$= \frac{1}{2 \times 10^5}[65 - 20 \times 0.3 + 85 \times 0.3]$$

$$= \frac{1}{2 \times 10^5}[65 - 6 + 25.5]$$

$$= 42.25 \times 10^{-5} = 4.225 \times 10^{-4}$$

Similarly, strain along y-axis $(\varepsilon_y) = \dfrac{\sigma_y}{E} - \mu \cdot \dfrac{\sigma_x}{E} - \mu \cdot \dfrac{\sigma_z}{E}$

$$= \frac{1}{2 \times 10^5}[20 - 65 \times 0.3 + 85 \times 0.3]$$

$$= \frac{1}{2 \times 10^5}[20 - 19.5 + 25.5]$$

$$= 13 \times 10^{-5} = 1.3 \times 10^{-4}$$

and, Strain along z-axis $(\varepsilon_z) = \dfrac{\sigma_z}{E} - \mu \cdot \dfrac{\sigma_x}{E} - \mu \cdot \dfrac{\sigma_y}{E}$

$$= \frac{1}{2.5}[-85 - 65 \times 0.3 + 20 \times 0.3]$$

$$= -5.525 \times 10^{-4} \qquad \textbf{Ans.}$$

PROBLEMS FOR PRACTICE

1. The state of stress at a point for a given reference xyz is given by the following array of form.

$$\begin{bmatrix} 15 & 8 & -6 \\ 8 & -12 & 5 \\ -6 & 5 & 8 \end{bmatrix} \text{MPa}$$

Determine the principal stresses.

2. The Cartesian components of stress at a point are given below:

$\sigma_x = 10 \; ; \sigma_y = 5 \; ; \sigma_z = 4$

$\tau_{xy} = 2 \; ; \tau_{yz} = -4 \; ; \tau_{xz} = -6 \text{ MPa}$

Determine the normal and shear stress on a plane whose direction cosines

are $\dfrac{1}{3}, -\dfrac{2}{3} ; \dfrac{2}{3}$.

3. The Cartesian components of stress at a point are given below:

$\sigma_x = 15 \; ; \sigma_y = \sigma_z = 8$

$\tau_{xy} = 6 \; ; \tau_{yz} = 4 \; ; \tau_{zx} = 4 \text{ MPa}$

Determine the normal and shear stresses on a plane whose direction cosines are $\dfrac{1}{\sqrt{3}} ; \dfrac{1}{\sqrt{3}} ; \dfrac{1}{\sqrt{3}}$.

ANSWERS

1. $\begin{bmatrix} 19.19 \text{ MPa} \\ 10.27 \text{ MPa} \\ 10.02 \text{ MPa} \end{bmatrix}$
2. $\begin{bmatrix} 5.1 \text{ MPa} \\ 4.17 \text{ MPa} \end{bmatrix}$
3. $\begin{bmatrix} 19.6 \text{ MPa} \\ 3.83 \text{ MPa} \end{bmatrix}$

— ❖❖ —

4

CENTROID AND CENTRE OF GRAVITY

4.1 CENTRE OF AREA 'OR' CENTROID

Centroid is applicable for plane geometrical figure such as rectangle; square, triangle etc. Centroid is the point at which the whole area of a plane figure is assumed to be concentrated. The centroid of an area is located at its geometrical centre.

4.2 CENTRE OF GRAVITY

The centre of gravity of a body is the point in the body through which the whole weight of the body acts. It is denoted by G.

4.3 APPLICATION OF CENTRE OF GRAVITY AND CENTROID

In Engineering practice, it may be required to determine the location of centroid, centre of gravity of the following cases:

1. Solid bodies and areas of regular shape like rectangular, triangular, and circular areas.
2. Solid bodies and plane figure of regular shape comprising two or more geometrical section.
3. Plane figures of irregular shape.
4. Solid bodies such as sphere; cone; hemisphere; cylinder or their combinations.

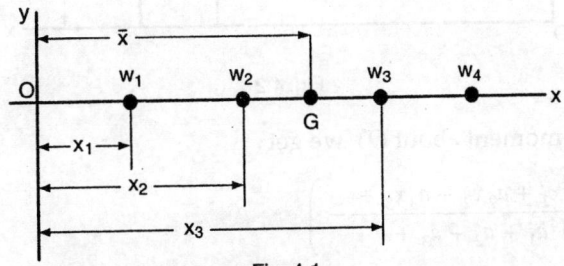

Fig. 4.1

N.B.: For 'plane area' we use term centroid. For figure where mass density is involved we use term centre of gravity.

4.4 DETERMINATION OF C.G.

Let us consider weight w_1, w_2, w_3 ... which are placed on axis ox. Their distances from O are x_1, x_2, x_3 respectively.

Let G is the C.G. of all these weights and its distance from O is $\bar{x}$.

Now, taking moment about O we have

$$(w_1 + w_2 + w_3 + \cdots)\,\bar{x} = w_1 x_1 + w_2 x_2 + w_3 x_3 + \cdots$$

$$\therefore \quad \bar{x} = \frac{w_1 x_1 + w_2 x_2 + w_3 x_3 + \cdots}{w_1 + w_2 + w_3 + \cdots}$$

$$= \frac{\Sigma w x}{\Sigma w}$$

$$= \frac{\Sigma w x}{W}$$

4.5 CENTROID OF PLANE AREA

If a plane area A is divided into strip 1, 2, 3 etc. and if these strip areas are a_1, a_2, a_3 ... each having its c.g. $(x_1, y_1); (x_2, y_2) (x_3, y_3)$ ... then the centroid of whole area $(a_1 + a_2 + a_3 + ...)$ is at G having co-ordinate $(\bar{x};\ \bar{y})$.

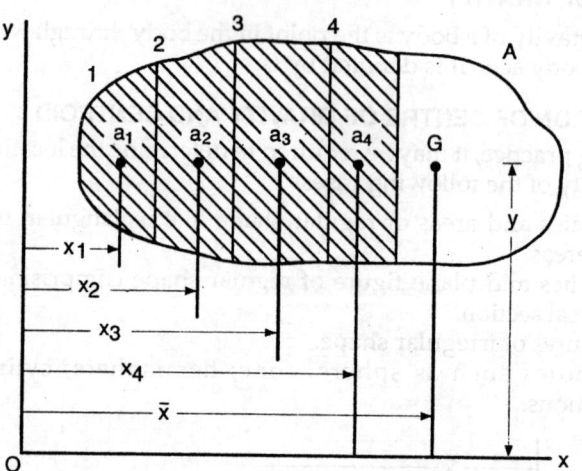

Fig. 4.2

Now, by taking moment about OY we get

$$\bar{x} = \left(\frac{a_1 x_1 + a_2 x_2 + a_3 x_3 + \cdots}{a_1 + a_2 + a_3 + \cdots} \right)$$

$$= \frac{\Sigma a x}{\Sigma a}$$

Taking moment about OX, we get,

$$\bar{y} = \frac{a_1 y_1 + a_2 y_2 + a_3 y_3 + \cdots}{a_1 + a_2 + a_3 + \cdots}$$

$$= \frac{\Sigma ay}{\Sigma a}$$

In general, $\bar{x} = \dfrac{\Sigma a_i x_i}{\Sigma a_i}$ and $\bar{y} = \dfrac{\Sigma a_i y_i}{\Sigma a_i}$

where, $i = 1; 2; 3; 4; ....$

$x_i =$ distance of C.G. of area a_i from axis OY.

and, $y_i =$ distance of C.G. of area a_i from axis OX.

The value of i depends upon the number of small area.

If the small areas are large in number (*i.e.* infinite) then the summation symbol in the above equation can be replaced by integration.

Let us consider that small areas are represented by dA instead of 'a'.

Then, $\bar{x} = \dfrac{\int x \cdot dA}{\int dA}$ and $\bar{y} = \dfrac{\int y \cdot dA}{\int dA}$

where, $\int x \cdot dA = \Sigma x_i \, a_i$

$\int dA = \Sigma a_i$

$\int y \cdot dA = \Sigma y_i \, a_i$

x and y are the distances of C.G. of area dA from axis OY and OX respectively.

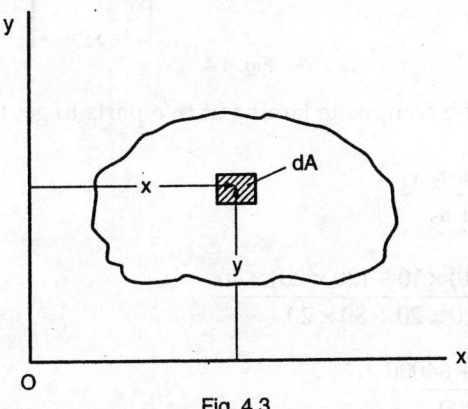

Fig. 4.3

Similarly centroid of volume of the body is

$$\bar{x} = \frac{\int x \, dv}{\int dv} \text{ and } \bar{y} = \frac{\int y \, dv}{\int dv} \text{ and } z = \frac{\int z \, dv}{dv}$$

where, x = distance of C.G. of small volume dv from yz-plane (or on axis OY)

$\quad\quad\quad y$ = distance of C.G. of small volume dv from xz plane (or on axis OX)

$\quad\quad\quad z$ = distance of C.G. of the small volume dv from xy plane.

Centroid of length of a curve 'or' line

$$\bar{x} = \frac{\int x \, dl}{\int dl} \; ; \bar{y} = \frac{\int y \, dl}{\int dl}$$

4.6 METHOD OF FINDING CENTROID OF A COMPOSITE FIGURE

The centroid of the composite area obtained by splitting them into the definite geometrical shape *i.e.* triangle, rectangle, circle, semi circle etc.

The second step in determining the position of the centroid involves taking the moments of the length, areas with respect to some axes. Therefore, reference axis (x and y axis) is chosen. Proper selection of axis makes the solution easier. If mass is involved use term centre of gravity.

EXAMPLE 1 *Determine the centroid of the lamina as shown in figure.*

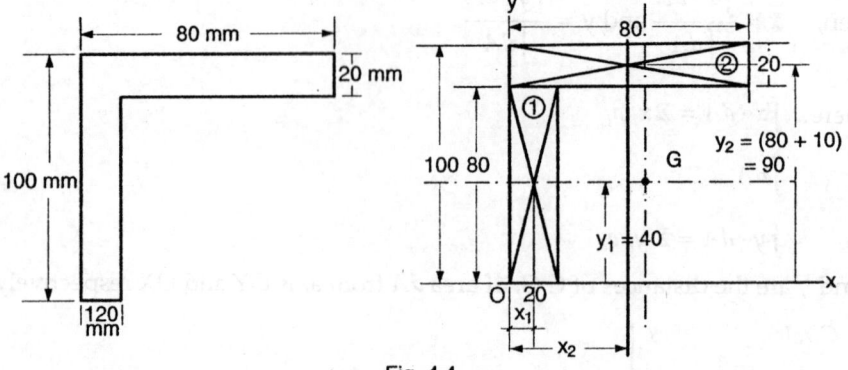

Fig. 4.4

SOLUTION Divide the composite lamina in two parts to get the desired $(\bar{x}; \bar{y})$.

$$\bar{x} = \left(\frac{a_1 x_1 + a_2 x_2}{a_1 + a_2} \right)$$

$$= \frac{(80 \times 20) \times 10 + (80 \times 20) \times 40}{80 \times 20 + 80 \times 20}$$

$$= \frac{16000 + 64000}{3200}$$

$$= \frac{\overset{25}{\cancel{80000}}}{\underset{2}{\cancel{3200}}}$$

$$\bar{x} = 25 \text{ mm}$$

$$\bar{y} = \left(\frac{a_1 y_1 + a_2 y_2}{a_1 + a_2} \right)$$

$$= \frac{1600 \times 40 + 1600 \times 90}{3200}$$

$$= \frac{64000 + 144000}{3200} = 65 \text{ mm} \quad \therefore \quad \left. \begin{array}{l} \bar{x} = 25 \text{ mm} \\ \bar{y} = 65 \text{ mm} \end{array} \right] \quad \textbf{Ans.}$$

4.7 CENTROID FOR PLANE LAMINA

(a) *A triangular lamina:*

$$\text{Area} = \left[\frac{1}{2} \times b \times h \right]$$

Distance of centroid from the base $= \left(\dfrac{h}{3} \right)$

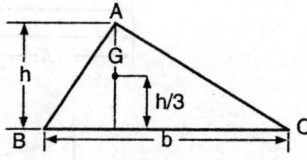

Fig. 4.5

(b) *Circle:*

$$\text{Area} = \frac{\pi d^2}{4}$$

Centroid is at the centre of the circle.

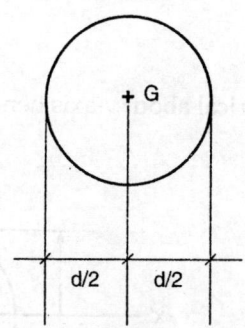

Fig. 4.6

(c) Square:

Area = a^2

Centroid at $\left(\dfrac{a}{2}\right)$ from each side.

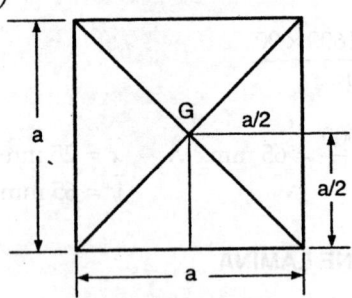

Fig. 4.7

(d) Rectangle:

Area = $L \times B$

Centroid at $\dfrac{L}{2}$ and $\dfrac{B}{2}$

i.e. $\bar{x} = \dfrac{L}{2}$

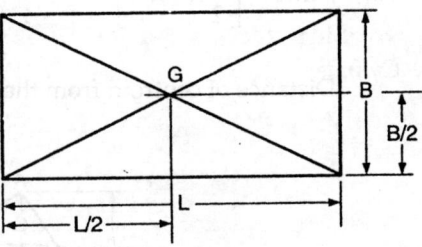

Fig. 4.8

and $\bar{y} = \dfrac{B}{2}$

(e) Trapezium:

Area = $\dfrac{1}{2} \times h \times (a + b)$

$\bar{x} = \left(\dfrac{a + 2b}{a + b}\right) \cdot \dfrac{h}{3}$

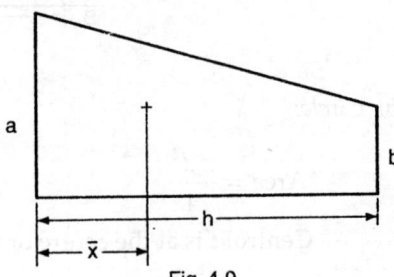

Fig. 4.9

(f) Semi-circle:

Semi-circle is symmetrical about y-axis hence $\bar{x} = 0$

$A = \dfrac{1}{2} \pi r^2$

$\bar{y} = \dfrac{4r}{3\pi}$ from AB

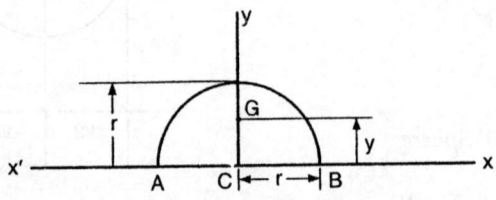

Fig. 4.10

(g) *Quadrant of Circle:*

$$A = \frac{1}{4}\pi r^2$$

$$\bar{x} = \frac{4r}{3\pi} = \bar{y}$$

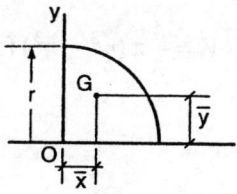

Fig. 4.11

4.8 C.G. FOR SOLID BODIES

(a) *Rod:*

$$V = \frac{\pi d^2}{4} \cdot L$$

$$\bar{x} = \left(\frac{L}{2}\right)$$

$$\bar{y} = 0$$

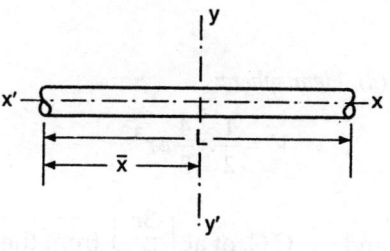

Fig. 4.12

Since, the rod is symmetrical about x-axis.

(b) *Cylinder:*

$$V = \pi r^2 h$$

$$= \frac{\pi D^2 h}{4}$$

$$\bar{y} = \frac{h}{2}$$

Since, the cylinder is symmetrical about y-axis, therefore, $\bar{x} = 0$

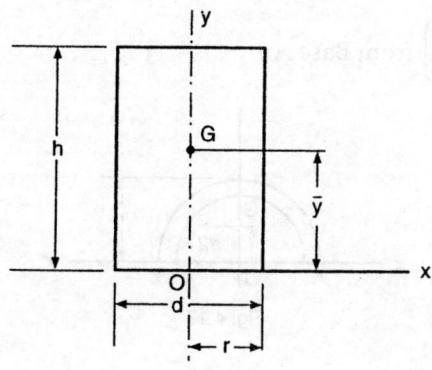

Fig. 4.13

(c) *Sphere:*

$$V = \frac{4}{3}\pi r^3 \text{ for solid sphere}$$

$$V = \frac{4}{3}\pi(r_0{}^3 - r_i{}^3) \text{ for hollow sphere C.G. at center}$$

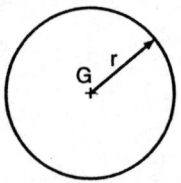

Fig. 4.14

(d) *Hemisphere:*

$$V = \frac{1}{2} \times \frac{4}{3}\pi r^3$$

and   C.G. of at $\left(\dfrac{3r}{8}\right)$ from the base

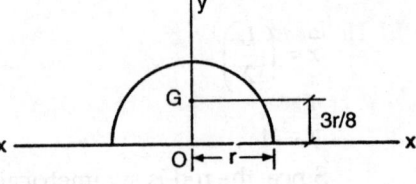

Fig. 4.15

∴ $\bar{y} = \left(\dfrac{3r}{8}\right)$

(e) *Quadrant of Sphere:*

$$V = \frac{1}{4} \times \frac{4}{3}\pi r^2$$

$$\text{C.G.}(\bar{x}, \bar{y}) = \left(\frac{3r}{8}; \frac{3r}{8}\right)$$

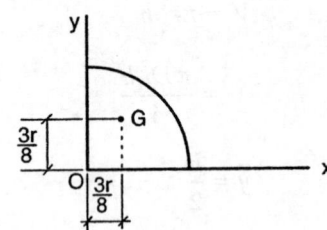

Fig. 4.16

(f) *Hollow hemisphere*

$$\text{C.G. is at } \left(\frac{r}{2}\right) \text{ from Base } AB$$

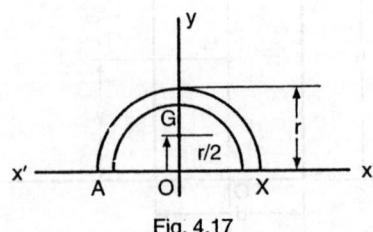

Fig. 4.17

(g) *Solid Cone:*

$$V = \frac{1}{3}\pi r^2 h$$

C. G at $\left(\dfrac{h}{4}\right)$ from the base.

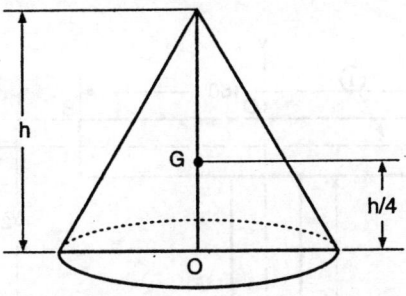

Fig. 4.18

(h) Hollow cone:

C.G. in at $\left(\dfrac{h}{3}\right)$ from base.

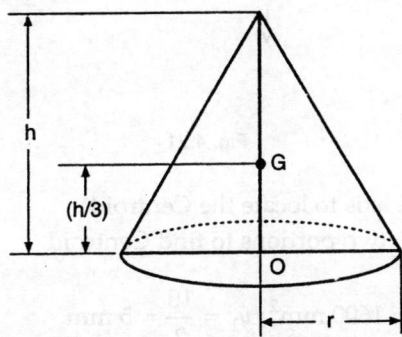

Fig. 4.19

EXAMPLE 1 *Determine the Centroid of the T-section shown in Fig. 4.20.*

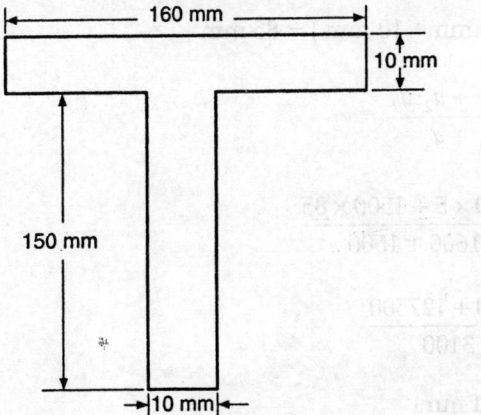

Fig. 4.20

SOLUTION Due to symmetry of the section, its Centroid lies at G on the y-axis i.e. $\bar{x} = 0$.

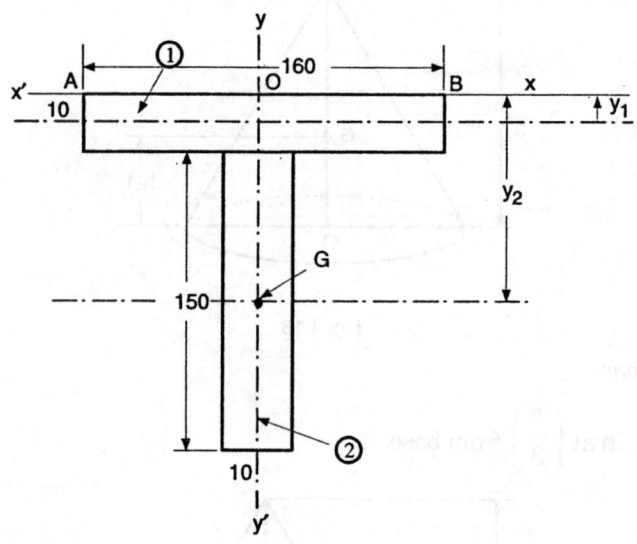

Fig. 4.21

Let *AB* as the reference axis to locate the Centroid.
Dividing *T*-section into two portions to find Centroid.

$$a_1 = 160 \times 10 = 1600 \text{ mm}^2; y_1 = \frac{10}{2} = 5 \text{ mm}$$

$$a_2 = 150 \times 10 = 1500 \text{ mm}^2;$$

$$y_2 = (75 \text{ mm} + 10 \text{ mm}) = 85 \text{ mm}$$

$$\bar{y} = \frac{a_1\,y_1 + a_2\,y_2}{a_1 + a_2}$$

$$= \frac{1600 \times 5 + 1500 \times 85}{1600 + 1500}$$

$$= \frac{8000 + 127500}{3100}$$

$$= 43.71 \text{ mm}$$

Hence, Centroid of T-section lies on the y-axis ($\bar{x}$ = 0)
and at 43.71 mm from the top face of the section   **Ans.**

EXAMPLE 2 *Find the centroid of the I-section shown in given figure.*

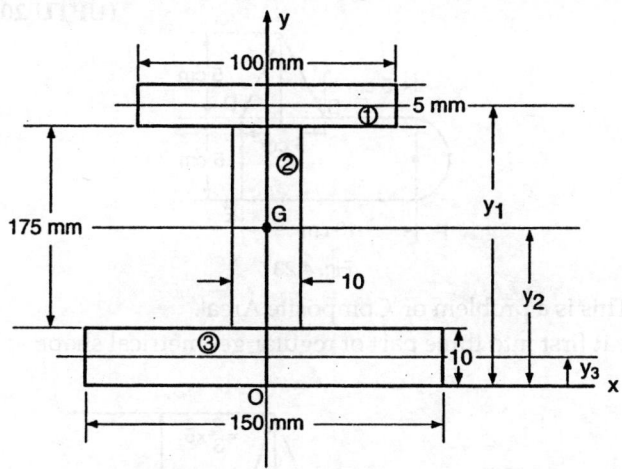

Fig. 4.22

SOLUTION Since, the section is symmetrical about y-axis. Hence, $\bar{x} = 0$. Therefore, only $\bar{y}$ should be calculated.

As discussed in Section 4.6, let us break the I-section into three rectangular parts.

Part	Area in (mm^2)	Distance of C.G. (in mm) from x-axis
Ist	$a_1 = 100 \times 5 = 500 \text{ mm}^2$	$y_1 = \left(10 + 175 + \dfrac{5}{2}\right) = 187.5 \text{ mm}$
IInd	$a_2 = 175 \times 10 = 1750 \text{ mm}^2$	$y_2 = \left(10 + \dfrac{175}{2}\right) = 97.5 \text{ mm}$
IIIrd	$a_3 = 150 \times 10 = 1500 \text{ mm}^2$	$y_3 = \dfrac{10}{2} = 5 \text{ mm}$

The y-coordinate of the centroid of the I-beam

$$\bar{y} = \frac{a_1\, y_1 + a_2\, y_2 + a_3\, y_3}{a_1 + a_2 + a_3}$$

$$= \frac{(500 \times 187.5) + (1750 \times 97.5) \times (1500 \times 5)}{500 + 1750 + 1500}$$

$$\bar{y} = 72.5 \text{ mm}$$

Hence, $\left. \begin{array}{l} \bar{x} = 0 \\ \bar{y} = 72.5 \ \text{mm} \end{array} \right]$ **Ans.**

EXAMPLE 3 *Determine the Centroid of the plane uniform lamina as shown in Figure.*

(UPTU 2001-02, 08-09)

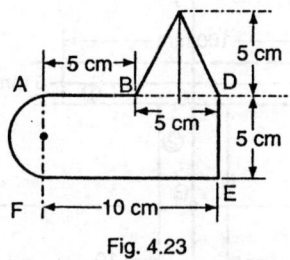

Fig. 4.23

SOLUTION   This is a problem of 'Composite Area'.

Let us divide it first into three part of regular geometrical shape as below:

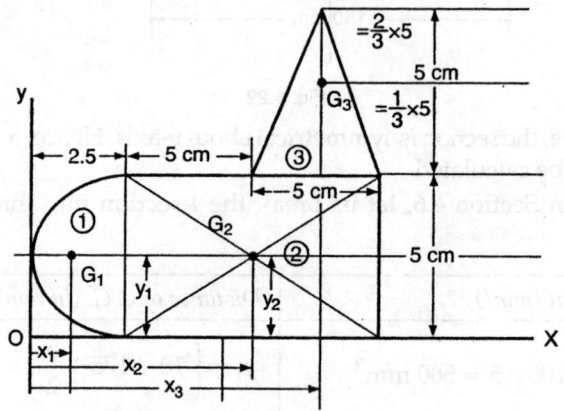

Fig. 4.24

For Portion 1   Area $(a_1) = \dfrac{\pi}{4} \times \dfrac{D^2}{2}$

$$= \dfrac{\pi}{4} \times \dfrac{4r^2}{2}$$

$$= \dfrac{\pi}{2} \times (2.5)^2$$

$$= 9.81 \text{ cm}^2$$

$x_1 = \left(2.5 - \dfrac{4r}{3\pi} \right)$

$ = \left(2.5 - \dfrac{4 \times 2.5}{3 \times 3.14} \right)$

$ = 1.44 \text{ cm}$

$$y_1 = \left(\frac{5}{2}\right) = 2.5 \text{ cm}$$

For Portion 2

$$\text{Area } (a_2) = 10 \times 5$$

$$= 50 \text{ cm}^2$$

$$y_2 = \left(\frac{5}{2}\right) = 2.5 \text{ cm} \; ; \; x_2 = 2.5 + \frac{10}{2} = 7.5 \text{ cm}$$

For Portion 3

$$\text{Area } (a_3) = \frac{1}{2} \times 5 \times 5 = 12.5 \text{ cm}^2$$

$$y_3 = \left(5 + \frac{5}{3}\right) = 6.66 \text{ cm}$$

$$x_3 = (2.5 + 5 + 2.5) = 10 \text{ cm}$$

$$\therefore \quad \bar{y} = \frac{a_1 y_1 + a_2 y_2 + a_3 y_3}{a_1 + a_2 + a_3}$$

$$= \frac{(9.81 \times 2.5) + (50 \times 2.5) + (12.5 \times 6.66)}{9.81 + 50 + 12.5}$$

$$\boxed{\bar{y} = 3.22 \text{ cm}} \quad \textbf{Ans.}$$

$$\bar{x} = \frac{a_1 x_1 + a_2 x_2 + a_3 x_3}{a_1 + a_2 + a_3}$$

$$= \frac{(9.81 \times 1.44) + (50 \times 7.5) + (12.5 \times 10)}{9.81 + 50 + 12.5}$$

$$= \frac{514.126}{72.31}$$

$$\boxed{\bar{x} = 7.11 \text{ cm}} \quad \textbf{Ans.}$$

4.9 CENTROID OF A SECTION WITH 'CUT OUT'

The centroid of a section with cut-out is found first then the cut-out section is subtracted to get the desired result.

If the area of the 'main section' and cut-out are a_1 and a_2 respectively and centroid distances are x_1, y_1 and x_2, y_2 from the reference lines then centroid of the remaining section is

$$\bar{x} = \frac{a_1 x_1 - a_2 x_2}{a_1 - a_2}$$

$$\text{and } \bar{y} = \frac{a_1 y_1 - a_2 y_2}{a_1 - a_2}$$

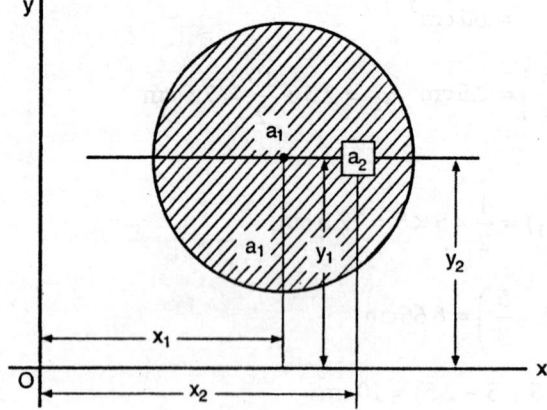

Fig. 4.25

EXAMPLE 1 *A square hole is punched out of a circular lamina, the diagonal of the square being the radius of the circle. Find the centroid of the remainder if r is the radius of circle.*

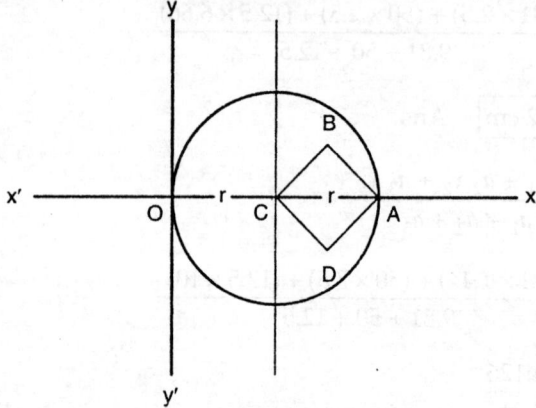

Fig. 4.26

SOLUTION As the given section is symmetric about OA, therefore, its centroid will be on diagonal OA.

Now, consider O as reference point (origin)

$$\bar{x} = \left(\frac{a_1 x_1 - a_2 x_2}{a_1 - a_2} \right)$$

$$a_1 = \pi r^2; x_1 = r$$

$$a_2 = \frac{r \times r}{2} = \frac{r^2}{2}; \, x_2 = r + \frac{r}{2}$$

$$\therefore \quad \overline{x} = \frac{\pi r^2 \times r - \left(\dfrac{r^2}{2} \times 1.5r \right)}{\pi r^2 - \dfrac{r^2}{2}}$$

$$\therefore \quad \overline{x} = 0.905 \, r$$
$$\text{and } \overline{y} = 0 \quad \bigg] \qquad \textbf{Ans.}$$

EXAMPLE 2 *Determine the centroid of the area of the circular sector OAB of radius r and central angle α as shown in figure.* **(M.T.U-2nd Semester 2011-12)**

SOLUTION Let us choose axes first,

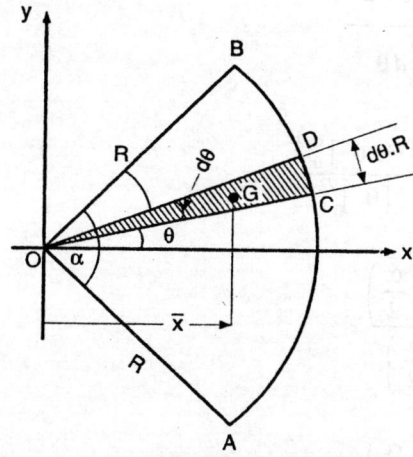

Fig. 4.27

The area *OAB* has been divided into large number of triangular element. The altitude of each is *R*

and   Base $= R \cdot d\theta$

Now, Area $(dA) = \dfrac{OC \times CD}{2}$ $\qquad \begin{bmatrix} CD = R \cdot d\theta \\ \because \theta = \dfrac{l}{R} \\ \therefore l = R\theta \end{bmatrix}$

$$= \frac{R \times R \, d\theta}{2}$$

$$x = OG \cos \theta$$

$$= \frac{2}{3} R \cos \theta$$

$$\bar{y} = \left(\frac{a_1\, y_1 + a_2\, y_2}{a_1 + a_2} \right) \qquad\qquad \left[OG = \frac{2}{3} R \right]$$

$$\bar{x} = \frac{\int x\, dA}{\int dA}$$

$$= \frac{2 \int_0^{\alpha/2} \frac{2}{3} R \cos\theta \cdot \left(\dfrac{R^2 d\theta}{2} \right)}{2 \int_0^{\alpha/2} \dfrac{R^2}{2} d\theta}$$

$$= \frac{\dfrac{R^3}{3} \int_0^{\alpha/2} \cos\theta\, d\theta}{\dfrac{R^2}{2} \int_0^{\alpha/2} d\theta}$$

$$= \frac{R^3}{3} \times \frac{2}{R^2} \frac{\left[\sin\theta \right]_0^{\alpha/2}}{\left[\theta \right]_0^{\alpha/2}}$$

$$= \frac{2R}{3} \cdot \frac{\sin\left(\dfrac{\alpha}{2} \right)}{\left(\dfrac{\alpha}{2} \right)}$$

$$= \frac{4R}{3\alpha} \cdot \sin\left(\frac{\alpha}{2} \right) \qquad \textbf{Ans.}$$

The area OAB is symmetrical about the x-axis, hence $\bar{y} = 0$.   **Ans.**

Special Cases:

(i) For a semi-circle, $\alpha = \pi = 180°$ hence

$$\bar{x} = \frac{4R}{3\pi} \cdot \sin\left(\frac{\pi}{2} \right)$$

$$= \frac{4R}{3\pi} \times \sin\left(\frac{180°}{2} \right)$$

$$= \frac{4R}{3\pi}$$

$$= 0.424\, R \ \ \textbf{Ans.}$$

(ii) For a quarter circle $\alpha = \dfrac{\pi}{2} = 90°$, Hence,

$$\bar{x} = \frac{4R}{3 \times \dfrac{\pi}{2}} \times \sin\left(\frac{\pi}{4}\right)$$

$$= \frac{8R}{3\pi} \times \frac{1}{\sqrt{2}}$$

$$= \frac{8R}{3 \times \dfrac{22}{7}} \times \frac{1}{\sqrt{2}}$$

$$= \frac{\overset{28}{56}R}{\underset{33}{66}} \times \frac{1}{\sqrt{2}}$$

$$= \frac{28^{14}}{33} R \times \frac{\sqrt{2}}{2}$$

$$= \frac{14\sqrt{2}}{33} R = \frac{14 \times 1.414}{33} = 0.599\,R$$

EXAMPLE 3 *Determine the centroid for the area bounded by the parabola* $y^2 = 4ax$ *and the line $x = 0$; $y = b$.*

SOLUTION Let us take a differential strip parallel to x-axis as shown in the given figure.

$$\therefore \qquad \bar{x} = \frac{\int x \cdot dA}{\int dA}$$

$$= \frac{\displaystyle\int_0^b \left(\frac{x}{2}\right) \cdot x\,dy}{\displaystyle\int_0^b x\,dy}$$

$$= \frac{\dfrac{1}{2}\displaystyle\int_0^b x^2 dy}{\displaystyle\int_0^b x\,dy}$$

$$= \frac{\dfrac{1}{2}\displaystyle\int_0^b (y^4/16a^2)\,dy}{\displaystyle\int_0^b (y^2/4a) \cdot dy}$$

$$= \frac{3b^2}{40a}$$

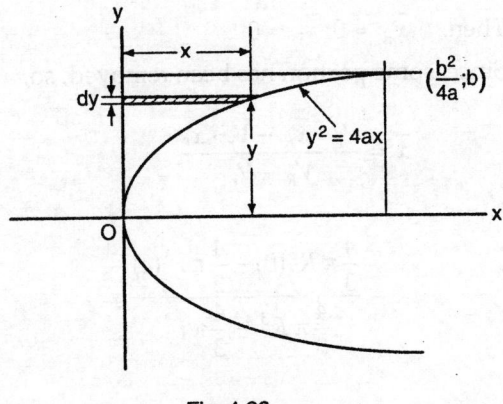

Fig. 4.28

In the same manner, $\bar{y} = \dfrac{\displaystyle\int_0^b y \cdot x\, dy}{\dfrac{b^3}{12a}}$

$$= \dfrac{\displaystyle\int_0^b (y^3/4a) \cdot dy}{\dfrac{b^3}{12a}}$$

$$= \dfrac{b^4/16a}{b^3/12a}$$

$$= \left(\dfrac{3}{4}\right) b$$

EXAMPLE 4 *A sphere of radius r is cut from a larger sphere of radius R. The distance between their centers is 'a'. Find the centroid of the remaining volume.*

SOLUTION Volume of larger sphere $V_R = \dfrac{4}{3}\pi R^3$

Volume of smaller sphere $V_r = \dfrac{4}{3}\pi r^3$

Let us assume that origin of the x, y and z axes is at the center of the larger sphere and positive x-axis is the line of centre of the two spheres.

Then, $\bar{x}_R = 0;\ \bar{x}_r = 0$

Since, some portion has been removed, so,

$$\bar{x} = \dfrac{V_R \cdot \bar{x}_R - V_r \cdot \bar{x}_r}{V_R - V_r}$$

$$= \dfrac{\dfrac{4}{3}\pi R^3(0) - \dfrac{4}{3}\pi r^3(a)}{\dfrac{4}{3}\pi R^3 - \dfrac{4}{3}\pi r^3}$$

$$= \dfrac{-ar^3}{R^3 - r^3}$$

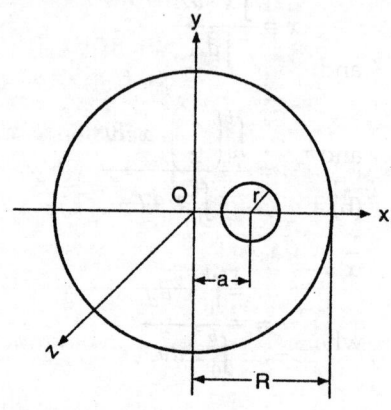

Fig. 4.29

.his follows that the centroid is on the line of centers and to the left the yz-plane at a distance of $\dfrac{ar^3}{(R^3 - r^3)}$.

HIGHLIGHTS

1. Centre of gravity of a body is the point through which the whole weight of the body acts.

2. Centroid is the point where the whole area of the lamina is assumed to be concentrated.

3. (a) Centroid of a composite figure *i.e.* a figure in which many shapes are integrated like below:

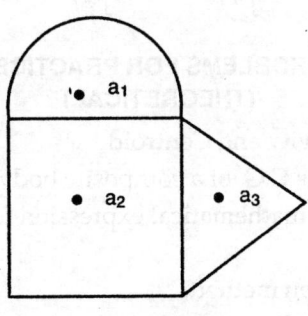

Fig. 4.30

$$\bar{x} = \frac{a_1 x_1 + a_2 x_2 + a_3 x_3 + \cdots}{a_1 + a_2 + a_3 + \cdots}$$

$$\bar{y} = \frac{a_1 y_1 + a_2 y_2 + a_3 y_3 + \cdots}{a_1 + a_2 + a_3 + \cdots}$$

where, $\bar{x}$ and $\bar{y}$ are the centroid of the body from the axis of reference.

$a_1, a_2, a_3 \cdots$ are areas of the section of body

and $x_1, x_2, x_3 \cdots$ are distance of the centroid of the areas $a_1, a_2, a_3 \cdots$ from y-axis

and $y_1, y_2, y_3 \cdots$ are distance of the centroid of the areas $a_1, a_2, a_3 \cdots$ from x-axis

(b) C.G. of Solid bodies:

$$\bar{x} = \frac{V_1 x_1 + V_2 x_2 + V_3 x_3 + \cdots}{V_1 + V_2 + V_3} \quad \text{and} \quad \bar{y} = \frac{V_1 y_1 + V_2 y_2 + V_3 y_3 + \cdots}{V_1 + V_2 + V_3}$$

where, $V_1, V_2, V_3 \cdots$ are volume of the solid bodies

and $\left. \begin{array}{c} x_1, x_2, x_3 \\ y_1, y_2, y_3 \end{array} \right]$ have the same meaning as above.

4. (a) Centroid of an area by integration is as below:

$$\bar{x} = \frac{\int x \cdot dA}{\int dA} \quad \text{and} \quad \bar{y} = \frac{\int y \cdot dA}{\int dA}$$

(b) Centroid of a curve line/straight line is given by

$$\bar{x} = \frac{\int x \cdot dL}{\int dL} \text{ and } \bar{y} = \frac{\int y \cdot dL}{\int dL}$$

(c) Centroid of volume

$$\bar{x} = \frac{\int x \cdot dV}{\int dV}; \ \bar{y} = \frac{\int y \cdot dV}{\int dV}; \ \bar{z} = \frac{\int z \cdot dV}{\int dV}$$

PROBLEMS FOR PRACTICE
(THEORETICAL)

1. Define Centre of Gravity and Centroid.
2. How will you find the C.G. of a composite body and C.G. of a remainder. Derive the necessary mathematical expression for the same.
3. Derive the C.G. of:
   (a) Area by integration method.
   (b) Straight or curved line by integration method.

(NUMERICAL)

1. Find the Centroid of L-section

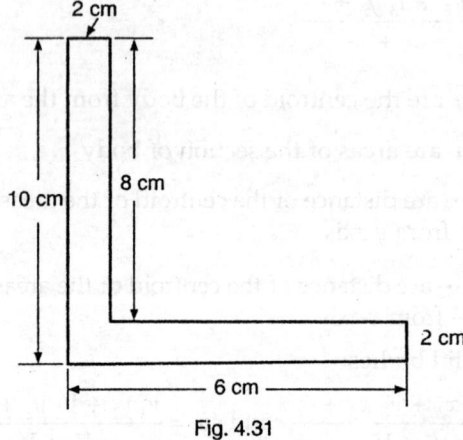

Fig. 4.31

2. Find the location of the centroid of the centreline of the weld pattern.

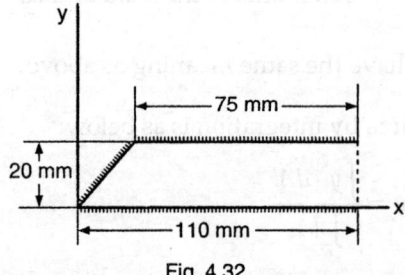

Fig. 4.32

3. The given figure shows the weld pattern on flat plate. Find location of the centroid of the centre length.

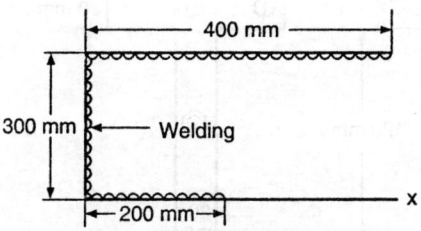

Fig. 4.33

4. A rectangular hole of 3 cm × 5 cm is cut from a rectangular lamina of 10 cm × 14 cm. Find the centroid of the remainder lamina.

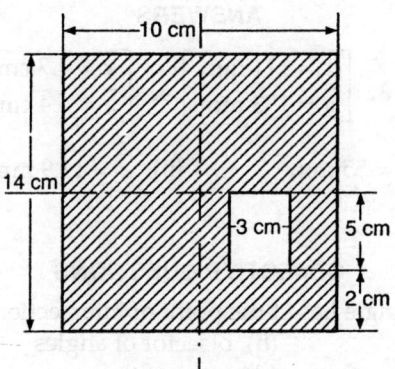

Fig. 4.34

5. Locate the centroid of the following figure with respect to the axes shown in the Figures 4.35 (a) and (b).

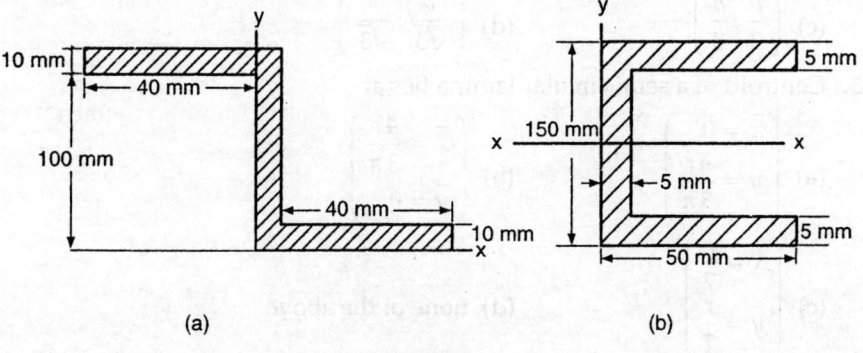

(a)　　　　　　　　　　　　　　　(b)

Fig. 4.35

6. Find the centroid of the *I*-section shown in Fig. 4.36.

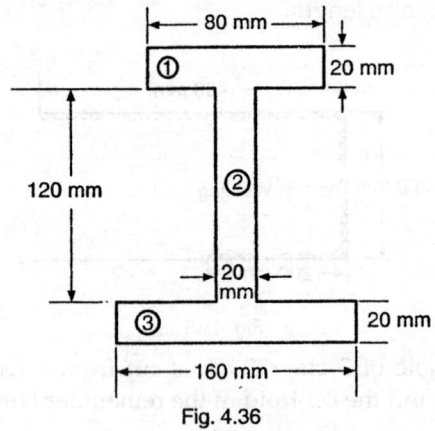

Fig. 4.36

ANSWERS

2. $\begin{bmatrix} \bar{x} = 54.1 \text{ mm} \\ \bar{y} = 8.45 \text{ mm} \end{bmatrix}$ 3. $\begin{bmatrix} \bar{x} = 111 \text{ mm} \\ \bar{y} = 183 \text{ mm} \end{bmatrix}$ 4. $\begin{bmatrix} \bar{x} = 4.7 \text{ cm} \\ \bar{y} = 6.4 \text{ cm} \end{bmatrix}$

5. (a) $\bar{x} = 5$ mm; $\bar{y} = 55$ mm (b) $\bar{x} = 11.9$ mm; $\bar{y} = 0$

6. $\bar{y} = 6.44$ mm

OBJECTIVE QUESTIONS

1. Centroid of a triangle lies at the point of intersection of
   (a) altitude (b) bisector of angles
   (c) median (d) none of these
2. The centroid of a right angled triangle with base '*b*' and height '*h*' is

   (a) $\left(\dfrac{2}{\sqrt{3}} h; \dfrac{1}{\sqrt{3}} b \right)$ (b) $\left(\dfrac{b}{h}; \dfrac{h}{2} \right)$

   (c) $\left(\dfrac{b}{3}; \dfrac{h}{3} \right)$ (d) $\left(\dfrac{b}{\sqrt{3}}; \dfrac{h}{\sqrt{3}} \right)$

3. Centroid of a semi circular lamina lies at

   (a) $\begin{pmatrix} \bar{x} = 0 \\ \bar{y} = \dfrac{4r}{3\pi} \end{pmatrix}$ (b) $\begin{pmatrix} \bar{x} = \dfrac{4r}{3\pi} \\ \bar{y} = 0 \end{pmatrix}$

   (c) $\begin{pmatrix} \bar{x} = \dfrac{r}{2} \\ \bar{y} = \dfrac{r}{2} \end{pmatrix}$ (d) none of the above

ANSWERS

1. (c)   2. (c)   3. (a)

— ❖❖ —

MOMENT OF INERTIA

5.1 INTRODUCTION

In the study of 'Strength of Material' we come across 'moment of inertia' in various chapters.

'Moment of Inertia' is an indication of the stiffness of a beam *i.e.* resistance to deflection when subjected to load. More is the moment of inertia more stiffer is the beam.

The deflection of beam is inversely proportional to the moment of inertia.

5.2 DEFINTION OF MOMENT OF INERTIA (M.I.)

The mathematical definition of moment of inertia $I = \int r^2 dA$, known as moment of inertia of area. The above mathematical form of moment of inertia indicates that an area is divided into small parts such as dA and each area is multiplied by the square of the distance (*i.e.* r^2) from the reference axis.

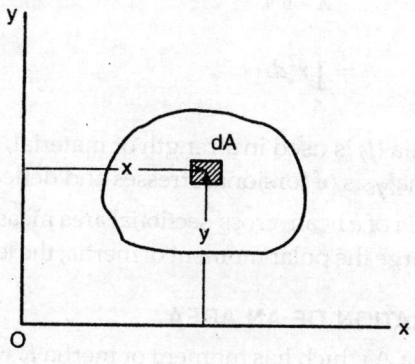

Fig. 5.1

In the Fig. 5.1 if the coordinates of the differential area dA is (x, y) the moment of inertia about x-axis is I_{XX} or $I_x = \int y^2\, dA$

and,   Moment of inertia about y-axis is or $I_y = \int x^2 dA$

The above M.I. of area is sometimes called the second moment of area (Area have no Inertia).

The unit of M.I. for any machine parts or structure is expressed in mm⁴.

The sign of I depends on the sign of area. A positive area is that area which adds to the area of figure and a negative area is one that reduces the area of figure. .

N.B. For a net area the moment of inertia must always be positive.

5.3 POLAR MOMENT OF INERTIA OF A PLANE AREA

If the area moment of inertia $I_x = \sum_i y_i^2\, A_i$ and $I_y = \sum_i x_i^2 A_i$ are added the result is

$$I_x + I_y = \sum_i (x_i^2 + y_i^2) \cdot A_i$$

From the Fig. 5.2 it may been observed that

$$x_i^2 + y_i^2 = r_i^2$$

where, r_i is the distance from the area element to the origin of the coordinates.

The polar moment of inertia J is defined as

$$J = \sum_i r_i^2 \cdot A_i$$

$$= (I_x + I_y)$$

The reference axis for J is an axis that is perpendicular to the xy-plane and acts through the origin of these coordinates.

The integral form will be $J = \lim_{A_i \to 0} \sum_i r_i^2\, dA$

$$= \int_A r^2 dA$$

Polar moment of inertia (J) is used in strength of material; mechanics where this form is used for the analysis of torsional stresses and deflection of shafts.

Polar moment of Inertia of a beam cross-sectional area measures the beams ability to resist torsion. The large the polar moment of inertia, the less the beam will twist.

5.4 RADIUS OF GYRATION OF AN AREA

Let us consider an area A which has moment of inertia I_x w.r.t. x-axis.

Let us consider this area A to be concentrated into thin strip parallel to x-axis.

If this area (concentrated strip) have the same M.I. (I_x) with respect to x-axis, the strip should be placed at a distance K_x from the x-axis and we have, $I_x = K_x^2 \cdot A$

$$\therefore \qquad K_x = \sqrt{\frac{I_x}{A}}$$

K_x is known as 'radius of gryration' with respect to x-axis.

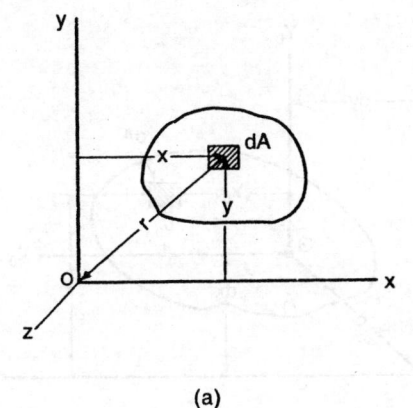

(a)

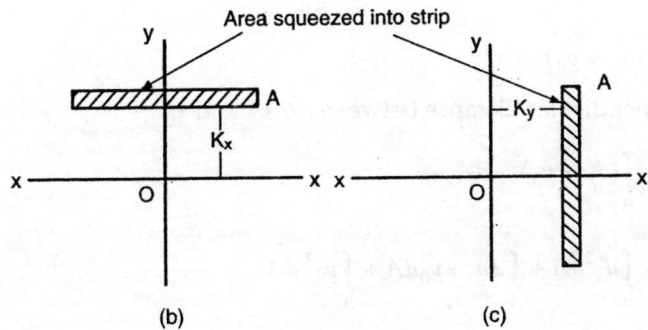

Fig. 5.2

Similarly, radius of gyration with respect to the y-axis.

$$K_y = \sqrt{\frac{I_y}{A}}$$

"The radius of gyration K is the effective distance where the entire area may be considered to be located with respect to the axis of rotation".

5.5 PARALLEL AXIS THEOREM (DISPLACEMENT OF THE AXIS PARALLEL TO ITSELF)

Let X, Y be the rectangular coordinates axes through any point 'O' in the plane of area A.

Let X_0, Y_0 be the corresponding parallel axes through the centroid G of the area. The area through the centroid of an area is also called the centroidal axes.

M.I. of the area 'A' about x-axis

$$I_X = \int y^2 dA$$

where, dA is an element at a distance 'y' from x-axis.

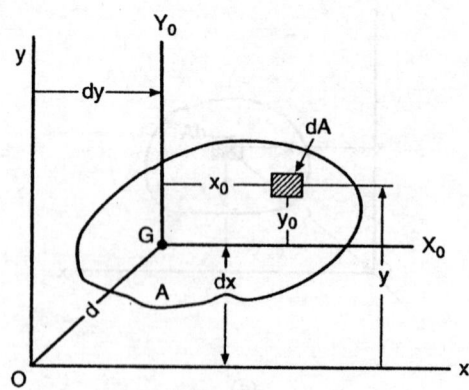

Fig. 5.3

But, $y = (d_x + y_0)$

d_x being perpendicular distance between axes x and x_0

$\therefore$ $I_x = \int_A (d_x + y_0)^2 \cdot dA$

$$= \int_A d_x^2 dA + \int_A 2d_x \cdot y_0 dA + \int_A y_0^2 \, dA$$

$$y_{OG} = \frac{\int_A y_0 \, dA}{A} = 0 \qquad\qquad \left[\begin{array}{l} x_0 \text{ and } y_0 \text{ pass through the} \\ \text{centroid of the area} \end{array} \right]$$

$$\int_A y_0 \, dA = 0$$

Hence, $I_x = d_x^2 \int_A dA + \int_A y_0^2 dA$

$$= A \cdot d_x^2 + I_{ox}$$

Similarly, $I_y = I_o y + A \cdot d^2 y$.

These two equations are called 'parallel axis' theorem or 'transfer theorem'.

5.6 THEOREM OF THE PERPENDICULAR AXIS

This theorem states that 'moment of inertia' of a lamina about an axis perpendicular to the plane of the lamina and passing through its C.G. is equal to the sum of the moment of interia of the lamina about two mutually perpendicular axes passing through its C.G.

Consider a lamina of area A. Let xx and yy be two mutually perpendicular axes being in the plane of the lamina passing through its centroid G.

zz is the axis which is perpendicular to the plane of the lamina passing through.G. *i.e.* through the point of intersection of xx and yy.

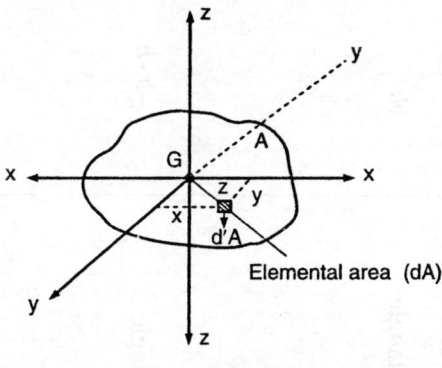

Fig. 5.4

Let an elementary area dA.

Let x, y and z are the perpendicular distances of the area dA from the respective axes.

$\therefore$ M.I. of the elementary area about zz axis $= dA \cdot z^2$

M.I. of the entire area about $zz = \Sigma dA \cdot z^2$

$$= \Sigma \, dA \, (x^2 + y^2)$$

$$= \Sigma \, dA \cdot x^2 + \Sigma \, dA \cdot y^2$$

$\therefore$ $I_{ZZ} = I_{YY} + I_{XX}$

5.7 MOMENT OF INERTIA OF PLANE FIGURES

S. No.	Figure	Description	Area	Moment of Inertia
1.		Rectangle	bh	$\left. \begin{aligned} I_{xx} &= \frac{bh^2}{12}; I_{X_1X_2} = \frac{bh^3}{12} \\ I_{yy} &= \frac{hb^2}{12}; I_{Y_1Y_2} = \frac{hb^3}{12} \\ J_G &= \frac{bh}{12}(b^2+h^2) \\ I_{p_1p_2} &= \frac{b^3h^3}{6(b^2+h^2)} \end{aligned} \right.$
2.		Triangle	$\dfrac{1}{2}b \cdot h$	$I_{xx} = \dfrac{bh^3}{36}; I_{X_1X_2} = \dfrac{bh^3}{12}$ $I_{yy} = \dfrac{hb^3}{48}$
3.		Right Angle Triangle	$\dfrac{1}{2}b \cdot h$	$I_{XX} = \dfrac{bh^3}{36}$ $I_{YY} = \dfrac{hb^3}{36}$

	Shape	Area	Moment of Inertia
4.	Circle	$\dfrac{\pi}{4}\cdot d^2$	$I_{xx} = \dfrac{\pi d^4}{64} = I_{yy}$ $J_G = \dfrac{\pi d^4}{32}$
5.	Ring	$\pi \cdot d \cdot t$	$I_{xx} = \dfrac{\pi t d^3}{8} = I_{yy}$ $J_G = \dfrac{\pi t d^2}{4}$
6.	Quarter circle	$\dfrac{\pi d^2}{16}$	$I_{xx} = 0.00344 d^4 = I_{yy}$ $I_{xx} = \pi\cdot\left(\dfrac{d}{4}\right)^4$
7.	Ellipse	πab	$I_{xy} = \dfrac{\pi a b^2}{4}$ $I_{yy} = \dfrac{\pi b a^2}{4}$ $J_G = \dfrac{\pi a b}{4}(a^2 + b^2)$

EXAMPLE 1 *Determine M.I. w.r.t xx and yy of the I-Beam shown in Figure.*

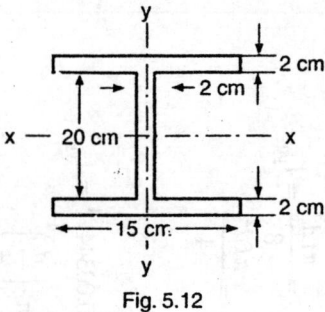

Fig. 5.12

SOLUTION We can solve this problem by various methods, let us discuss the method I.

Method I:

In this method, we will divide the I-beam into two parts flange (1) and web (2).

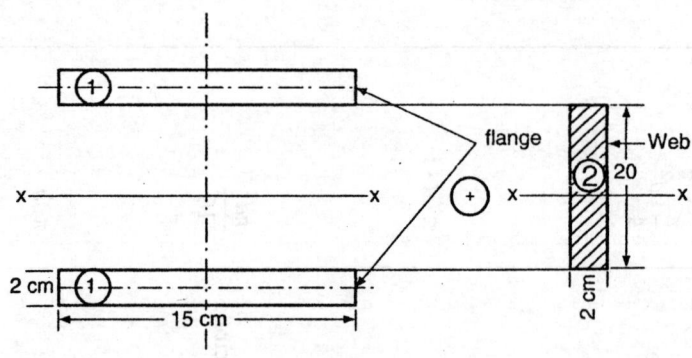

Fig. 5.13

i.e.   2 × moment of inertia of flange about x-x.

         +

Moment of inertia of web about xx.

$\therefore$ $I_{xx} = 2 \times \left[\dfrac{15 \times 2^3}{12} + (15 \times 2) \times 11^2 \right] + \dfrac{2 \times 20^3}{12}$

           $= 7280 \text{ cm}^4 + 1333 \text{ cm}^4$

           $= 8613 \text{ cm}^4$ **Ans.**

Method II:

In this method, we evaluate M.I. of the rectangle 15 × 24 and subtract the M.I. of the shaded rectangle.

Hence, $I_{xx} = \dfrac{15 \times 24^3}{12} - 2 \times \dfrac{6.5 \times 20^3}{12}$

           $= 8613 \text{ cm}^4$ **Ans.**

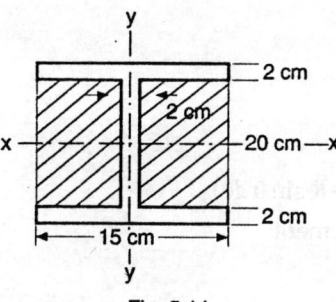

Fig. 5.14

Similarly, by method (I)

$I_{yy} = I_{yy}$ of web + I_{yy} of 2 flanges

$$= \frac{20 \times 2^3}{12} + 2 \times \left(\frac{2 \times 15^3}{12} \right)$$

$$= (13.3 + 1125) \, \text{cm}^4$$

$$= 1138.3 \, \text{cm}^4$$

N.B: (i) Method adopted in (I) can be used to find the M.I. of any composite body.

(ii) Method (II) is not suitable everywhere.

Students are advised to choose Method (I) to find the M.I. of any composite Area/Body. For non symmetrical section, first cg is computed then by applying parallel axis theorem, MOI about the desired axis can be known.

EXAMPLE 2 *Determine the moment of inertia of a 'circular area' about the centroidal axes.*

SOLUTION Consider an elementary strip at a distance 'y' from x-axis of thickness dy.

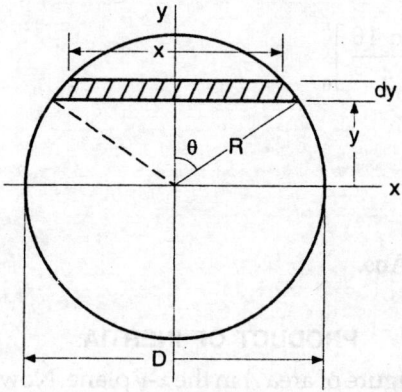

Fig. 5.15

Area of the element $= x \, dy$

But, $x = 2 (R \sin \theta)$

and $y = R \cos \theta$

$\therefore$ $dy = - R \sin \theta \, d\theta$

$dA = x \, dy$

$= 2 R \sin \theta \cdot (- R \sin \theta \, d\theta)$

Moment of Inertia of the element

$DI_x = \int y^2 dA$

$= \int (R \cos \theta)^2 \cdot (-2R^2 \sin^2 \theta \, d\theta)$

$\therefore$ $\overline{I_x} = \int d \, I_x$

$= \int_{\theta=-\pi}^{\theta=0} -2R^4 \cdot \cos^2 \theta \cdot \sin^2 \theta \, d\theta$

$= -2R^4 \int_{-\pi}^{0} \cos^2 \theta \cdot \sin^2 \theta \, d\theta$

$= 2R^4 \int_{0}^{\pi} \left(\frac{1 + \cos 2\theta}{2} \right) \cdot \left(\frac{1 - \cos 2\theta}{2} \right) d\theta$

$= \frac{R^4}{2} \int_{0}^{\pi} (1 - \cos^2 2\theta) \, d\theta$

$= \frac{R^4}{2} \int_{0}^{\pi} \left[1 - \left(\frac{1 + \cos 4\theta}{2} \right) \right] d\theta$

$= \frac{R^4}{2} \int_{0}^{\pi} (1 - \cos 4\theta) \, d\theta$

$= \frac{R^4}{4} \left[\theta - \frac{\sin 4\theta}{4} \right]_{0}^{\pi}$

$= \frac{\pi R^4}{4}$

$= \frac{\pi D^4}{64}$ **Ans.**

PRODUCT OF INERTIA

Let us consider a plane figure of area A in the x-y plane. Now, let us further divide the area into infinitesimal areas. Then product of inertia

$I_{xy} = \int_{A} xy \, dA$

Hence, product of Inertia is obtained by multiplying each element dA of the area A by its coordinates x and y and then inegrating over the entire area.

So, we observed that product of inertia

$$I_{xy} = \int_A xy \, dA$$

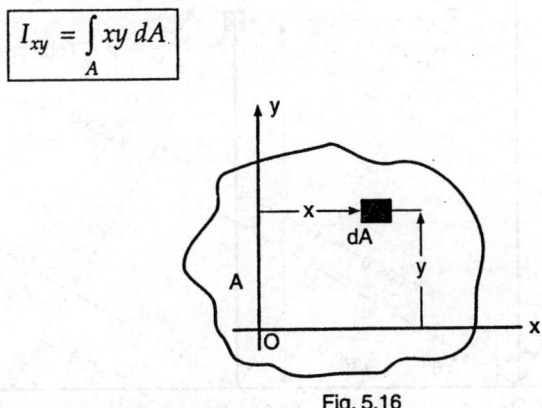

Fig. 5.16

It should be noted that

(i) Product of inertia (I_{xy}) for a positive area may be either positive or negative or zero depending upon distance x and y which could be positive, negative or zero.

(ii) Product of inertia (I_{xy}) is zero when either one or both of x and y axes are axis of symmetry.

For example, let us observe the section of a channel as shown below. We find that the given section of channel is symmetrical about x-axis so $I_{xy} = 0$ for the entire area.

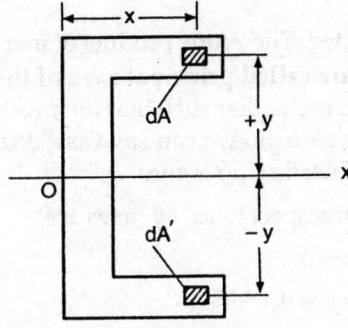

Fig. 5.17

$$\left[\begin{aligned} \text{Here, } I_{xy} &= \int (x)(y) \, dA + \int (x)(-y) \, dA' \\ &= 0 \end{aligned} \right] \qquad (\text{As } dA = dA' \text{ taken for analysis})$$

ROTATION OF AXES
PRINCIPAL AXES AND PRINCIPAL MOMENTS OF INERTIA

So far, we saw that for an area A and the coordinate axes ox and oy.

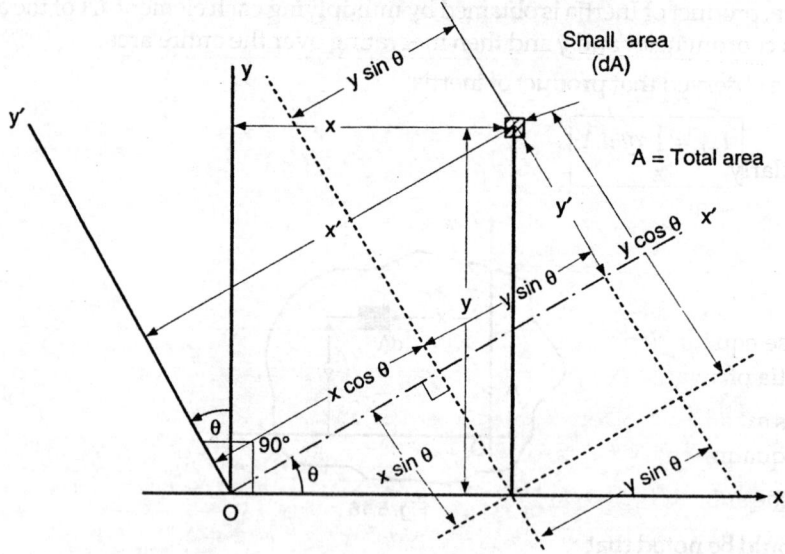

Fig. 5.18

$$I_{xx} = \int_A y^2 \, dA$$

$$I_{yy} = \int_A x^2 \, dA$$

$$I_{xy} = \int_A xy \, dA$$

Now, let the axes are rotated. Therefore, product of inertia will also change.

The axes after rotation are called principal axes of the area. The two principal axes are perpendicular to each other such that the product of inertia of the given area w.r. to these axes is zero. So we can say that "**Principal axes are the axes about which product of Inertia (I_{xy}) is zero**".

Now, the coordinate with respect to $ox'\, oy'$ axes are

$$x' = x\cos\theta + y\sin\theta$$

$$y' = -x\sin\theta + y\cos\theta$$

where, θ is the CCW rotation of the axes.

$$\therefore \quad I_{xx'} = \int_A (y')^2 \, dA$$

$$= \int_A (-x\sin\theta + y\cos\theta)^2 \, dA$$

$$= I_{yy}\sin^2\theta + I_{xx}\cos^2\theta - 2I_{xy}\sin\theta\cos\theta$$

$$= I_{yy}\cdot\left(\frac{1-\cos2\theta}{2}\right) + I_{xx}\left(\frac{1+\cos2\theta}{2}\right) - 2I_{xy}\sin\theta\cdot\cos\theta$$

$$= \left(\frac{I_{xx} + I_{yy}}{2}\right) + \left(\frac{I_{xx} - I_{yy}}{2}\right)\cos 2\theta - I_{xy}\sin 2\theta \qquad ...(1)$$

Similarly, $I_{yy'} = \left(\frac{I_{xx} + I_{yy}}{2}\right) + \left(\frac{I_{yy} - I_{xx}}{2}\right)\cos 2\theta + I_{xy}\sin 2\theta \qquad ...(2)$

and $\qquad I_{x'y'} = \frac{I_{xx} - I_{yy}}{2}\sin 2\theta + I_{xy}\cos 2\theta \qquad ...(3)$

These equations permits us to determine the moment of inertia and product of inertia of an area about any set of axes with an origin O.

Axes *ox'* and *oy'* corresponding to zero value of product of inertia can be obtained by equating eqn. (3) to zero.

Let the angle is denoted by θ_m.

∴ From each (3) equating it to zero

$$0 = \frac{I_x - I_y}{2}\sin 2\theta_m + I_{xy}\cos 2\theta_m$$

or $\qquad \boxed{\tan 2\theta_m = (-)\dfrac{2 I_{xy}}{I_x - I_y}} \qquad ...(4)$

Above expression can be used to find the direction of the principal axes through O.

This equation defines two values of $2\theta_m$ which are 180° apart. Thus, the values of θ_m are $\left(\dfrac{180}{2}\right)^{\circ} = 90°$ apart.

The moment of inertia about these axes are called 'principal moment of inertia' and are given by

$$I_{max} = \frac{I_x + I_y}{2} + \sqrt{\left(\frac{I_x - I_y}{2}\right)^2 + (I_{xy})^2} \qquad ...(5)$$

$$I_{min} = \frac{I_x + I_y}{2} - \sqrt{\left(\frac{I_x - I_y}{2}\right)^2 + (I_{xy})^2} \qquad ...(6)$$

The principal axes also represent the two axes for which moment of inertia are maximum and minimum.

Equations (1) to (6) are valid for any point located inside or outside the given area.

EXAMPLE 3 *Determine the product of inertia of a rectangular area about the x and y axis.*

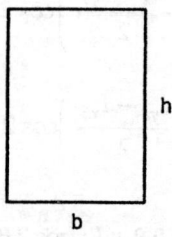

Fig. 5.19

SOLUTION Let us consider an element of thickness dy located at a distance y from the x-axis.

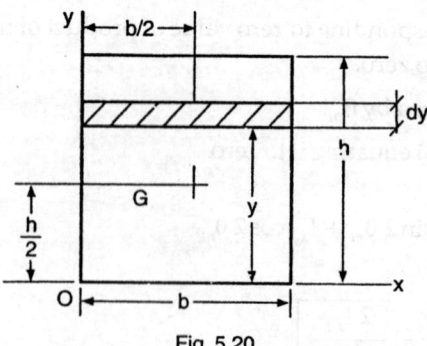

Fig. 5.20

Area of the element $= b \cdot dy$

$$dI_{xy} = (b \cdot dy) \cdot \frac{b}{2} \cdot y$$

$$\therefore \qquad I_{xy} = \int \frac{b^2}{2} \cdot y \cdot dy$$

$$= \frac{b^2}{2} \cdot \left[\frac{y^2}{2} \right]_0^h$$

$$= \frac{b^2 \cdot h^2}{4} \quad \textbf{Ans.}$$

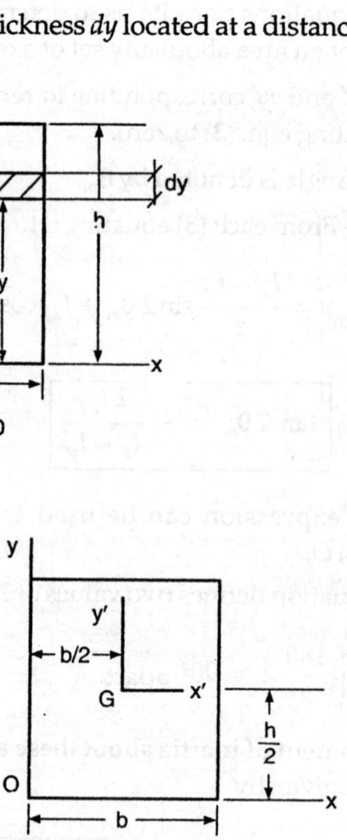

Fig. 5.21

We can solve it by applying parallel axes theorem also.

$$I_{xy} = I_{x'y'} + A \cdot \left(\frac{h}{2} \right) \cdot \left(\frac{b}{2} \right)$$

$I_{x'y'} = 0$; x' and y' being the axes of symmetry

$A = b \cdot h$

$$\therefore \qquad I_{xy} = 0 + b \cdot h \cdot \frac{hb}{4} = \frac{b^2 h^2}{4} \quad \textbf{Ans.}$$

EXAMPLE 4 *Determine the product of inertia (I_{xy}) of the L-section.*

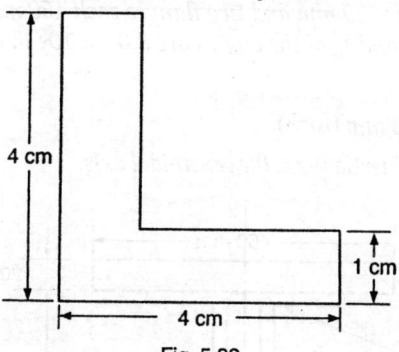

Fig. 5.22

SOLUTION Let us divide the L-section in two parts (1) and (2).

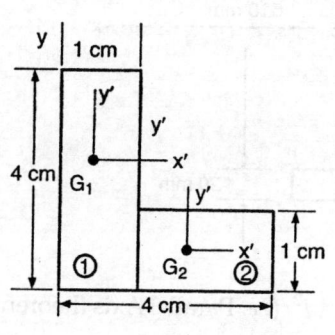   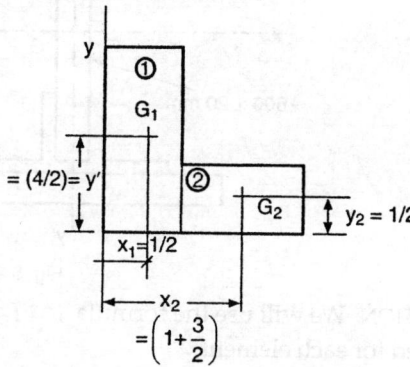

Fig. 5.23

Applying parallel axis theorem

For portion (1) $I_{xy} = I_{x'y'} + A_1 \cdot x_1\, y_1$

$$= 0 + (4 \times 1) \cdot \frac{1}{2} \cdot \frac{4}{2}$$

$$= 4 \text{ cm}^4 \qquad \left[\begin{array}{l} I_{x'y'} = 0 \text{ as } x' \text{ and } y' \text{ are} \\ \text{the axes of symmetry} \end{array} \right]$$

For portion (2) $I_{xy} = I_{x'y'} + A_2 \cdot x_2\, y_2$

$$= 0 + (3 \times 1) \cdot \left(1 + \frac{3}{2}\right) \cdot \frac{1}{2}$$

$$= 0 + 3 \times \frac{5}{2} \times \frac{1}{2} = \frac{15}{4} \text{ cm}^4 \qquad \left[\begin{array}{l} I_{x'y'} = 0 \text{ as } x' \text{ and } y' \text{ are} \\ \text{the axes of symmetry} \end{array} \right]$$

Hence, product of inertia (I_{xy}) of the total area.

$$I_{xy} = \left(4 + \frac{15}{4}\right) \text{cm}^4 = \left(\frac{31}{4}\right) \text{cm}^4 \textbf{ Ans.}$$

EXAMPLE 5 *A Girder is composed of four angles of size 150 × 150 × 3 mm and conneted to the web plate 600 mm × 20 mm and two flanges each 460 mm × 20 mm as shown in figure 5.24. In figure I_x and I_y of the angles are $8.05 × 10^6$ mm⁴ each; the area of angle = 3730 mm².*

$$\bar{x} \text{ and } \bar{y} = 42.3 \text{ mm (each).}$$

Evaluate the moment of inertia w.r.t. the centroidal axis.

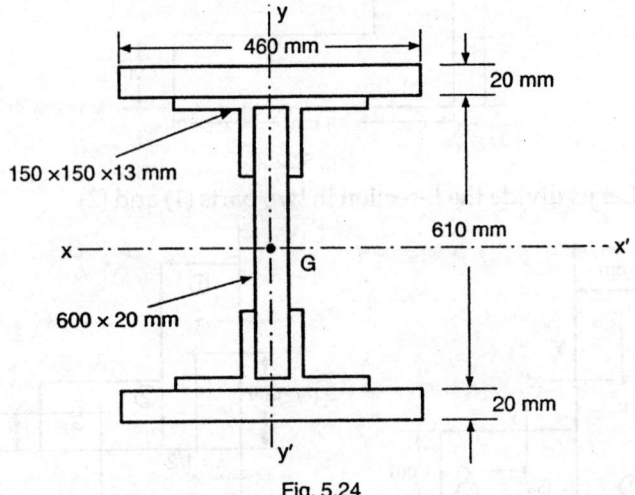

Fig. 5.24

SOLUTION We will use the formula $I = I_G + Ad^2$ (*i.e.* Parallel Axis theorem will be used for each element).

For web (plate) we have,

$$I_{web} = \frac{20 × (600)^3}{12} + (20 × 60) × (0)^2$$

$$= 360 × 10^6 \text{ mm}^4$$

For two numbers flange plates

$$I_{flange} = 2 \left[\frac{40 (20)^3}{12} + (460 × 20) (315)^2 \right]$$

$$= 1830 × 10^6 \text{ mm}^4$$

For four angles $I_{angle} = 4 \left[8.05 × 10^6 + 3730 (305 - 42.3)^2 \right]$

$$= 1060 × 10^6 \text{ mm}^4$$

$\therefore \qquad I_{Total} = I_{Web} + I_{flange} + I_{angle}$

$$= [360 + 1830 + 1060] 10^6$$

$$= 3250 × 10^6 \text{ mm}^4 \qquad \textbf{Ans.}$$

EXAMPLE 6 *For the z-section, the M.I. w.r.t x and y axes are given by* $I_x = 1548\ cm^4$ *and* $I_y = 2668\ cm^4$. *Evaluate the principle axes of the section about O and also find the values of the principal moment of inertia.*

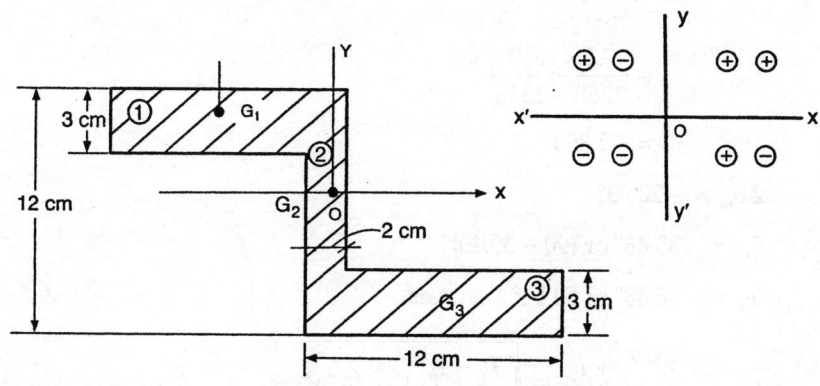

Fig. 5.25

SOLUTION Areas of z-section may be considered to be made up of three rectangles (1), (2) and (3) with their centroids at G_1, G_2 and G_3 respectively.

In rectangle (2) G_2 and O are coinciding.

Area = (cm)²	Distance of centroid from x and y axes	
	$\bar{x}$ (cm)	$\bar{y}$ (cm)
For portion (1) = 12 × 3 = 36	$\bar{x}_1 = -5$	$\bar{y}_1 = +4.5$
For portion (2) = 2 × 6 = 12	$\bar{x}_2 = 0$	$\bar{y}_2 = 0$
For portion (3) = 12 × 3 = 36	$\bar{x}_3 = +5$	$\bar{y}_3 = -4.5$

'Product of Inertia' of total z-section

$$I_{xy} = [\Sigma\ xy\ dA]$$

$$= 36 \times (-5)(4.5) + 0 + 36 \times (5)(-4.5)$$

$$= -1620\ cm^4$$

If x or y axes is the axis of symmetry then product of Inertia Vanishes.
It is given that

$$I_x = 1548\ cm^4$$

$$I_y = 2668\ cm^4$$

For the **direction of principal axes** applying formula,

$$\tan 2\,\theta_m = \frac{2I_{xy}}{I_y - I_x}$$

$$= \frac{-2 \times 1620}{2268 - 1548}$$

$$= -2.893$$

$$2\,\theta_m = -70.93°$$

$$\theta_m = -35.46° \text{ or } (90 - 35.46)°$$

$$\therefore \quad \theta_m = -35.46° \text{ or } 54.54° \qquad \textbf{Ans.}$$

$$I_{max,\, min} = \frac{I_x + I_y}{2} \pm \sqrt{\left(\frac{I_x - I_y}{2}\right)^2 + (I_{xy})^2}$$

$$= \frac{1548 + 2668}{2} \pm \sqrt{\left(\frac{1548 - 2668}{2}\right)^2 + (1620)^2}$$

$$= 2108 \pm 1714$$

$$\therefore \quad I_{max} = 2108 + 1714$$

$$= 3822 \text{ cm}^4 \quad \textbf{Ans.}$$

and $\quad I_{min} = 2108 - 1714$

$$= 394 \text{ cm}^4 \quad \textbf{Ans.}$$

I_{max} and I_{min} are the values of principal moment of Inertia.

5.8 MOMENT OF INERTIA OF MASS (REGID BODY)

M.I. of a system of particle about a line is given as $I = \Sigma m_i\, r_i^2$.

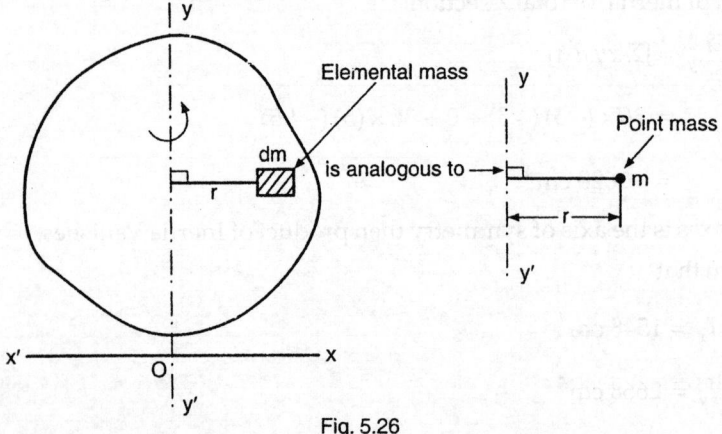

Fig. 5.26

The mass moment of inertia is a measure of resistance to the rotational acceleration of the mass of the body.

M.I. of the body in the above figure with respect to oy is defined as

$$I = \int r^2 dm$$

where dm = mass of the element of the body located at a distance r from the axis oy

The radius of gyration (k) of the body with respect to yy' is given by the relation

$$I = mk^2$$

$\therefore \qquad k = \sqrt{\dfrac{I}{m}}$ \hfill (Expressed in metre)

5.9 PARALLEL AXIS THEOREM

Let us consider a body of mass 'm'. Let the moment of inertia of the body w.r.t. axis YGY' passing through the centre of gravity G of the body be $\bar{I}$. Therefore, the moment of inertia (I) of the body with respect to the axis RS which is parallel to the centroidal axis YGY' and at a distance d from it is given by

$$I = \bar{I} + md^2$$

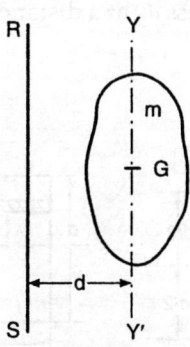

Fig. 5.27

(a) Mass M.I. of a uniform Rod about a perpendicular bisector

Consider a uniform rod of mass M and length l. I about AB is to be calculated. Take an element dx of the rod between distance x and $(x + dx)$ from the origin O.

Mass per unit length of the rod $= \dfrac{M}{l}$

So mass of the element $= \left(\dfrac{M}{l}\right) dx.$

M.I. of the element about AB, $dI = \left(\dfrac{M}{l}dx\right) \cdot x^2$

M.I. of the entire rod about AB,

$$I = \int_{-l/2}^{+l/2} \left(\frac{M}{l}\, dx \right) \cdot x^2$$

$$= \frac{2M}{l} \int_0^{l/2} x^2\, dx$$

$$= \frac{2M}{l} \left[\frac{x^3}{3} \right]_0^{l/2}$$

$$= \frac{\overset{1}{\cancel{2}} M}{3l} \times \frac{l^3}{\underset{4}{\cancel{8}}}$$

$$I = \frac{Ml^2}{12}$$

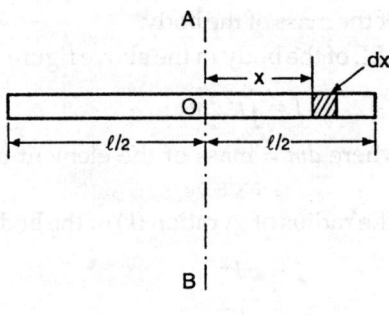

Fig. 5.28

(b) Mass M.I. of a rectangular plate about xx passing through the C.G. of plate

Let us take an element of thickness dy at a distance of y. From xx'. Hence, area of element $= b \cdot dy$.

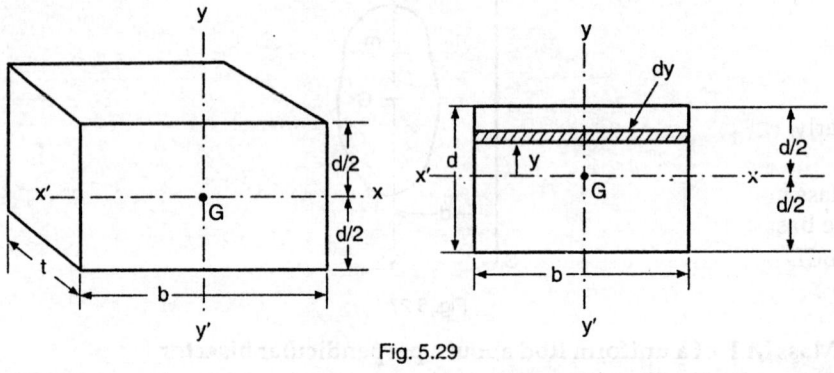

Fig. 5.29

Mass of the element $(dm) = \rho \times$ Volume of element

$$= \rho \times [b \times dy \times t]$$

$$= \rho \cdot b \cdot t\, dy \qquad \left[\begin{array}{l} \rho = \text{density of plate material} \\ \text{and } t = \text{thickness} \end{array} \right]$$

Mass moment of inertia of the element about xx-axis

$$= \text{Mass of the element} \times y^2$$

$$= (\rho \cdot b \cdot t\, dy) \times y^2$$

$$= \rho\, b\, t\, y^2 dy$$

Mass moment of inertia of the plate will be obtained by integrating

$\therefore \qquad (I_{xx})_{\text{mass}} = \int_{-d/2}^{d/2} \rho b t \, y^2 dy$

$\qquad\qquad\qquad = \rho b t \int_{-d/2}^{d/2} y^2 \cdot dy$

$\qquad\qquad\qquad = \rho b t \times 2 \int_0^{d/2} y^2 dy$

$\qquad\qquad\qquad = 2\rho b t \left[\dfrac{y^3}{3} \right]_0^{d/2}$

$\qquad\qquad\qquad = \dfrac{\cancel{2}\rho b t}{3} \times \dfrac{d^3}{\underset{4}{\cancel{8}}}$

$\qquad\qquad\qquad = \dfrac{\rho b t}{12} \times d^3$

$\qquad\qquad\qquad = \dfrac{b d^3}{12} \times \rho t$

$\therefore \qquad (I_{xx})_{\text{mass}} = (\rho b d t) \cdot \dfrac{d^2}{12}$

$\qquad\qquad\qquad = M \cdot \dfrac{d^2}{12}$

Similarly, $(I_{yy})_{\text{mass}} = M \cdot \dfrac{b^2}{12}$

(c) Mass moment of Inertia of the rectangular plate about line passing through the base

Let $ABCD$ be a rectangular plate having width $= b$

$\qquad\qquad\qquad\qquad\qquad\qquad\qquad$ thickness $= t$

and $\qquad\qquad\qquad\qquad\qquad\qquad$ depth $= d$

and $\qquad\qquad\qquad\qquad\qquad$ denisty of plate material $= \rho$

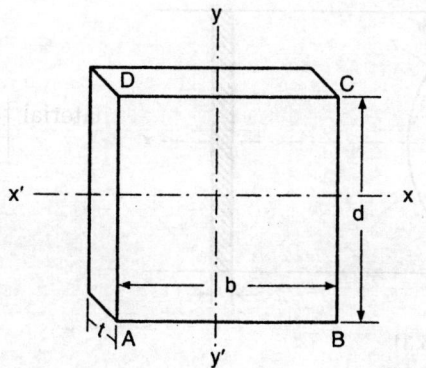
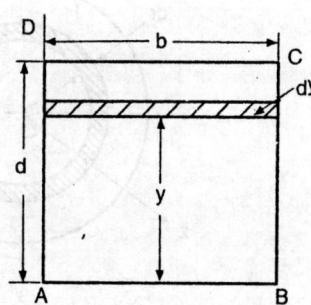

Fig. 5.30

Our aim is to find mass moment of inertia about AB.

Now,　　　　　Area of strip $(dA) = b.\,dy$

Volume of the strip $(dV) = dA \cdot t$

$$= b \cdot dy \cdot t$$

Mass of the strip (dm) = Density $\times$ Volume of strip

$$= \rho \cdot b \cdot t \cdot dy$$

Now, mass moment of inertia about AB

$$= \int y^2 dm$$

$$= \int_0^d y^2 \cdot \rho b t \, dy$$

$$= \int_0^d \rho b t \cdot y^2 dy$$

$$= \rho b t \int_0^d y^2 dy$$

$$= \rho b t \left[\frac{y^3}{3} \right]_0^d$$

$$= \frac{\rho b t}{3} \times d^3$$

$$= \frac{\rho b t d}{3} \times d^2$$

$$(I_{AB})_{\text{mass}} = \frac{M d^2}{3}$$

(d) Mass moment of Inertia of a circular plate

The figure shows a circular plate of radius R and thickness $'t'$

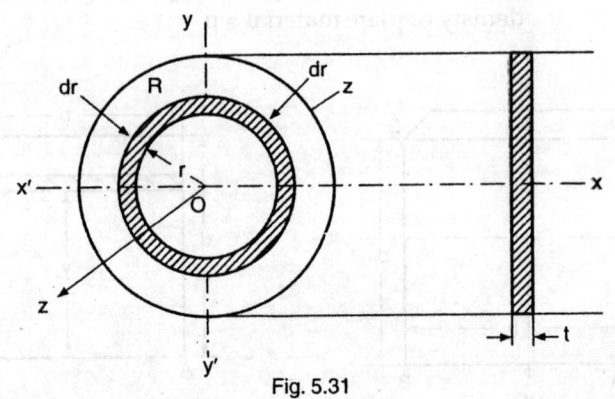

Fig. 5.31

To find M.I., let us consider an elementary circular ring of radius 'r' and width 'dr'.

Area of ring $(dA) = 2\pi r\,dr$

Volume of ring $(dV) = 2\pi r\,dr \cdot t$

Mass of ring $(dM) = \rho\,(2\pi r\,dr \cdot t)$

∴ Mass moment of inertia of the circularing about zz (which is ⊥, to plate)

$$= dM \times r^2$$

$$= \rho \cdot 2\pi r\,dr \cdot t \times r^2$$

$$= \rho \cdot t \cdot 2\pi r^3 dr$$

∴ Mass moment of inertia of the circular plate about zz-axis is given by

$$(I_{zz})_{mass} = \int_0^R \rho \cdot t \cdot 2\pi r^3 dr$$

$$= 2\pi\rho t \int_0^R r^3 dr$$

$$= 2\pi\rho \cdot t \left[\frac{r^4}{4}\right]_0^R$$

$$= \frac{2\pi\rho t}{4} \times R^4$$

$$= \pi\rho \cdot t \cdot \frac{R^2}{2}$$

$$= (\rho \times \pi R^2 \times t) \times \frac{R^2}{2}$$

∴ $$(I_{zz})_{mass} = \frac{MR^2}{2}$$

Now, $I_{zz} = I_{xx} + I_{yy}$, by perpendicular axis theorem

∴ $$I_{xx} = I_{yy} = \left(\frac{I_{zz}}{2}\right) \qquad (I_{xx} = I_{yy} \text{ due to symmetry})$$

$$= \frac{MR^2}{4}$$

(e) Mass Moment of Inertia of a Hollow Circular Cylinder

Let R_i = inside radius of cylinder

R_o = outside radius of cylinder

L = length

M = mass of cylinder

ρ = density of material of the cylinder

To achieve the desired goal, let us consider a circular ring of radius 'r' and width dr.

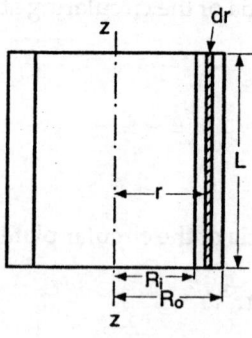

Fig. 5.32

Therefore, mass of the element $(dm) = \rho \times 2\pi r\, dr \cdot L$

M.I. of the circular ring about zz-axis = $(\rho \times 2\pi r\, dr \times L) \times r^2$

Hence, mass moment of inertia of the entire hollow circular cylinder will be obtained by integrating between R_i to R_o.

$\therefore \qquad (I_{zz})_{mass} = \int_{R_i}^{R_o} (\rho \times 2\pi r\, dr \times L) \cdot r^2$

$$= \rho 2\pi L \int_{R_i}^{R_o} r^3 dr$$

$$= 2\pi \rho L \left[\frac{r^4}{4} \right]_{R_i}^{R_o}$$

$$= \frac{2\pi \rho L}{4} \left[R_o^4 - R_i^4 \right]$$

$$= \frac{\pi \rho L}{2} (R_o^2 - R_i^2)(R_o^2 + R_i^2)$$

$$= \left[\rho \times \pi (R_o^2 - R_i^2) L \right] \times \frac{(R_o^2 + R_i^2)}{2}$$

$$= \frac{M \cdot (R_i^2 + R_o^2)}{2} \qquad \left[\begin{array}{l} \text{Mass of hollow cylinder} \\ = \rho \pi (R_o^2 - R_i^2) L \end{array} \right]$$

$\therefore \qquad (I_{xx})_{mass} = (I_{yy})_{mass} = \dfrac{I_{zz}}{2} = \dfrac{M (R_i^2 + R_o^2)}{4}$

Mass Moment of Inertia of Various Bodies

S. No.	Object	Moment of Inertia
1.	Slender Rod 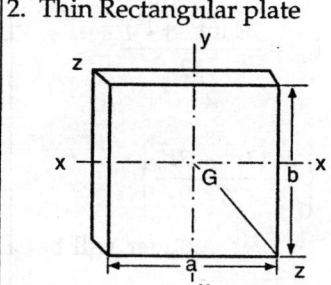	$I_{xx} = \dfrac{Ml^2}{12}; I_{yy} = 0$ $I_{x_1 x_2} = \dfrac{Ml^2}{3};$ $I_{zz} = I_{xx} + I_{yy}$ $= \dfrac{Ml^2}{12} + 0 = \dfrac{Ml^2}{12}$
2.	Thin Rectangular plate 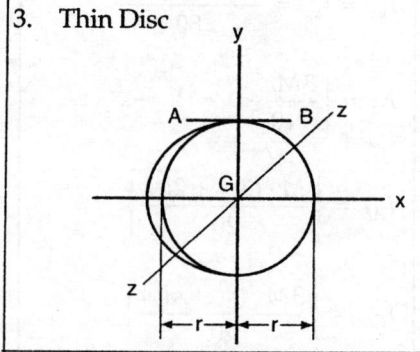	$I_{xx} = I_x = \dfrac{Mb^2}{12}$ $I_{yy} = I_y = \dfrac{Ma^2}{12}$ $I_{zz} = I_z = \dfrac{M(a^2 + b^2)}{12}$
3.	Thin Disc 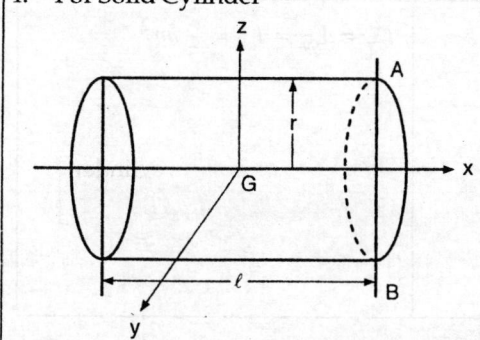	$I_{xx} = I_{yy} = \dfrac{Mr^2}{4}$ $I_z = 2I_{xx} = 2I_{yy}$ $= \dfrac{Mr^2}{2}$ $I_{AB} = \dfrac{3Mr^2}{2}$
4.	For Solid Cylinder	$I_{xx} = \dfrac{Mr^2}{2}$ $I_{yy} = I_{zz} = \dfrac{M(3r^2 + l^2)}{12}$ $I_{AB} = \dfrac{M(3r^2 + 4l^2)}{12}$

5. Thin hoop 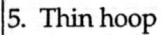 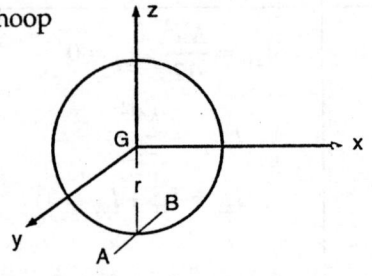	$I_{xx} = I_{zz} = \dfrac{M r^2}{2}$ $I_{yy} = Mr^2$ $I_{AB} = 2Mr^2$
6. For thin cylinderical sheet 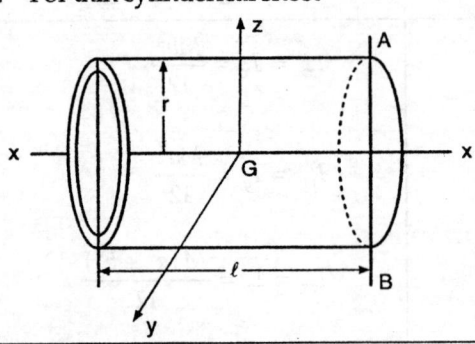	$I_{xx} = Mr^2$ $I_{yy} = I_{zz} = \dfrac{M(6r^2 + l^2)}{12}$ $I_{AB} = \left\{ \dfrac{M(3r^2 + 2l^2)}{6} \right\}$
7. Right Circular Cone 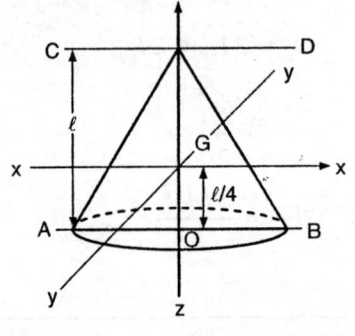	$I_{yy} = I_{xx} = \dfrac{3M(4r^2 + l^2)}{80}$ $I_{zz} = \left\{ \dfrac{3Mr^2}{10} \right\}$ $I_{AB} = \left\{ \dfrac{M \cdot (3r^2 + 2l^2)}{20} \right\}$ $I_{CD} = \left\{ \dfrac{3M \cdot (r^2 + 4l^2)}{20} \right\}$
8. Sphere 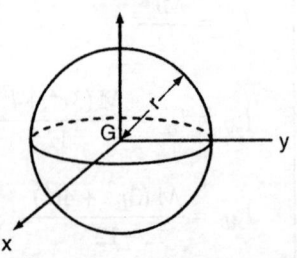	$I_{xx} = I_{yy} = I_{zz} = \dfrac{2}{5} mr^2$

9. Spherical sheet

$$I_{xx} = I_{yy} = I_{zz} = \frac{2}{3}mr^2$$

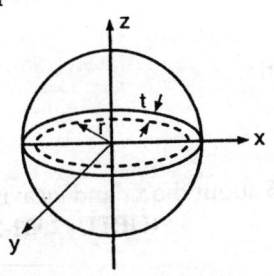

HIGHLIGHTS

1. Moment of Inertia of an area (or mass) about an axis is the product of area (or mass) and square of the distances of the C.G. of the area or mass from that axis.

   Mathematically

   $$I_{Area} = \int r^2 dA$$

   $$I_{mass} = \int r^2 dm$$

   what dA and dm are the elementary area and mass respectively.

2. Radius of gyration $(k) = \sqrt{\dfrac{I}{A}}$

   So, $k_{xx} = \sqrt{\dfrac{I_{xx}}{A}}$, $k_{yy} = \sqrt{\dfrac{I_{yy}}{A}}$

3. 'Perpendicular axis theorem' is $I_{zz} = I_{xx} + I_{yy}$ where I_{xx} and I_{yy} and I_{zz} are the M.I. along the x-axis, y and z-axis respectively.

4. Parallel axis theorem

   I about any arbitrary axis $= I_G + Ad^2$

   where, I_G = M.I. of the given area about an axis passing through C.G.

   d = distance of the arbitrary axis from C.G.

   A = Area of the section.

PROBLEMS FOR PRACTICE
(THEORETICAL)

1. Define Moment of Inertia.
2. Explain parallel axis theorem and perpendicular axis theorem.
3. Derive expression for M.O.I. of the following
   (i) Rectangular lamina

    (ii) Circular lamina

    (iii) Semi circular lamina

    (iv) Thin ring

  4. Define radius of gyration and product of inertia.

(NUMERICAL)

1. Find the moment of inertia of ISA $100 \times 75 \times 6$ about the xx and yy axis.

(UPTU- 2001-2002)

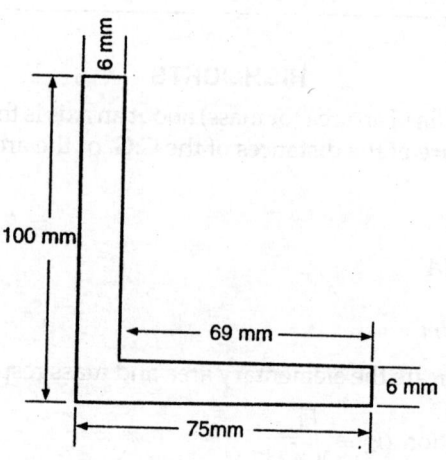

Fig. 5.42

2. Determine I_{xy} and $I_{xG . yG}$ for the angle section shown.

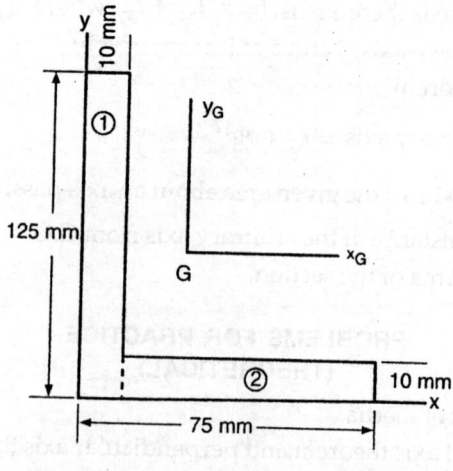

Fig. 5.43

3. Find the moment of inertia about the horizontal axis through the C.G. of the section shown in Fig. 5.44.

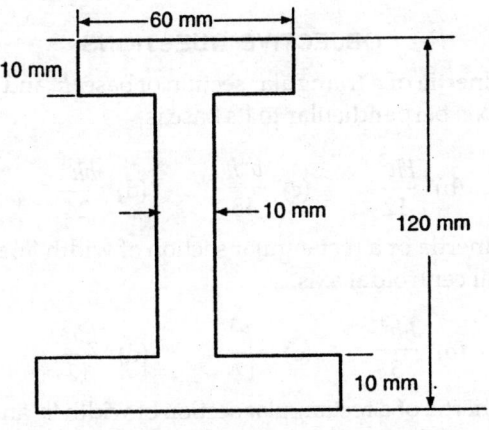

Fig. 5.44

4. For the angle shown in given figure, find:
   (i) I_{xx}
   (ii) I_{yy}
   (iii) Polar moment of inertia about an axis through G.
   (iv) Product of inertia about xx and yy axes.

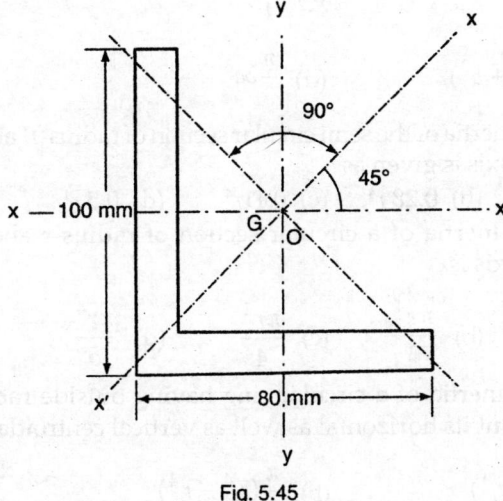

Fig. 5.45

ANSWERS

1. $\begin{bmatrix} I_{xx} = 1042.37 \times 10^3 \text{ mm}^4 \\ I_{yy} = 510.54 \times 10^3 \text{ mm}^4 \end{bmatrix}$

2. $\begin{bmatrix} I_{xx} = 52.8 \times 10^4 \text{ mm}^4 \\ I_{xG} \cdot y_G = -92 \times 10^4 \text{ mm}^4 \end{bmatrix}$

4. (i) 290.67 cm^4 (ii) 162.677 cm^4
   (iii) 453.334 cm^4 (iv) -120 cm^4

OBJECTIVE QUESTIONS

1. Moment of Inertia of a triangular section of base 'b' and height 'h' about the centroidal axis perpendicular to its base is

   (a) $\dfrac{bh^3}{36}$ (b) $\dfrac{bh^3}{12}$ (c) $\dfrac{b^3h}{48}$ (d) $\dfrac{bh^3}{24}$

2. Moment of Inertia or a rectangular section of width 'b' and height 'h' about its horizontal centroidal axis is

   (a) $\dfrac{bh^3}{3}$ (b) $\dfrac{hb^3}{3}$ (c) $\dfrac{bh^3}{12}$ (d) $\dfrac{hb^3}{12}$

3. Moment of Inertia of a rectangular section of width 'b' and depth 'd' about its vertical centroidal axis is

   (a) $\dfrac{bd^3}{12}$ (b) $\dfrac{db^3}{12}$ (c) $\dfrac{bd^3}{3}$ (d) $\dfrac{db^3}{3}$

4. Moment of inertia of an elliptical section with major axis '$2a$' and minor axis '$2b$' about its horizontal centroidal axis is given as

   (a) $\dfrac{\pi}{4}ba^3$ (b) $\dfrac{\pi}{4}ab^3$

   (c) $\dfrac{\pi ab}{4}(a^2 + b^2)$ (d) $\dfrac{\pi}{3}\,va^3$

5. Moment of inertia of the semi circular section of radius 'r' about its horizontal. Centroidal axis is given as
   (a) $0.35\, r^4$ (b) $0.28\, r^4$ (c) $0.11 r^4$ (d) $0.5\, r^4$

6. Moment of Inertia of a circular section of radius r about its horizontal centroidal axis is

   (a) $\dfrac{\pi r^4}{2}$ (b) $\dfrac{\pi r^4}{3}$ (c) $\dfrac{\pi r^4}{4}$ (d) $\dfrac{\pi r^4}{5}$

7. Moment of Inertia of a circular ring having outside radius r_o and inside radius r_i about its horizontal as well as vertical centroidal axis is

   (a) $\dfrac{\pi}{2}(r_0{}^4 - r_i{}^4)$ (b) $\dfrac{\pi}{4}(r_0{}^4 - r_i{}^4)$

   (c) $\dfrac{\pi}{3}(r_0{}^4 - r_i{}^4)$ (d) $\dfrac{\pi}{5}(r_0{}^4 - r_i{}^4)$

8. Moment of Inertia of a quadrant about its xx-axis is given by
   (a) $0.055\, r^4$ (b) $0.04\, r^4$ (c) $0.06\, r^4$ (d) r^4

9. The moment of inertia about a principal axis is called
   (a) mass moment of inertia

   (b) second moment of area

   (c) principal moment of inertia

   (d) none of the above

10. If the product of Inertia (I_{xy}) is zero then the two axes (x and y) are called

   (a) centroidal axes   (b) major and minor axes

   (c) principal axes   (d) none of the above

11. Moment of inertia of a triangle section of base 'b' and height 'h' about its base is

   (a) $\dfrac{bh^3}{12}$ (b) $\dfrac{bh^3}{24}$ (c) $\dfrac{bh^3}{36}$ (d) $\dfrac{bh^3}{48}$

ANSWERS

1. (c)	2. (c)	3. (b)	4. (b)	5. (c)	6. (c)
7. (b)	8. (a)	9. (c)	10. (c)	11. (a)	

— ❖❖ —

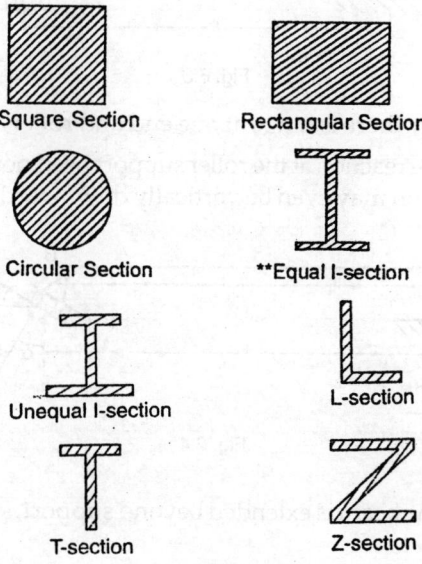

SHEARING FORCE AND BENDING MOMENT

6.1 WHAT IS BEAM

Beam is essentially a piece of structure which carries transverse loads, i.e. load perpendicular to it's axis. Transverse load causes bending and shear in the beam.

Beams are subjected to variety of loading pattern including normal concentrated loads, inclined concentrated loads; uniformly distributed loads, varying distributed loads; moments etc.

Beams are made up of non-metal, that is wood, concrete* or metal, i.e. steel, aluminium etc.

Beams may be of the following type section:

Square Section

Rectangular Section

Circular Section

**Equal I-section

Unequal I-section

L-section

T-section

Z-section

Fig. 6.1

The type of section depends upon the requirements of strength, stability etc.

---

*In concrete beam, the transverse reinforcement is used to prevent bending moment while vertical reinforcement is used to prevent the shear stresses caused due to loading.
**I-beam resist both bending and shear, that is why I-beam is preferred in most of the work of engineering.

Beam Support

Beams are classified according to the manner in which they are supported. The distance between two supports is called **Span** of the beam. If there is one support we write with the letter l or L and if there are more than one span we write $l_1, l_2, l_3,$ or L_1, L_2, L_3.

In the case of cantilever we take distance (l) between fixed end and free end. Beams are classified as follows:

Cantilever

A beam having one end fixed and other free is known as cantilever as shown in Fig. 6.2. Cantilever is fixed in a wall or column at one end and the other end is free.

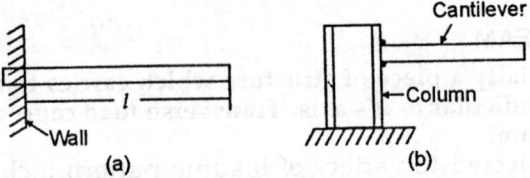

(a)   (b)

Fig. 6.2

Simply Supported beam

A beam resting freely on the supports at its both end is known as simply supported beam.

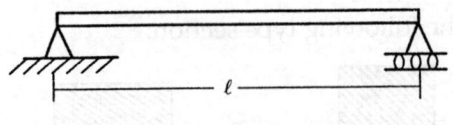

Fig. 6.3

In such beam normally there is hinge at one end and roller at the other end.

It may be noted that the reaction at the roller support need not be vertical but it may be inclined. The reaction may even be vertically downward also.

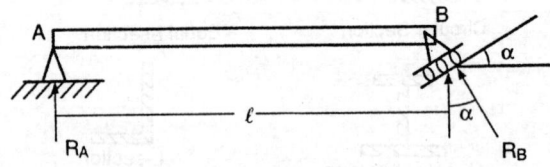

Fig. 6.4

Overhanging Beam

If the end portion of the beam is extended beyond support, such beam is known as overhanging beam.

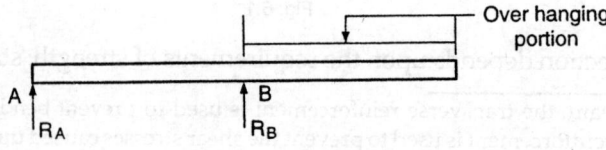

Fig. 6.5

Fixed Beam

A beam whose both ends are fixed or built in wall, is known as fixed beam.

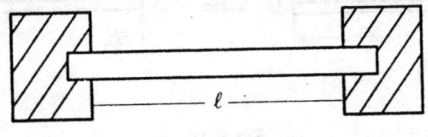

Fig. 6.6

Continuous Beam

A beam having more than two supports are known as continuous beam.

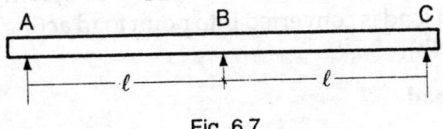

Fig. 6.7

Propped Cantilever Beam

When a support is provided at some suitable point of a cantilever beam in order to resist the deflection of the beam, it is known as propped cantilever beam.

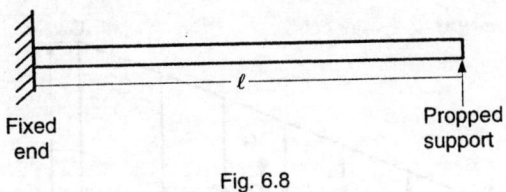

Fig. 6.8

6.2 TYPES OF LOAD

Beams are commonly loaded with the following four types of loads:

   (i) Concentrated or point load
  (ii) Uniformly distributed load
 (iii) Uniformly varying load
 (iv) Oblique load

Concentrated or Point Load (W)

A concentrated load is one which is considered to act at a point. The load is denoted by Newton (N) 'or' Kilo Newton (kN).

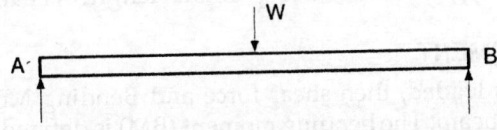

Fig. 6.9

Practically, point load cannot be placed on a beam. When a weight is kept on a beam, it covers some area (small). But for calculation purpose we consider it acting at a point.

Uniformly distributed load (w)

A uniformly distributed load is one which is spread over a beam in such a manner that rate of loading w is uniform along the length.

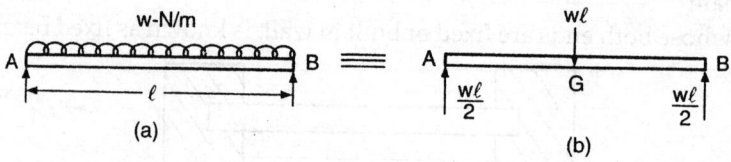

Fig. 6.10

The rate of loading is expressed as w N/m.

Uniformly distributed load is written as u.d.l. For solving problem the total uniformly distributed load is converted into point load acting at the centre of u.d.l. as shown in Fig. 6.10 (b).

Uniformly Varying load

A uniformly varying load is one which is spread over a beam in such a manner that rate of loading varies from point to point along the beam as shown in Fig. 6.11.

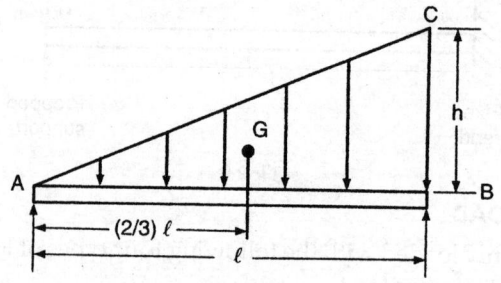

Fig. 6.11

Total load = Area of triangle ABC

$$= \frac{1}{2} \times l \times h$$

The total load is acting at a distance of $\frac{2}{3}$ of total length of beam from left end.

6.3 BENDING MOMENT

When the beam is loaded, then shear force and Bending Moment occurs at each section of the beam. The bending moment (BM) is defined as the algebraic sum of moments of the forces about the section taken on either side of the section.

6.4 SHEARING FORCE (F OR F_s)

The shearing force at a section of a beam is defined as the resultant transverse force acting on either side of the section and trying to shear the beam across the section.

For equilibrium, of the beam the resultant force on the two side of the section will be of equal magnitude and opposite in sense.

The shearing force at the section can therefore, be computed by taking the algebraic sum of all the transverse force acting on the beam either to the left or to the right of section.

A SFD (Shear Force Diagram) shows the variation of the shear force along the length of the beam.

6.5 PROCEDURE FOR DRAWING SFD AND BMD

1. Draw the load diagram showing all the load acting on the beam.
2. Put the left end of the beam at origin and its axis parallel to x-axis.
3. y-axis is perpendicular to x-axis.
*4. **Start from left side.** Find reaction force by applying $\Sigma F_y = 0$ and taking moment about any support will give you reaction at support.
5. Take an imaginary section at a distance x from origin.
   Find $F(x)$ then put the various value of x and get the profile of shear force. Similarly find $M(x)$. Put the various value of x to get the profile of moment diagram.

N.B: Students are advised to start the solution pertaining to SFD and BMD as per procedure to prevent mistakes completely.

6.6 SIGN CONVENTION

(i) The shear force at any point of a beam is positive when the external forces (loads and reactions) acting on the beam tend to shear off the beam at that point as shown in the figure.

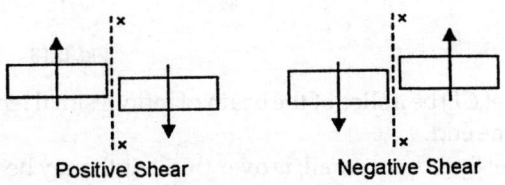

Positive Shear   Negative Shear

(ii) The positive values of shear force and B.M are plotted above the base line and negative value below the base line (*i.e.* x-axis).

(iii) The SFD will increase or decrease suddenly *i.e.* by a vertical straight line at section where there is a vertical point load.

(iv) The shear force between any two vertically load will be constant and hence the SFD between two vertical loads will be horizontal.

(v) The bending moment at the two supports of a simply supported beam and at free end of a cantilever is zero.

(vi) The point where the bending moment changes from sagging to hogging i.e. (+) to (−) is called **point of contraflexure.**

(vii) When the loads applied on the beam are not perpendicular to the axis of beam then loading is resolved axially and transversely to the beam. The

---

*In the case of cantilever start from the free end.

transverse component of load produces shear force and bending moment whereas axial component produces push or pull.

Sign convention for bending moment can also be determined in the following manner:

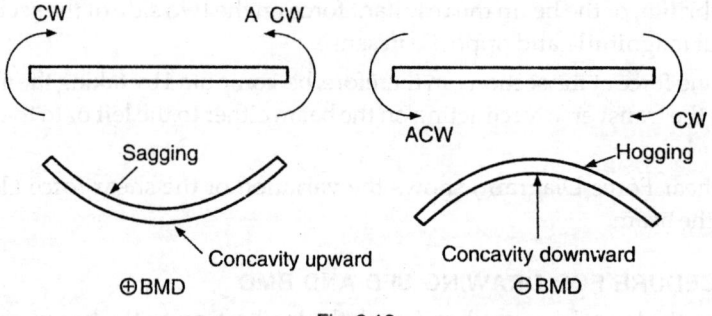

Fig. 6.12

6.7 RELATION BETWEEN *W*, *F* AND *M*

Let us consider a beam subjected to a load whose intensity per unit length w varies as a continuous function of x.

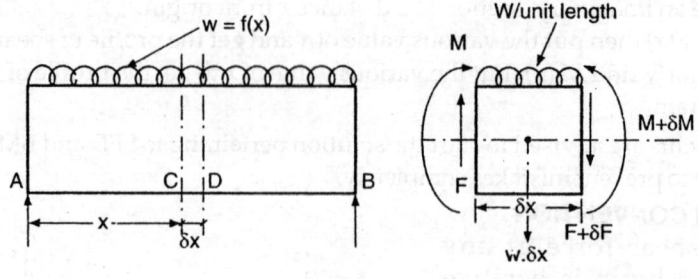

Fig. 6.13

Let CD be a slice of the beam of infinitesimal length δx, located at a distance x from one end.

As δx is very small, w over this length may be taken as constant.

For equilibrium of this beam slice, sum of the vertical forces and moment about any point say D has to be zero.

i.e. $\qquad F - w \cdot \delta x - (F + \delta F) = 0$ ...(1)

and $\qquad M + F \cdot \delta x - w \cdot \delta x \cdot \dfrac{\delta x}{2} - (M + \delta M) = 0$ ...(2)

From (1) $w = -\left(\dfrac{dF}{dx}\right)$ ...(3)

From (2) neglecting smaller term $\dfrac{w \cdot \delta x^2}{2}$

$\qquad F \cdot \delta x - \delta M = 0$

or, $F = \dfrac{\delta M}{\delta x}$

In the limit

$$F = \left(\dfrac{dM}{dx} \right)$$ ...(4)

Hence, the rate of change of B.M. is equal to the shear force.

It can be seen from eqn. (3) and (4) that if w is a continuous function of x, the shear force and bending moment can be determined by integration.

The constant of integration can be determined from the known conditions along the beam.

If w = constant i.e. the loading is uniformly distributed then integrating eqn. (3) and (4) gives.

$$F = -wx + A$$

and, $M = \int F \, dx$

$$= -w \cdot \dfrac{x^2}{2} + Ax + B$$

where A and B are constant of integration.

(i) For the portion of the beam carrying no load i.e. $w = 0$,

$$F = A$$

and $M = Ax + B$

(ii) For the portion of the beam where shear force is zero i.e. $F = 0$, integrating equation (4) gives

$$M = \text{constant}$$

(iii) The point where shear force changes sign through zero i.e. $F = 0$ we have from eqn. (4)

$$\dfrac{dM}{dx} = 0$$

which is the condition for M to be maximum or minimum.

N.B: It should be remembered that the above relations and conclusions are valid only when w is continuous function of x and there is no discontinuities like concentrated load.

6.8 EXAMPLES ON CONCENTRATED LOAD

EXAMPLE 1 *A cantilever of length 'l' carries a concentrated load W at its free end. Draw the S.F and B.M diagram.*

SOLUTION Let us take an imaginary section at a distance x from the free end and consider the origin in the left.

Hence shear force $F_x = -w$ and is constant along the whole length for all value of x.

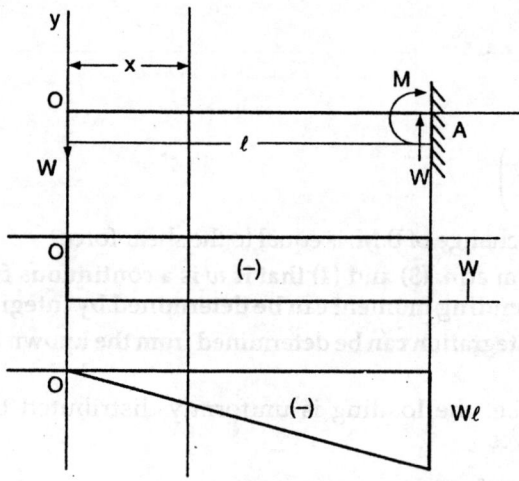

Fig. 6.14

B.M.

$$M_x = -Wx \qquad \text{(hogging)}$$

At $x = 0, M_o = 0$

At $x = l, M_A = -Wl$

EXAMPLE 2 *Simply supported beam subjected to Eccentric point load.*
SOLUTION We will determine reaction at support *i.e.* R_A and R_B.
Taking moment about B,

$$R_A \times l = W \times b$$

$$R_A = \left(\frac{W \cdot b}{l} \right)$$

Applying condition of **equilibrium** $\Sigma F_y = 0$, we get

$$R_A + R_B = W$$

$$R_B = W - R_A$$

$$= W - \frac{W_b}{l}$$

$$= W \left(\frac{L - b}{l} \right)$$

$$= \frac{W}{l} \times a$$

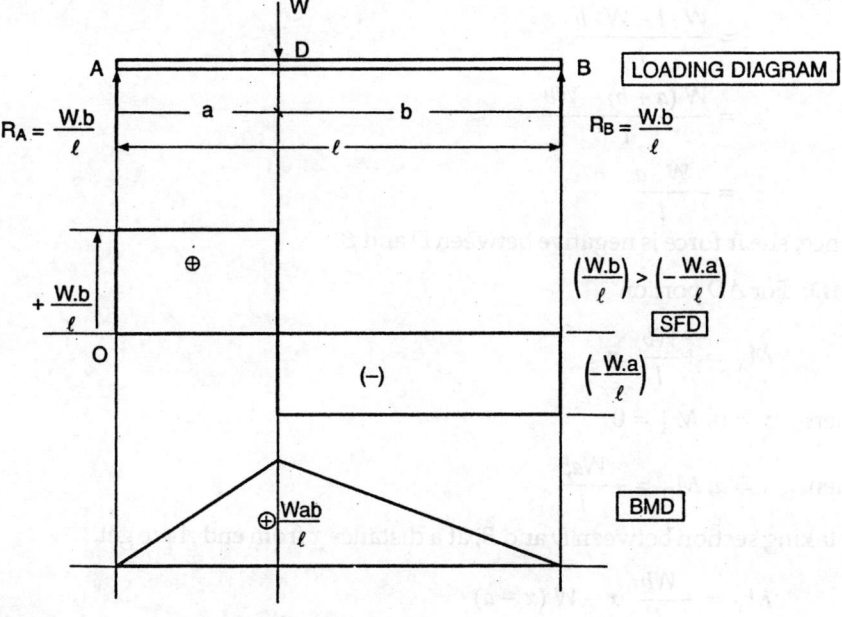

Fig. 6.15

SFD: For AD portion

Consider an imaginary section between A and D

$$F_X = + R_A = + \frac{Wb}{l}$$

Shear force is constant between A and D

Now, taking section between D and B, we get

$$F_x = R_A - W$$

$$= + \frac{W \cdot b}{l} - W$$

$$= \frac{Wb - WL}{l}$$

$$= \frac{W\cancel{b} - Wa - W\cancel{b}}{l}$$

$$= -\frac{W}{l} \cdot a.$$

$$R_B = W - R_A$$

$$= W - \frac{W \cdot b}{l}$$

$$= \frac{W \cdot l - W \cdot b}{l}$$

$$= \frac{W(a+b) - Wb}{l}$$

$$= -\frac{W \cdot a}{l}$$

Hence, shear force is negative between D and B.

BMD: For AD portion

$$M_X = +\frac{Wb}{l} \cdot x$$

when $x = 0, M_A = 0$

when $x = a; M_D = +\frac{Wab}{l}$

By taking section between D and B, at a distance x from end A we get,

$$M_X = +\frac{Wb}{l} \cdot x - W(x-a)$$

when $x = 0$ than $M_D = +\frac{Wab}{l}$

when $x = l$ then $M_B = +\frac{Wb\cancel{l}}{\cancel{l}} - W(l-a)$

$$= W \cdot \cancel{b} - W\cancel{b} = 0$$

EXAMPLE 3 *Simply supported beam with point load at mid of beam:*

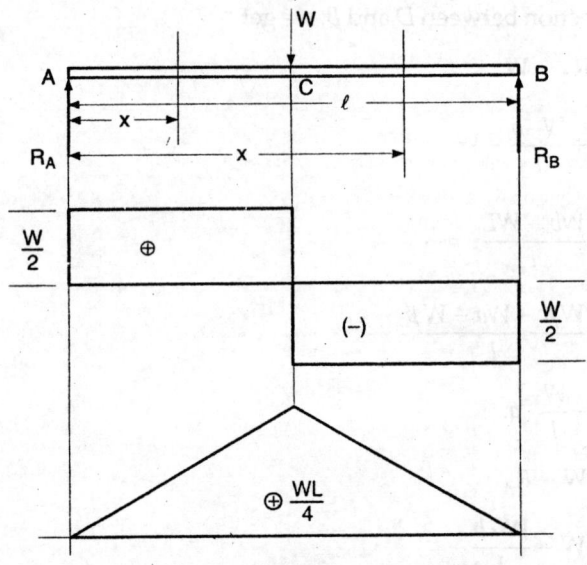

Fig. 6.16

SOLUTION First reaction force R_A and R_B are to be determined. By taking moments of all the forces about A we get,

$$R_B \times L = W \times \frac{l}{2}$$

$$R_B = \frac{W}{2}$$

Applying condition of equilibrium $\Sigma F_y = 0$ we get,

$$R_A + R_B = W$$

or, $$R_A = W - R_B$$

$$= W - \frac{W}{2}$$

$$= \left(\frac{W}{2} \right)$$

SFD: Between A and C

$$F_x = +\frac{W}{2}$$

Between C and B

$$F_x = R_A - W$$

$$= +\frac{W}{2} - W$$

$$= -\frac{W}{2} \text{ constant}$$

Hence, SF is constant between C and B having a value of $-\left(\dfrac{W}{2} \right)$.

BMD: Between A and C

$$M_X = +R_A \cdot x \qquad\qquad\qquad \text{(Sagging moment is +ve)}$$

$$= \frac{W}{2} \cdot x$$

when $x = 0, \ M_A = 0$

when $x = \dfrac{l}{2}; \ M_C = \dfrac{W}{2} \cdot \dfrac{l}{2}$

$$= \frac{Wl}{4}$$

By taking section between C and B at a distance x from A

$$M_X = +R_A x - W\left(x - \frac{l}{2}\right)$$

$$= +\frac{W}{2}x - W\left(x - \frac{l}{2}\right)$$

At $\quad x = \dfrac{l}{2}, M_C = +\dfrac{W}{2} \cdot \dfrac{l}{2} - W \cdot 0$

At $\quad x = l, M_C = +\dfrac{W}{2}l - W\left(l - \dfrac{l}{2}\right)$

$$= \frac{Wl}{2} - \frac{Wl}{2}$$

$$= 0$$

+ values of SFD and BMD are plotted above the base line.
− values of SFD and BMD are plotted below the base line.

EXAMPLE 4 *Cantilever subjected to UDL over it entire length:*

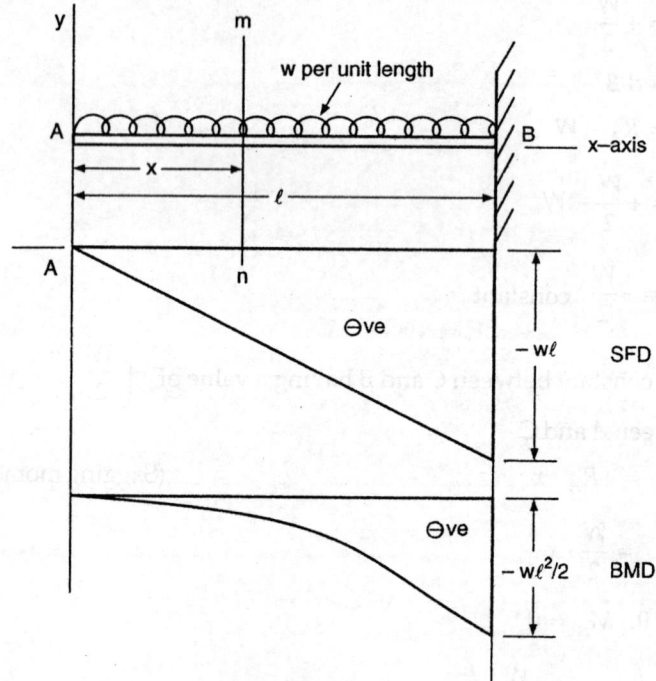

Fig. 6.17

SOLUTION Let us start from the left portion of beam. Let us take an imaginary section $m\,n$ at a distance x from A.

SFD: Then $F_x = -w \cdot x$ \qquad\qquad (hogging is occurring, so moment is −ve)

At $x = 0$ $F_A = 0$

At $x = 1$, $F_B = -w \cdot L$

Now, $M_X = -w \cdot x \cdot \dfrac{x}{2}$

$$= -\dfrac{wx^2}{2}$$

For $x = 0$, $M_A = 0$

For $x = 1$, $M_B = -\left(\dfrac{wl^2}{2} \right)$

EXAMPLE 5 *Cantilever subjected to uniformly Varying load :*

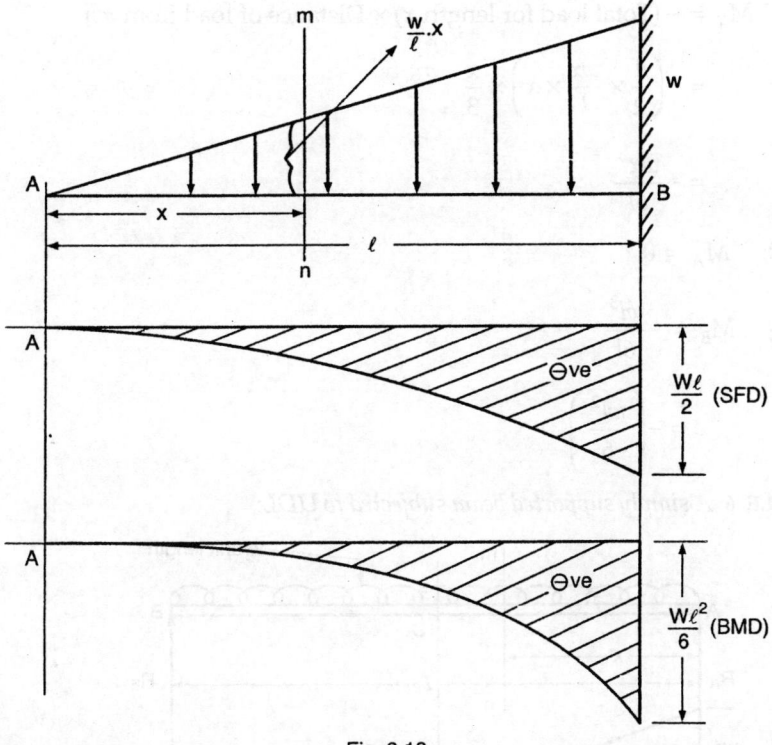

Fig. 6.18

N.B: In the case of 'cantilever' the imaginary section *mn*, should be taken from the free end as shown below.

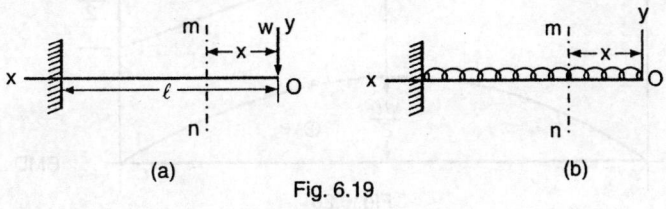

(a)   (b)

Fig. 6.19

SOLUTION As discussed before, let us take an imaginary section *mn*, at a distance *x* from origin (*O*) *i.e. A*.

then $\quad F_X = -\dfrac{1}{2} \cdot \dfrac{wx}{l} \cdot x$

$\qquad\quad = -\left(\dfrac{wx^2}{2l}\right)$

At $x = 0, \quad F_A = 0$

At $x = l, \quad F_B = -\dfrac{wl^2}{2l}$

At a distance *x* from free end

$\qquad M_X = -(\text{Total load for length } x) \times \text{Distance of load from } mn$

$\qquad\qquad = -\left(\dfrac{1}{2} \times \dfrac{wx}{l} \times x\right) \times \dfrac{x}{3}$

$\qquad\qquad = -\dfrac{wx^3}{6l}$

At $x = 0; \quad M_A = 0$

At $x = l; \quad M_B = -\dfrac{wl^3}{6l}$

$\qquad\qquad = -\left(\dfrac{wl^2}{6}\right)$

EXAMPLE 6 *A simply supported beam subjected to UDL:*

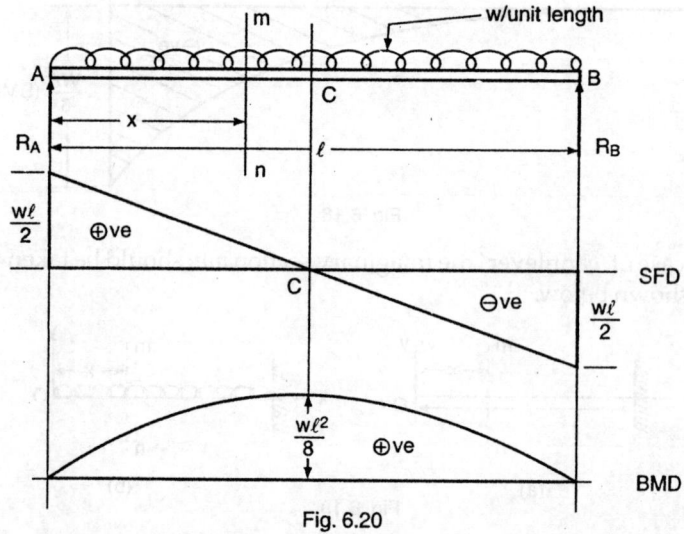

Fig. 6.20

SOLUTION By summertry $R_A = R_B = \dfrac{wl}{2}$

Shear Force

Let us consider a section of the beam at a distance x from A.

Then $\quad F_X = R_A - w \cdot x$

$$= \frac{wl}{2} - wx$$

At $x = 0$, $F_A = \dfrac{wl}{2}$

At $x = l$, $F_B = -\dfrac{wl}{2}$

Shear force (F_x) is zero at x value given by

$$0 = \frac{wl}{2} - wx$$

$$x = \frac{l}{2}$$

So for $x = \dfrac{l}{2}$, shear force = zero.

Hence, maximum B.M. will occur at this point.

Bending Moment

$$M_x = R_A \cdot x - (wx) \cdot \frac{x}{2}$$

$$= \frac{wl \cdot x}{2} - \frac{wx^2}{2}$$

At $x = 0$, $B.M = M_A = 0$

At $x = l$, $B.M = M_B = 0$

At $x = \dfrac{l}{2}$; $BM = M_C = \dfrac{wl}{2} \cdot \dfrac{l}{2} - \dfrac{w}{2} \cdot \left(\dfrac{l}{2} \right)^2$

$$= \frac{wl^2}{4} - \frac{wl^2}{8}$$

$\therefore \qquad M_C = \dfrac{2wl^2 - wl^2}{8} = \dfrac{wl^2}{8}$ **Ans.**

$$\boxed{\therefore M_{max} = \frac{wl^2}{8}}$$

EXAMPLE 7 *Draw the shear force and bending moment diagram for the beam as shown in Fig. 6.21.*

SOLUTION Support-Reaction at A and B:

Using $\Sigma M_A = 0$

$$R_B \times 4 = \frac{1}{2} \times 2 \times 3 \times \left(\frac{2}{3} \times 2 \right) + 2 \times 1 \times \left(3 + \frac{1}{2} \right)$$

$$= 4 + 2 \times \frac{7}{2}$$

$$= 11 \text{ kN}$$

$$R_B = \left(\frac{11}{4} \right) = 2.75 \text{ kN} \uparrow$$

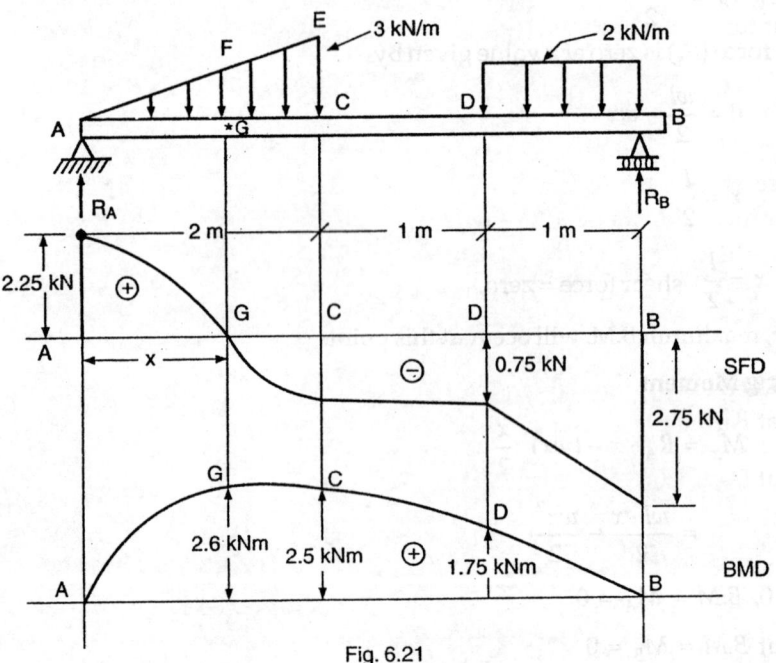

Fig. 6.21

Further, $R_A + R_B = \dfrac{1}{2} \times 2 \times 3 + 2 \times 1$

$$= 3 + 2 = 5 \text{ kN} \uparrow$$

$$R_A = 5 - R_B$$

$$= 5 - 2.75 = 2.25 \text{ kN} \uparrow$$

Calculation for Shear Force

SF at $A = R_A = 2.25 \text{ kN}$

To find rate of loading from similar triangles ACE and AGF.

---

*C.G. of portion AFG (acting here at $\dfrac{2}{3}x$ from A or $\dfrac{x}{3}$ from G)

$$\frac{AC}{EC} = \frac{AG}{FG}$$

$$\left(\frac{2}{3}\right) = \frac{x}{FG}$$

$$FG = \left(\frac{3x}{2}\right)$$

Now, $F(x) = R_A - \dfrac{1}{2} \times x \times \dfrac{3x}{2}$

$$= 2.25 - \frac{3x^2}{4} \qquad \qquad \qquad \ldots(I)$$

By putting the value of x, we can get the profile of shearing force for the portion AC.
Shear force (F) will be zero when

$$0 = 2.25 - \frac{3x^2}{4}$$

∴ $x = 1.732$ m

Hence, shear force is zero at a distance 1.732 m from A.
Shear force at C can be computed by putting $x = 2$ in eqn. (I).

∴ $F(2) = 2.25 - \dfrac{3}{4} \times (2)^2$

$$= 2.25 - 3 = -0.75 \text{ kN}$$

*B.M.D (For Portion BD)
B.M at B (M_B) = 0

B.M at D is, $M_D = R_B \times 1 - 2 \times 1 \times \dfrac{1}{2}$

$$= 2.75 \times 1 - 1$$

$$= 1.75 \text{ kNm}$$

B.M at C is, $M_C = R_B \times 2 - 2 \times 1 \times \left(1 + \dfrac{1}{2}\right)$

$$= 2.75 \times 2 - \cancel{2} \times 1 \times \frac{3}{\cancel{2}}$$

$$= 5.50 - 3$$

$$= 2.5 \text{ kNm}$$

---

*In a complex problem, it is better if we start from right side along with left side to get the desired result considering the sign convention for moment.
N.B.: Students are advised to use graph paper of good quality to plot the graph of SFD and BMD (assuming suitable scale).

Maximum B.M occurs at G, given by $M_G = R_A \times x - \left(\dfrac{1}{2} \times x \times \dfrac{3}{4} x \right) \times \left(\dfrac{1}{3} x \right)$

Hence, $M_G = R_A \times 1.732 - \left(\dfrac{1}{2} \times 1.732 \times \dfrac{3}{2} \times 1.732 \right) \left(\dfrac{1}{3} \times 1.732 \right)$

$$= 2.25 \times 1.732 - 1.298 = 2.599$$

$$= 2.6 \text{ kNm}$$

B.M at A is $M_A = 0$.

EXAMPLE 8 *Simply supported beam subjected to uniformly varying load:*

SOLUTION   Total load $= \dfrac{1}{2} w.l$ acting $\left(\dfrac{2}{3} l \right)$ from A or $\left(\dfrac{l}{3} \right)$ from B.

Consider a section $m - n$ at a distance x from A.

First, let us find out R_A and R_B.

Taking moment about B and equating it to zero

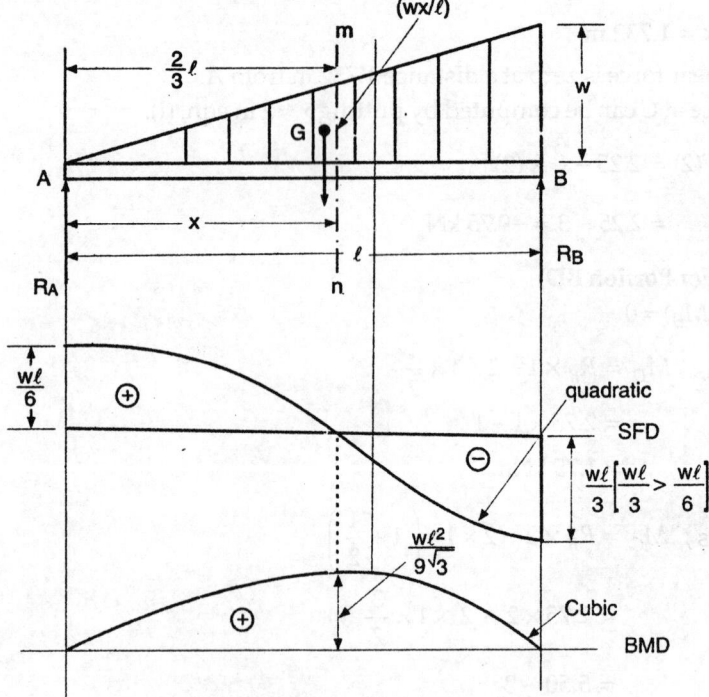

Fig. 6.22

$$R_A \cdot l = \left(\dfrac{1}{2} \cdot w \cdot l \right) \times \dfrac{l}{3}$$

$$R_A = \dfrac{1}{6} w \cdot l$$

$$R_B = \frac{1}{2}w \cdot l - \frac{wl}{6}$$

$$= \left(\frac{wl}{3}\right)$$

*SFD: $F_X = R_A - \frac{1}{2} \cdot \frac{wx}{l} \cdot x$

$$= \left(\frac{wl}{6} - \frac{wx^2}{2l}\right)$$

At $x = 0$, $F_A = \frac{wl}{6}$

At $x = l$, $F_B = \frac{wl}{6} - \frac{w}{2l} \times l^2$

$$= \frac{wl}{6} - \frac{wl}{2}$$

$$= -\left(\frac{wl}{3}\right)$$

If $\qquad F_X = 0$

then, $\qquad \dfrac{wl}{6} = \dfrac{wx^2}{2l}$

$\therefore \qquad x = \dfrac{l}{\sqrt{3}}$

So for $x = \dfrac{l}{\sqrt{3}} = 0.577\, l$ shear force will be zero.

Bending Moment

At section mn,

$$M_X = R_A \cdot x - \frac{wx^2}{2l} \times \frac{x}{3}$$

$$= \frac{wlx}{6} - \frac{wx^3}{6l}$$

This equation shows that B.M varies between A and B according to cubic law.
Maximum B.M occurs at a point where $SF = 0$.

$\Rightarrow \qquad x = \dfrac{l}{\sqrt{3}}$

---

* We can write F_X or $F(x)$.

$$\therefore \qquad M_{max} = \frac{wl}{6} \times \frac{l}{\sqrt{3}} - \frac{w}{6l} \times \left[\frac{l}{(3)^{1/2}} \right]^3$$

$$= \frac{wl^2}{6\sqrt{3}} - \frac{w}{6l} \times \frac{l^3}{(3)^{3/2}}$$

$$= \frac{wl^2}{6\sqrt{3}} - \frac{wl^2}{18\sqrt{3}}$$

$$\boxed{M_{max} = \frac{wl^2}{9\sqrt{3}}}$$

EXAMPLE 9 *A simply supported beam carrying uniformly varying load from zero at each end to w per unit length at the centre.*

SOLUTION   Let R_A and R_B be the reaction at A and B respectively.

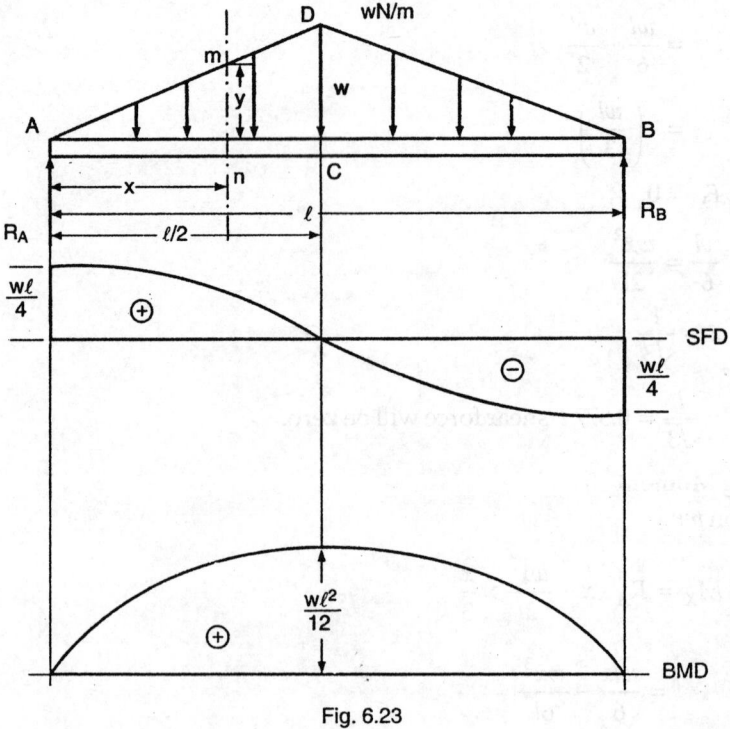

Fig. 6.23

Total load on the beam $= \dfrac{1}{2} \times L \times w$ Newton.

Since the load is symmetrical .

Hence, $R_A = R_B = \dfrac{wL}{4}$ Newton

SFD:

Let us take section *m-n* at a distance x from the point A **support.**

We must know that what is the load intensity at a distance x. For this we take two similar triangles Amn and ADC.

We have,

$$\frac{y}{x} = \frac{w}{l/2}$$

$$\therefore \qquad y = \left(\frac{2w}{l}\right) x \ i.e. \ w_x = \left(\frac{2w}{l}\right) \cdot x.$$

So, we have evaluated the load intensity at a distance x (w_x) from support A.

Now, by using formula,

Shear force at a distance x will be

$$F_x = -\int w_x \cdot dx \qquad\qquad\qquad\qquad ...(1)$$

$$= -\int \left(\frac{2w}{l}\right) \cdot x \, dx$$

$$= -\frac{2w}{l} \int x \, dx$$

$$= -\frac{2w}{l} \times \frac{x^2}{2} + C_1 \qquad\qquad\qquad ...(2)$$

where, C_1 is constant of integration.

B.C are At $x = 0$, $F_X = R_A \Rightarrow C_1 = R_A = \dfrac{wl}{4}$

$$\therefore \qquad F_x = -\frac{wx^2}{l} + \frac{wl}{4}$$

where $x = \dfrac{l}{2}$,

$$F_C = -\frac{w}{l} \times \frac{l^2}{4} + \frac{w}{4} \times l$$

$$= -\frac{wl}{4} + \frac{wl}{4}$$

$$= 0$$

i.e. shear force (F_C) is zero at the center.

BMD:

$$M_x = \int F_x \cdot dx$$

$$= \int \left(-\frac{w}{l}x^2 + \frac{wl}{4}\right) dx$$

$$= -\frac{w}{l} \cdot \frac{x^3}{3} + \frac{wl}{4}x + C_2$$

where, C_2 is constant of Integration.

At $x = 0$, $M_A = 0 \Rightarrow C_2 = 0$

$\therefore \qquad M_X = -\dfrac{w}{3l}x^3 + \dfrac{wl}{4}x$

When $x = \dfrac{l}{2}$ than $M_{max} = -\dfrac{w}{3l} \cdot \left(\dfrac{l}{2}\right)^3 + \dfrac{wl}{4}\left(\dfrac{l}{2}\right)$

$$= -\dfrac{wl^2}{24} + \dfrac{wl^2}{8}$$

$$= \dfrac{wl^2}{8} - \dfrac{wl^2}{24}$$

$$= \dfrac{3wl^2 - wl^2}{24}$$

$$\boxed{\therefore M_{max} = \dfrac{wl^2}{12}}$$

6.9 BEAM WITH INCLINED LOADING

When a beam is subjected to a load P which is inclined at an angle θ with the axis of the beam, the load P can be resolved into two components:

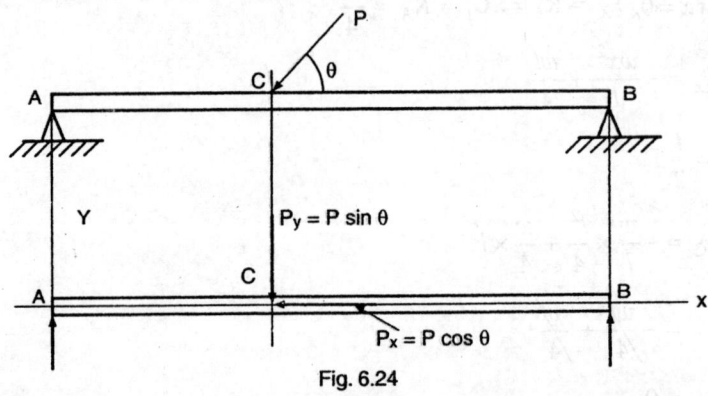

Fig. 6.24

(i) Transverse (or vertical) component $P_y = P \sin \theta$

(ii) Axial (or horizontal component) $P_x = P \cos \theta$

The transverse component will produce 'shear force' and 'bending moment' whereas the axial component will produce pull or push.

Therefore, the beam at any section has to resist:

(i) Shear force

(ii) Bending moment

(iii) Axial force which may be push or pull.

EXAMPLE 1 *Construct the axial thrust, shear force and bending moment diagram for the following loaded beam.*

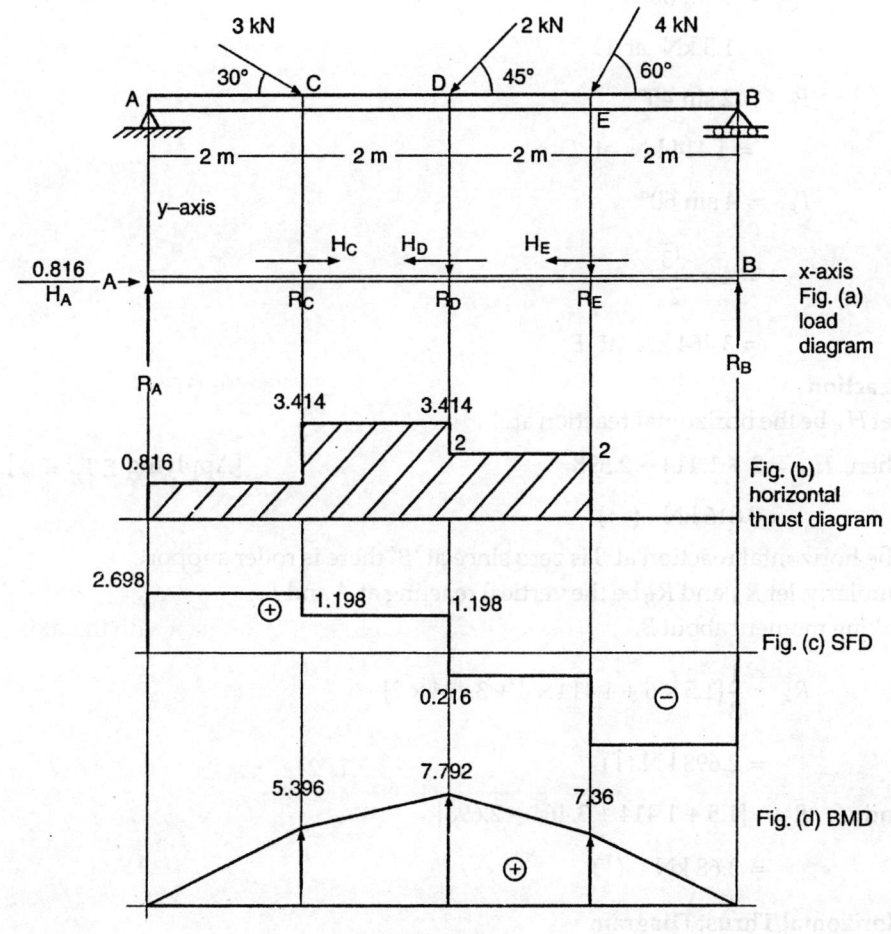

Fig. 6.25

SOLUTION Resolving the load horizontally and vertically
We have,
Load component along x-axis

$$P_{CX} = 3 \cos 30°$$

$$= 2.598 \text{ kN at } C$$

$$P_{DX} = 2 \cos 45°$$

$$= 1.414 \text{ kN at } D$$

$$P_{EX} = 4 \cos 60°$$

$$= 2 \text{ kN at } E$$

Load components along y-axis are

$$P_{CY} = 3 \sin 30°$$

$$= 1.5 \, \text{kN} \quad \text{at} \quad C$$

$$P_{DY} = 2 \sin 45°$$

$$= 1.414 \, \text{kN} \quad \text{at} \quad D$$

$$P_{EY} = 4 \sin 60°$$

$$= 4 \times \frac{\sqrt{3}}{2}$$

$$= 3.464 \, \text{kN} \quad \text{at} \quad E.$$

Reaction

Let H_A be the horizontal reaction at A.

Then, $H_A = 2 + 1.414 - 2.598$ [Applying $\Sigma F_X = 0$]

$$= 0.816 \, \text{kN} \quad (\rightarrow)$$

The horizontal reaction at B is zero since at 'B' there is roller support.

Similarly, let R_A and R_B be the vertical reacting at A and B.

Taking moment about B,

$$R_A = \frac{1}{8}[1.5 \times 6 + 1.414 \times 4 + 3.464 \times 2]$$

$$= 2.698 \, \text{kN} \, (\uparrow)$$

and $R_B = [1.5 + 1.414 + 3.464 - 2.698]$

$$= 3.68 \, \text{kN} \quad (\uparrow)$$

Horizontal Thrust Diagram

For AC, horizontal thrust $H_T = 0.816$ kN

For CD, horizontal thrust $H_T = 0.816 + 2.598$

$$= 3.414 \, \text{kN}$$

For DE, horizontal thrust $H_T = 0.186 + 2.598 - 1.414$

$$= 2 \, \text{kN}$$

For EB, horizontal thrust $H_T = 0.816 + 2.598 - 1.414 - 2$

$$= 0$$

The profile of horizontal thrust is shown in diagram.

SFD

The SFD is shown in the figure.

BMD

For AC: $M(x) = 2.698 \, x$ varies linearly

At $x = 0$, $M_A = 0$

At $x = 2$, $M_C = 2.698 \times 2$
$$= 5.396 \text{ kNm}$$

For CD: $\quad M(x) = R_A \cdot x - P_{cy} \cdot (x - 2)$ varies linearly
$$= 2.698\,x - 1.5\,(x - 2)$$

At $x = 2$m, $M_C = 2.698 \times 2 = 5.396$ kN m

At $x = 4$m, $M_D = 2.698 \times 4 - 1.5\,(4 - 2) = 7.792$ kN m

For DE: $\quad M(x) = 2.698x - P_{Cy}\,(x - 2) - P_{Dy}\,(x - 4)$

$$= 2.698x - 1.5\,(x - 2) - 1.414\,(x - 4)$$

At $x = 4$m, $M_D = 7.792$ kN m

At $x = 6$m; $M_E = 7.36$ kN m

For EB: $\quad M(x) = 2.698x - 1.5\,(x - 2) - 1.414\,(x - 4) - 3.464\,(x - 6)$

At $x = 6$ m; $M_E = 7.36$ kN m

At $x = 8$ m; $M_B = 0$

B.M.D is shown in Fig. 6.25.

6.10 TABLE FOR MAXIMUM 'SHEAR FORCE' AND 'BENDING MOMENT' IN STANDARD CASE

S. No.	Loading	Maximum shear force (F_{max})	Maximum moment (M_{max})
1.	W / L	W	WL (fixed end)
2.	w/unit length / L	wL	$\dfrac{wL^2}{2}$ (fixed end)
3.	W / a · b / L / $L = a + b$	$\dfrac{W \cdot b}{a + b}$ when $a = b$ then $F_{max} = \dfrac{W}{2}$	$\dfrac{Wab}{a + b}$ $M_{max} = \dfrac{W \cdot L}{4}$
4.	w/unit length / L	$\dfrac{w \cdot L}{2}$	$\dfrac{wL^2}{8}$

Cantilever with Several Point Load

EXAMPLE 1 *Draw SFD and BMD of the loaded Beam.*

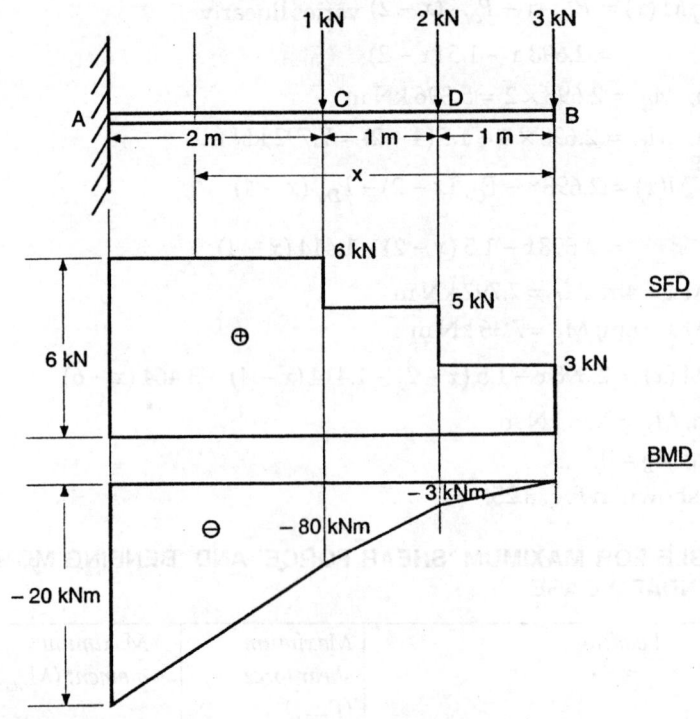

Fig. 6.26

SOLUTION **Shear Force Analysis:**

Between B and D:

$$F_x = 3 \text{ kN}$$

Between D and C:

$$F_x = (3+2) = 5 \text{ kN}$$

Between C and A:

$$F_x = 3+2+1 = 6 \text{ kN}$$

Shear force will consist of several rectangle.

Bending Moment Analysis:

Between B and D:

$$M(x) = -3x \text{ linear}$$

at B, $x = 0$, hence $M_B = 0$

at D, $x = 1$, hence $M_D = -3 \times 1 = -3 \text{ kN m}$

Between D and C:

$$M(x) = -3x - 2(x-1) \text{ linear} = -5x + 2$$

at $D, x = 1,$ $\therefore$ $M_D = -3$

at $C, x = 2,$ $\therefore$ $M_C = -5 \times 2 + 2 = -8$ kN m

Between C and A:

$M(x) = -3x - 2(x-1) - 1(x-2)$

at $C, x = 2,$ $\therefore$ $M_C = -3 \times 2 - 2 \times 1 = -6 - 2 = -8$ kN m

at $A, x = 4,$ $\therefore$ $M_A = -3 \times 4 - 2 \times 3 - 1 \times 2$

$= -12 - 6 - 2 = -20$ kN m **Ans.**

EXAMPLE 2 *Draw SFD and BMD of the loaded Beam.*

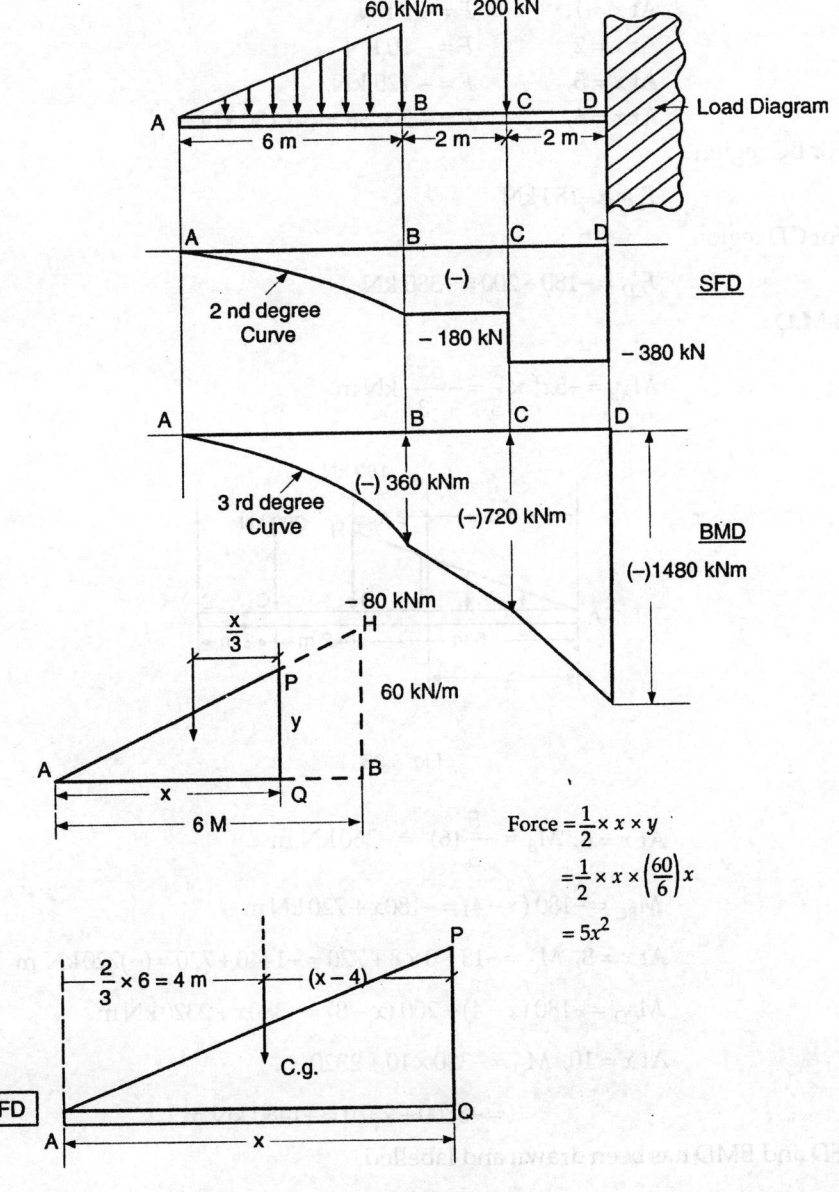

Fig. 6.27

SOLUTION

$$\text{Force} = \frac{1}{2} \times x \times y$$

$$= \frac{1}{2} \times x \times \left(\frac{60}{6}\right) x = 5x^2$$

For the region AB, $F_{AB} = -5x^2$ kN

At $x = 0$,	$F = 0$
At $x = 1$,	$F = -5$ kN
At $x = 2$,	$F = -10$ kN
At $x = 5$,	$F = -125$ kN
At $x = 6$,	$F = -5 \times 36 = (-) 180$ kN

For BC region

$$F_{BC} = -180 \text{ kN}$$

For CD region

$$F_{CD} = -180 - 200 = -380 \text{ kN}$$

B.M.D.:

$$M_{AB} = -5x^2 \times \frac{x}{3} = -\frac{5x^3}{3} \text{ kN m}$$

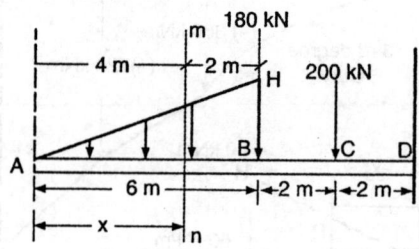

Fig. 6.28

At $x = 6$, $M_B = -\frac{5}{3}(6)^3 = -360$ kN m

$M_{BC} = -180(x-4) = -180x + 720$ kN m

At $x = 8$, $M_C = -18 - 0 \times 8 + 720 = -1440 + 720 = (-)720$ kN m

$M_{CD} = -180(x-4) - 200(x-8) = -380x + 2320$ kN m

At $x = 10$, $M_D = -380 \times 10 + 2320$

$$= -3800 + 2320 = -1480 \text{ kN m}$$

SFD and BMD has been drawn and labelled.

EXAMPLE 3 *Draw SFD and BMD of the loaded beam given in figure 6.29.*

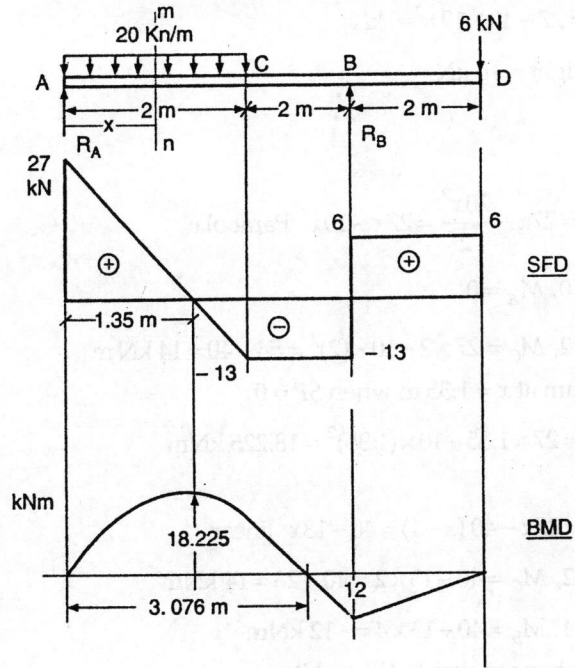

Fig. 6.29

SOLUTION   We have,

$$R_A + R_B = 20 \times 2 + 6 = 46 \text{ kN}$$

Taking moment about B

$$R_A \times 4 - 20 \times 2 \times (1+2) + 6 \times 2 = 0$$

$$R_A = \frac{120-12}{4} = \frac{\overset{27}{\cancel{108}}}{\cancel{4}} = 27 \text{ kN} \uparrow$$

$$R_B = 46 - 27 = 19 \text{ kN} \uparrow$$

SFD:

Taking imaginary section *mn* at a distance *x* in *AC*, we have

For *AC* $F(x) = R_A - 20x = 27 - 20x$ linear

At $x = 0$; $F_A = 27 \text{ kN}$

At $x = 2$; $F_C = 27 - 20 \times 2 = 27 - 40 = -13 \text{ kN}$

For *SF* is zero when $x = \dfrac{27}{20} = 1.35$ m from *A*

For *CB*

$$F(x) = 27 - 40 = -13 \text{ kN}$$

$$F(C) = -13 \text{ kN (left)}$$

For *BD*

$$F(x) = 27 - 40 + 19 = +6 \text{ kN}$$

$$F(B) \text{ right} = +6 \text{ kN}$$

BMD:
For AC

$$M(x) = 27x - \frac{20x^2}{2} = 27x - 10x^2 \text{ Parabola}$$

At $x = 0$, $M_A = 0$

At $x = 2$, $M_C = 27 \times 2 - 10 \times (2)^2 = 54 - 40 = 14 \text{ kNm}$

B.M. is maximum at $x = 1.35$ m when $SF = 0$

$$\therefore \qquad M_{max} = 27 \times 1.35 - 10 \times (1.35)^2 = 18.225 \text{ kNm}$$

For *CB*

$$M(x) = 27x - 40(x-1) = 40 - 13x \text{ linear}$$

At $x = 2$, $M_C = 40 - 13 \times 2 = 40 - 26 = 14 \text{ kNm}$

At $x = 4$, $M_B = 40 - 13 \times 4 = -12 \text{ kNm}$

Therefore, *BM* changes sign in *CB* and its value is zero at

$$x = \left(\frac{40}{13}\right) = 3.076 \text{ m from } A.$$

SFD and *BMD* has been drawn in figure.

EXAMPLE 4 *A simply supported beam of 9m span is loaded as shown in Fig. 6.30. Draw the SFD and BMD including principal values.*

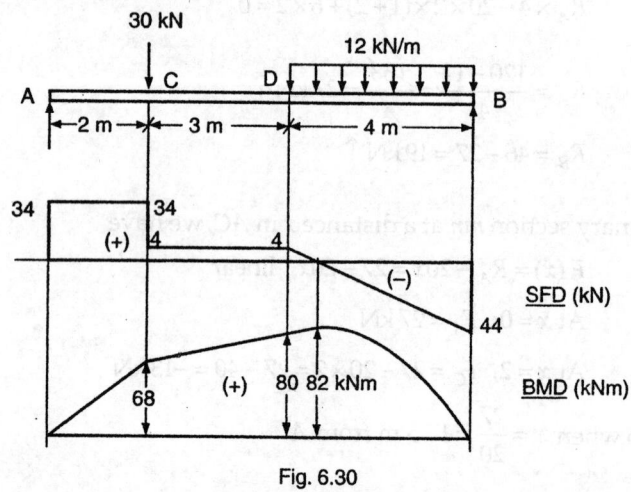

Fig. 6.30

SOLUTION We have,

$$R_A + R_B = 30 + 12 \times 4 = 30 + 48 = 78 \text{ kN}$$

$\Sigma M_B = 0$ gives:

$$R_A \times 9 = 30 \times 7 + 12 \times 4 \times 2$$

$$\therefore \quad R_A = \frac{30 \times 7 + 12 \times 4 \times 2}{9}$$

$$= \frac{210 + 96}{9} = \frac{306}{9} = 34 \text{ kN} \uparrow$$

SFD:

For *AC*,

$$F(x) = 34 \text{ kN (Constant)}$$

$$F_A = F(x) = 34 \text{kN}$$

$$F_C = 34 \text{ kN}$$

For *CD*,

$$F(x) = 34 - 30 = 4 \text{kN}$$

For *DB*,

$$F(x) = 34 - 30 - 12 \, (x - 5)$$

$$= 64 - 12x \text{ linear}$$

At $x = 5$; $F_D = 64 - 12 \times 5 = 4 \text{kN}$

At $x = 9$; $F_B = 64 - 12 \times 9 = 64 - 108 = -44 \text{ kN}$

Therefore, SF changes sign in DB and is zero at $x = \dfrac{64}{12} = 5.33$ from *A*

BMD:

For *AC*,

$$M(x) = 34x$$

At $x = 0$, $M_A = 0$

At $x = 2$, $M_C = 34 \times 2 = 68 \text{ kN m}$

For *CD*,

$$M(x) = 34x - 30 \, (x - 2) = 4x + 60 \text{ linear}$$

At $x = 2$, $M_C = 4 \times 2 + 60 = 68 \text{ kNm}$

At $x = 5$, $M_D = 4 \times 5 + 60 = 80 \text{ kNm}$

For *DB*,

$$M(x) = 34x - 30 \, (x - 2) + \frac{12}{2} (x - 5)^2$$

$$= 4x + 60 + 6 \, (x - 5)^2, \text{ parabolic}$$

At $x = 5$m, $M_D = 4 \times 5 + 60 = 80$ kNm

At $x = 9$m, $M_B = 4 \times 9 + 60 + 6(9-5)^2 = 0$

B.M. will be maximum at $x = 5.33$ where *SF* is zero.

$\therefore$ $\quad M_{max} = 4 \times 5.33 + 60 + 6(5.33-5)^2$

$\qquad\qquad = 21.32 + 60 + 6 \times (0.33)^2 = 81.97 \simeq 82$kNm **Ans.**

EXAMPLE 5 *Draw SFD and BMD of the following loaded beam.*

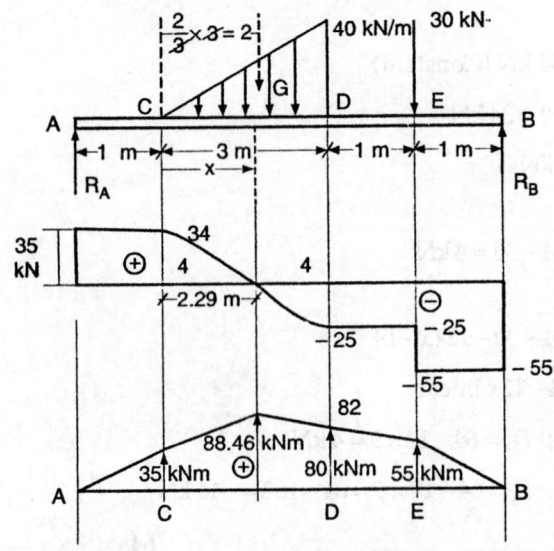

Fig. 6.31

SOLUTION

$$R_A + R_B = \frac{1}{2} \times 3 \times \underset{20}{\cancel{40}} + 30 \simeq 90 \text{ kN}$$

Taking moment about *B*

$$R_A \times 6 - \frac{1}{2} \times 3 \times \underset{20}{\cancel{40}} (1+1+1) - 30 \times 1 = 0$$

$$6R_A = 180 + 30 = 210$$

$$R_A = \frac{310}{6} = 35 \text{ kN} \uparrow$$

$$R_B = (90-35) = 55 \text{ kN} \uparrow$$

Shear Force Analysis:

For *AC*,

$$F_A = 35 \text{ kN}$$

For *CD*,

$$F(x) = R_A - \frac{1}{2} \times x \times \frac{40}{3} x = 35 - \frac{20x^2}{3}$$

At $x = 0$, shear force $F = 35$

At $x = 1$, shear force $F = 35 - \frac{20}{3} = \frac{105-20}{3} = \frac{85}{3} = 28.3 \text{ kN}$

At $x = 2$, $F = 35 - \frac{20 \times 4}{3} = \frac{25}{3} = 8.33 \text{ kN}$

At $x = 3$, $F = 35 - \frac{20}{3} \times (3)^2 = 35 - 60 = -25 \text{ kN}$

Bending Moment Analysis:

For *AC*,

BM at $A = 0$

BM at $C = 35 \times 1 = 35 \text{ kNm}$.

For *CD*,

$$M(x) = 35(1+x) - \left(\frac{1}{2} \times x \times \frac{40x}{3} \right) \times \frac{x}{3}$$

$$= 35 + 35x - \frac{20x^3}{9}$$

At $x = 0$, $M_C = 35 \text{ kN m}$

At $x = 1$, $M = 35 + 35 - \frac{20}{9} = 70 - \frac{20}{9}$

$$= \frac{610}{9} = 67.77 \text{ kN m}$$

At $x = 3$, $M_D = 35 \times 4 \times - \frac{1}{9} \times 20 \times (3)^3$

$$= 140 - \frac{1}{9} \times 20 \times 27 = 140 - 60 = 80 \text{ kN m}$$

At zero shear, $35 - \frac{20x^2}{3} = 0$

$$x = \sqrt{\frac{3 \times 35}{20}} = 2.29 \text{ m}$$

At zero shear M will be maximum

$$\therefore \qquad M_{max} = 35\,(1+2.29) - \frac{20}{9} \times (2.29)^3$$

$$= 115.15 - 26.68 = 88.47 \text{ kN m}$$

$$M_E = -55 \text{ kN m}$$

$$M_B = 0$$

SFD and BMD has been drawn in figure.   **Ans.**

EXAMPLE 6 *Draw SFD and BMD of the following loaded beam*

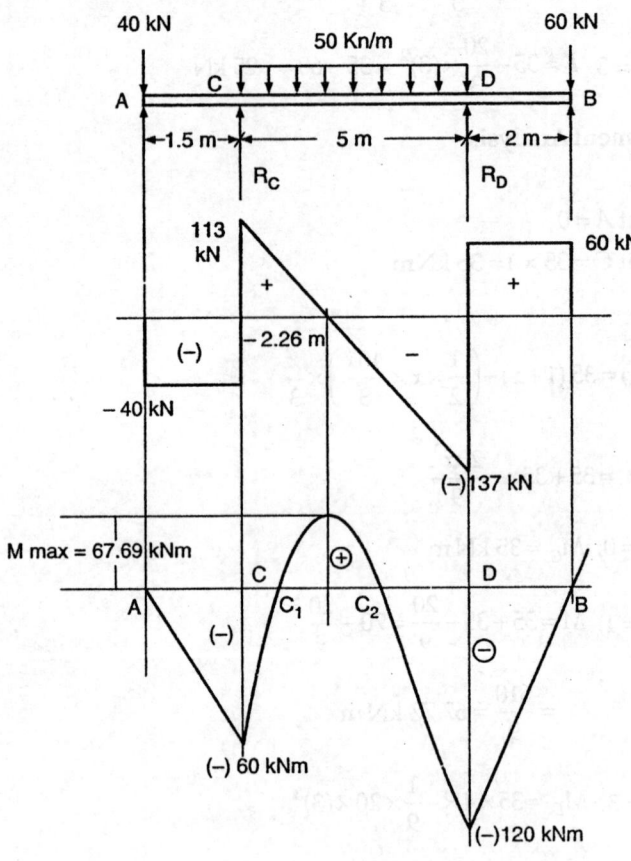

Fig. 6.32

SOLUTION

$$\Sigma F_y = 0 \text{ gives}$$

$$R_C + R_D = 40 + 50 \times 5 + 60 = 350 \text{ kN}$$

$$\Sigma M_D = 0 \text{ gives}$$

$$R_C \times 5 + 60 \times 2 = 40 \times 6.5 + (50 \times 5) \times 2.5$$

$$R_C \times 5 + 120 = 260 + 625$$

$$R_C = \left(\frac{885-120}{5}\right) = \left(\frac{765}{5}\right) = 153 \text{ kN} \uparrow$$

$$R_D = 350 - 153 = 197 \text{ kN} \uparrow$$

SFD Analysis

$$F_A = (-)40 \text{ kN}; \ F_C = 103 - 40 = 113 \text{ kN}$$

$$F(x) = F_C - 50x = 113 - 50x$$

$$F(D) = 113 - 50 \times 5 = 113 - 250 = (-)137 \text{ kN}$$

SF, $F(x)$ will zero at $x = \dfrac{113}{50} = 2.26 \text{ m}$

On the right side of D, $F(D) = -137 + 197 = 60 \text{ kN}$

BMD analysis:

$$M(A) = 0$$

$$M(C) = 40 \times 1.5 = 60 \text{ kNm}$$

For CD portion:

$$M(x) = -40\,(1.5 + x) + 153x - 50x \cdot \frac{x}{2}$$

$$= -60 - 40x + 153x - 25x^2$$

$$= -60 + 113x - 25x^2$$

At $x = 2.26$ m, M will be maximum

$$\therefore \quad M_{max} = -60 + 113 \times 2.26 - 25 \times (2.26)^2$$

$$= -60 + 225.38 - 127.69 = 67.69 \text{ kN m}$$

At $x = 5$m, $M_D = -60 + 113 \times 5 - 25 \times (5)^2$

$$= -60 + 565 - 625 = -60 - 60 = -120 \text{ kN m}$$

For $M(x)$ to be zero,

$$-60 + 113x - 25x^2 = 0$$

on $x^2 - 4.52x + 2.4 = 0$

$$\therefore \quad x = \frac{4.52 \pm \sqrt{(4.52)^2 - 4 \times 2.4 \times 1}}{2}$$

$$= 2.26 \pm 1.645 = 2.905 \text{ or } 0.615$$

*Points of contraflexure are 0.615 m and 3.905 m from C.

Points of contraflexures are shown by C_1, and C_2 in B.M.D. in the figure.

---

*Here at C_1 and C_2, B.M. changes it's sign so these are called as points of contraflexure.

EXAMPLE 7 *Draw SFD and BMD of the following loaded beam*   **(UPTU 2007)**

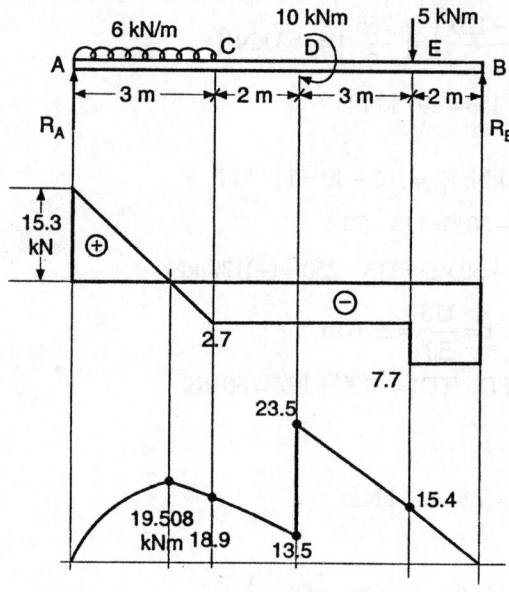

Fig. 6.33

SOLUTION   We have

$$R_A + R_B = 6 \times 3 + 5 = 23 \text{ kN}$$

$$\Sigma M_B = 0 \text{ gives}$$

$$R_A \times 10 - 6 \times 3 (1.5 + 2 + 3 + 2) + 10 - 5 \times 2 = 0$$

$$R_A = 10 - 18 \times 8.5 + 10 - 10 = 0$$

$$R_A = \left[\frac{18 \times 8.5}{10} \right] = 15.3 \text{ kN} \uparrow$$

Shear Force Analysis:

For *AC* part

$$F(x) = R_A - 6x = 15.3 - 6x$$

At $x = 0$, $F_A = 15.3$ kN

At $x = 3$, $F_C = 15.3 - 6 \times 3 = -2.7$ kN

Shear force will be zero at $x = \left(\dfrac{15.3}{6} \right) = 2.55$ m

For *CE* part

$$F(x) = 15.3 - 6 \times 3 = -2.7 \text{ kN}$$

For *EB* part

$$F(x) = -2.7 - 5 = -7.7 \text{ kN}$$

Bending Moment Analysis:

For *AC* part

$$M(x) = 15.3x - 6x \cdot \frac{x}{2} = 15.3x - 3x^2 \quad \text{Parabola}$$

Maximum moment will occur when $SF = 0$
i.e. at $x = 2.55$ m

Hence, $M_{max} = 15.3 \times 2.55 - 3 \times (2.55)^2$

$$= 39.015 - 19.507 = 19.508 \text{ kN m}$$

At $x = 3$m, $M_C = 15.3 \times 3 - 3 \times (3)^2$

$$= 45.9 - 27 = 18.9 \text{ kNm}$$

For *CD* part

$$M(x) = 15.3x - 6 \times 3 (x - 1.5)$$
$$= 15.3x - 18x + 27 = -2.7x + 27$$

At $x = 3$m, $M_C = -2.7 \times 3 + 27 = 18.9$ kNm

At $x = 5$m, $M_D = -2.7 \times 5 + 27 = 13.5$ kNm

For *DE* part

$$M(x) = 15.3x - 6 \times 3 (x - 1.5) + 10 = -2.7x + 37$$

At $x = 5$m, $M_D = -2.7 \times 5 + 37 = 23.5$ kNm

At $x = 8$m, $M_E = -2.7 \times 8 + 37 = -21.6 + 37 = 15.4$ kNm

For *EB* part

$$M(x) = 15.3x - 6 \times 3 (x - 1.5) + 10 - 5 (x - 8)$$
$$= -2.7x + 37 - 5x + 40 = -7.7x + 77$$

At $x = 8$, $M_E = -7.7 \times 8 + 77 = -61.6 + 77 = 15.4$ kNm

At $x = 10$, $M_B = 0$

SFD and BMD after labelling has been shown in figure.

HIGHLIGHTS

1. (a) The diagram which shows the variation of shear force along the length of beam is called S.F.D. Similarly the diagram which shows the variation of B.M. along the length of a beam is known as B.M.D.

   (b) Shear force at a section is the resultant vertical force either to the right or to the left of the section.

2. Bending moment at a section is the algebraic sum of the moments of all forces either to the left or the right of the section.

3. Positive shear force will occur when left position moves upward with respect to right portion.

Negative shear force will occur when left portion moves downwards with respect to right portion.

4. For B.M. left clockwise and right anticlockwise are taken as positive and vice versa as negative.

5. The S.F. diagram suddenly changes at a section for a vertical point load. The S.F. diagram between two vertical load, remains constant.

6. The S.F. diagram for u.d.l between two points will be inclined straight line and B.M. diagram will be parabolic.

7. For uniformly varying load S.F. diagram and B.M. diagram will be parabolic and cubic parabolic respectively.

8. Maximum B.M. occurs where S.F. change sign i.e. S.F. passes through zero value.

9. The point where B.M. changes sign is known as point of contraflexure 'or' point of inflection.

10. When a beam is subjected to a moment at a section, the S.F. remains constant, but B.M. changes suddenly in magnitude equal to the moment.

11. For inclined loads, vertical component will be taken only for calculating S.F. and B.M. and horizontal components only will be taken for calculating axial force.

12. When a beam is subjected to a couple at a section then B.M. changes suddenly at the section but S.F. remains unaltered at the section.

PROBLEM FOR PRACTICE

1. Draw SFD and BMD for the following loaded beam.

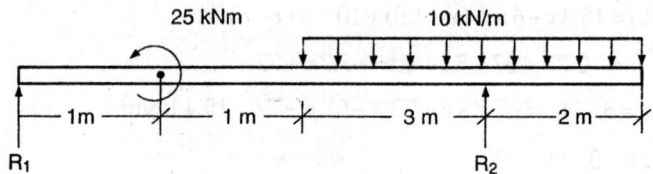

Fig. 6.34

2. Draw SFD and BMD for the following loaded beam.

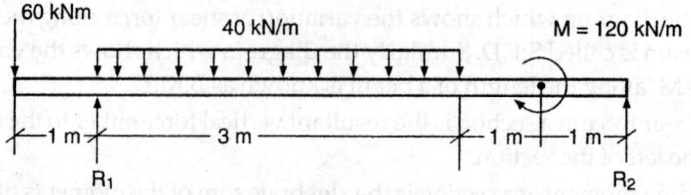

Fig. 6.35

3. A beam 25 m long is supported at A and B and loaded as shown in the figure.

Sketch the SF and BM diagram and find:
  (a) The position and magnitude of maximum B.M.
  (b) The position of the point of contraflexure.

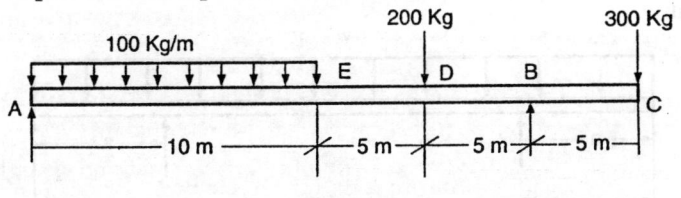

Fig. 6.36

4. Draw the SFD and BMD for a simply supported beam of length 8 m and carrying a uniformly distributed load of 10 kN/m for a distance of 4 m as shown in figure.

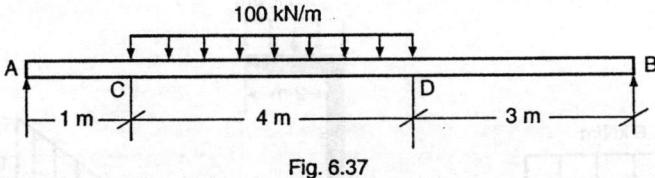

Fig. 6.37

5. Draw the SFD and BMD diagram for the beam. Also calculate the position and magnitude of maximum bending moment.

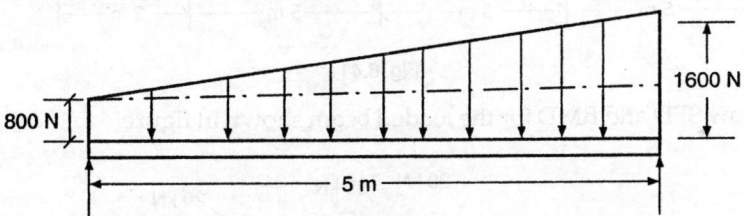

Fig. 6.38

6. A beam ABCD is supported by a roller at A and a hinge at D. The beam is subjected to load as shown in figure.

Draw the shear force and bending moment diagram for the beam ABCD only.

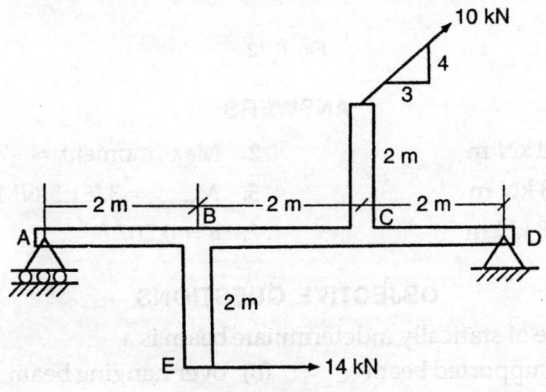

Fig. 6.39

7. A beam of length 'l' carrying a uniformly distributed load 'w' over its whole length is supported on two symmetrical supports.

Locate the position of the supports to keep the maximum BM as low as possible.

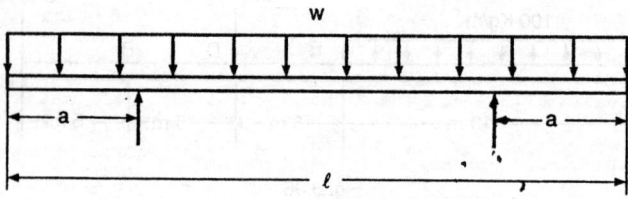

Fig. 6.40

8. Draw SFD and BMD for the beam as shown in the figure.

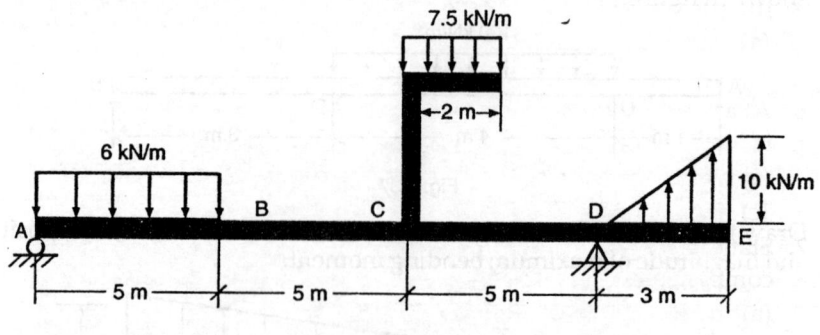

Fig. 6.41

9. Draw SFD and BMD for the loaded beam shown in figure.

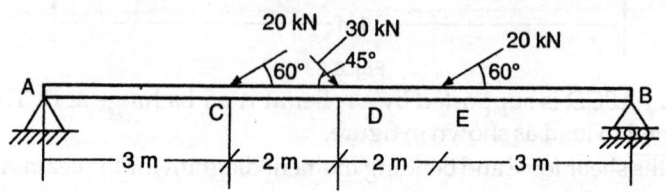

Fig. 6.42

ANSWERS

1. $M_{max} = -20$ kN m
2. Max. moment = -72 kN m
3. $M_{max} = 258$ kN m
5. $M_{max} = 3761.5$ NM
6. $M_{max} = -28$ kN m
7. $a = 0.207\ l$

OBJECTIVE QUESTIONS

1. The example of statically indeterminate beam is a
   (a) simply supported beam
   (b) over hanging beam
   (c) fixed beam
   (d) cantilever

2. The type of load that is applied to a beam through knife edge is
   (a) concentrated load
   (b) uniformly distributed load
   (c) uniformly increasing load
   (d) parabolically increasing load
3. Maximum bending moment in the case of simply supported beam of span '*L*' and subjected to a central load *W* is
   (a) *WL*
   (b) $\dfrac{WL}{2}$
   (c) $\dfrac{WL}{4}$
   (d) $\dfrac{WL}{8}$
4. A 'point of contraflexure' is a point where
   (a) shear force is zero
   (b) shear force is maximum
   (c) bending moment is zero
   (d) bending moment is maximum
5. For any part of the beam between two concentrated loads, the shear force diagram is a
   (a) horizontal straight line
   (b) vertical straight line
   (c) sloping straight line
   (d) parabola
6. At a point on the beam where shear force change sign, the bending moment is
   (a) zero
   (b) maximum
   (c) increasing
   (d) decreasing
7. Statically determinate beams have the following number of unknown reaction components
   (a) two
   (b) three
   (c) four
   (d) five
8. Statically indeterminate beams have the following number of unknown reaction components
   (a) less than three
   (b) equal to three
   (c) more than three
   (d) none of the above
9. Which of the following is statically determinate beam?
   (a) simple beam
   (b) overhanging beam
   (c) cantilever beam
   (d) all the above
10. Which of the following is statically indeterminate beam?
    (a) propped cantilever beam
    (b) fixed beam
    (c) continuous beam
    (d) all the above
11. Which of the following is known as simple supports?
    (a) roller and fixed supports
    (b) hinge and fixed supports
    (c) roller and hinge supports
    (d) none of the above
12. Which of the following is true about a continuous beam?
    (a) it is supported on three or more roller supports
    (b) it is supported on three or more hinge supports
    (c) it is supported on the hinge support and two or more roller supports
    (d) none of these
13. In a cantilever carrying a load whose intensity varies uniformly from zero at the free end to *w* per unit run at the fixed end, the S.F. diagram will change according to the following law
    (a) a linear law
    (b) a parabolic law
    (c) cubic law
    (d) none of the above

14. Bending moment at supports in the case of simple supported beams is always
    (a) less than unity   (b) more than unity
    (c) zero   (d) none of the above

15. In a simply supported beam carrying a uniformly distributed load 'w' per unit run over the whole span. The maximum B.M is equal to

    (a) $\dfrac{wl^2}{4}$ (b) $\dfrac{wl^3}{6}$ (c) $\dfrac{wl^2}{8}$ (d) $\dfrac{wl^3}{8}$

16. In a simply supported beam carrying a load whose intensity varies uniformly from zero at one end to 'w' per unit run at the other end the maximum B.M is equal to

    (a) $\dfrac{wl^2}{8}$ (b) $\dfrac{wl^2}{12}$ (c) $\dfrac{wl^2}{24}$ (d) $\dfrac{wl^3}{9\sqrt{3}}$

17. The point of contraflexure is also called
    (a) the point of inflexion   (b) a virtual hinge
    (c) both (a) and (b)   (d) none of the above

18. In case of a loaded cantilever, maximum B.M. occurs at the point where
    (a) S.F. is zero   (b) S.F. is maximum
    (c) cantilever beam   (d) none of the above

19. For the shear force to be uniform throughout the span of a simply supported beam, it should carry
    (a) U.D.L over its entire span
    (b) a point load at its mid point
    (c) a couple any where in the span
    (d) two concentrated load equally spaced.

ANSWERS

1. (c)	2. (a)	3. (c)	4. (c)	5. (a)	6. (b)
7. (b)	8. (c)	9. (d)	10. (d)	11. (c)	12. (c)
13. (b)	14. (c)	15. (c)	16. (d)	17. (a)	18. (b)
19. (c)					

— ❖❖ —

BENDING STRESS IN BEAM

7.1 INTRODUCTION

When external load acts on a beam, then shear force and bending moments are set up at all section of the beam. Owing to shearing force and bending moment, the beam undergoes deformation and stresses are induced in the beam.

The stresses developed by bending moment are known as 'bending stresses'or flexural stresses.

Pure bending refers to the loading of beam so that the beam is absolute free from shear force and is subjected to only constant bending moment.

Most real beams are subjected to shear loading in combination of the bending moment.

7.2 PURE BENDING

If the length of a beam is subjected to a constant bending moment and no shear, then that length of the beam is said to be in pure bending or simple bending.

Portion B to C is under pure bending or simple bending.

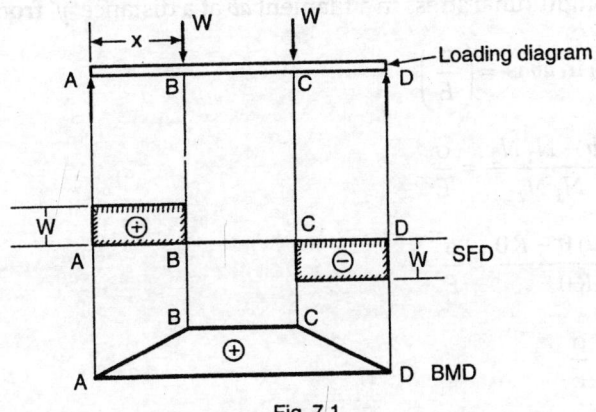

Fig. 7.1

7.3 ASSUMPTION MADE IN SIMPLE BENDING

(i) The material is homogenous, isotropic and has the same value of Young Modulus (E) in tension and compression.

(ii) The beam is initially straight and all the longitudinal filament bend into circular are with a common centre of curvature.

(iii) The transverse section which were plane before bending, remain plain after bending also.

(iv) The radius of curvature is large compared with the dimensions of the cross-section.

(v) The material of the beam obey's Hook's law and is stressed within its elastic limit.

(vi) Each layer of the beam is free to expand 'or' contract independently of the layer, above or below it.

7.4 BENDING EQUATION

Figure 7.2 shows a length of beam under the action of bending moment M.

O is the centre of curvature and R is the radius of curvature of the neutral surface $N_1 N_2$.

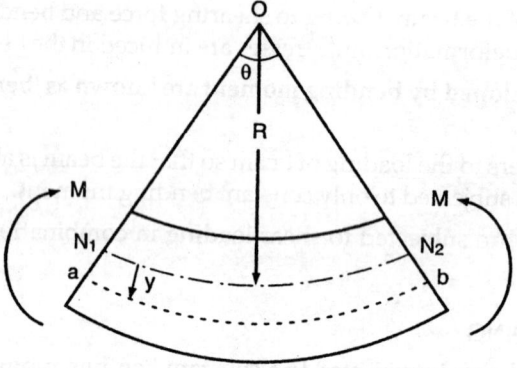

Fig. 7.2

The beam subtends an angle θ at O.

Let σ be the longitudinal stress in a filament ab at a distance 'y' from $N_1 N_2$.

Then strain (ε) in ab is $= \left(\dfrac{\sigma}{E} \right)$

$$\varepsilon = \frac{ab - N_1 N_2}{N_1 N_2} = \frac{\sigma}{E}$$

$$\frac{(R+y)\theta - R\theta}{R\theta} = \frac{\sigma}{E}$$

$$\frac{y\theta}{R\theta} = \frac{\sigma}{E}$$

$$\therefore \qquad \boxed{\dfrac{\sigma}{E} = \dfrac{y}{R}}$$

$$\therefore \qquad \sigma = E \times \dfrac{y}{R}$$

Since E and R are constant therefore stress in any layer is directly proportional to the distance of the layer from the neutral layer.

Consider an elementary area δA of the beam section at a distance y from the neutral axis $N_1\, N_2$.

Force on this area $= \sigma \times \delta A$

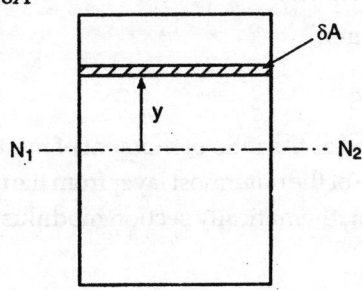

Fig. 7.3

where, σ = stress induced on this elementary strip area δA due to bending.

From the equation $\sigma = \dfrac{E}{R} \times y$

$\therefore \qquad$ Force on this strip area $= \left(\dfrac{E}{R} \times y \right) \times \delta A$

$\therefore \qquad$ Moment of resistance offered by the elementary area

$$\text{about } N_1\, N_2 = \left(\dfrac{E}{R} \times y \times \delta A \right) \times y$$

$\therefore \qquad$ Total moment of resistance offered by the beam section $= \dfrac{E}{R} \int y^2\, \delta A$

Let M = External moment offered on the beam section.

For equilibrium

$$M = \dfrac{E}{R} \int y^2 dA$$

$$= \dfrac{E}{R} \times I$$

$$\therefore \qquad \dfrac{M}{I} = \dfrac{E}{R}$$

But $\qquad \dfrac{E}{R} = \dfrac{\sigma}{y}$

$$\therefore \qquad \frac{M}{I} = \frac{\sigma}{y} = \frac{E}{R}$$

This equation is known as 'bending equation' based on the theory of pure bending.

where M—expressed in N mm

σ—expressed in N/mm^2

I—expressed in mm^4

y—expressed in mm

E—expressed in N/mm^2

R—expressed in mm.

7.5 SECTION MODULUS

Section modulus is defined as the ratio of moment of inertia of a section about the neutral axis to the distance of the outermost layer from the neutral axis. It is denoted by the symbol Z. Hence mathematically section modulus is expressed by,

$$Z = \frac{I}{y_{max}}$$

where I = Moment of Inertia about neutral axis.

and y_{max} = Distance of the outermost layer from the neutral axis.

$$\frac{M}{I} = \frac{\sigma}{y}$$

The stress σ will be maximum when y is maximum.

Hence the above equation can be written as

$$\frac{M}{I} = \frac{\sigma_{max}}{y_{max}}$$

$$\therefore \qquad M = \sigma_{max} \times \frac{I}{y_{max}}$$

$$M = \sigma_{max} \times Z$$

Here M is the maximum bending moment (or moment of resistance offered by the section).

Hence, moment of resistance offered by the section is maximum when section modulus Z is maximum.

Therefore section modulus represents the strength of the section.

7.6 SECTION MODULUS FOR VARIOUS BEAM SECTION

1. Rectangular Section

M.I. through its $CG = \dfrac{bd^3}{12}$

Distance of outermost layer from N.A is given by

$$y_{max} = \left(\frac{d}{2}\right)$$

∴ Section modulus is given by

$$Z = \frac{I}{y_{max}}$$

$$= \frac{bd^3/12}{d/2}$$

$$= \left(\frac{bd^2}{6}\right)$$

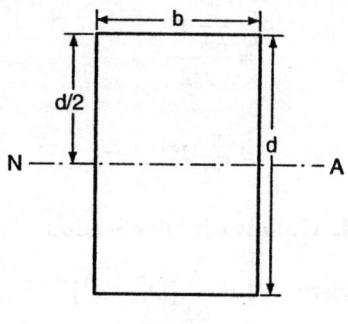

Fig. 7.4

2. Hollow Rectangular Section
For hollow rectangular section,

$$I = \frac{BD^3}{12} - \frac{bd^3}{12}$$

$$= \frac{1}{12}[BD^3 - bd^3]$$

$$y_{max} = \frac{D}{2}$$

∴ $$Z = \frac{I}{y_{max}}$$

$$= \frac{\frac{1}{12}[BD^3 - bd^3]}{D/2}$$

$$= \frac{1}{6D}[BD^3 - bd^3]$$

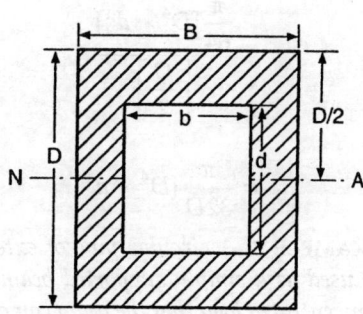

Fig. 7.5

3. Circular Section
For a circular section

$$I = \frac{\pi}{64}d^4$$

and, $y_{max} = \left(\dfrac{d}{2}\right)$

$\therefore$ $Z = \left[\dfrac{I}{y_{max}}\right]$

$= \dfrac{\dfrac{\pi}{64}d^4}{d/2}$

$= \dfrac{\pi}{32}d^3$

4. Hollow Circular Section

Here, $I = \dfrac{\pi}{64}[D^4 - d^4]$

and $y_{max} = \dfrac{D}{2}$

$\therefore$ $Z = \dfrac{I}{y_{max}}$

$= \dfrac{\dfrac{\pi}{64}[D^4 - d^4]}{\left[\dfrac{D}{2}\right]}$

$= \dfrac{\pi}{32D}[D^4 - d^4]$

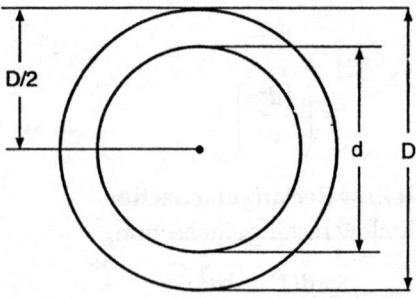

Fig. 7.6

EXAMPLE 1 *A circular pipe of external diameter 100 mm and 80 mm respectively is used as a simply supported beam. The span of the beam is 4 metre. Find the safe concentrated load that the beam can carry at the midspan if the permissible stress in the beam is 120 N/mm².*

SOLUTION Given external dia (D_o) = 100 mm.

Internal diameter = (D_i) = 80 mm.

$\sigma_{permissible} = 120 \text{ N/mm}^2$

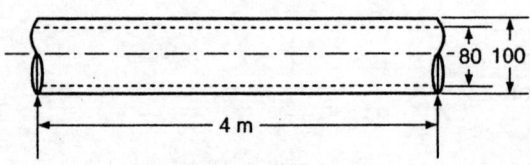

Fig. 7.7

Distance from the N.A. axis to the extreme fibre

$$y_{max} = \left(\frac{D}{2}\right)$$

$$= \left(\frac{100}{2}\right)$$

$$= 50 \text{ mm}$$

Moment of Inertia $(I) = \dfrac{\pi}{64}(D_0^4 - D_i^4)$

$$= 2.898 \times 10^6 \text{ mm}^4$$

Section Modulus $(z) = \dfrac{I}{y_{max}}$

$$= \left[\frac{2.898 \times 10^6}{50}\right]$$

$$= 57960 \text{ mm}^3$$

Moment of Resistance $= \sigma \cdot z$

$$= 120 \times 57960 = \frac{N}{mm^2} \times mm^3$$

$$= 6.96 \times 10^6 \text{ N-mm}$$

Let W is the concentrated load in newton

$\therefore \qquad M_{max} = \dfrac{W \cdot l}{4}$

$$= \frac{W \times \cancel{4}}{\cancel{4}}$$

$$= W \text{ N.meter} = W \times 10^3 \text{ N-mm}$$

Equating maximum bending moment to moment of resistance.

$$M_{max} = M \cdot R$$

$$W \times 10^3 = 6.96 \times 10^6$$

$\therefore \qquad W = 6960 \text{ Newton} \qquad \textbf{Ans.}$

EXAMPLE 2 *Compare the weight of two equally strong beams of circular sections made up of the same material. One beam is of solid circular section and other to hollow circular section for which the ratio of inside and outside diameters is (3/5).*

SOLUTION   Let diameter of solid beam $= D$

Inside diameter of hollow beam $= D_i$

and   Outside diameter of hollow beam $= D_o$

The section modulus for the solid beam is, $Z_S = \dfrac{\pi}{32} D^3$

The section modulus for the hollow beam is

$$Z_H = \frac{\pi D_0^{\,3}}{32}\left[1 - \left(\frac{D_i}{D_o}\right)^4\right]$$

$$= \frac{\pi D_0^{\,3}}{32}\left[1 - \left(\frac{3}{5}\right)^4\right] \qquad\qquad \left\{ \because \frac{D_i}{D_o} = \frac{3}{5}\ \text{given} \right\}$$

$$= \frac{544}{625} \times \frac{\pi}{32} D_o^{\,3}$$

Since the beam are of equal strength, hence their section moduli are equal.

i.e. $Z_S = Z_H$

or, $\dfrac{\pi}{32} D^3 = \left(\dfrac{544}{625}\right)\dfrac{\pi}{32} D_o^{\,3}$

On simplification, we find

$$\left(\frac{D}{D_o}\right) = 0.954$$

Now, owing to the same material for the beam, the ratio of their weights is equal to the ratio of their cross-sectional area.

Let W_S = weight of solid beam

W_H = weight of hollow beam.

$$\therefore \qquad \left(\frac{W_S}{W_H}\right) = \frac{\dfrac{\pi}{4} D^2}{\dfrac{\pi}{4}(D_o^{\,2} - D_i^{\,2})}$$

$$= \frac{D^2}{D_o^{\,2} - D_i^{\,2}}$$

$$= \frac{D^2}{D_0^{\,2}\left[1 - \left(\dfrac{D_i}{D_o}\right)^2\right]}$$

Substituting the values of $\left(\dfrac{D_i}{D_o}\right)$ and $\left(\dfrac{D}{D_o}\right)$ we get

$$\frac{W_S}{W_H} = \frac{(0.954)^2}{\left[1 - \left(\dfrac{3}{5}\right)^2\right]}$$

$$\frac{W_S}{W_H} = 1.422$$

∴ $W_S = 1.422\, W_H$ **Ans.**

EXAMPLE 3 *A rolled steel joist of I-section has the dimensions as shown in Fig. 7.8. This beam of I-section carries a u.d.l of 40 kN/m run on a span of 10 metre. Evaluate the maximum stress produced due to bending.*

SOLUTION M.I. about the neutral axis $= \dfrac{200 \times (400)^3}{12} - \dfrac{(200 - 10) \times (360)^3}{12}$

$$= 327946666 \text{ mm}^4$$

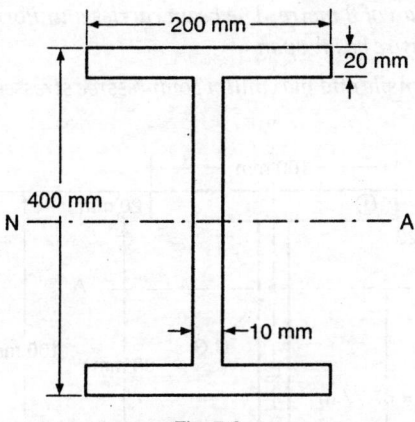

Fig. 7.8

Maximum B. M. is given by $M_{max} = \dfrac{Wl^2}{8}$

$$= \frac{40000 \times 10^2}{8}$$

$$= 500000 \text{ Nm}$$

$$= 5 \times 10^8 \text{ Nmm}$$

Now, By relation $\dfrac{M}{I} = \dfrac{\sigma}{y}$

$$\sigma_{max} = \left[\frac{M}{I} \times y_{max}\right]$$

$$= \frac{5 \times 10^8}{327946666} \times 200 \qquad\qquad [\because y_{max} = 200 \text{ mm}]$$

$$= 304.9 \text{ N/mm}^2 \qquad \textbf{Ans.}$$

Evaluation of bending stress for unsymmetrical section

We know that the neutral axis passes through the geometrical centre of the section for symmetrical section. But in the case of unsymmetrical section (*e.g.* L section; T section) the neutral axis does not pass through the geometrical centre of the section. Therefore, the value of *y* for the topmost layer or the bottom layer of the section from the neutral axis will not be the same.

For finding the bending stress in the beam the bigger value of *y* is taken for calculation. Since the neutral axis passes through the centre of gravity of the section, therefore, while solving the problem of unsymmetrical section, first of all, the centre of gravity is calculated.

EXAMPLE 4 *A C.I. beam is in the shape of T-section as shown in figure. The beam is simply supported on a span of 8 metre. The beam carries a uniformly distributed load of 1.5 kN/m length on the entire beam-span.*

Evaluate the maximum tensile and maximum compressive stresses.

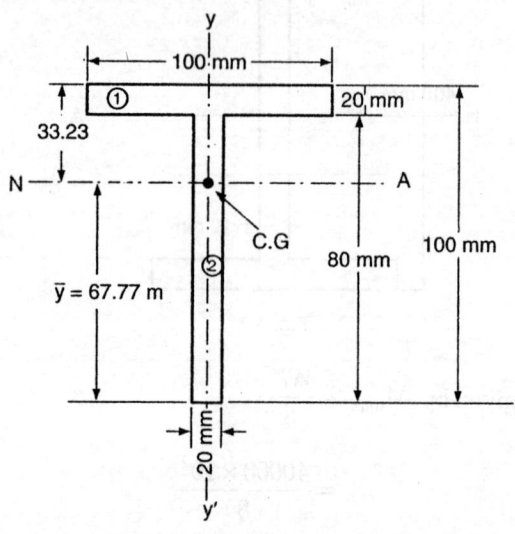

Fig. 7.9

SOLUTION As the given section is unsymmetrical, so first of all we will find out C.G. lying on the *y*-axis.

Let $\quad \bar{y}$ = distance of the C.G. of the section from the bottom.

$$\therefore \qquad \bar{y} = \left(\frac{A_1 y_1 + A_2 y_2}{A_1 + A_2} \right)$$

$$= \frac{(100 \times 20) \times \left(80 + \dfrac{20}{2}\right) + (80 \times 20) \times \dfrac{80}{2}}{(100 \times 20) + (80 \times 20)}$$

$$= \left(\frac{180000 + 64000}{2000 + 1600}\right)$$

$$= \left(\frac{244000}{3600}\right)$$

$$= 67.77 \text{ mm}$$

Therefore, Neutral Axis lies at a distance of 67.77 mm from the bottom face or $(100 - 67.77) = 33.23$ mm from the top face.

M.I. of the section about N.A. is given by

$$I = (I_1 + I_2)$$

where, I_1 = M.I. of the flange about N.A.

and, I_2 = M.I. of the web about N.A.

I_1 = M.O.I of top flange about N.A.

= M.O.I of the top flange about its *e.g.* + $A_1 d_1^2$

(By Parallel Axis theorem)

$$= \frac{100 \times 20^3}{12} + (100 + 20) \times (32.23 - 10)^2$$

(where d_1 = distance of its C.G. from N.A.)

$$= 66666.7 + (100 \times 20) \times (22.23)^2$$

$$= 1055012.5 \text{ mm}^4$$

I_2 = Moment of Inertia of web about N.A.

= M.I. of web about its C.G. + $A_2 d_2^2$

$$= \frac{20 \times 80^3}{12} + (80 \times 20) \times (67.77 - 40)^2$$

(where d_2 = distance of its C.G. from N.A.)

$$= 853333.3 + 1233876.6$$

$$= 2087209.9 \text{ mm}^4$$

$\therefore \qquad I = (I_1 + I_2)$

$\qquad\qquad = (1055012.5 + 2087209.9)$

$\qquad\qquad = 3142222.4 \text{ mm}^4$

$\therefore \qquad$ Max. B.M.,

$\qquad M_{max} = \dfrac{wl^2}{8}$ Since the beam carries u.d.l 1.5 kN/m

$\qquad\qquad = \dfrac{1500 \times 8^2}{8} \text{ N metre}$

$\qquad\qquad = 12 \times 10^6 \text{ N metre}$

$\qquad\qquad = 12 \times 10^9 \text{ Nmm}$

By relation, $\dfrac{M}{I} = \dfrac{\sigma}{y}$

$\qquad \sigma = \left(\dfrac{M}{I}\right) \times y$

From this relation we find that when y is more σ will be more i.e. $\sigma = f(y)$.

$\therefore \qquad$ Maximum tensile stress =

$\qquad \sigma_t(\text{max}) = \dfrac{12 \times 10^6}{3142222.4} \times 67.77$

$\qquad \boxed{\sigma_t(\text{max}) = 258.81 \text{ N/mm}^2} \qquad$ **Ans.**

$\therefore \qquad$ Maximum compressive stress =

$\qquad \sigma_c(\text{max}) = \dfrac{M}{I} \times y$

$\qquad\qquad = \dfrac{12 \times 10^6}{3142222.4} \times 32.23$

$\qquad \sigma_{c\,(\text{max})} = 123.06 \text{ N/mm}^2 \qquad$ **Ans.**

7.7 COMPOSITE BEAM (FLITCHED BEAM)*

A beam made up of two 'or' more different material assumed to be rigidly connected together and behaving like a single piece is known as composite beam.

Let us consider a composite beam with the two materials denoted by the suffixes 1 and 2.

---

*Flitched beams 'or' composite beams are used when one material, if used alone, requires large cross sectional area which is not suitable to the space available and also to reinforce the beam at region of high bending moment or to equalise the strength of the beam in tension or compression.

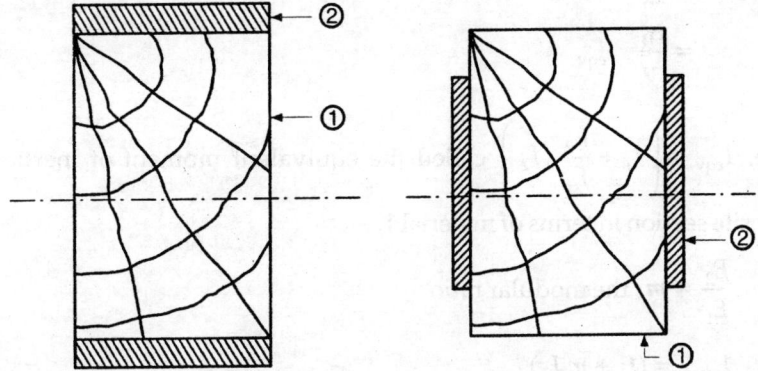

Fig. 7.10

As the two are rigidly connected together, the strains in both will be equal.
Therefore, at any common surface, strain will be same for both material

i.e. $\qquad \varepsilon_1 = \varepsilon_2$

or, $\qquad \dfrac{\sigma_1}{E_1} = \dfrac{\sigma_2}{E_2}$

or, $\qquad \dfrac{\sigma_1}{\sigma_2} = \dfrac{E_1}{E_2}$ $\hspace{3cm}$ ...(1)

Now, from the bending equation,

$$\text{Moment of resistance } M = \left(\frac{\sigma}{y} \right) \cdot I$$

$\therefore \qquad M_1 = \dfrac{\sigma_1 I_1}{y}$

and $\qquad M_2 = \dfrac{\sigma_2 I_2}{y}$

where, y is the distance of the common surface. From the neutral axis.

$\therefore \qquad$ Total moment of resistance of the composite section

$$M = M_1 + M_2$$

$$= \frac{\sigma_1 I_1}{y} + \frac{\sigma_2 I_2}{y} \hspace{3cm} ...(2)$$

Substituting the value of σ_2 from (1) into (2)

$$M = \frac{\sigma_1 I_1}{y} + \left(\sigma_1 \cdot \frac{E_2}{E_1} \right) \cdot \frac{I_2}{y}$$

$$= \frac{\sigma_1}{y} \left[I_1 + \frac{E_2}{E_1} \cdot I_2 \right]$$

$$= \frac{\sigma_1}{y} \cdot I_{eqv}$$

where, $I_{eqv} = \left(I_1 + \frac{E_2}{E_1} \cdot I_2 \right)$ called the equivalent moment of inertia of the composite section in terms of material 1.

If $\qquad \frac{E_2}{E_1} = m,$ the modular ratio

then $\qquad I_{equ1} = (I_1 + m\,I_2)$ $\qquad$ ...(3)

Similarly, the equivalent moment of inertia of the composite section in terms of material 2 is given by

$$I_{eqv2} = \left(I_2 + \frac{1}{m} \cdot I_1 \right) \qquad \qquad ...(4)$$

Equations (3) and (4) provide us with a very simple method of finding bending stresses in the composite sections.

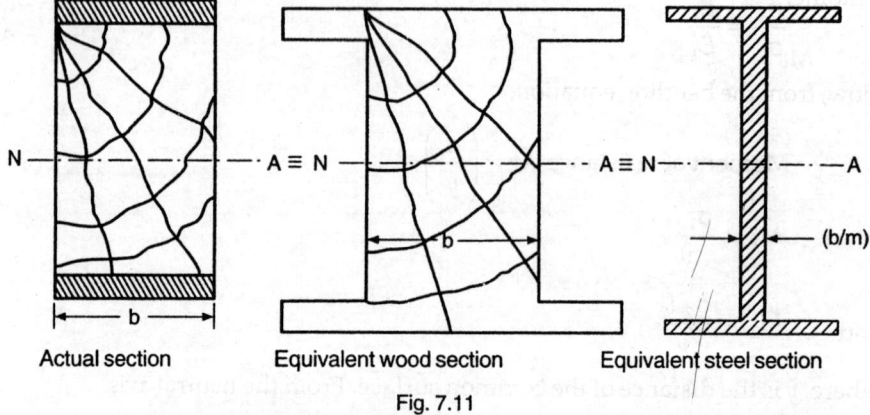

| Actual section | Equivalent wood section | Equivalent steel section |

Fig. 7.11

EXAMPLE 5 *A composite beam is made by placing two steel plates, 12 mm thick and 240 mm deep, one each on both sides of a wooden section 90 mm wide and 240 mm deep. Determine the moment of resistance of the section of the beam.*

Take $\left(\dfrac{E_S}{E_w} \right) = 15,$ *the stress in the wood should not exceed 7 MPa.*

SOLUTION Modular Ratio $(m) = \dfrac{\sigma_S}{\sigma_W} = \dfrac{E_S}{E_W} = 15$

Steel in wood $(\sigma_W) = 7$ MPa

$$= 7 \times 10^6 \text{ Pa}$$

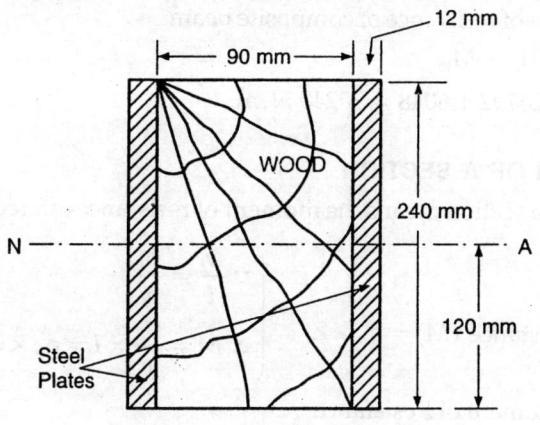

Fig. 7.12

Steel in steel plate $(\sigma_S) = m \times \sigma_W$

$$= 15 \times 7 \times 10^6 \text{ Pa}$$

$$= 105 \times 10^6 \text{ Pa}$$

The moment of resistance of the steel plate M_s is given by

$$M_S = \sigma_S \times \frac{I_S}{y}$$

$$= \sigma_S \times \left(2 \times \frac{td^3}{12} \right) \times \frac{1}{(d/2)}$$

$$= \frac{\sigma_S \cdot t \cdot d^2}{3}$$

$$= \frac{105 \times 10^6 \times 12 \times 10^{-3} \times (240 \times 10^{-3})^2}{3}$$

$$= 24192 \text{ N.m}$$

The moment of resistance of the wooden section is M_w given by

$$M_w = \sigma_w \cdot \frac{I_w}{y}$$

$$= \sigma_w \cdot \frac{bd^3}{12} \cdot \frac{1}{(d/2)}$$

$$= \frac{\sigma_w bd^2}{6}$$

$$= \frac{7 \times 10^6 \times 90 \times 10^{-3} \times (240 \times 10^{-3})^2}{6} \text{N.m}$$

$$= 6048 \text{ Nm}$$

∴   Moment of resistance of composite beam

$(M) = M_S + M_W$

$= 24192 + 6048 = 30240 \text{ N.m}$

7.8 STRENGTH OF A SECTION

The strength of a section means the moment of resistance offered by the section.

Moment of Resistance $(M) = \sigma_b \times Z$
$$\left(\begin{array}{l} \because \dfrac{M}{I} = \dfrac{\sigma_b}{y} \\[2mm] \therefore M = \dfrac{\sigma_b}{y} \times I = \sigma_b \times Z \end{array} \right)$$

where M = Moment of Resistance

σ_b = Bending stress

Z = section Modulus.

Moment of resistance depends upon the section modulus. Therefore, the section modulus represents the strength of the section.

Higher the value of Z, stronger will be the section.

7.9 BEAM OF UNIFORM STRENGTH

A beam in which every section along the longitudinal axis has the same maximum bending stress is called the beam of uniform strength.

EXAMPLE 6 *Prove that the ratio of depth to width of the strongest beam that can be cut from a circular log of diameter 'd' is 1.414. Calculate the depth and width of the strongest beam that can be cut of a cylindrical log of wood whose diameter is 300 mm.*

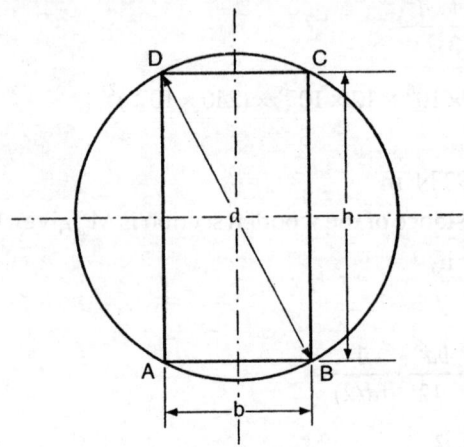

Fig. 7.13

SOLUTION Let the dia. of log = d

Let *ABCD* be the strongest rectangular section which can be cut out of the cylindrical log.

Let b = width of the strongest section

d = depth of the strongest section.

Hence, Section modulus $(z) = \dfrac{I}{y}$

$$= \left(\dfrac{\dfrac{bh^3}{12}}{\dfrac{h}{2}} \right)$$

$$= \dfrac{bh^2}{6} \qquad \qquad \dots (1)$$

From $\triangle BCD$, $b^2 + h^2 = d^2$

$\therefore \qquad h^2 = (d^2 - b^2)$

Now, substituting the value of h^2 in equation (1) we get

$$Z = \dfrac{b}{6}(d^2 - b^2)$$

$$= \dfrac{1}{6}(bd^2 - b^3) \qquad \qquad \dots (2)$$

Now, for the beam to be strongest, the section modulus should be maximum.

For section modulus (Z) to be maximum

$$\dfrac{dZ}{db} = 0$$

or, $\qquad \dfrac{d}{db}\left[\dfrac{bd^2 - b^3}{6} \right] = 0$

or, $\qquad \dfrac{d^2 - 3b^2}{6} = 0$

or, $\qquad d^2 = 3b^2 \qquad \qquad \dots (3)$

From triangle BCD, $d^2 = b^2 + h^2$

Putting the value of d^2 in equation (3) we have

$$b^2 + h^2 = 3b^2$$

$$h^2 = 2b^2$$

$$h = \sqrt{2}b$$

$$\boxed{\dfrac{h}{b} = \sqrt{2} = 1.414. \textbf{ Proved}}$$

Now, from equation (3)

$$d^2 = 3b^2$$

$$3b^2 = d^2 = (300)^2$$

$$b^2 = \left(\frac{\cancel{90000}^{\,30000}}{\cancel{3}}\right)$$

$$b = \sqrt{30000}$$

$$= \sqrt{3} \times 100$$

$$= 1.732 \times 100 \text{ mm}$$

$$= 173.200 \text{ mm}$$

$$\boxed{b = 173.2 \text{ mm}} \qquad \textbf{Ans.}$$

$$\therefore \qquad h = \sqrt{2} \times b = 1.414 \times 173.2$$

$$\boxed{h = 249.95 \ \text{mm}} \qquad \textbf{Ans.}$$

EXAMPLE 7 *A timber beam of 3 metre span carries a uniformly distributed load of 5 kN/m and a point load 1 kN at the centre of the span. If the permissible bending stress be 100 N/mm², find the section taking depth as twice the breadth.*

(UPTU 2006-07)

SOLUTION

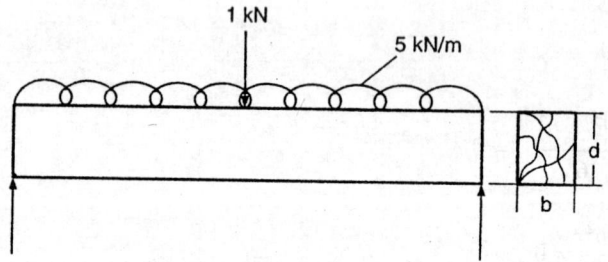

Fig. 7.14

Given $W = 1 \text{ kN}$

$\qquad w = 5 \text{ kN/m}$

$\qquad \sigma_b = 100 \text{ N/mm}^2$

$$\text{Maximum Bending Moment} = \left(\frac{wl^2}{8} + \frac{Wl}{4}\right) = \frac{5 \times (3)^2}{8} + \frac{1 \times 3}{4}$$

$$= \frac{45}{8} + \frac{3}{4} = 6.375 \text{ kNm}$$

$$= 6375 \times 10^3 \text{ Nmm}$$

By formula, $I = \dfrac{b.d^3}{12}$

Given, $d = 2b$

Hence, $I = \dfrac{b \times (2b)^3}{12} = \dfrac{8b^4}{12} = \dfrac{2}{3}b^4$

Now, by formula,

$$\dfrac{M}{I} = \dfrac{\sigma_b}{y}$$

$$\dfrac{6375 \times 10^3}{\dfrac{2b^4}{3}} = \dfrac{100}{\left(\dfrac{d}{2}\right)}$$

or, $\quad \dfrac{6375 \times 3000}{2b^3} = 100 \qquad\qquad\qquad \left[As \dfrac{d}{2} = b \right]$

or, $\quad b = \left(\dfrac{6375 \times 3000}{2 \times 100} \right)^{1/3} = 44$ mm **Ans.**

Hence, $d = 2b = 88$ mm **Ans.**

7.10 DESIGN OF BEAM FOR BENDING STRESS

The process of designing a beam requires
  (i) Type of structure (airplane, automobile, bridge, building or whatever)
 (ii) The materials to be used
(iii) Loads to be supported
 (iv) The environmental condition
  (v) Costs to be paid

From the view of strength, the task ultimately reduces to select the shape and size of the beam such that actual stress in the beam do not exceed the allowable stress for the material.

While designing a beam to resist bending stress, we normally begin by calculating the required section modulus (Z). To ensure that allowable stress is not exceeded, we must choose a beam that provides a section modulus (Z) as large as obtained from equation $Z = \dfrac{M_{max}}{\sigma_{allowable}}$.

We usually select a beam that provides the least cross-sectional area (A) and still providing the required Section Modulus (Z).

Beams are constructed in a great variety of shapes and size to suit the requirement. Very large beams are fabricated by welding.

Beams of standard size can be supplied by dealers and manufactures. Readily available shape for the beam are wide flange beam, I-beam, angles, channels, rectangular beams and tubes.

HIGHLIGHTS

1. The stress produced due to constant bending moment (with zero shear force) is known as bending Stress or flexural stress.
2. The bending equation is given by

$$\frac{M}{I} = \frac{\sigma}{y} = \frac{E}{R}$$

3. The bending stress in any layer is directly proportional to the distance of the layer from the neutral axis (N.A) and so at N.A. the bending stress is zero.
4. The neutral axis of a symmetrical section (*e.g.* circular; rectangular or square I-section) lies at a distance of $(d/2)$ from the outer most layer of the section where d = depth of the section.
5. If the top layer of any section is subjected to compressive stress, then tensile stress will be developed in bottom layer.
6. Section Modulus $(z) = \dfrac{I}{y_{max}}$

For rectangular section $z = \dfrac{bd^2}{6} = \dfrac{1}{6D}[BD^3 - bd^3]$

For circular section $= \dfrac{\pi D^3}{32}$

For hollow circular section $= \dfrac{\pi}{32D}[D^4 - d^4]$

7. For finding bending stress in an unsymmetrical section first their C.G. is to be obtained. This gives the position of N.A. The bigger value of y is used in bending equation.
8. A beam made up of two or more different materials assumed to be rigidly connected together and behaving like a single unit, is known as a composite beam or flitched beam.
9. The strain at the common surface of a composite beam is same *i.e.*
$\varepsilon_1 = \varepsilon_2$

$$\therefore \quad \frac{\sigma_1}{E_1} = \frac{\sigma_2}{E_2}$$

10. The moment of resistance offered by the section is known as the strength of the section.

PROBLEMS FOR PRACTICE
(THEORETICAL)

1. Derive the bending equation.
2. What is neutral axis?
3. What is moment of resistance of a section?
4. Define 'section modulus'.

5. What is the meaning strength of a section?
6. How do you find bending stress in unsymmetrical section.

(NUMERICAL)

1. A copper strip (E_c = 105 GPa) and an aluminium strip (E_{al} = 75 GPa) are bonded together to form the composite bar. Knowing that the bar is bent about a horizonal axis by a couple of moment 35 N.M, determine the maximum stress in the aluminium strip and the copper strip.

2. A steel pipe and an aluminium pipe are securely bonded together to form the composite beam as shown in figure. The modulus of elasticity is 210 GPa for the steel and 70 GPa for the aluminium. Knowing that the composite beam is bent by the couples of moment 500 N.m, determine the maximum stress (a) in the aluminium (b) in the steel.

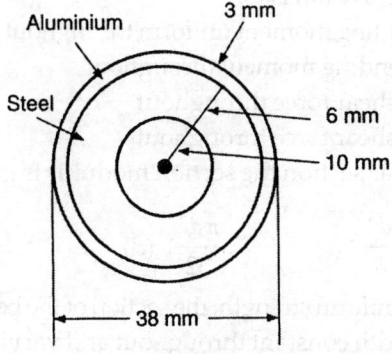

Fig. 7.15

3. The design of a reinforced concrete beam is said to be balanced if the maximum stress in the steel and concrete are equal, respectively, to the allowable stresses σ_s and σ_c. Show that to achieve a balanced design, the distance x from the top of the beam to the neutral axis must be

$$x = \frac{d}{1 + \dfrac{\sigma_s \cdot E_c}{\sigma_c \cdot E_s}}$$

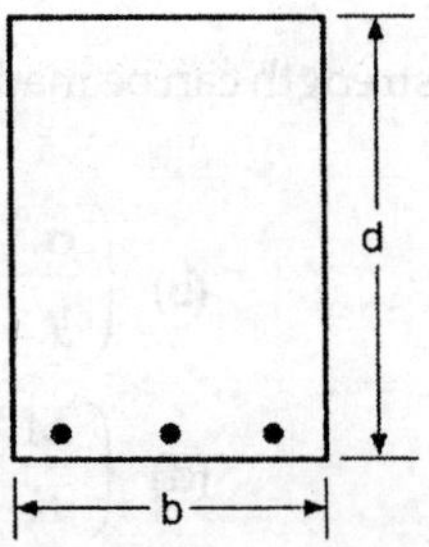

Fig. 7.16

ANSWERS

1. − 56 MPa; 66.4 Mpa   **2.** (a) 52.3 MPa   (b) 132.1 MPa

OBJECTIVE QUESTIONS

1. A beam is said to be under pure bending if:
   (a) shear force is zero
   (b) bending moment is constant but
   (c) rate of loading is uniform
   (d) none of the above
2. The strength of the beam depends on:
   (a) bending moment   (b) section modulus
   (c) C.G. of the section   (d) its weight
3. The effect of arching a beam is to:
   (a) to make the bending moment uniform throughout
   (b) to reduce the bending moment throughout
   (c) to increase the shear force throughout
   (d) to increase the shear force throughout
4. In the case of circular section the section modulus is given as:

   (a) $\dfrac{\pi d^2}{16}$ (b) $\dfrac{\pi d^3}{16}$ (c) $\dfrac{\pi d^3}{32}$ (d) $\dfrac{\pi d^3}{64}$

5. To get the beam of uniform strength, the section of the beam may be varied by:
   (a) keeping the width constant throughout and varying the depth
   (b) **keeping the depth constant throughout the length and varying the width**
   (c) varying both *i.e.* width and depth in a suitable manner
   (d) all the above
6. The most common ways of keeping the beam of uniform strength by:
   (a) keeping the width uniform and varying the depth
   (b) keeping the depth uniform and varying the width
   (c) varying both width and depth
   (d) none of the above
7. Circular beams of uniform strength can be made by varying diameter in such a way that:

   (a) $\left(\dfrac{M}{Z}\right)$ is constant   (b) $\left(\dfrac{\sigma}{y}\right)$ is constant

   (c) $\left(\dfrac{E}{R}\right)$ is constant   (d) $\left(\dfrac{M}{R}\right)$ is constant

8. In a section subjected to bending moment M its moment of resistance:

(a) is greater than
(b) is smaller than M
(c) is equal to M
(d) can be greater than or equal to M

9. Reinforced concrete beams are designed on the assumption that concrete cannot take any

(a) tensile stress
(b) compressive stress
(c) tensile load
(d) compressive load

10. A rectangular timber beam is cut-out of a cylinderical log of diameter D. The depth of the strongest timber beam is:

(a) $\sqrt{\dfrac{1}{2}D}$
(b) $\sqrt{\dfrac{2}{3}D}$
(c) $\sqrt{\dfrac{5}{8}D}$
(d) $\sqrt{\dfrac{3}{4}D}$

11. A simply supported beam of span 'l' carries load W at mid point. The breadth 'b' of the beam along the entire span is constant.

Given σ_a = allowable stress for a beam of uniform strength, the depth of the beam at any cross-section at a section at a distance x from the support will be:

(a) $\dfrac{\sigma Wx}{\sigma_a \cdot b}$
(b) $\sqrt{\dfrac{\sigma Wx}{\sigma_a \cdot b}}$
(c) $\dfrac{3Wx}{\sigma_a \cdot b}$
(d) $\sqrt{\dfrac{3Wx}{\sigma_a \cdot b}}$

12. A cantilever of constant depth carries a uniformly distributed load on the whole span. To make the maximum stress at all sections the same the breadth of the section at a distance from the free end should be proportional to:

(a) x
(b) $\sqrt{x}$
(c) x^2
(d) x^3

13. Neutral axis in the case of a beam subjected to bending:
(a) may coincide with its centroidal axis
(b) always coincides with its centrodial axis
(c) should not coincide with its centroidal axis
(d) never coincides with its centroidal axis

ANSWERS

1. (b)	2. (b)	3. (b)	4. (c)	5. (d)	6. (a)
7. (a)	8. (c)	9. (a)	10. (b)	11. (d)	12. (c)
13. (b)					

COMBINED STRESSES
(Direct Stress and Bending Stress)

8.1 INTRODUCTION

When several types of loadings are superimposed on the same point in a section, it is known as combined loading. We have already discussed earlier that applied load develops stress so here also as a result of combined loading combined stresses are developed in a machine member or structure.

The basic type of loading are:

  (i) Axial loading

  (ii) Torsional loading

 (iii) Flexural loading

Due to axial loading (Tensile or Compressive) axial stress or normal stress is developed in the member of a machine or structure.

Due to torsional loading torsional shear stress is developed in the member of a machine or structure.

Due to flexural loading *i.e.*, by bending moment, flexural stress or bending stress is developed in the member.

The axial stress or normal stress (σ_a) or $(\sigma_n) = \dfrac{P}{A}$

Torsional stress $(\tau) = \dfrac{T \cdot r}{J}$ and

Flexural stress or bending stress $(\sigma_b) = \dfrac{M}{I} \cdot y$

There are four possible combination of loading:

  (i) Axial and flexural

  (ii) Axial and torsional

 (iii) Torsional and flexural

 (iv) Axial, torsional and flexural acting simultaneously.

Hence, it is important to find their combined effect.

To memorise we can adopt the following sketch as shown in Fig. 8.1.

Some examples of combined loading are as follows:

1. A short column with eccentric loading have axial compression and bending effect.

2. A beam when subjected to load(s) has bending moment and shear force at the same time.

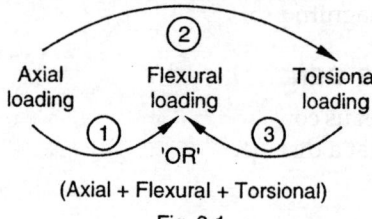

3. A shaft supporting an overhanging flywheel is simultaneously under bending and torsion.

In this chapter we will focus on the type one loading *i.e.*, **Axial and Flexural**. The rest we will study in the chapter of torsion.

8.2 COLUMN SUBJECTED TO ECCENTRIC LOAD

When a short column is subjected to a vertical load which is axial, then compressive stress occurs uniformly throughout the entire section at the base as shown in Fig. 8.2. However, when the load is eccentric *i.e.* little away from the centre of gravity, then bending moment also develops in the column that induces bending stress. Therefore, we can say that the column is subjected to combined loading comprising direct stress and bending stress shown in Fig. 8.3.

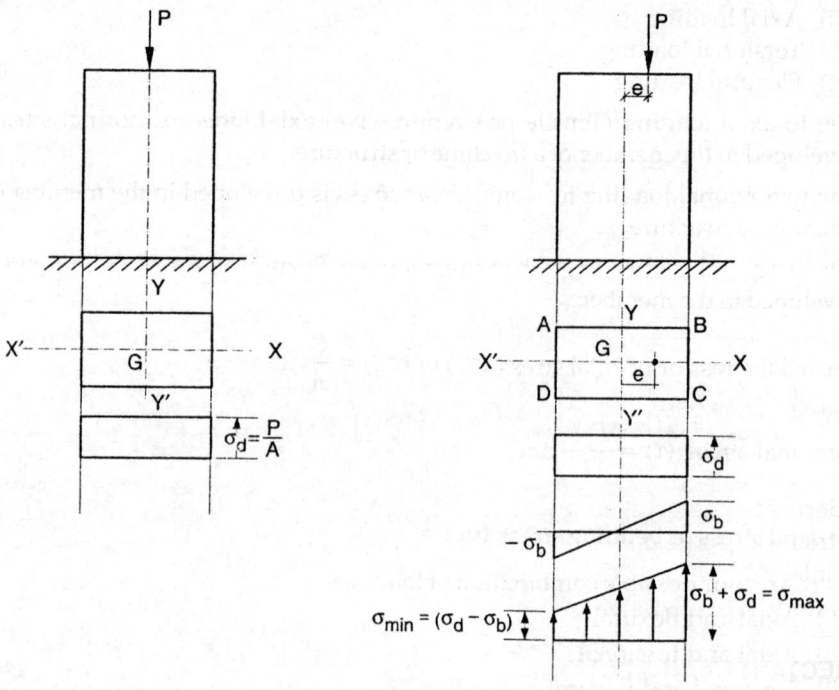

Fig. 8.2   Fig. 8.3

It is observed that the nature of resultant stress will always be positive on the load side of the body while on the opposite side, the resultant will depend on the magnitude of σ_d and σ_b.

8.3 GENERALISED ECCENTRIC LOADING

Let us consider a arbitratory, section of a body subjected to eccentric load P which is at a distance e_x from XX' axis and e_y from YY' axis.

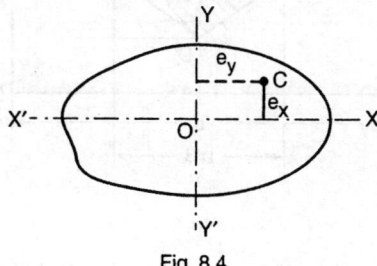

Fig. 8.4

So, like previous discussion the body will have moments about XX' axis and YY' axis.

Therefore, resultant stress (σ_R) at point C is given by the following expression.

σ_R = Direct stress + Bending stresses along x and y axes.

$\therefore \qquad \sigma_R = \dfrac{P}{A} \pm \Sigma \dfrac{M}{I} \times$ Distance of the load from the neutral axis

$$= \frac{P}{A} \pm \frac{M_{xx}}{I_{xx}} \times y \pm \frac{M_y}{I_{yy}} \times x$$

$$= \frac{P}{A} \pm \frac{M_{xx}}{A \cdot r_x^2} \times y \pm \frac{M_{yy}}{A \cdot r_y^2} \times x$$

$$(\because I = A \cdot r^2 \text{ where } r \text{ is the radius of gyration})$$

$$= \frac{P}{A} \pm \frac{P \cdot e_x \cdot y}{A \cdot r_x^2} \pm \frac{P \cdot e_y \cdot x}{A \cdot r_y^2}$$

$$= \frac{P}{A}\left[1 \pm \frac{e_x \cdot y}{r_x^2} \times y \pm \frac{e_y \cdot x}{r_y^2} \right]$$

This derivation of resultant stress is needed to know the maximum value of the eccentricities so that no resultant tensile stresses occur in the material which is weak intension *i.e.,* concrete.

Let us study the rectangular section first.

8.4 RECTANGULAR SECTION

Let us study the eccentric loading for rectangular section of short column having length b and width d.

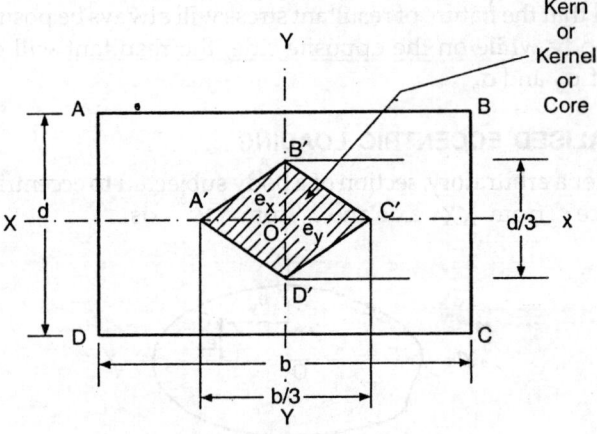

Fig. 8.5

By the generalised expression of eccentric loading the resultant stress at the point of loading in a concrete column is given by

$$(\sigma_R) = \frac{P}{A}\left[1 \pm \frac{e_x \cdot y}{r_x^2} \pm \frac{e_y \cdot x}{r_y^2}\right]$$

Here, $x = \dfrac{b}{2}$ and $y = \dfrac{d}{2}$

$$r_x^2 = \frac{I_{xx}}{A}$$

$$= \frac{bd^3}{12} \times \frac{1}{bd} = \frac{d^2}{12}$$

and $\qquad r_y^2 = \dfrac{I_{yy}}{A}$

$$= \frac{db^3}{12} \times \frac{1}{bd} = \frac{b^2}{12}$$

Hence, $\quad \sigma_R = \dfrac{P}{A}\left[1 \pm \dfrac{e_x \cdot \dfrac{d}{2}}{\dfrac{d^2}{12}} \pm \dfrac{e_y \cdot \dfrac{b}{2}}{\dfrac{b^2}{12}}\right]$

$$= \frac{P}{A}\left[1 \pm \frac{6e_x}{d} \pm \frac{6e_y}{b}\right]$$

For no tension, $\pm\left(\dfrac{6e_x}{d} + \dfrac{6e_y}{b}\right) \le 1$

When $\quad e_x = 0 \Rightarrow e_y \leq \dfrac{b}{6}$

When $\quad e_y = 0 \Rightarrow e_x \leq \dfrac{d}{6}$

So, the no tension zone will be are $A'B'C'D'$. **The shaded area is known as Kern; Kernel or Core of the section.**

This is known as **'middle third rule'** for rectangular section.

8.5 CIRCULAR SECTION

We know that resultant stress $(\sigma_R) = \dfrac{P}{A}\left[1 \pm \dfrac{e_x \cdot y}{r_x^2} \pm \dfrac{e_y \cdot x}{r_y^2}\right]$

Due to symmetry $x = y = \dfrac{d}{2}$

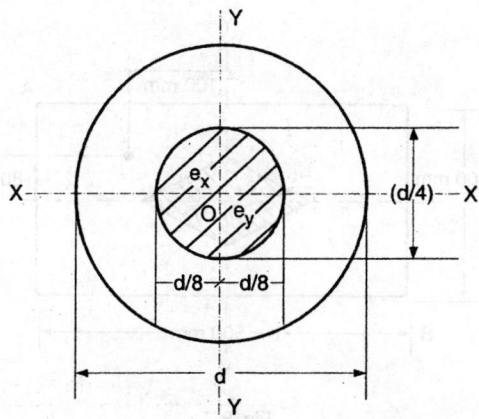

Fig. 8.6

$\Rightarrow \qquad r_x^2 = r_y^2 = \dfrac{I}{A} \qquad\qquad \left[\because I = A \cdot r^2\right]$

$$= \dfrac{\pi}{64}d^4 \times \dfrac{1}{\dfrac{\pi}{4}d^2} = \dfrac{d^2}{16}$$

Hence, $\quad \sigma_R = \dfrac{P}{A}\left[1 \pm \dfrac{e_x \cdot \dfrac{d}{2}}{\dfrac{d^2}{16}} \pm \dfrac{e_y \cdot \dfrac{d}{2}}{\dfrac{d^2}{16}}\right]$

$$= \dfrac{P}{A}\left[1 \pm \dfrac{8e_x}{d} \pm \dfrac{8e_y}{d}\right]$$

For no tension, $\pm\left(\dfrac{8e_x}{d} + \dfrac{8e_y}{d}\right) \leq 1$

When $\quad e_x = 0 \Rightarrow e_y \leq \pm\dfrac{d}{8}$

When $\quad e_y = 0 \Rightarrow e_x \leq \pm\dfrac{d}{8}$

So for no tension to occur in the section, the load should be applied within one fourth of diameter of the circle. The no tension zone is shown by shaded area. This is known as **middle quarter rule**.

EXAMPLE 1 *A rectangular masonary column has a cross-section 500 mm × 400 mm and is subjected to a vertical compressive load of 100 kN applied at point P. Determine the value of the maximum stress produced in the section. Is the section at any point is subjected to tensile stress?*   **(UPTU 2005-06 3rd Sem.)**

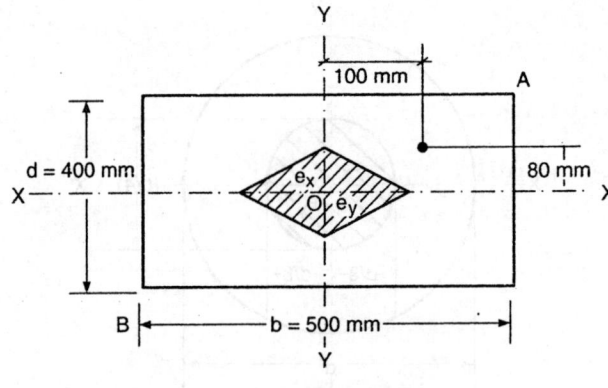

Fig. 8.7

SOLUTION Given $b = 500$ mm; $d = 400$ mm; $e_x = 80$ mm; $e_y = 100$ mm and $P = 100$ kN.

Objective: To compute σ_{max} and σ_{min}

Resultant stress (σ_R) = Direct Stress + Bending Stresses

$$= \sigma \pm \sigma_{bx} \pm \sigma_{by}$$

$$= \frac{P}{A} \pm \frac{M_{xx}}{Z_{xx}} \pm \frac{M_{yy}}{Z_{yy}} \qquad \left[Z = \text{Section Modulus} = \frac{I}{y}\right]$$

Now, $\quad \dfrac{P}{A} = \dfrac{100 \times 10^3}{20 \times 10^4}$ N/mm^2

$$= 0.5 \text{ N/mm}^2$$

$$M_x = P \cdot e_x$$

$$= 100 \times 10^3 \times 80 = 8 \times 10^6 \text{ N mm}$$

$$M_y = P \cdot e_y$$

$$= 100 \times 10^3 \times 100$$

$$= 10 \times 10^6 \text{ N mm}$$

$$Z_{xx} = \frac{I_{xx}}{y}$$

$$= \frac{bd^3}{12} \Big/ \frac{d}{2} \qquad\qquad \left(\text{Here, } y = \frac{d}{2} \right)$$

$$= \frac{bd^3}{12} \times \frac{2}{d} = \frac{bd^2}{6}$$

$$= \frac{500 \times (400)^2}{6} = 12.33 \times 10^6 \text{ mm}^3$$

$$Z_{yy} = \frac{I_{yy}}{x}$$

$$= \frac{db^3}{12} \times \frac{2}{b} \qquad\qquad \left(\because x = \frac{b}{2} \right)$$

$$= \frac{db^2}{6}$$

$$= \frac{400 \times (500)^2}{6} = 16.66 \times 10^6 \text{ mm}^3$$

Since the load P is acting in the first quadrant *i.e.*, near corner A, the maximum compressive stress is developed at A and tensile stress will be developed at B.

Resultant stress at A $(\sigma_A) = \sigma + \sigma_{bx} + \sigma_{by}$

$$= \frac{P}{A} + \frac{M_{xx}}{Z_{xx}} + \frac{M_{yy}}{Z_{yy}}$$

$$= \frac{100 \times 10^3}{20 \times 10^4} + \frac{8 \times 10^6}{13.33 \times 10^6} + \frac{10 \times 10^6}{16.66 \times 10^6}$$

$$= 0.5 + 0.6 + 0.6$$

$$= 1.7 \text{ N/mm}^2 \text{ (Maximum)}$$

Resultant stress at B $(\sigma_B) = \sigma - \sigma_{bx} - \sigma_{by}$

$(B$ is in IVth quadrant where x and y both are $-$ve)

$$= 0.5 - 0.6 - 0.6$$

$$= 0.7 \text{ N/mm}^2 \text{ (Minimum)}$$

N.B.: (a) While computing stress here, care should be taken for the sign of x and y as following.

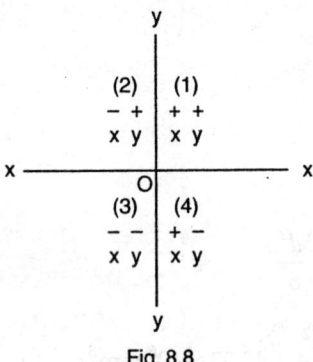

Fig. 8.8

(b) Further, opposite nature stress will develop in the opposite quadrant. So, if compressive stress develops in the Ist quadrant, then tensile stress will develop in the IIIrd quadrant.

EXAMPLE 2 *A rectangular bar 60 mm × 50 mm is subjected to a pull of 100 kN in such a way that it is parallel to the bar axis and is 10 mm away from x-axis.*

Evaluate the values of stresses produced and plot a diagram showing the variation of stress across the bar section.

SOLUTION Q is the point on y-axis where the tensile load 10 kN is acting.

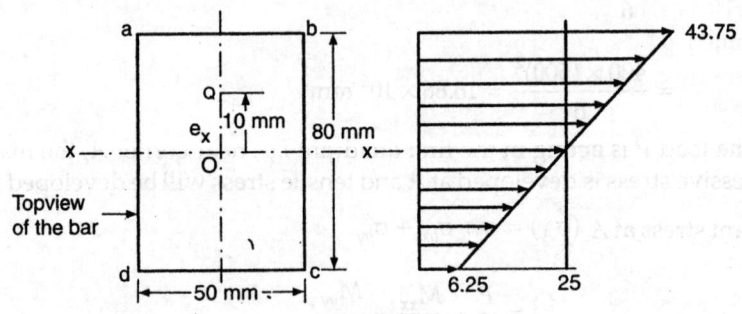

Fig. 8.9

Direct stress $(\sigma_d) = \dfrac{P}{A}$

$$= \frac{100 \times 10^3}{80 \times 50}$$

$$= \frac{1000}{40}$$

$$= 25 \text{ N/mm}^2$$

Bending stress $(\sigma_b) = \pm \dfrac{(P \cdot e_x) \cdot y}{I_x}$

$$= \pm \frac{(100 \times 10^3 \times 10) \times 40}{\dfrac{50 \times (80)^3}{12}}$$

$$= \pm 18.75 \text{ N/mm}^2$$

Here bending stress $(\sigma_b) = +18.75 \text{ N/mm}^2$ $\left(\begin{array}{l}\text{A positive quantity}\\ \text{being in Ist Quadrant}\end{array}\right)$

Hence, at the top, resultant stress $= 25 + 18.75$

$$= 43.75 \text{ N/mm}^2$$

$$= 43.75 \text{ MPa} \quad \text{(Tensile)}$$

And, at the bottom, resultant stress $= 25 - 18.5$

$$= 6.52 \text{ MPa} \quad \text{(Tensile)}$$

Let us study the combined stresses for a helicopter shaft. The rotor shaft of a helicopter drives the rotor blade that provides the lifting force to support the helicopter in the air. As a consequence, the shaft is subjected to a combination of torsion and axial loadings.

EXAMPLE 3 *For a 50 mm diameter shaft of a helicopter transmitting torque T = 2.4 kN·m, and a tensile force P = 125 kN·m, determine the maximum tensile, compressive and shear stresses in the shaft respectively.*

SOLUTION The stresses in the rotor shaft of a helicopter are produced by the combined action of two forces, *i.e.* axial force P and the torque T. Therefore, the stresses, at any point on the surface of the shaft consists of tensile stress σ_o, shear stress τ_o as shown in the figure.

y-axis is parallel to the longitudinal axis of the shaft.

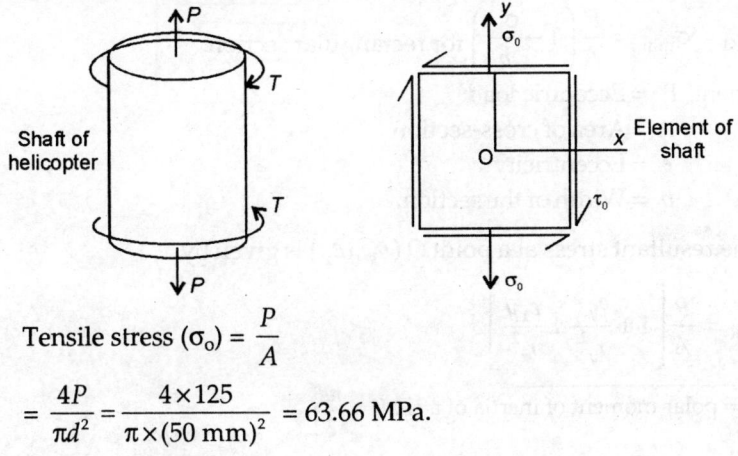

Tensile stress $(\sigma_o) = \dfrac{P}{A}$

$$= \frac{4P}{\pi d^2} = \frac{4 \times 125}{\pi \times (50 \text{ mm})^2} = 63.66 \text{ MPa.}$$

Shear stress $(\tau_o) = \dfrac{T.r}{{}^*I_P} = \dfrac{16T}{\pi d^3} = \dfrac{16 \times 2.4}{\pi \times (50)^3} = 97.78$ MPa.

The stresses σ_o and τ_o act directly on cross-section of the shaft.

Principle stress, $\sigma_{1,2} = \dfrac{\sigma_x + \sigma_y}{2} \pm \sqrt{\left(\dfrac{\sigma_x - \sigma_y}{2}\right)^2 + \tau^2_{xy}}$

$\qquad = \dfrac{0 + 64.00}{2} \pm \sqrt{\left(\dfrac{0 - 64.00}{2}\right)^2 + (97.78)^2}$

$\qquad = 32 \pm 103$

Substituting $\sigma_x = 0$, $\sigma_y = \sigma_o = 0 = 63.66$ MPa $= 64$ MPa (let)

$\qquad \tau_{xy} = + \tau_o = + 97.78$ MPa

$\qquad \sigma_{1,2} = 32 \pm 103$ MPa

$\qquad \sigma_1 = 135$ MPa   (max. tensile) in rotor shaft

$\qquad \sigma_2 = -71$ MPa   (max. compressive stress) in rotor shaft

$\qquad \tau_{max} = \sqrt{\left(\dfrac{\sigma_x - \sigma_y}{2}\right)^2 + \tau^2_{xy}}$

$\qquad \tau_{max} = 103$ MPa.

HIGHLIGHTS

1. The axial load produces direct stress (σ_d).
2. Eccentric load produces direct stress and bending stress (σ_b)
3. The maximum and minimum stress at a point in a section which is subjected to load which is eccentric to y-axis is given by

   σ_{max} = Direct stress + Bending stress

   $\qquad = \dfrac{P}{A}\left(1 + \dfrac{\sigma_e}{b}\right)$ for rectangular section

   and $\sigma_{min} = \dfrac{P}{A}\left(1 - \dfrac{\sigma_e}{b}\right)$ for rectangular section.

   where, P = Eccentric load
   $\qquad A$ = Area of cross-section
   $\qquad e$ = Eccentricity
   $\qquad b$ = Width of the section.

4. The resultant stress at a point $Q(e_y, e_x)$ is given by

   $\sigma_R = \dfrac{P}{A}\left[1 \pm \dfrac{e_y x}{r_y^2} \pm \dfrac{e_x y}{r_x^2}\right]$

$^*I_p$ or J = polar moment of inertia of a shaft $= \dfrac{\pi d^4}{32}$

where, r_x and r_y are the radii of gyration about x and y axes respectively.

$$I_x = A \cdot r_x^2$$

$$I_y = A \cdot r_y^2$$

5. For a rectangular section, there will be no tensile stress if the load is on the either axis within the middle third of section.

6. For a circular section of diameter 'd' there will be no tensile stress if the load lies in a circle of diameter $(d/4)$ with centre 'O' of the main circular section. This is known as middle quarter rule for circular section.

7. For no tensile stress, eccentricity (e) is given by,

$$e \leq \frac{d}{8} \text{ for circular section}$$

$$\leq \frac{1}{8d_o}(d_o^2 + d_i^2) \text{ for hollow circular section with diameter } d_o \text{ (external) and}$$

d_i (internal)

$$\leq \frac{b}{6} \text{ and } \frac{d}{6} \text{ for rectangular section}$$

$$\leq \frac{\text{One side of square}}{6} \text{ for square section}$$

PROBLEMS FOR PRACTICE

1. A hollow cast iron column of rectangular section 60 cm × 40 cm overall and 50 cm × 20 cm internally carries a load of 1800 kN which is off the geometric axis by 10 cm in the vertical plane bisecting the thickness. Calculate the extreme intensities of stress induced in the section.

2. A short column of external diameter 50 cm and internal diameter 30 cm carries an eccentric load of 100 kN. Find the greatest ecentricity which the load can have without producing tension on the cross-section.

OBJECTIVE QUESTIONS

1. An eccentric load W with eccentricity e is equivalent to:
   - (a) an axial load W
   - (b) a moment equal to $W \times e$
   - (c) both (a) and (b)
   - (d) none of the above

2. 'Middle third rule' is valid in the case of:
   - (a) rectangular section
   - (b) circular section
   - (c) hexagonal section
   - (d) any section

3. In the case of a circular section, no 'reverse stress' condition is given by:
   - (a) middle third rule
   - (b) middle quarter rule
   - (c) parallel axis theorem
   - (d) bending equation

4. For no tension in the section, the ecentricity must not exceed:

   (a) $\dfrac{K^2}{d}$ (b) $\dfrac{2K^2}{d}$ (b) $\dfrac{4K^2}{d}$ (d) $\dfrac{K}{\sqrt{d}}$

   where, d = depth of the section

   K = radius of gyration.

ANSWERS

1. (c)   2. (a)   3. (b)   4. (b)

— ❖❖ —

9

SHEAR STRESSES IN BEAMS

9.1 INTRODUCTION

In chapter 6 we studied that when a beam is subjected to a transverse load 'shear force' and 'bending moment' are produced at every section of the beam. We had neglected the shear stress, because this is very small as compared to bending stress.

But, in actual practice when a beam is subjected to a transverse load, shear force and bending moment are produced at each section of the beam and we can not ignore shear stress.

In this chapter we will study the distribution of shear stress across the various sections (*e.g.* rectangular section, circular section, I-section, T-section etc.).

9.2 SHEAR STRESS DISTRIBUTION

Shear stress distribution will be based on the following assumption:

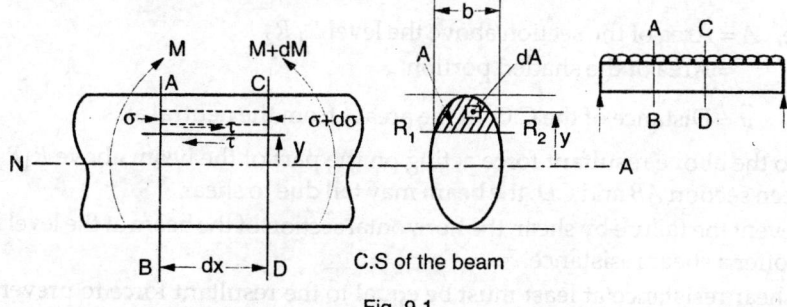

Fig. 9.1

(i) The material is homogenous, isotropic and elastic.

(ii) The modulii of elasticity in tension and compression are equal i.e. $E_t = E_c$.

(iii) The shear stress is constant along the beam width.

(iv) The presence of shear stress does not affect the distribution of bending stresses.

Let us consider a beam subjected to uniformly distributed load.

Let $\quad M =$ B.M. at AB

and $\quad F =$ S.F. at B

$\sigma =$ bending stress at AB

$(M + dM) =$ B.M. at CD

and $\quad (F + dF) =$ S.F. at CD

$(\sigma + d\sigma) =$ bending stress at CD

Let I is the moment of Inertia of the section about Neutral axis.

Our aim is to find the shear stress on the section AB at a distance 'y' from the neutral axis.

Bending stress at a distance y from the N.A. on the section AB due to B.M (M),

$$\sigma = \frac{M}{I} \cdot y$$

Similarly, bending stress on the section CD

$$(\sigma + d\sigma) = \frac{(M + dM)}{I} \cdot y$$

$\therefore \quad$ Resultant longitudinal force on area A

$$= \int (\sigma + d\sigma)\, dA - \int \sigma \cdot dA$$

$$= \int \frac{dM \cdot y}{I} \cdot dA$$

$$= \frac{dM}{I} \int y \cdot dA$$

$$= \frac{dM}{I} \times A \times \bar{y} \qquad \left[\because \int y\, dA = A \times \bar{y} \right] \qquad \ldots(1)$$

where, $A =$ Area of the section above the level $R_1 R_2$

$\qquad\quad =$ Area of the shaded portion.

and $\quad \bar{y} =$ Distance of the C.G. of the area A from the neutral axis.

Due to the above resultant force acting on the part of the beam above $R_1 R_2$ and between section AB and CD, the beam may fail due to shear.

To prevent the failure by shear, the horizontal section of the beam at the level $R_1 R_2$ must offer a shear resistance.

This shear resistance at least must be equal to the resultant force to prevent the failure due to shear.

$\therefore \qquad$ Shear resistance 'or' shear force at the level $R_1 R_2$

$$= \frac{dM}{I} \times A \times \bar{y} \qquad \ldots(2)$$

Let τ = Intensity of horizontal shear at level $R_1 R_2$

and, b = width of the beam at the level $R_1 R_2$

$\therefore$ Area = $b \times dx$

Shear force due to τ

     = Shear stress $\times$ Shear Area

     = $\tau \times b \times dx$ ...(3)

Equating (2) and (3)

$$\tau \times b \times dx = \frac{dM}{I} \times A \times \bar{y}$$

$\therefore$
$$\tau = \frac{dM}{I} \times \frac{A \times \bar{y}}{b \times dx}$$

$$= \frac{dM}{dx} \times \frac{A \times \bar{y}}{I \times b}$$

$$= F \times \frac{A\bar{y}}{I \cdot b} \qquad \left[\because \frac{dM}{dx} = \text{shear force} = F \right]$$

9.3 SHEAR STRESS DISTRIBUTION FOR RECTANGULAR SECTION

The given figure shows a rectangular section of a beam of width 'b' and depth 'd'.
Let F is the shear force acting at the section.

Let us consider a level EF at a distance y from the neutral axis.

Now, shear stress $\tau = F \cdot \dfrac{A \cdot \bar{y}}{b \times I}$ ...(1)

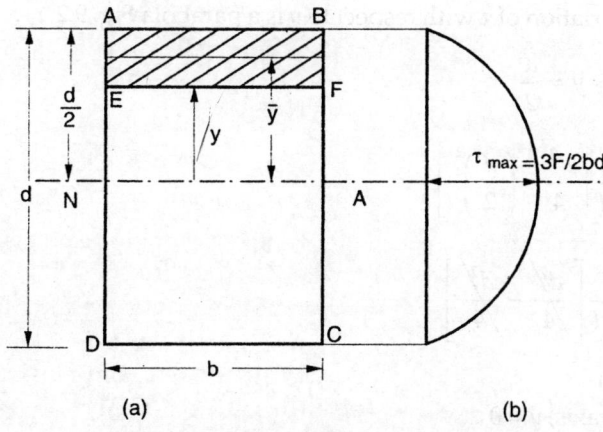

Fig. 9.2

where, A = Area of the section above y (Shaded Area)

$$= \left(\frac{d}{2} - y \right) \times b$$

$\bar{y}$ = distance of the C.G. of Area A from neutral axis

$$= y + \frac{1}{2} \left(\frac{d}{2} - y \right)$$

$$= y + \frac{d}{4} - \frac{y}{2}$$

$$= \left(\frac{y}{2} + \frac{d}{4} \right)$$

$$= \frac{1}{2} \left(y + \frac{d}{2} \right)$$

b = width of the section

I = moment of inertia of the whole section about N.A.

Substituting these values in equation (1) we get

$$\tau = F \cdot \frac{\left(\frac{d}{2} - y \right) \times \cancel{b} \times \frac{1}{2} \left(y + \frac{d}{2} \right)}{\cancel{b} \times I}$$

$$= \frac{F}{2I} \left(\frac{d^2}{4} - y^2 \right) \qquad \qquad ...(2)$$

From eqn. (2) we observe that τ increase as y decreases.

Further, the variation of τ with respect to y is a parabola Fig. 9.2.

At the top edge $y = \dfrac{d}{2}$

$$\therefore \qquad \tau = \frac{F}{2I} \left[\frac{d^2}{4} - \left(\frac{d}{2} \right)^2 \right]$$

$$= \frac{F}{2I} \left[\frac{\cancel{d^2}}{\cancel{4}} - \frac{\cancel{d^2}}{\cancel{4}} \right]$$

$$= 0$$

At the neutral axis, $y = 0$

$$\therefore \qquad \tau = \frac{F}{2I} \left(\frac{d^2}{4} - 0 \right)$$

$$= \frac{Fd^2}{8I}$$

$$= \frac{Fd^2}{8 \times \dfrac{bd^3}{12}}$$

$$= \frac{\overset{3}{\cancel{12}}\, Fd^2}{\underset{2}{\cancel{8}}\, bd^3}$$

$$= \frac{1.5F}{bd} \qquad \qquad \dots(3)$$

$$\tau_{\text{average}} = \frac{F}{b \times d}$$

$\therefore \qquad \tau = 1.5 \times \tau_{\text{average}} \qquad \qquad \dots(4)$

Equation (4) gives the shear stress at the neutral axis where $y = 0$. This stress is also the maximum shear stress.

$\therefore \qquad \boxed{\tau_{\max} = 1.5\, \tau_{\text{average}}}$

EXAMPLE 1 *A beam 100 mm wide and 150 mm deep in cross-section is simply supported and carries a uniformly distributed load over its entire span of 2 metre. If the allowable stresses for the beam material are 30 MPa in bending and 2 MPa in shear, calculate the maximum load which the beam can carry.*

SOLUTION Let the intensity of load is w N/m.

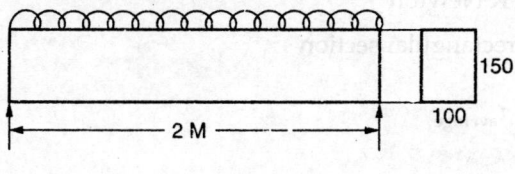

Fig. 9.3

Now, maximum B.M $(M) = \dfrac{wl^2}{8}$

$$= \frac{w \times 2^2}{8}$$

$$= \left(\frac{w}{2}\right) \text{Nm}$$

and,   Maximum shear force (F) at the support $= \dfrac{wl}{2} = \dfrac{w \times 2}{2} = w$

Maximum bending stress $(\sigma_{max}) = \dfrac{M}{I} \cdot y$

$$= \frac{0.5w}{\left(\dfrac{100}{1000}\right)\left(\dfrac{150}{1000}\right)^3 \times \dfrac{1}{12}} \times \frac{75}{1000}$$

$$= \frac{0.5\,w \times 12 \times 0.075}{0.1 \times (0.15)^3}$$

$$= 1333.33 \; w \; \text{N/m}^2$$

Stress $\sigma_{allowable}$ (given) $= 30 \, \text{MPa}$

$$= 30 \times 10^6 \, \text{Pa}$$

$$= 30 \times 10^6 \, \text{N/m}^2$$

Equating these two stress

$$1333.33 \, w = 30 \times 10^6$$

$$w = \left(\frac{30 \times 1000000}{1333.33}\right)$$

$$= 22500.05 \, \text{Newton}$$

$$= 22.5 \, \text{K Newton}$$

We know that for rectangular section

$$\tau_{max} = \frac{3}{2} \, \tau_{average}$$

$$= \frac{3}{2} \times \frac{F}{bd}$$

$$= \frac{3}{2} \times \frac{w}{\left(\dfrac{100}{1000}\right) \times \left(\dfrac{150}{1000}\right)}$$

$$= \frac{1.5 \times w}{0.1 \times 0.15}$$

$$= 99.9 \, w$$

$$\simeq 100 \, w \, \text{N/m}^2$$

Shear stress $\tau_{\text{allowable}}$ (given) = 2 MPa

$$= 2 \times 10^6 \, \text{Pa}$$

$$= 2 \times 10^6 \, \text{N/m}^2$$

Equating these two shear stresses

$$100 \, w = 2 \times 10^6$$

$$w = \frac{2 \times 10^6}{100}$$

$$= 2 \times 10^4 \, \text{Newton}$$

$$= 20 \, \text{kN}$$

∴   Allowable load is the minimum of the two values.

∴   Weight ($w_{\text{allowable}}$) = 20 kN/mtr.

9.4 STRESS DISTRIBUTION IN I-SECTION

I-section is widely used in engineering practice *e.g.* in construction of bridges, railway lines etc. The *I*-shape beam resists both bending as well as shear.

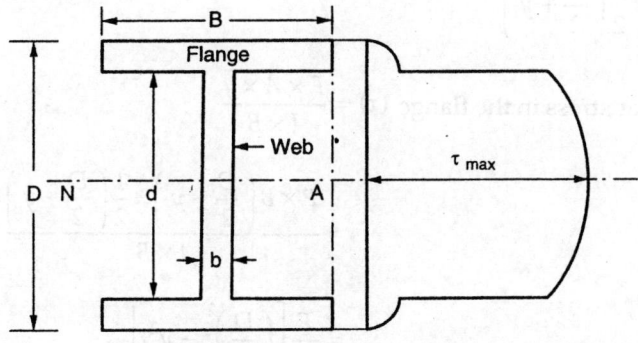

Fig. 9.4

The bending is taken mostly by the flanges, whereas the web takes most of the shear.

In the case of I-section, the shear stress distribution in the web and shear stress distribution in the flange are calculated separately.

9.5 (a) SHEAR STRESS DISTRIBUTION IN THE FLANGE

Let us consider a section at a distance y from the N.A. in the flange.

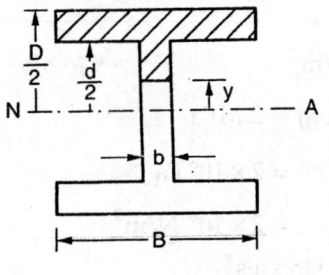

Fig. 9.5

Shaded area of flange $A = B \cdot \left(\dfrac{D}{2} - y \right)$

Distance of the C.G. of the shaded area from the neutral axis is given by

$$\bar{y} = y + \frac{1}{2}\left(\frac{D}{2} - y \right)$$

$$= y + \frac{D}{4} - \frac{y}{2}$$

$$= \frac{D}{4} + \frac{y}{2}$$

$$= \frac{1}{2}\left(\frac{D}{2} + y \right)$$

$\therefore$ Shear stress in the flange $(\tau) = \dfrac{F \times A \times \bar{y}}{I \times B}$

$$= \frac{F \times B\left(\dfrac{D}{2} - y \right) \times \dfrac{1}{2}\left(\dfrac{D}{2} + y \right)}{I \times B}$$

$$= \frac{F}{2I}\left[\left(\frac{D}{2} \right)^2 - y^2 \right]$$

$$= \frac{F}{2I}\left[\frac{D^2}{4} - y^2 \right] \qquad \qquad ...(3)$$

From the above equation it is evident that $\tau = f\left(\dfrac{1}{y} \right)$ i.e. with the increase of y

shear stress decreases.

For the upper edge of the flange

$$y = \frac{D}{2}$$

∴   Shear stress $(\tau) = \frac{F}{2I}\left[\frac{D^2}{4} - \frac{D^2}{4}\right]$

$$= 0$$

For the lower edge of the flange, $y = \frac{d}{2}$

∴ $\tau_{flange} = \frac{F}{8I}(D^2 - d^2)$

(b) SHEAR STRESS DISTRIBUTION IN THE WEB

Here, $A\bar{y}$ = Moment of flange area about N.A. + Moment of the shaded area of the web about the N.A.

$$= B\left(\frac{D}{2} - \frac{d}{2}\right) \times \frac{1}{2}\left(\frac{D}{2} + \frac{d}{2}\right) + b\left(\frac{d}{2} - y\right) \times \frac{1}{2}\left(\frac{d}{2} + y\right)$$

$$= \frac{B}{8}(D^2 - d^2) + \frac{b}{2}\left(\frac{d^2}{4} - y^2\right)$$

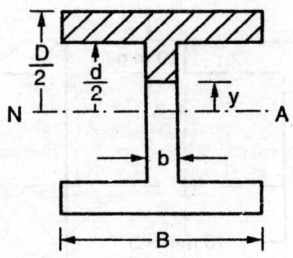

Fig. 9.6

Shear stress in the web (τ_{web}) is

$$\tau_{web} = \frac{FA\bar{y}}{Ib}$$

$$= \frac{F}{Ib}\left[\frac{B}{8}(D^2 - d^2) + \frac{b}{2}\left(\frac{d^2}{4} - y^2\right)\right] \qquad \ldots(1)$$

At the neutral axis, $y = 0$ and hence shear stress is maximum.

$$\therefore \quad \tau_{max} = \frac{F}{Ib}\left[\frac{B}{8}(D^2 - d^2) + \frac{b}{2} \times \frac{d^2}{4}\right]$$

$$= \frac{F}{Ib}\left[\frac{B(D^2 - d^2)}{8} + \frac{bd^2}{8}\right]$$

At the junction of top of the web and bottom of flange we have $y = \dfrac{d}{2}$

Therefore, shear stress is given by eqn. (1)

$$\tau_{max} = \frac{F}{I \times b}\left[\frac{B(D^2 - d^2)}{8} + \frac{b}{2}\left(\frac{d^2}{4} - \frac{d^2}{4}\right)\right]$$

$$= \frac{F B(D^2 - d^2)}{8\,Ib}$$

N.B: *The shear stress at the junction of the flange and the web changes abruptly.*

EXAMPLE 2 *The I-section beam is loaded such that at a certain section, there is bending moment of 75 kNm together with a vertical shearing force.*

Calculate the value of shearing force if the maximum stress in the beam is not to exceed 120 MPa.

SOLUTION Shearing stress $(\tau) = \dfrac{FA\overline{y}}{bI}$

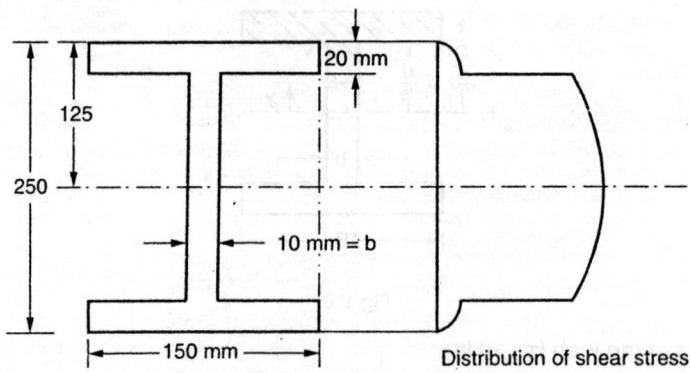

Fig. 9.7

$$I = \left[\frac{150 \times 250^3}{12} - \frac{140 \times 210^3}{12}\right]$$

$$= (1.953 - 1.080)\, 10^8$$

$$= 0.873 \times 10^8 \text{ mm}^4$$

At the top of web

$$b = 10 \text{ mm}$$

$$A\overline{y} = 150 \times 20 \times 115$$

$$= 345000 \text{ mm}^3$$

$$\therefore \quad \tau = \frac{F \times 345000}{10 \times 0.873 \times 10^8}$$

$$= \frac{F \times 345}{1000 \times 873}$$

$$= \frac{F}{2530.4} \text{ N/mm}^2$$

If σ_b is the bending stress at the top of the web, where, $y = 105$ mm

then, $\quad \sigma_b = \dfrac{M}{I} \cdot y$

$$= \frac{75 \times 10^3 \times 10^3}{0.873 \times 10^8} \times (10)^5$$

$$= \frac{75 \times 105}{87.300}$$

$$= 90.20 \text{ N/mm}^2$$

$$\sigma_{max} = \frac{\sigma_b}{2} + \sqrt{\left(\frac{\sigma_b}{2}\right)^2 + \tau^2}$$

$$120 = \frac{90.20}{2} + \sqrt{\left(\frac{90.20}{2}\right)^2 + \left(\frac{F}{2530.4}\right)^2}$$

or, $\quad 120 - 45.10 = \sqrt{(45.10)^2 + \left(\dfrac{F}{2530.4}\right)^2}$

or, $\quad 74.9 = \sqrt{(45.10)^2 + \left(\dfrac{F}{2530.4}\right)^2}$

or, $\quad 75 = \sqrt{(45.10)^2 + \left(\dfrac{F}{2530.4}\right)^2}$

or,$\quad 75 \times 75 = (45.10)^2 + \left(\dfrac{F}{2530.4} \right)^2$

or,$\quad 75 \times 75 - (45.10)^2 = \dfrac{F^2}{(2530.4)^2}$

or,$\quad F^2 = (2530.4)^2 \, [(75)^2 - (45.10)^2]$

or,$\quad F^2 = (2530.4)^2 \times [5625 - 2034]$

$\qquad = (2530.4)^2 \times 3591$

$\quad F = 2530.4 \times 59.92$

$\qquad = 151634.1 \text{ Newton}$

$\therefore \qquad F = 151.6 \text{ kN} \qquad\qquad$ **Ans.**

9.6 SHEAR STRESSES IN CIRCULAR SECTION

Shear stress $(\tau) = \dfrac{F A \bar{y}}{b I}$

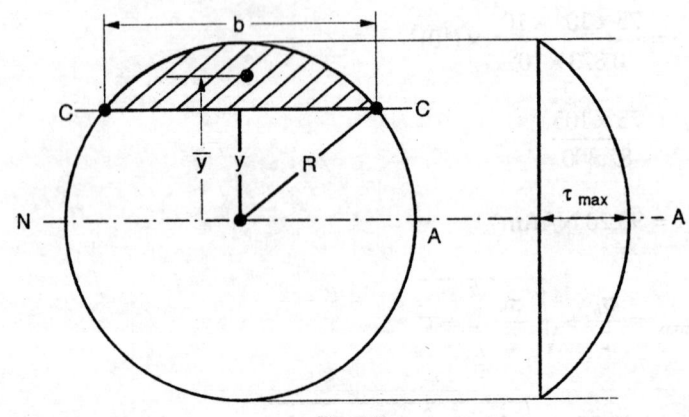

Fig. 9.8

$A \cdot \bar{y} = b^3/12$ and $I = \dfrac{\pi R^4}{4}$

$A \cdot \bar{y} = \dfrac{b^3}{12}$ and $I = \dfrac{\pi R^4}{4}$

$\tau = \dfrac{F \times \dfrac{b^3}{12}}{b \times \dfrac{\pi R^4}{12}}$

$\quad = \dfrac{F b^2}{3 \pi R^4}$

$A \cdot \bar{y} = $ Moment of shaded Area about the N.A.

$\quad = \int_y^R b \cdot dA = \int_y^R b \cdot (y \cdot dy)$

$b = 2\sqrt{R^2 - y^2}$

$b^2 = 4 \, (R^2 = y^2)$

$2b \cdot db = -8y \cdot dy \quad$ when $y = y; b = b$

$b \cdot db = -4 \cdot y \, dy \quad$ when $y = R; b = 0$

Hence, $A \cdot \bar{y} = (-)\dfrac{1}{4}\int_b^0 b \cdot db = \dfrac{1}{4}\int_0^b b \cdot db = \dfrac{b^3}{12}$

$$= \frac{4}{3} \cdot \frac{F}{\pi R^4} \cdot \left(\frac{b}{2}\right)^2$$

Now, $$\left(\frac{b}{2}\right)^2 = (R^2 - y^2)$$

$\therefore$ $$\tau = \frac{4}{3} \cdot \frac{F}{\pi R^4} \cdot (R^2 - y^2)$$

$$= \frac{4}{3} \cdot \frac{F}{\pi R^2} \left(1 - \frac{y^2}{R^2}\right)$$

τ is maximum when $y = 0$ *i.e.* τ is maximum at neutral axis.

$\therefore$ $$\tau_{max} = \frac{4}{3} \cdot \frac{F}{\pi R^2}$$

$$\tau_{average} = \frac{F}{\pi R^2}$$

$$\boxed{\therefore \tau_{max} = \frac{4}{3} \tau_{average}}$$

9.7 SHEAR STRESSES IN TRIANGULAR SECTION

The N.A. of $\triangle ABC$ will be at the C.G. of the triangle and C.G. of the triangle is at a

distance of $\left(\dfrac{2h}{3}\right)$ from the top.

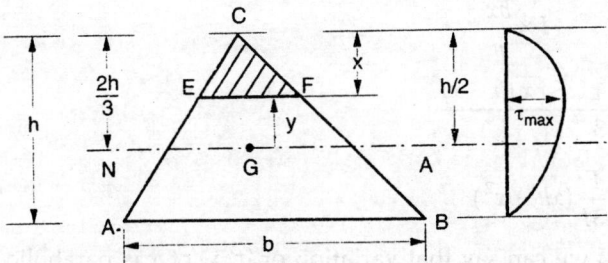

Fig. 9.9

Therefore, N.A will be at a distance of $\left(\dfrac{2h}{3}\right)$ from the top.

Let us consider a level EF at a distance y from the N.A.

Hence, the shear stress at this level is given by

Let us consider a level EF at a distance y from the N.A.

Hence, the shear stress at this level is given by

$$\tau = \frac{F A \bar{y}}{I \times b} \qquad \qquad ...(1)$$

$A\bar{y}$ = Moment of the shaded area bout the N.A.

= Area of the triangle CEF × distance of the C.G. of triangle CEF from N.A.

$$= \left(\frac{1}{2} \times EF \times x \right) \times \left(\frac{2h}{3} - \frac{2x}{3} \right)$$

$$= \left(\frac{1}{2} \times \frac{bx}{h} \times x \right) \times \frac{2}{3} (h - x) \qquad \begin{bmatrix} \triangle\, CEF \text{ and} \triangle\, CAB \text{ are similar} \\ \therefore \dfrac{EF}{AB} = \dfrac{x}{h} \\ \dfrac{EF}{b} = \dfrac{x}{h} \\ \therefore EF = \dfrac{b \cdot x}{h} \end{bmatrix}$$

$$= \frac{1}{2} \times \frac{bx^2}{h} \times \frac{2}{3} (h - x)$$

$$= \frac{1}{3} \times \frac{bx^2}{h} \times (h - x)$$

Substituting the value of $A \cdot \bar{y}$ in eqn. (1)

$$\tau = \frac{F \times \dfrac{1}{3} \dfrac{bx^2}{h} (h - x)}{I \times \dfrac{bx}{h}}$$

$$= \frac{1}{3} \cdot \frac{F \cdot x (h - x)}{I}$$

$$= \frac{F}{3I} (xh - x^2) \qquad \qquad ...(2)$$

From eqn. (2) we can say that variation of 'τ' w.r.t x is parabolic. At top $x = 0$ therefore, τ is also zero.

At the bottom $x = h$ so again τ is zero.

At the N.A, $x = \dfrac{2h}{3}$ and hence the shear at the N.A. becomes,

$$\tau \text{ at N.A} = \frac{F}{3 I_{NA}} \left[\frac{2h}{3} \times h - \left(\frac{2h}{3} \right)^2 \right]$$

$$= \frac{F}{3\,I_{NA}} \left[\frac{2h^2}{3} - \frac{4h^2}{9} \right]$$

$$= \frac{F}{3\,I_{NA}} \times \left(\frac{\sigma h^2 - 4h^2}{9} \right)$$

$$= \frac{F}{3\,I_{NA}} \times \frac{2h^2}{9}$$

$$= \frac{2}{27} \times \frac{Fh^2}{I_{NA}}$$

But $\qquad I_{NA} = \dfrac{bh^3}{36}$

$\therefore \qquad \tau = \dfrac{2}{27} \times \dfrac{Fh^2}{\left(\dfrac{bh^3}{36} \right)}$

$$= \frac{2}{27} \times \frac{36\,Fh^2}{bh^3}$$

$$= \frac{8}{3} \cdot \left(\frac{F}{b \cdot h} \right)$$

Maximum Shear Stress (τ_{max})

Shear stress at any depth $x = \dfrac{F}{3I}(xh - h^2)$

The maximum shear stress will be obtained by differentiating equation (2) w.r.t x and equating it to zero.

$\therefore \qquad \dfrac{d}{dx}\left[\dfrac{F}{3I_G}(xh - x^2) \right] = 0$

$$\frac{F}{3I_G}(h - 2x) = 0$$

But $\qquad \dfrac{F}{3I_G} \neq 0$

$\therefore \qquad (h - 2x) = 0$

$$\therefore \qquad x = \left(\frac{h}{2}\right)$$

$$\therefore \qquad \tau_{max} = \frac{F}{3I_G}\left[\frac{h}{2} \times h - \left(\frac{h}{2}\right)^2\right]$$

$$= \frac{Fh^2}{12I_G}$$

$$= \frac{Fh^2}{\cancel{12}} \times \frac{\cancel{36}^{3}}{bh^3}$$

$$= \left(\frac{3F}{bh}\right) \qquad \textbf{Ans.}$$

EXAMPLE 3 *T-section beam shown in the figure is subjected to shear force of 15 kN. Draw the profile of shear stress.* **(Similar Problem UPTU 2014-15)**

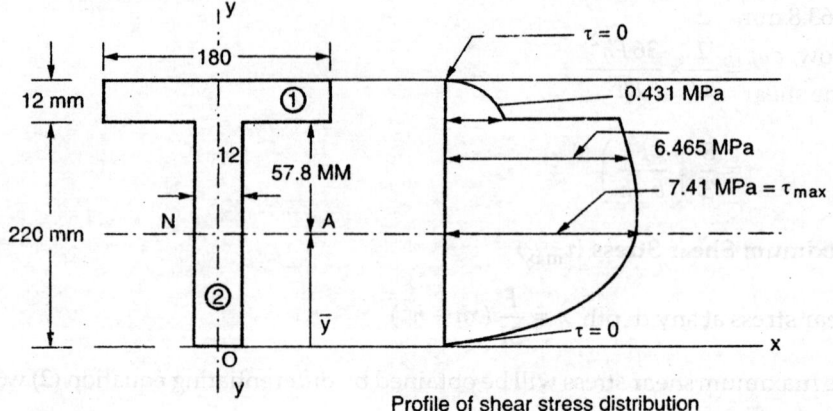

Profile of shear stress distribution

Fig. 9.10

SOLUTION Since the section is symmetrical about y-axis, therefore $\bar{x} = 0$.
Let us divide the T-section into part (1) and (2) to find out $\bar{y}$.

For part (1)

Area $\quad A_1 = 180 \times 12$

$\qquad = 2160 \text{ mm}^2$

Distance of C.G. from x-axis

$$y_1 = 220 + \frac{12}{2}$$

$$= 226 \text{ mm}$$

For part (2)

Area $\quad A_2 = 220 \times 12$

$$= 2640 \text{ mm}^2$$

Distance of its C.G. from x-axis

$$y_2 = \left(\frac{220}{2}\right) = 110 \text{ mm}.$$

Now, $\quad \bar{y} = \left(\dfrac{A_1 y_1 + A_2 y_2}{A_1 + A_2}\right)$

$$= \left(\frac{2160 \times 226 + 2640 \times 100}{2160 + 2640}\right)$$

$$= 162.2 \text{ mm}.$$

Therefore, N.A. is at a distance of 162.2 mm from the bottom of the web.

M.I. about N.A is found to be $= 2.66 \times 10^{-5} \text{ mm}^4$

Hence, distance of the centroid of the flange from the N.A. is $(220 - 162.2 + 6)$ mm
$= 63.8$ mm.

Now, τ at the top of flange is zero.

The shear stress at the lower part of flange is

$$\tau_{\text{lower flange}} = \frac{F A \bar{y}}{b \cdot I}$$

$$= \frac{15 \times 10^3 \times (180 \times 12 \times 10^{-6}) \times (63.8 \times 10^{-3})}{(180 \times 10^{-3}) \times (2.66 \times 10^{-5}) \times 10^6}$$

$$= 0.431 \text{ MPa}$$

$A\bar{y}$ for flange and web above N.A.

$$= \left(180 \times 12 \times 63.8 + 57.8 \times 12 \times \frac{57.8}{2}\right) \times 10^{-9} \text{ m}^3$$

$$= 1.578 \times 10^{-4} \text{ m}^3$$

Now,

$$\tau_{\text{max}} = \frac{F \cdot A \cdot \bar{y}}{b \cdot I}$$

$$= \frac{(15 \times 10^3) \times 1.578 \times 10^{-4}}{(12 \times 10^{-3}) \times (2.66 \times 10^{-5})} \times \frac{1}{10^6} \text{ MPa}$$

$$= 7.41 \text{ MPa}$$

Shear stress at the junction of flange and web is

$$= 0.431 \times \frac{180}{12}$$

$$= 6.465 \text{ MPa}$$

The shear stress at the bottom of the web is zero.

The profile of shear stress distribution is shown in Fig. 9.10.

EXAMPLE 4 *A beam of square section is placed in such a manner that one of its diagonal is horizontal.*

The beam is subjected to shear force F at a section. Find the maximum shear in the cross-section of the beam and draw the profile of shear distribution for the section.

SOLUTION Let the side of square section is '*a*'

Let us assume shear stress at a distance *x* from the apex. Then,

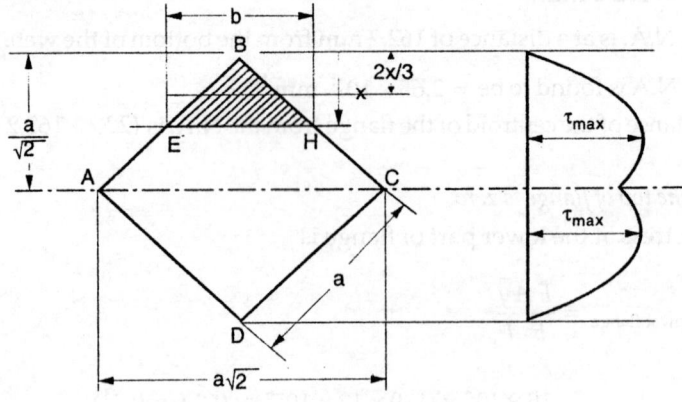

Fig. 9.11

$$A\bar{y} = \left(\frac{1}{2} b \cdot x \right) \left(\frac{a}{\sqrt{2}} - \frac{2x}{3} \right) \qquad \begin{bmatrix} A.\bar{y} = \text{Moment of the shaded} \\ \text{Area about } NA \end{bmatrix}$$

$$= \left(\frac{1}{2} \times 2x \times x \right) \left(\frac{a}{\sqrt{2}} - \frac{2x}{3} \right)$$

$$= x^2 \left(\frac{a}{\sqrt{2}} - \frac{2x}{3} \right) \qquad \begin{bmatrix} \Delta \ BEH \text{ and } \Delta \ BAC \text{ are similar} \\ \therefore \frac{EH}{x} = \frac{AC}{a/\sqrt{2}} \\ \frac{b}{x} = \frac{a\sqrt{2}}{a/\sqrt{2}} \\ \therefore \ b = 2x \end{bmatrix}$$

$$I = 2 \times \Delta\ ABC's\ \text{M.I. about } AC$$

$$= 2 \left[\frac{\sqrt{2}a \times \left(\dfrac{a}{\sqrt{2}} \right)^3}{12} \right]$$

$$= \left(\frac{a^4}{12} \right)$$

∴ $\tau = \dfrac{F\,A\,\overline{y}}{b \cdot I}$ by formula

$$= \frac{Fx^2 \left(\dfrac{a}{\sqrt{2}} - \dfrac{2x}{3} \right)}{2x \times \dfrac{a^4}{12}}$$

$$= \frac{6F}{a^4} \left[\frac{a}{\sqrt{2}} x - \frac{2}{3} x^2 \right] \qquad \qquad ...(1)$$

For τ to be max, $\dfrac{d\tau}{dx} = 0$

∴ $\dfrac{d}{dx} \left\{ \dfrac{6F}{a^4} \left(\dfrac{a}{\sqrt{2}} x - \dfrac{2}{3} x^2 \right) \right\} = 0 \Rightarrow x = \dfrac{3a}{4\sqrt{2}}$

Putting value of x in eqn. (1)

$$\boxed{\tau_{max} = \frac{9}{8} \cdot \frac{F}{a^2}} \qquad \textbf{Ans.}$$

EXAMPLE 5 *A beam of triangular cross-section is subjected to a shear force of 40 kN. The base of the section is 250 mm and height 200 mm. The beam is placed with its base horizontal. Find the maximum shear stress and the shear stress at the N.A.*

SOLUTION $F = 40\ \text{kN} = 40 \times 10^3\ \text{N}$

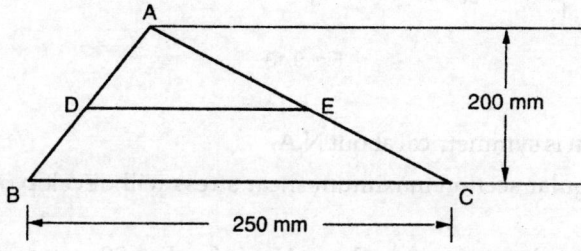

Fig. 9.12

By formula, $\tau_{max} = \dfrac{3F}{bh}$

$$= \dfrac{3 \times 4 \times 10^4}{250 \times 200}$$

$$= \dfrac{12\cancel{0}}{5\cancel{0}}$$

$$= 2.4 \text{ N/mm}^2 \qquad \textbf{Ans.}$$

Shear stress (τ) at N.A. $= \dfrac{8F}{3bh}$

$$= \dfrac{8 \times 4 \times 10^4}{3 \times 250 \times 200}$$

$$= \dfrac{32\cancel{0}}{15\cancel{0}}$$

$$= 2.13 \text{ N/mm}^2 \qquad \textbf{Ans.}$$

N.B: *In the case of triangular section shear stress is not maximum at the N.A.*

EXAMPLE 6 *For the given section which is subjected to shear force of 100 kN, evaluate the maximum shear stress.*

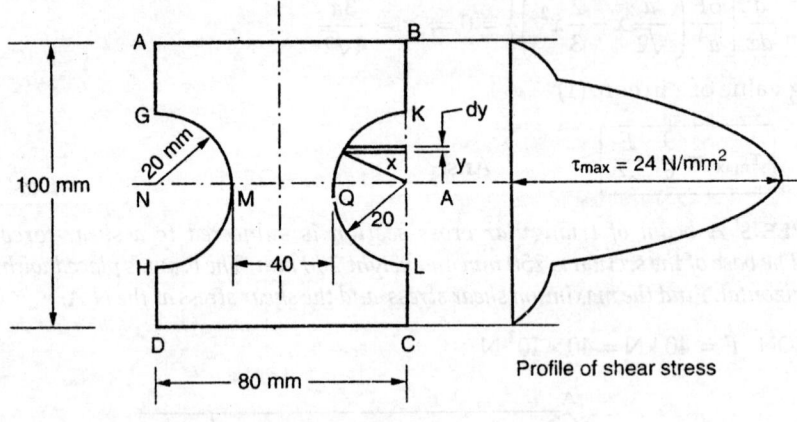

Fig. 9.13

SOLUTION

Here, the section is symmetrical about N.A.

For this rectangular section maximum shear stress will develop on the neutral axis (N.A.).

Here, the two quadrants of circle above N.A. of radius 20 mm combine to form semicircle fo radius 20 mm above N.A.

$$\therefore \qquad I = \frac{\overset{20}{\cancel{80}} \times 100^3}{\underset{3}{\cancel{12}}} - \frac{\pi}{64}(40)^4$$

$$= \frac{20 \times 100^3}{3} - \frac{22}{7 \times \cancel{64}} \times \frac{\overset{4}{\cancel{256}} \times 10^4}{1}$$

$$= \frac{2 \times 10^7}{3} - \frac{88}{7} \times 10^4$$

$$= 10^4 \left[\frac{2 \times 10^3}{3} - \frac{88}{7} \right]$$

$$= 10^4 \left[\frac{7 \times 2 \times 10^3 - 3 \times 88}{21} \right]$$

$$= 10^4 \left[\frac{21000 - 264}{21} \right]$$

$$= 10^4 \times 987.43 \text{ mm}^4$$

Now, $\quad A\overline{y}$ = Moment of Area above N.A.

= (Moment of Area of rectangle 80 × 50 above N.A.) – (Moment of Area of circular portion between KQ about N.A.)

$$= \cancel{80} \times 50 \times \frac{50}{\cancel{2}} - \int_0^{20} 2 \cdot x \cdot dy \cdot y$$

$$= 100,000 - \int_0^{20} 2 \times \sqrt{400 - y^2} \times y \times dy \qquad \left(\because x = \sqrt{400 - y^2} \right)$$

$$= 10^5 - \int_0^{20} -\sqrt{400 - y^2}\,(-2y) \cdot dy$$

$$= 10^5 + \int_0^{20} \sqrt{400 - y^2}\,(-2y)\,dy$$

$$= 10^5 + \left[\frac{(400 - y^2)^{3/2}}{3/2} \right]_0^{20}$$

$$= 10^5 + \frac{2}{3} \left[(400 - 20^2)^{3/2} - (400 - 0^2)^{3/2} \right]$$

$$= 10^5 + \frac{2}{3} \left[0 - (20^{\cancel{2}})^{3/\cancel{2}} \right]$$

$$= 10^5 + \frac{2}{3}[-8000]$$

$$= 100000 - \frac{16000}{3}$$

$$= \frac{30,0000 - 16000}{3}$$

$\therefore \qquad A \cdot \overline{y} = 94666.66 \text{ mm}^4$

Now, $\quad \tau_{max} = \tau$ at N.A.

$$= \frac{F \cdot A \cdot y}{b \cdot I}$$

$$= \frac{100 \times 10^3 \times 94666.66}{40 \times 10^4 \times 987.33} \qquad [b \text{ at N.A.} = 80 - (2 \times 20) = 40 \text{ mm}]$$

$$= \left[\frac{94666.66}{4 \times 987.33} \right]$$

$$= 23.97 \text{ N/mm}^2$$

$\therefore \qquad \tau_{max} \simeq 24 \text{ N/mm}^2 \qquad$ **Ans.**

9.8 STRESSES IN WIDE FLANGE BEAM

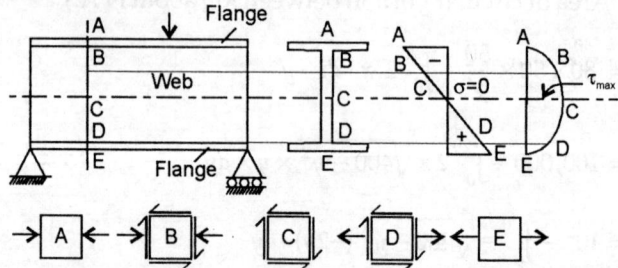

The largest principal stresses usually occur at the top and bottom of beam (point A and E), where the stresses obtained from the flexural formula have their largest value. However, depending upon the relative magnitude of B.M. and shear force, the largest stresses sometimes occur in the web where it meets the flange (points B and D).

The explanation lies in the fact that the normal stresses at B and D are only slightly smaller than those at A and E, where as the shear stresses (which are zero at point A and E) may be significant at points B and D because of this web. The maximum shear stress (τ_{max}) acting on a cross-section of wide flange occur at the Neutral Axis (NA). However, the maximum shear stresses acting on inclined plane usually occur at the top and bottom of the beam (points A and E) or in the web where it meets the flange (points B and D) because of the presence of normal stresses.

HIGHLIGHTS

1. The stress produced in a beam which is subjected to shear force is known as shear stress.

2. The shear stress at a fibre in a section of a beam is given by $\tau = \dfrac{F \times A \times \bar{y}}{I \times b}$

   where, F = Shear force at a given section

   A = Area of the section above the fibre

   $\bar{y}$ = Distance of C.G. of area A from the N.A.

   I = M.I. of the whole section about N.A.

   b = Actual width at the fibre

3. The shear stress distribution across a rectangular section is parabolic and is given by

   $$\tau = \dfrac{F}{2I}\left(\dfrac{d^2}{4} - y^2\right)$$

   where, d = depth of the beam

   y = distance fo the fibre from N.A.

4. The maximum shear stress is at the N.A. for a rectangular section is given by $\tau_{max} = 1.5\,\tau_{av}$.

5. The shear stress distribution for a circular section is given by

   $$\tau = \dfrac{F}{3I}(R^2 - y^2)$$

6. The shear stress is maximum at the N.A. for a circular section is given by

   $$\tau_{max} = \dfrac{4}{3} \times \tau_{average}$$

7. The shear stress distribution on I-section is parabolic. But at the junction of web and flange, the shear stress changes abruptly.

8. The shear stress distribution for unsymmetrical section is obtained after calculating the position of N.A.

9. The shear stress distribution diagram for a composite section is drawn by calculating the shear stress at important points.

OBJECTIVE QUESTIONS

1. In case of a rectangular section:

   (a) $\tau_{max} = \dfrac{1}{2}\,\tau_{max}$

   (b) $\tau_{max} = \dfrac{1}{2}\,\tau_{mean}$

   (c) $\tau_{max} = \dfrac{3}{2}\,\tau_{mean}$

   (b) none of the above

2. In case of a circular section:

   (a) $\tau_{max} = \dfrac{3}{2}\,\tau_{mean}$

   (b) $\tau_{max} = \tau_{mean}$

   (c) $\tau_{max} = \dfrac{2}{3}\,\tau_{mean}$

   (b) $\tau_{max} = \dfrac{4}{3}\,\tau_{mean}$

3. In the case of I-section beam, maximum shear stress is at:
   (a) the junction of the top flange and web
   (b) middle of the web
   (c) either (a) or (b)
   (d) none of the above

4. In the I-section of a beam subjected to transverse shear force (F), the maximum stress is developed:
   (a) at the centre of the web
   (b) at the top edge of the top flange
   (c) at the bottom edge of the top flange
   (d) none of the above

ANSWERS

1. (c)   2. (d)   3. (b)   4. (a)

DEFLECTION OF BEAMS

10.1 INTRODUCTION

In this chapter, we will learn how to compute the deflection of beam under a given loading pattern. When any transverse load*(s) are applied to beam, its longitudinal axis deflects from its initial position. At any section of the beam, there is thus transverse shift called 'deflection' and rotation of the beam is called 'slope'.

As an engineer or designer one must see that deflection should be within limit. If the deflection of beam is above the design limit, misalignment between driver and driven (in the case of rotating equipment) will take place which will disrupt the operation of the machine.

Although there are certain machine elements where deflection is the only criteria *e.g.* leaf spring; shock absorber etc. but **in most cases excessive deflection of machine parts; beams etc. are avoided.**

A loaded beam deflects by an amount that depends on several factors including:
— magnitude and types of loading
— the span of the beam
— the material properties of the beam (modulus of elasticity)
— the moment of inertia
— the beam type (simple, cantilever, overhanging, continuous)

Deflection may or may not be critical. **Critical deflection should be avoided by suitable design.**

Deflection(s) are denoted by the variable $'y'$ measured perpendicular to the original neutral axis. Upward deflections are positive, downward deflections are negative. The variable $'x'$ denotes the horizontal position on the beam measured from one of the supports (from LHS or RHS).

To minimise the deflection of a beam one should choose a material with the highest modulus of elasticity (E) and one should design the shape to have the largest moment of inertia (I).

---

*If the loads are inclined then it is resolved into x and y components to get the transverse load. The y-component is the transverse load in the oblique loading.

The deflection formulae are valid only for the cases, where the cross section of the beam is uniform for its entire length.

There are several methods which are used to determine slope and deflection of the beam. These are the following:

(i) By moment curvature relation or Double Integration Method

(ii) By Macaulay's method

(iii) By moment area method

(iv) By method of superposition

(v) By energy method

The last one i.e. (v) will be discussed in the separate chapter, i.e. Ch. 13.

From Bending relation

$$\frac{M}{I} = \frac{E}{R}$$

$$\therefore \quad \frac{1}{R} = \frac{M}{EI}$$

10.2 DIFFERENTIAL EQUATION OF THE DEFLECTED BEAM

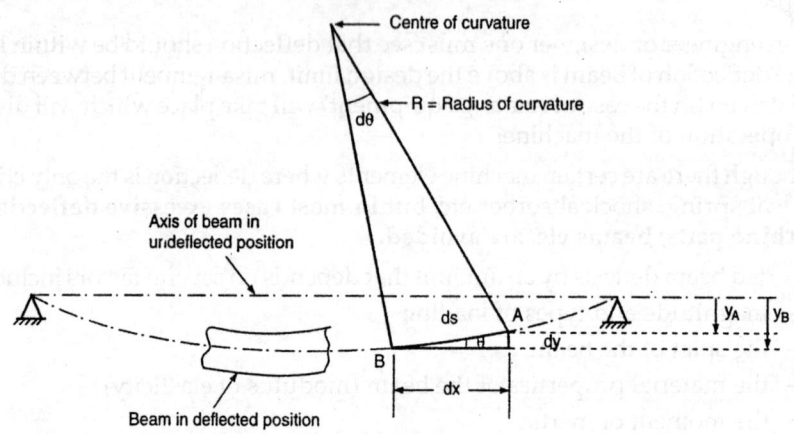

Fig. 10.1

We know that

$$(\text{Slope}), \tan \theta = \left(\frac{dy}{dx} \right)$$

$$\theta = \left(\frac{dy}{dx} \right) \qquad\qquad \left[\begin{array}{l} \text{As } \theta \text{ is small} \\ \therefore \tan \theta \approx \theta \end{array} \right]$$

$$\therefore \quad \frac{d\theta}{dx} = \frac{d^2 y}{dx^2} \qquad\qquad\qquad\qquad\qquad ...(1)$$

From above figure $ds = R \cdot d\theta$

$\therefore \qquad \dfrac{1}{R} = \dfrac{d\theta}{ds} \approx \dfrac{d\theta}{dx}$ $[ds \approx dx]$

$\therefore \qquad \dfrac{1}{R} = \dfrac{d}{dx}\left(\dfrac{dy}{dx}\right) \quad$ or $\quad \dfrac{1}{R} = \dfrac{d^2y}{dx^2}$

From the chapter of bending

$$\dfrac{\sigma}{y} = \dfrac{M}{I} = \dfrac{E}{R} \qquad \therefore \quad \dfrac{1}{R} = \dfrac{M}{EI}$$

$$\therefore \qquad \dfrac{d^2y}{dx^2} = \dfrac{M}{EI}$$

$$\boxed{EI \cdot \dfrac{d^2y}{dx^2} = M} \qquad\qquad ...(2)$$

(where M represents the bending moment at a distance x from one end of beam and so written as $M(x)$ since M is a function of x)

M may be positive when beam is sagging

M may be negative when beam is hogging

Equation (2) is called the curvature–moment relation 'or' the differential equation of flexure or governing equation for elastic curve.

The term EI is known as flexural rigidity.

Integrating eqn. (2) twice we get the deflection of beam (y) as a function of x at point (s) along the axis of the beam and by putting different value of 'x', we get the specific value of deflection (s) along the length of the beam.

$$EI \cdot \dfrac{dy}{dx} = \int M \, dx + A$$

and $\qquad EIy = \int \left(dx \int M \, dx\right) + Ax + B$

A and B are constant of integration which can be known by applying boundary condtion.

---

*We can use y'' instead of $\dfrac{d^2y}{dx^2}$ and y' instead of $\dfrac{dy}{dx}$.

So, $\qquad EI \dfrac{d^2y}{dx^2} = M(x)$

or, $\qquad EI\, y'' = M(x) \quad$ or, $\quad EI\, y' = \int M(x) \, dx + A$

and $\qquad EI\, y = \int \left(dx \int M(x) \, dx\right) + Ax + B$

So, we get the general equation of deflection y as a function of x.

We know that $w = -\left(\dfrac{dF}{dx}\right)$

and $\quad F = \dfrac{dM}{dx}$

$\therefore \qquad w = -\dfrac{d^2M}{dx^2}$

Substituting the value of $M = EI \cdot \dfrac{d^2y}{dx^2}$

$$F = \dfrac{d}{dx}\left(EI \cdot \dfrac{d^2y}{dx^2} \right)$$

$$= EI \cdot \dfrac{d^3y}{dx^3}$$

and $\qquad w = -\dfrac{d^2}{dx^2}\left(EI \cdot \dfrac{d^2y}{dx^2} \right)$

$$= -EI \cdot \dfrac{d^4y}{dx^4}$$

In the above expression F = shear force

$\qquad\qquad\qquad\qquad w$ = load distribution per unit length

10.3 DEFLECTION OF A SIMPLY SUPPORTED BEAM CARRYING A POINT LOAD AT THE CENTRE

By symmetry $R_A = R_B = \dfrac{W}{2}$

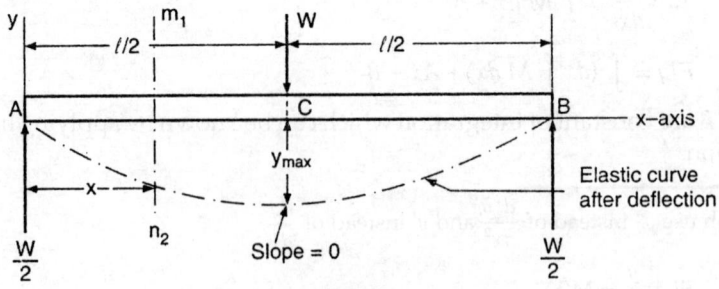

Fig. 10.2

Let us consider a section $m_1\, n_2$ at a distance x from A.

Then, B.M at this section $M(x) = R_A \cdot x$

$$= \dfrac{W}{2} \cdot x$$

By curvature moment relation $M = EI \cdot \dfrac{d^2y}{dx^2}$

Now, equating these two M, we get

$$EI \cdot \frac{d^2y}{dx^2} = \frac{W}{2} \cdot x \qquad \qquad ...(1)$$

After integrating, we get

$$EI \cdot \frac{dy}{dx} = \frac{Wx^2}{4} + C_1 \qquad \qquad ...(2)$$

where, C_1 is constant of integration, the value of which can be obtained from boundary condition.

Now, B.C. are

$$\text{At } x = \frac{l}{2}; \text{Slope} \left(\frac{dy}{dx} \right) = 0$$

$$\therefore \qquad 0 = \frac{W}{4} \cdot \left(\frac{l}{2} \right)^2 + C_1$$

$$\therefore \qquad C_1 = -\left(\frac{Wl^2}{16} \right)$$

Substituting C_1 in eqn. (2) we get

$$EI \cdot \frac{dy}{dx} = \frac{Wx^2}{4} - \frac{Wl^2}{16} \qquad \qquad ...(3)$$

Again integrats

$$\therefore \qquad EIy = \frac{W}{4} \cdot \frac{x^3}{3} - \frac{Wl^2}{16} x + C_2 \qquad \qquad ...(4)$$

At $x = 0, y = 0 \Rightarrow C_2 = 0$

$$\therefore \qquad EIy = \frac{W}{4} \cdot \frac{x^3}{3} - \frac{Wl^2}{16} x$$

Also, at $x = \dfrac{l}{2}; y = y_{max} = y_c$

$$\therefore \qquad EI \cdot y_{max} = \frac{W}{4} \cdot \left(\frac{l}{2} \right)^3 \cdot \frac{1}{3} - \frac{W \cdot l^2}{16} \times \frac{l}{2}$$

$$= \frac{Wl^3}{32 \times 3} - \frac{Wl^3}{32}$$

$$= \frac{Wl^3 - 3Wl^3}{96}$$

$$= -\frac{2Wl^3}{96}$$

$$= -\frac{Wl^3}{48}$$

$$\therefore \qquad y_{max} = -\left[\frac{Wl^3}{48EI}\right] \qquad \textbf{Ans.}$$

(–) sign indicates that deflection is downward.

The above expression can be used as a formula for a beam (simply supported) and loaded at centre.

10.4 (a) EXPRESSION FOR SLOPE AND DEFLECTION FOR A CANTILEVER BEAM CARRYING UNIFORMLY DISTRIBUTED LOAD (w) PER UNIT LENGTH OVER THE ENTIRE SPAN

Let us consider section *mn* at a distance *x* from the end *B*.

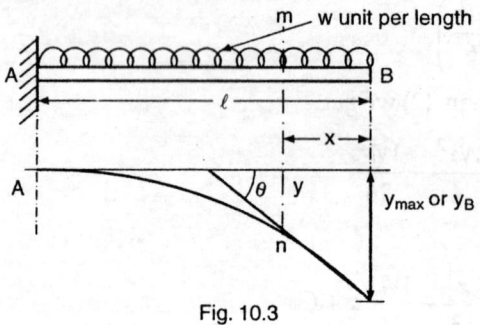

Fig. 10.3

Then, $\qquad M(x) = -\frac{wx^2}{2}$

or, $\qquad EI \cdot \frac{d^2y}{dx^2} = -\frac{wx^2}{2}$

Integrating, we get

$$EI \cdot \left(\frac{dy}{dx}\right) = -\frac{w}{6}x^3 + C_1 \qquad\qquad \text{...(1)}$$

Again, integrating

$$EIy = -\frac{w}{6} \cdot \frac{x^4}{4} + C_1x + C_2 \qquad\qquad \text{...(2)}$$

Boundary conditions are

At $x = l; \dfrac{dy}{dx} = 0$

$\therefore$ From (1) $C_1 = \dfrac{wl^3}{6}$

From (2) $EIy = -\dfrac{w}{24}x^4 + \dfrac{wl^3}{6}x + C_2$

At $x = l; y = 0$

$\therefore \qquad 0 = -\dfrac{wl^4}{24} + \dfrac{wl^4}{6} + C_2$

$\therefore \qquad C_2 = \dfrac{wl^4}{24} - \dfrac{wl^4}{6}$

$\qquad\qquad = \dfrac{wl^4 - 4wl^4}{24}$

$\qquad\qquad = -\dfrac{wl^4}{8}$

$\therefore \qquad y = \dfrac{1}{EI}\left[-\dfrac{wx^4}{24} + \dfrac{wl^3 x}{6} - \dfrac{wl^4}{8} \right]$ From (2)

At $\qquad x = 0, y = y_{\text{max}} = -\left[\dfrac{wl^4}{8EI} \right] \qquad$ **Ans.**

(b) EXPRESSION FOR SLOPE AND DEFLECTION FOR A CANTILEVER BEAM CARRYING CONCENTRATED LOAD W AT THE FREE END.

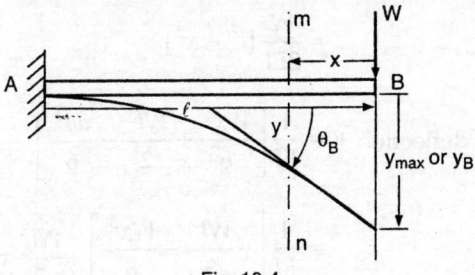

Fig. 10.4

At any section mn

$$M(x) = -W \cdot x$$

or $\qquad EI \cdot \dfrac{d^2 y}{dx^2} = -W \cdot x \qquad\qquad\qquad …(1)$

Integrating (1), we get

$$EI \cdot \frac{dy}{dx} = -W \cdot \frac{x^2}{2} + C_1 \qquad \qquad \dots(2)$$

Again, integrating (2), we get

$$EIy = -\frac{W}{2} \cdot \frac{x^3}{3} + C_1 x + C_2 \qquad \qquad \dots(3)$$

B.C. are

At $x = l$, $\dfrac{dy}{dx} = 0$

Also at $x = l$; $y = 0$

From (2), we get

$$0 = -\frac{W \cdot l^2}{2} + C_1$$

$$C_1 = \left(\frac{Wl^2}{2} \right)$$

From (3)

$$0 = -\frac{Wl^3}{6} + C_2 + \frac{Wl^3}{2}$$

$$\therefore \qquad C_2 = \left(\frac{Wl^3}{6} - \frac{Wl^3}{2} \right) = -\frac{Wl^3}{3}$$

$$\therefore \qquad \text{Equation of slope} \left(\frac{dy}{dx} \right) = \frac{1}{EI} \left[\frac{Wl^2}{2} - \frac{Wx^2}{2} \right]$$

$$= \frac{W}{2EI} [l^2 - x^2]$$

$$\text{Equation of deflection } y = \frac{1}{EI} \left[\frac{Wx^3}{6} + \frac{Wl^3}{2} - \frac{wl^3}{6} \right]$$

$$= \frac{1}{EI} \left[-\frac{Wl^3}{3} - \frac{Wx^3}{6} \right] + \frac{Wl^2}{2} x$$

At free end $x = 0$ $\Rightarrow$ $y_{max} = \dfrac{(-) Wl^3}{3EI} \downarrow$ **Ans.**

Beam subjected to multiple concentrated loads (two point load)

EXAMPLE 1 *Compute the maximum deflection for the loaded beam given in Fig. 10.5.*

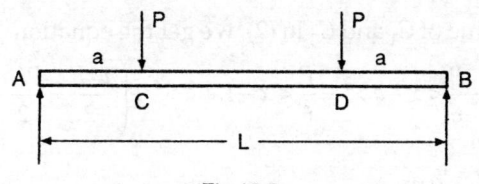

Fig.10.5

SOLUTION

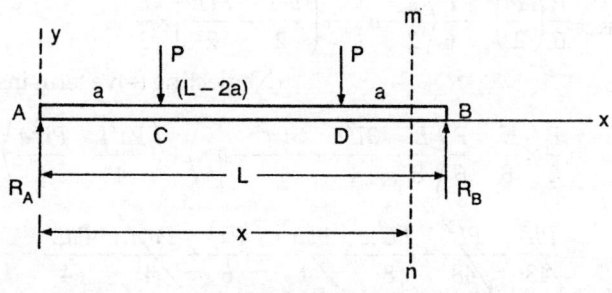

Fig.10.5 (a)

Let us take an imaginary section mn at a distance x from A.

Then $\qquad M(x) = R_A.x - P<x-a> - P<x-L+a>$

By symmetry, $R_A = R_B = P$

Hence, $M(x) = P.x - P<x-a> - P<x-L+a>$

As $\qquad M(x) = EIy''$

So, $\qquad EIy'' = P.x - P<x-a> - P<x-L+a>$

Integrating, we get

$$EIy' = \frac{Px^2}{2} - \frac{P}{2}<x-a>^2 - \frac{P}{2}<x-L+a>^2 + C_1 \qquad \ldots(1)$$

Again, integrating, we get

$$EIy = \frac{Px^3}{6} - \frac{P}{6}<x-a>^3 - \frac{P}{6}<x-L+a>^3 + C_1 x + C_2 \qquad \ldots(2)$$

BC are

At $x=0$, $y=0 \Rightarrow C_2 = 0$

At $x=L$, $y=0 \Rightarrow$ from (2)

$$0 = \frac{PL^3}{6} - \frac{P}{6}<L-a>^3 - \frac{P}{6}a^3 + C_1 L$$

$$= \frac{PL^3}{6} - \frac{P}{6}(L^3 - 3L^2 a + 3La^2 - a^3) - \frac{Pa^3}{6} + C_1 L$$

$$C_1 = -\frac{PLa}{2} + \frac{Pa^2}{2}$$

Substituting the value of C_1 and C_2 in (2), we get the equation

$$EIy = \frac{Px^3}{6} - \frac{P}{6}<x-a>^3 - \frac{P}{6}<x-L+a>^3 + \left(\frac{a^2 P}{2} - \frac{PLa}{2}\right)x$$

At $x = \frac{L}{2}$; $y = y_{max}$

$\therefore$
$$EIy_{max} = \frac{P}{6}\left(\frac{L}{2}\right)^3 - \frac{P}{6}\left\langle\frac{L}{2}-a\right\rangle^3 + \left(\frac{a^2 P}{2} - \frac{PLa}{2}\right)\times\frac{L}{2}$$

(Neglecting (−)ve term inside bracket)

$$= \frac{P}{6}\times\frac{L^3}{8} - \frac{P}{6}\left(\frac{L^3}{8} - \frac{3L^2 a}{4} + \frac{3La^2}{2} - a^3\right) + \left(\frac{Pa^2 L}{4} - \frac{PL^2 a}{4}\right)$$

$$= \frac{PL^3}{48} - \frac{PL^3}{48} + \frac{PL^2 a}{8} - \frac{PLa^2}{4} + \frac{Pa^3}{6} + \frac{Pa^2 L}{4} - \frac{PaL^2}{4}$$

$$= \frac{Pa^3}{6} - \frac{PaL^2}{8}$$

$$= \frac{1}{24}\left(\frac{4Pa^3 - 3PaL^2}{1}\right)$$

$$= -\frac{Pa}{24}\left(3L^2 - 4a^2\right)$$

$$*y_{max} = -\frac{Pa}{24EI}\left(3L^2 - 4a^2\right) \quad \textbf{Ans.}$$

EXAMPLE 2 *Compute y_{max} in the loaded beam as shown in Fig. 10.6.*

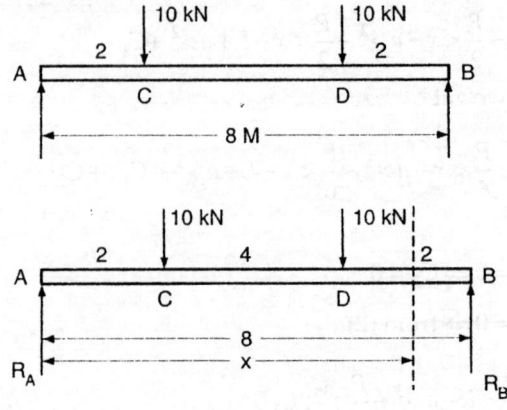

Fig. 10.6

SOLUTION

By symmetry $R_A = R_B = 10$ kN

---

*Reader should remember this formula to solve the Objective Question asked in various competition Examinations.

Now, $M(x) = R_A.x - 10 < x-2 > -10 < x-6 >$

or $EIy'' = 10x - 10 < x-2 > -10 < x-6 >$

Integrating, we get

$$EIy' = \frac{10x^2}{2} - \frac{10}{2} < x-2 >^2 - \frac{10}{2} < x-6 >^2 + C_1 \qquad \ldots(1)$$

Again, integrating, we get

$$EIy' = \frac{5}{3}x^3 - \frac{5}{3} < x-2 >^3 - \frac{5}{3} < x-6 >^3 + C_1 x + C_2 \qquad \ldots(2)$$

BC at $x = 0, y = 0 \Rightarrow C_2 = 0$

and, at $x = 8, y = 0 \Rightarrow$ from (2)

$$0 = \frac{5}{3}(8)^3 - \frac{5}{3}(8-2)^3 - \frac{5}{3}(8-6)^3 + C_1 8$$

$$0 = \frac{5}{3} \times 64 \times 8 - \frac{5}{3} \times 36 \times 6 - \frac{5}{3} \times 8 + C_1 \times 8$$

$$\Rightarrow \qquad C_1 = -60$$

Substituting the value of C_1 and C_2 in eqn. (2), we get

$$EIy = \frac{5}{3}x^3 - \frac{5}{3} < x-2 >^3 - \frac{5}{3} < x-6 >^3 - 60x$$

We see that $x = 4m, y = y_{max}$ ***Alternatively**

$$\therefore \qquad EIy_{max} = \frac{5}{3} \times 64 - \frac{5}{3} \times 8 - 60 \times 4 \qquad \qquad ** y_{max} = (-)\frac{Pa}{24EI}(3L^2 - 4a^2)$$

$$= -\frac{440}{3} \qquad \qquad \qquad = (-)\frac{10 \times 2}{24EI}(3 \times 8^2 - 4 \times 2^2)$$

$$y_{max} = -\left(\frac{440}{3EI}\right) \qquad \textbf{Ans.} \qquad \qquad = (-)\frac{440}{3EI}$$

10.5 DEFLECTION OF A SIMPLY SUPPORTED BEAM SUBJECTED TO U.D.L. W OVER THE ENTIRE SPAN L   [UPTU 2002-03]

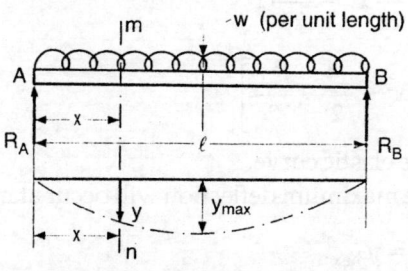

Fig. 10.7

*This formula can be used only when points loads are equal and at equidistance from supports.

**This formula can be used to solve the objective questions in competition examinations and to check the answer in university examination.

Total load on the entire span = $w \cdot l$

$$\therefore \qquad R_A = R_B = \frac{wl}{2} \text{ by symmetry}$$

Let us take a section mn at a distance x from A.
Then

$$M(x) = \frac{wl}{2} x - wx \cdot \frac{x}{2}$$

or,
$$EI \cdot \frac{d^2y}{dx^2} = \frac{wl}{2} x - \frac{wx^2}{2} \qquad \qquad ...(1)$$

On integrating

$$EI \cdot \frac{dy}{dx} = \frac{wl}{2} \cdot \frac{x^2}{2} - \frac{w}{2} \cdot \frac{x^3}{3} + C_1 \qquad \qquad ...(2)$$

Again, on integrating equation (2)

$$EIy = \frac{wl}{4} \cdot \frac{x^3}{3} - \frac{w}{6} \cdot \frac{x^4}{4} + C_1 x + C_2 \qquad \qquad ...(3)$$

At $x = 0, y = 0 \Rightarrow C_2 = 0$

At $x = l; y = 0 \Rightarrow 0 = \frac{wl}{4} \cdot \frac{l^3}{3} - \frac{w}{6} \cdot \frac{l^4}{4} + C_1 \cdot l$

$$C_1 = \frac{wl^3}{24} - \frac{wl^3}{12}$$

$$= \frac{wl^3 - 2wl^3}{24}$$

$$= -\frac{wl^3}{24}$$

Substituting the value of C_1 in eqn. (3)

$$EIy = \frac{wlx^3}{12} - \frac{w}{24}x^4 - \frac{wl^3}{24}x$$

$$\therefore \qquad y = \frac{w}{12EI}\left[lx^3 - \frac{x^4}{2} - \frac{l^3 x}{2} \right]$$

This equation gives the elastic curve.
Now, by symmetry the maximum deflection will occur at mid of the span.

Therefore, at $x = \frac{l}{2}; y = y_{max}$.

$$\therefore \qquad y_{max} = \frac{w}{12EI}\left[l\left(\frac{l}{2}\right)^3 - \frac{1}{2}\left(\frac{l}{2}\right)^4 - \frac{l^3}{2}\left(\frac{l}{2}\right) \right]$$

$$= \frac{w}{12EI}\left[\frac{l^4}{8} - \frac{l^4}{32} - \frac{l^4}{4}\right] = \frac{w}{12EI}\left[\frac{4l^4 - l^4 - 8l^4}{32}\right] = -\left(\frac{5wl^4}{384\,EI}\right)$$

N.B.: The above expression can be used to find y_{max} when w, l, E and I are given, w = load per unit length.

10.6 MACAULAY'S METHOD (THEORY)

Macaulay devised a simple method to compute moment at any arbitrary section of the beam when the beam is subjected to varieties of load *i.e.* concentrated; UDL; triangular; couple etc.

Consider a beam AB subjected to varieties of load *i.e.* concentrated load (w); moment (M_0); UDL $(w_0$ per unit length).

Let us first find moment equation by SFD and BMD chapter of the following loaded beam.

Taking imaginary section at a distance x from A for AC, CD, DE, EF and FB in turn.

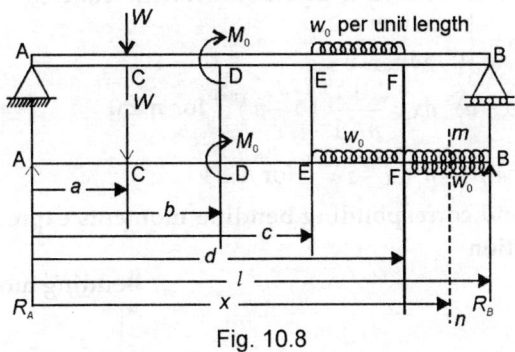

Fig. 10.8

Between

A and C: $M(x) = R_A \cdot x$

C and D: $M(x) = R_A \cdot x - W(x - a)$

D and E: $M(x) = R_A \cdot x - W(x - a) + M_0(x - b)$

E and F: $M(x) = R_A \cdot x - W(x - a) + M_0(x - b) - \frac{w_0}{2}(x - c)^2$

F and B: $M(x) = R_A \cdot x - W(x - a) + M_0(x - b) - \frac{w_0}{2}(x - c)^2 + \frac{w_0}{2}(x - d)^2$

Therefore, if we follow this method, five moment curvature equations would have to be solved with 10 constants of integration, the value of which can be achieved by boundary conditions, which will be too lengthy.

To solve such problem, Macaulay's devised a method to find the deflection equation $y(x)$ due to single and multiple loads (viz concentrated, moment, UDL, triangular and so on) by adopting singularity function $f_n(x) = \langle x - a \rangle^n$

$$\text{for } n \geq 0,\ \langle x - a \rangle^n = \begin{cases} (x-a)^n & \text{when } x \geq 0 \\ 0 & \text{when } x < 0 \end{cases}$$

We note that whenever quantity between brackets is positive or zero, the brackets should be replaced by ordinary parentheses and whenever that quantity is negative, the bracket is equal to zero.

Further, $n = 0$ for moment

$n = 1$ for concentrated load

$n = 2$ for uniformly distributed load

The three singularity functions corresponding to $n = 0, 1, 2$ have been plotted in Fig. 10.9(a).

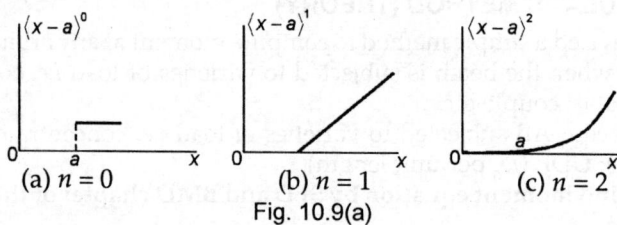

(a) $n = 0$ (b) $n = 1$ (c) $n = 2$

Fig. 10.9(a)

We observe that function $\langle x - a \rangle^0$ is discontinuous at $x = a$ and is in the shape of a step, therefore, it is referred to as the step function and so

$$\langle x - a \rangle^0 = \begin{cases} 1 & \text{when } x \geq a \\ 0 & \text{when } x < a \end{cases}$$

Also, $\int \langle x - a \rangle^n \, dx = \dfrac{1}{n+1} \langle x - a \rangle^{n+1}$ for $n \geq 0$

and $\dfrac{d}{dx} \langle x - a \rangle^n = n \langle x - a \rangle^{n-1}$ for $n \geq 1$

Basic loadings and corresponding bending moments expressed in terms of singularity function

| (I) | Loading | Bending moment |

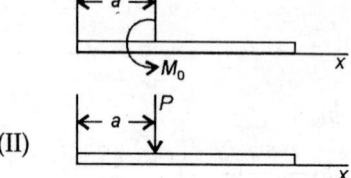
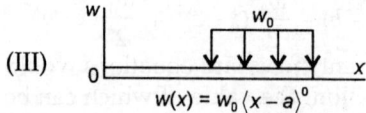
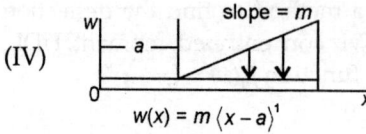

(II)

(III)

$w(x) = w_0 \langle x - a \rangle^0$

(IV)

$w(x) = m \langle x - a \rangle^1$

(V)

$w(x) = m \langle x - a \rangle^n$

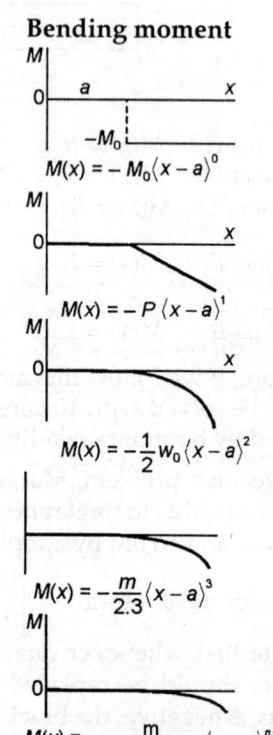

$M(x) = - M_0 \langle x - a \rangle^0$

$M(x) = - P \langle x - a \rangle^1$

$M(x) = - \dfrac{1}{2} w_0 \langle x - a \rangle^2$

$M(x) = - \dfrac{m}{2.3} \langle x - a \rangle^3$

$M(x) = - \dfrac{m}{(n+1)\,(n+2)} \langle x - a \rangle^{n+2}$

Fig. 10.9(b)

In Macaulay's method—only one moment curvature equation is written for a section close to the right hand end of the beam *i.e.* **leaving the extreme right hand side support so as to cover the bending moment for the entire length of the beam.**

Let us see how the problem becomes easy when we apply Macaulay's method to a beam subjected to various loadings.

First of all, the UDL was extended upto the last support. Since extra load was added to the beam so it has to be neutralised by applying load (w_0) from downward upto the last right side support.

We take an imaginary section mn so as to cover all the loads except R_B.
Now,

$$M(x) = R_A.x - W*\langle x-a \rangle + M_0 \langle x-b \rangle^0 - \frac{w_0}{2} \langle x-c \rangle^2 + \frac{w_0}{2} \langle x-d \rangle^2$$

or, $EI \cdot \dfrac{d^2 y}{dx^2} = R_A.x - W \langle x-a \rangle + M_0 \langle x-b \rangle^0 - \dfrac{w_0}{2} \langle x-c \rangle^2 + \dfrac{w_0}{2} \langle x-d \rangle^2$

or, $EIy'' = R_A.x - W \langle x-a \rangle + M_0 \langle x-b \rangle^0 - \dfrac{w_0}{2} \langle x-c \rangle^2 + \dfrac{w_0}{2} \langle x-d \rangle^2$

Now integrating both sides,

$$EIy' = R_A \cdot \frac{x^2}{2} - \frac{W}{2} \langle x-a \rangle^2 + M_0 \langle x-b \rangle - \frac{w_0}{6} \langle x-c \rangle^3 + \frac{w_0}{6} \langle x-d \rangle^3 + C_1$$
$$...(I)$$

Again integrating both sides

$$EI.y = R_A \cdot \frac{x^3}{6} - \frac{W}{6} \langle x-a \rangle^3 + \frac{M_0}{2} \langle x-b \rangle^2 - \frac{w_0}{24} \langle x-c \rangle^4 + \frac{w_0}{24} \langle x-d \rangle^4$$
$$+ C_1 x + C_2 \qquad\qquad ...(II)$$

Applying boundary condition, we scan find out the constants of integration *i.e.* C_1 and C_2.

Here B.C. are,

At $x = 0, y = 0 \implies C_2 = 0$ and At $x = l, y = 0$

or $0 = R_A \cdot \dfrac{l^3}{6} - \dfrac{W}{6} \langle l-a \rangle^3 + \dfrac{M_0}{2} \langle l-b \rangle^2 - \dfrac{w_0}{24} \langle l-c \rangle^4 + \dfrac{w_0}{24} \langle l-d \rangle^4 + C_1 l$

Thus C_1 can be calculated.

After finding C_1 and C_2 and substituting the values in Eqs. (I) and (II), we can get the equation of slope and deflection respectively.

EXAMPLE 1 *Derive the deflection at C for a simply supported beam of span 'l' with concentrated load W acting at 'a' distance (other than in the middle).*

Further, if load W acts in the centre of the beam then find maximum deflection. Use Macaulay's method.

SOLUTION   As imaginary section mn is taken at a distance x from A.

$\therefore \qquad\qquad M(x) = R_A \cdot x - W \langle x-a \rangle \quad$ or $\quad EI \cdot \dfrac{d^2 y}{dx^2} = \dfrac{Wb}{l} x - W \langle x-a \rangle$

Integrating, $EI \cdot \dfrac{dy}{dx} = \dfrac{Wb}{2l} x^2 - \dfrac{W}{2} \langle x-a \rangle^2 + C_1$

---

*Pointed brackets are same as the ordinary brackets like ( ) or [ ] except that their content are set equal to zero for any value of x less than a, b, c, d,... etc.

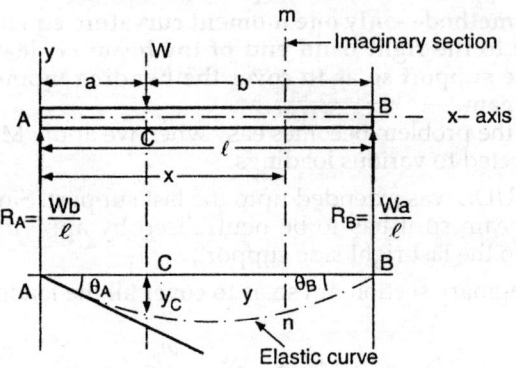

Fig. 10.10

Again, integrating

$$EI \cdot y = \frac{Wb}{6l} \cdot x^3 - \frac{W}{6}\langle x - a\rangle^3 + C_1 x + C_2 \qquad \dots(2)$$

Applying boundary condition

At $x = 0$, $y = 0 \Rightarrow C_2 = 0$ from (2)

At $x = l$, $y = 0$ hence from (2)

$$0 = \frac{Wbl^3}{6} - \frac{Wb^3}{6} + C_1 l$$

$$C_1 = -\frac{Wb}{6l}\langle l^2 - b^2\rangle$$

$$\therefore \qquad y = \frac{1}{EI}\left\{\frac{Wb}{6l}x^3 - \frac{W}{6}\langle x - a\rangle^3 - \frac{Wb}{6l}\langle l^2 - b^2\rangle x\right\} \qquad \dots(3)$$

This is the general equation of deflection.

Now, deflection at a particular point can be found out by substituting the distance of that particular point from the origin A in the Fig. 10.10.

Hence, deflection at C can be evaluated by substituting $x = a$ in eqn. (2).

$$\therefore \qquad y_C = \frac{1}{EI}\left\{\frac{Wb}{6l}a^3 - \frac{Wb}{6l}(l^2 - b^2)a\right\}$$

$$= \frac{Wb}{6EIl}\left\{a^3 - (l^2 - b^2)a\right\}$$

$$= \frac{Wb}{6EIl}\left\{a^3 - (l + b)\cdot a^2\right\}$$

$$= \frac{Wba^2}{6EIl}\left\{a - l - b\right\}$$

$$= \frac{Wba^2}{6EII}\left\{ \not{l} - \not{l} - b - b \right\} \qquad\qquad \left[\because l = a + b\right]$$

$$\boxed{y_C = -\left(\frac{W a^2 b^2}{3EII}\right)}$$

If the load is acting at the centre of beam than $a = b = \dfrac{l}{2}$ and we get the maximum deflection.

$$\therefore \qquad y_{max} = -\frac{W}{3 \cdot EII} \times \frac{l^2}{4} \times \frac{l^2}{4}$$

$$= -\left[\frac{W l^3}{48 EI}\right] \qquad \textbf{Ans.}$$

EXAMPLE 2 *Determine the equation of elastic curve and maximum deflection in the beam as shown in Fig. 10.11. Express the result in terms of E and I.*

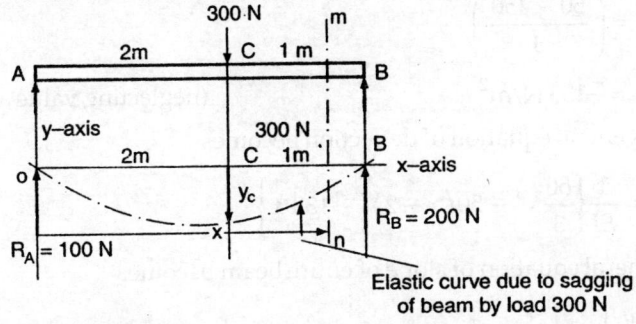

Fig. 10.11

SOLUTION $\Sigma F_y = 0$ gives

$$R_A + R_B = 300$$

Taking moment about A

$$300 \times 2 = R_B \times 3$$

$$\therefore \qquad R_B = \frac{600}{3} = 200\,\text{N}$$

Hence, $R_A = 100\,\text{N}$

Take an imaginary section mn at a distance x from the origin.

Hence, moment equation as a function of x becomes

$$M(x) = R_A \cdot x - 300 \langle x - 2 \rangle$$

---

*This formula can be used to find the deflection at a point (not in the centre) of a simply supported beam having single point load or concentrated load, distances a and b must be known.

$$EI \cdot \frac{d^2y}{dx^2} = 100x - 300\langle x - 2\rangle \text{ Nm} \qquad \ldots(1)$$

Integrating (1), we get

$$EI \cdot \frac{dy}{dx} = 50x^2 - 150\langle x - 2\rangle^2 + C_1 \text{ Nm}^2 \qquad \ldots(2)$$

Again, integrating (2), we get

$$EIy = \frac{50}{3}x^3 - 50\langle x - 2\rangle^3 + C_1 x + C_2 \text{ Nm}^3 \qquad \ldots(3)$$

B.C. are

At $x = 0; y = 0 \Rightarrow C_2 = 0$ (Ignoring negative value)

At $x = 3; y = 0$

Hence, from equation (3)

$$0 = \frac{50}{3}(3)^3 - 50\langle 3 - 2\rangle^3 + C_1 \cdot 3$$

$$\therefore \quad C_1 = \left(\frac{50 - 450}{3}\right)$$

$$\simeq -133 \text{ N/m}^2 \qquad \text{(neglecting value after decimal)}$$

Hence, the general equation of deflection becomes

$$y = \frac{1}{EI}\left\{\frac{50}{3}x^3 - 50\langle x - 2\rangle^3 - 133 x\right\}$$

and, the general equation of slope of entire beam becomes

$$\left(\frac{dy}{dx}\right) = \frac{1}{EI}\left\{50x^2 - 150\langle x - 2\rangle^2 - 133\right\}$$

From the given figure we observe that maximum deflection will occur in the segment AC.

Now, for segment AC

Slope equation up to segment AC

$$\left(\frac{dy}{dx}\right) = \frac{1}{EI}\{50x^2 - 133\} \qquad \ldots(4)$$

and, deflection $(y) = \frac{1}{EI}\left\{\frac{50}{3}x^3 - 133x\right\} \qquad \ldots(5)$

Now, at maximum deflection, slope is zero

$$\therefore \quad \frac{1}{EI}\{50x^2 - 133\} = 0$$

But $EI \neq 0$

$$\therefore \qquad 50x^2 - 133 = 0$$

$$\therefore \qquad x = \sqrt{\frac{133}{50}} = 1.630 \text{ metre}$$

So, we observe that at $x = 1.63$ metre, maximum deflection will take place.
Hence, substituting the value of x in eqn (5), we get

$$y_{max} = \frac{1}{EI}\left\{\frac{50}{3} \times (1.63)^3 - 133\,(1.63)\right\}$$

$$= -\frac{1}{EI} \times 144.61 \text{ metre}$$

Since, deflection in beam produced is normally small hence deflection should be expressed in mm.

$$\therefore \qquad y_{max} = -\frac{1}{EI} \times 0.1446 \text{ mm} \qquad \textbf{Ans.}$$

N.B.: Now, substituting the value of E and I of the given beam we can get the numerical value of deflection of beam.

EXAMPLE 3   *Find ymax for the loaded beam shown in Fig. 10.12.*

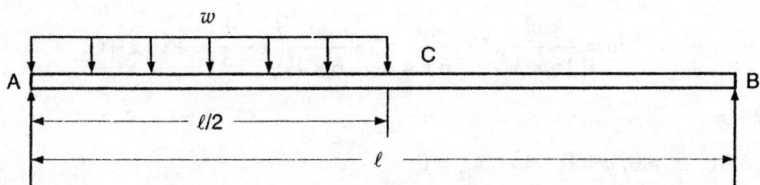

Fig. 10.12

SOLUTION As discussed in Fig. 10.6, the U.D.L w is extended up to B. Since extra load has been added between C and B, so, it has to be made zero by applying load from downward between C and B as shown in the figure below.

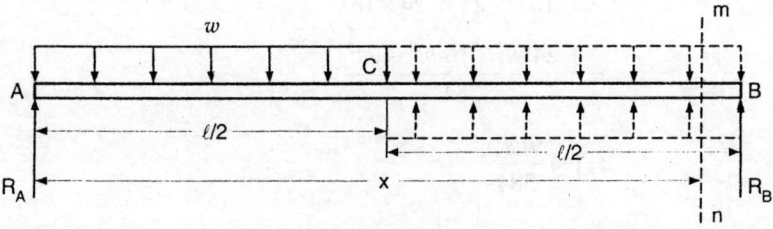

Fig. 10.13

$$R_A + R_B = \frac{wl}{2}$$

$$\Sigma M_B = 0 \text{ gives } R_A \cdot l - \frac{wl}{2}\left(\frac{l}{4} + \frac{l}{2}\right) = 0$$

or

$$R_A \cdot l = \frac{wl}{2} \times \frac{3l}{4}$$

$$= \frac{3wl}{8}$$

Taking section *mn* at a distance *x* from *A*, we get

$$M(x) = R_A \cdot x \frac{wx^2}{2} + \frac{w}{2}\left\langle x - \frac{l}{2} \right\rangle^2$$

or

$$EIy'' = \frac{3wl}{8} x - \frac{wx^2}{2} + \frac{w}{2}\left\langle x - \frac{l}{2} \right\rangle^2$$

Integrating, we get

or

$$EIy' = \frac{3wl}{8} \times \frac{x^2}{2} - \frac{w}{2 \times 3} x^3 + \frac{w}{2 \times 3}\left\langle x - \frac{l}{2} \right\rangle^3 + C_1 \qquad \text{...(1)}$$

Again, integrating

$$EIy = \frac{3wl}{16 \times 3} x^3 - \frac{w}{6 \times 4} x^4 + \frac{w}{6 \times 4}\left\langle x - \frac{l}{2} \right\rangle^4 + C_1 x + C_2 \qquad \text{...(2)}$$

BC are

At $\quad x = 0, y = 0 \quad \Rightarrow \quad C_2 = 0$

At $\quad x = l, y = 0$

$$= \frac{3wl}{48_{16}} \times l^3 + \frac{w}{24} \times \frac{l^4}{16} + C_1 \cdot l - \frac{wl^4}{24}$$

$\Rightarrow$

$$C_1 = -\frac{wl^3}{16} + \frac{wl^3}{24} - \frac{wl^3}{24 \times 16}$$

$\Rightarrow$

$$= \frac{-24wl^3 + 16wl^3 - wl^3}{384}$$

$$= (-) \frac{9wl^3}{384}$$

$\therefore$

$$EIy = \frac{3wl}{48} x^3 - \frac{wx^4}{24} + \frac{w}{24}\left\langle x - \frac{l}{2} \right\rangle^4 - \frac{9wl^3}{384} x \qquad \text{...(3)}$$

Now putting $x = \dfrac{l}{2}$ in eqn. (3) to get y_{max}

$\therefore \quad EIy_{max} = \dfrac{3wl}{48} \times \left(\dfrac{l}{2}\right)^3 - \dfrac{w}{24}\left(\dfrac{l}{2}\right)^4 - \dfrac{9wl^3}{384} \times \dfrac{l}{2}$

$$= \dfrac{3wl^4}{384} - \dfrac{wl^4}{384} - \dfrac{9wl^4}{384 \times 2}$$

$$= \dfrac{6wl^4 - 2wl^4 - 9wl^4}{2 \times 384}$$

$$= (-)\dfrac{5wl^4}{768}$$

$\therefore \quad y_{max} = (-)\dfrac{1}{EI}\left(\dfrac{5wl^4}{768}\right) \qquad \textbf{Ans.}$

EXAMPLE 4   *Compute y_{max} in the loaded beam, shown in Fig. 10.14.*

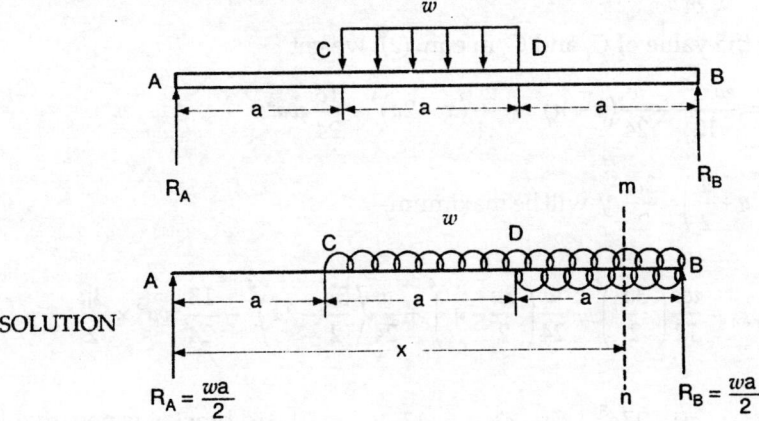

SOLUTION

Fig. 10.14

By symmetry $= R_A = R_B = \dfrac{wa}{2}$

Following Macaulay's method,

We have, $M(x) = R_A \cdot x - \dfrac{w}{2}<x-a>^2 + \dfrac{w}{2}<x-2a>^2$

$$EIy'' = \dfrac{wa}{2}x - \dfrac{w}{2}<x-a>^2 + \dfrac{w}{2}<x-2a>^2$$

Integrating, we get

$$EIy' = \frac{wa}{2} \times \frac{x^2}{2} - \frac{w}{6} <x-a>^3 + \frac{w}{2} <x-2a>^3 + C_1 \qquad \text{...(1)}$$

Again, integrating, we get

$$\therefore \qquad EIy = \frac{wa}{4} \times \frac{x^3}{3} - \frac{w}{24}\langle x-a\rangle^4 + \frac{w}{24}\langle x-2a\rangle^4 + C_1 x + C_2 \qquad \text{...(2)}$$

BC   At $x = 0, y = 0 \Rightarrow C_2 = 0$

At $x = 3a, y = 0 \Rightarrow$

$$0 = \frac{wa}{12} \times (3a)^3 - \frac{w}{24}(2a)^4 + \frac{w}{24}(a)^4 + C_1 \times 3a$$

$$= \frac{wa}{12} \times 27a^3 - \frac{w}{24} \times 16a^4 + \frac{w}{24}a^4 + 3C_1 a$$

$$\therefore \qquad C_1 = \frac{9wa^3}{12} + \frac{w}{72} \times 16a^3 - \frac{w}{72} \times a^3$$

$$= -\left(\frac{13}{24}\right)wa^3$$

Substituting the value of C_1 and C_2 in eqn. (2), we get

$$EIy = \frac{wax^3}{12} - \frac{w}{24}\langle x-a\rangle^4 + \frac{w}{24}\langle x-2a\rangle^4 - \frac{13}{24}wa^3 x$$

For $\quad x = \left(a + \frac{a}{2}\right) = \frac{3a}{2}, y$ will be maximum,

$$\therefore \qquad EIy_{\max} = \frac{wa}{12}\left(\frac{3a}{2}\right)^3 - \frac{w}{24}\left(\frac{3a}{2} - a\right)^4 + \frac{w}{24}\left\langle\frac{3a}{2} - 2a\right\rangle^4 - \frac{13}{24}wa^3 \times \frac{3a}{2}$$

$$= \frac{wa}{12} \times \frac{27a^3}{8} - \frac{w}{24} \times \frac{a^4}{16} + 0 - \frac{13}{16}wa^4 \qquad \left[\begin{array}{l}\text{3rd bracket is negative}\\ \text{hence neglected}\end{array}\right]$$

$$= (\div)\frac{-205}{384}wa^4$$

$$= (-)\, 0.5338\, wa^4$$

$$\therefore \qquad y_{\max} = (-)\frac{0.5338\, wa^4}{EI} \qquad \textbf{Ans.}$$

EXAMPLE 5   *A simply supported beam 3 m long is loaded as shown in the figure below. Calculate deflection at a point 2 metre from A. Given $E = 80$ GPa; $I = 800 \times 10^4$ mm^4.*

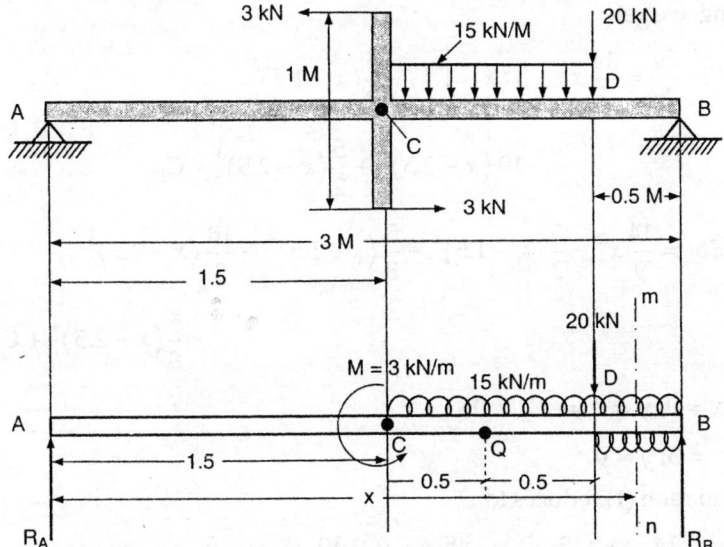

Fig. 10.15 Equivalent load diagram

SOLUTION   As per procedure discussed earlier, u.d.l was extended up to extreme right end of the beam to solve the problem by Macauley's method.

Since, the u.d.l was extended extra, so, it has to be neutralised by applying load (as per rating given) from downward of the beam upto DB.

Two loads (3 kN each) acting opposite to each other separated by a distance (1 M) will constitute a moment (anticlockwise), whose magnitude is 3 kNm and has been shown by arrow anticlockwise and so negative.

Taking moment about B, we have

$$R_A \times 3 - 3 - 15 \times 1 \times (0.5 + 0.5) - 20 \times 0.5 = 0$$

$$R_A = \left(\frac{28}{3}\right) kN$$

Applying Macaulay's Method we have

$$M(x) = EI\frac{d^2y}{dx^2} = R_A \cdot x - 3\langle x - 1.5\rangle^0 - \frac{15}{2}\langle x - 1.5\rangle^2 - 20\langle x - 2.5\rangle + \frac{15}{2}\langle x - 2.5\rangle^2$$

$$EI\frac{d^2y}{dx^2} = \frac{28}{3}x - 3\langle x - 1.5\rangle^0 - \frac{15}{2}\langle x - 1.5\rangle^2 - 20\langle x - 2.5\rangle$$

$$+\frac{15}{2}\langle x - 2.5\rangle^2$$

Integrating, we get

$$EI \cdot \frac{dy}{dx} = \frac{14}{3}x^2 - 3\langle x - 1.5 \rangle - \frac{5}{2}\langle x - 1.5 \rangle^3$$

$$-10\langle x - 2.5 \rangle^2 + \frac{5}{2}\langle x - 2.5 \rangle^3 + C_1$$

and

$$EIy = \frac{14}{9}x^3 - \frac{3}{2}\langle x - 1.5 \rangle^2 - \frac{5}{8}\langle x - 1.5 \rangle^4 - \frac{10}{3}\langle x - 2.5 \rangle^3$$

$$+\frac{5}{8}\langle x - 2.5 \rangle^4 + C_1 x + C_2$$

Now, at $x = 0$, $y = 0 \Rightarrow C_2 = 0$

Also, at $x = 3$; $y = 0$

Hence, equation (1) reduces to

$$0 = \frac{14}{9}(3)^3 - \frac{3}{2}(1.5)^2 - \frac{5}{8}(1.5)^4 - \frac{10}{3}(0.5)^3 + \frac{5}{8}(0.5)^4 + 3\,C_1$$

$\therefore$ $C_1 = -11.67$

$\therefore$ $$EIy = \frac{14}{9}x^3 - \frac{3}{2}\langle x - 1.5 \rangle^2 - \frac{5}{8}\langle x - 1.5 \rangle^4 - \frac{10}{3}\langle x - 2.5 \rangle^3$$

$$+\frac{5}{8}\langle x - 2.5 \rangle^4 - 11.67\,x \quad \text{...(I)}$$

$\therefore$ Deflection at Q which is 2 m from origin *i.e.* left corner A of the beam

$$EI \cdot y_Q = \frac{14}{9}(2)^3 - \frac{3}{2}\langle 0.5 \rangle^2 - \frac{5}{8}\langle 0.5 \rangle^4 - 11.67 \times 2$$

$$= \frac{14 \times 8}{9} - \frac{3 \times 0.25}{2} - \frac{5 \times 0.0625}{8} - 23.34$$

Since, for $x = 2 < 2.5$ hence the last two terms of eqn (I) will be neglected.

$\therefore$ $$y_Q = \frac{1}{EI}\left[\frac{14 \times 8}{9} - \frac{0.75}{2} - 23.34\right]$$

$$= \frac{1}{(80 \times 10^6) \times (800 \times 10^{-8})} \times [12.44 - 0.375 - 23.34]\,\text{m}$$

$$= -0.0176\,\text{m}$$

$$= (-)\,17.6\,\text{mm} \downarrow \qquad \textbf{Ans.}$$

EXAMPLE 6 *Find the equation of elastic curve of a cantilever beam supporting a uniformly distributed load of intensity w_0 over part of its length as shown in figure.*

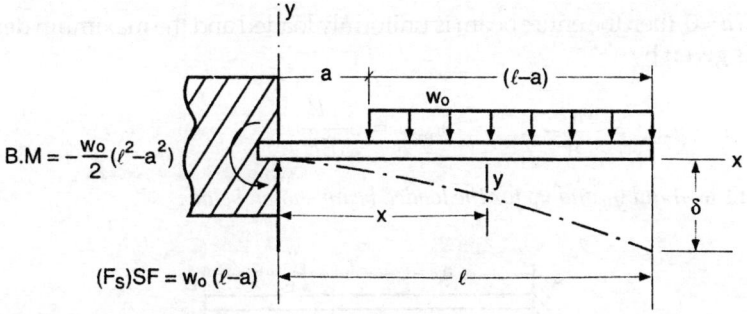

B.M $= -\dfrac{w_0}{2}(\ell^2 - a^2)$

(F_S)SF $= w_0\,(\ell - a)$

Fig. 10.16

SOLUTION

At the wall, $F_S = w_0\,(l - a)$

and $\quad M = -w_0\,(l - a)\left(a + \dfrac{l - a}{2}\right)$

$$= -\dfrac{w_0}{2}(l^2 - a^2)$$

Now, in terms of general moment equation, the differential equation of the elastic curve becomes.

$$M(x) = EI \cdot \dfrac{d^2y}{dx^2} = w_0 \langle l - a \rangle\, x - \dfrac{w_0}{2}\langle l^2 - a^2 \rangle - \dfrac{w_0}{2}\langle x - a \rangle^2 \qquad \text{...(1)}$$

Integraing equation (1)

$$EI \cdot \left(\dfrac{dy}{dx}\right) = w_0 \langle l - a \rangle \cdot \dfrac{x^2}{2} - \dfrac{w_0}{2} \times \langle l^2 - a^2 \rangle\, x - \dfrac{w_0}{6}\langle x - a \rangle^3 + C_1 \qquad \text{...(2)}$$

Now, at $x = 0, \dfrac{dy}{dx} = 0 \Rightarrow C_1 = 0$

$\therefore \qquad EI \cdot \left(\dfrac{dy}{dx}\right) = w_0 \langle l - a \rangle \cdot \dfrac{x^2}{2} - \dfrac{w_0}{2}\langle l^2 - a^2 \rangle\, x - \dfrac{w_0}{6}\langle x - a \rangle^3 \qquad \text{...(3)}$

Integrating eqn. (3), we get

$$EIy = w_0 \langle l - a \rangle \cdot \dfrac{x^3}{6} - \dfrac{w_0}{4}\langle l^2 - a^2 \rangle\, x^2 - \dfrac{w_0}{24}\langle x - a \rangle^4 + C_2 \qquad \text{...(4)}$$

At $x = 0;\, y = 0 \Rightarrow C_2 = 0$

$\therefore \qquad EIy = w_0 \langle l - a \rangle \cdot \dfrac{x^3}{6} - \dfrac{w_0}{4}\langle l^2 - a^2 \rangle\, x^2 - \dfrac{w_0}{24}\langle x - a \rangle^4$

The value of the maximum deflection occurs at the free end, i.e. at $x = l$, $y = y_{max}$.

$\therefore \qquad EI \cdot y_{max} = \dfrac{w_0 \langle l - a \rangle}{8}\left(l^3 + l^2 a + la^2 - \dfrac{a^3}{3}\right)$ **Ans.**

N.B: If $a = 0$, then the entire beam is uniformly loaded and the maximum deflection (y_{max}) is given by

$$EI \cdot y_{max} = \frac{w_0 \, l^4}{8} \quad \therefore \quad y_{max} = \frac{w_0 \, l^4}{8 \, EI}$$

EXAMPLE 6 *Find y_B and y_C for the loaded beam shown below.*

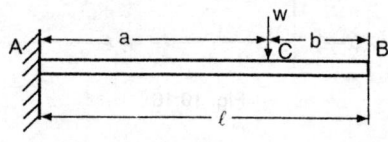

Fig. 10.17

SOLUTION Let us take an imaginary section *mn* at a distance '*x*' from the end *A*.

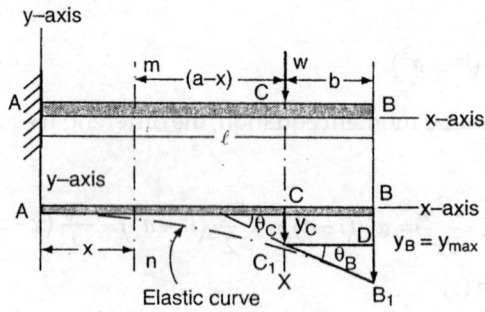

Fig. 10.18

B.M equation for *AC* will be

$$M(x) = -w(a - x) \qquad\qquad [M = f(x)]$$

or

$$EI \cdot \frac{d^2 y}{dx^2} = -w(a - x)$$

Intergrating both side w.r.t *x*

$$EI \cdot \frac{dy}{dx} = -\frac{w}{2}(a - x)^2 + C_1 \qquad\qquad \ldots(1)$$

Again, integrating both side w.r.t *x*

$$EIy = -\frac{w}{6}(a - x)^3 + C_1 x + C_2 \qquad\qquad \ldots(2)$$

C_1 and C_2 are constant of integration and can be obtained from boundary condition.

B.C. are

$$\text{At } x = 0; \text{Slope}\left(\frac{dy}{dx}\right) = 0 \Rightarrow C_1 = \frac{wa^2}{2}$$

and   At $x = 0$; deflection $(y) = 0 \Rightarrow C_2 = -\dfrac{wa^3}{6}$

Substituting the value of C_1 and C_2 in the eqn. (1) and (2), we get,

$$\text{Slope}\left(\frac{dy}{dx}\right) = \frac{1}{EI}\left\{-\frac{w}{2}(a-x)^2 + \frac{wa^2}{2}\right\} \qquad \qquad ...(3)$$

and   Deflection $(y) = \dfrac{1}{EI}\left\{-\dfrac{w}{6}(a-x)^3 + \dfrac{wa^2}{2}x - \dfrac{wa^3}{6}\right\}$ ...(4)

The above general equations are valid for AC portion only.

To find the specific value of slope and deflection at C, we put $x = a$, in equation (3) and (4)

$$\therefore \qquad \left(\frac{dy}{dx}\right)_C = \theta_C = \frac{wa^2}{2EI} \qquad \text{From eqn. (3)}$$

and $y_C = \dfrac{wa^3}{3\,EI}$ From eqn. (4)

θ_B and y_B

From ΔB_1C_1D, $\tan\theta_B = \dfrac{DB_1}{b}$

$$DB_1 = b \cdot \theta_B \qquad\qquad\qquad\qquad \text{[}\tan\theta_B = \theta_B \text{ for small angle]}$$

$$= b \cdot \theta_C \qquad\qquad\qquad\qquad\qquad (\because \theta_B = \theta_C)$$

$$= b \cdot \frac{wa^2}{2EI}$$

Deflection at B is maximum and is given by

$$y_B = y_{max} = BD + DB_1$$

$$= y_C + DB_1$$

$$= \frac{wa^3}{3EI} + \frac{wa^2 b}{2EI}$$

$$= \frac{wa^2}{6EI}(2a + 3b) \qquad\qquad \textbf{Ans.}$$

EXAMPLE 8 *Derive the expression for slope and deflection for a cantilever subjected to clockwise moment (M) at its free end.*

SOLUTION

Taken section mn at a distance 'x' from fixed end

Here, $M(x) = -M$ $\left(\begin{array}{l}\text{Negative B.M, as the applied moment}\\\text{is producing hogging in beam}\end{array}\right)$

$$EI \cdot \frac{d^2y}{dx^2} = -M$$

Integrating both sides w.r.t x

$$EI \cdot \frac{dy}{dx} = -M \cdot x + C_1 \qquad \qquad ...(1)$$

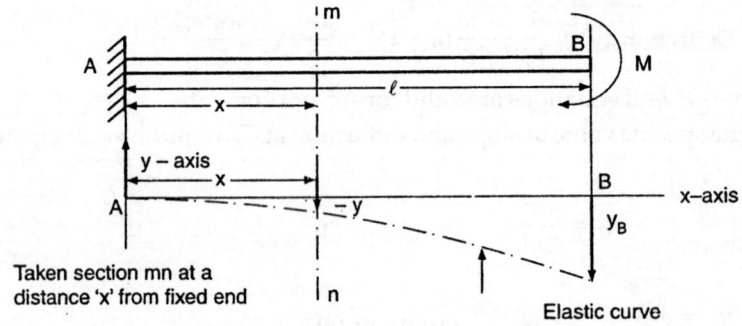

Fig. 10.19

Again, integrating

$$E \cdot I \cdot y = (-) M \cdot \frac{x^2}{2} + C_1 x + C_2 \qquad \qquad ...(2)$$

At $x = 0, \dfrac{dy}{dx} = 0 \Rightarrow C_1 = 0$

Also,   At $x = 0; y = 0 \Rightarrow C_2 = 0$

$\therefore$ Eqn. (1) reduces to $\left(\dfrac{dy}{dx}\right) = -\dfrac{M \cdot x}{EI}$

$\therefore$ $y = (-)\dfrac{M \cdot x^2}{2EI}$

For deflection at B (y_B), putting $x = l$, we get

$$y_B = (-)\frac{M \cdot l^2}{2EI} \ (\downarrow) \qquad \textbf{Ans.}$$

EXAMPLE 9 *A simply supported beam 6 m long is subjected to a uniformly varying load from 15 kN/metre run at one end to 60 kN/metre run at the other. Determine the deflection at the centre if flexural rigidity of the beam section is 2×10^9 Nm². Assume any missing data.*   **[I.E.S. 1991]**

SOLUTION

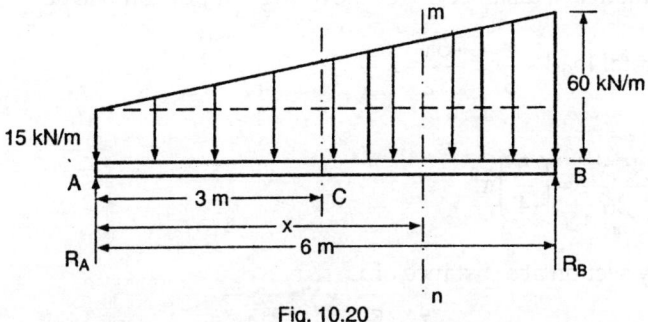

Fig. 10.20

Taking moment about 'B' and equating it to zero *i.e.* $\Sigma M_B = 0$

$$R_A \times 6 - \frac{15 \times 6^2}{2} - \left(\frac{1}{2} \times 45 \times 6\right) \times \frac{6}{3} = 0$$

$$R_A = 90 \text{ kN}$$

Let us take an imaginary section *mn* at a distance *x* from *A*.

Now, if we look at the figure, we find that it is composed of two parts as below.

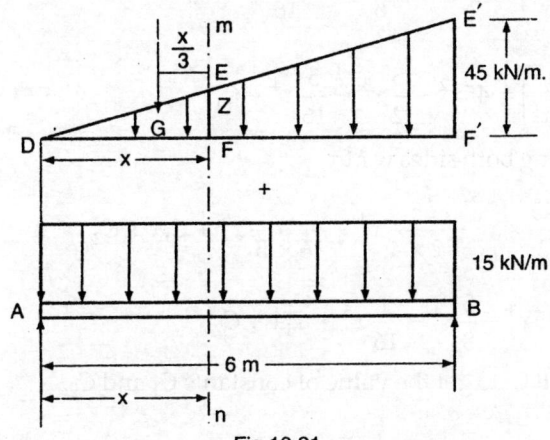

Fig.10.21

Now, for triangular portion $DE'F'$, we should find the load intensity at a distance *x*.

Let load intensity is Z, $\therefore \dfrac{z}{x} = \dfrac{45}{6}$ $\therefore z = \dfrac{45x}{6}$

$\therefore$ Total load on triangular portion *DEF*

$$= \frac{1}{2} \times x \times Z$$

$$= \frac{1}{2} \times x \times \frac{45x}{6}$$

$$= \frac{45x^2}{12} \text{ acting at a distance of } \left(\frac{x}{3}\right) \text{ from end } EF.$$

Hence, moment at a distance 'x' for the triangular portion will be

$$= \text{total load} \times \frac{x}{3} = \frac{45x^2}{12} \times \frac{x}{3}$$

$$= \frac{\overset{5}{\cancel{45}} \, x^3}{\underset{4}{\cancel{36}}} = \left(\frac{5}{4}\right) x^3$$

Now, at any section at a distance of x.

$$M(x) = 90x - (15x) \cdot \frac{x}{2} - \frac{5}{4} x^3$$

or $\qquad EI \cdot \left(\dfrac{d^2y}{dx^2}\right) = 90x - \dfrac{15x^2}{2} - \dfrac{5}{4} x^3$

Integrating both sides, we get, w.r.t x

$$EI \cdot \left(\frac{dy}{dx}\right) = \frac{90}{2} x^2 - \frac{\overset{5}{\cancel{15}}}{\underset{2}{\cancel{6}}} x^3 - \frac{5}{16} x^4 + C_1$$

∴ $\qquad EI \cdot \left(\dfrac{dy}{dx}\right) = 45x^2 - \dfrac{5}{2} x^3 - \dfrac{5}{16} x^4 - C_1$ $\qquad\qquad$ ...(1)

Again, integrating both sides w.r.t x

$$EIy = \frac{45}{3} \times x^3 - \frac{5}{2 \times 4} x^4 - \frac{\cancel{5}}{16 \times \cancel{5}} x^5 + C_1 x + C_2$$

∴ $\qquad EIy = 15x^3 - \dfrac{5}{8} x^4 - \dfrac{1}{16} x^5 + C_1 x + C_2$ $\qquad\qquad$ ...(2)

Now, applying B.C. to get the value of constants C_1 and C_2.

B.C. are

At $x = 0$, $y = 0 \Rightarrow C_2 = 0$

At $x = 6$, $y = 0 \Rightarrow 0 = 15 \times (6)^3 - \dfrac{5}{8}(6)^4 - \dfrac{1}{16}(6)^5 + C_1 \times 6$

$$6\,C_1 = (-)\,15 \times (6)^3 + \frac{5}{8}(6)^4 + \frac{1}{16}(6)^5$$

∴ $\qquad C_1 = (-)\,15 \times 6^2 + \dfrac{5}{6}(6)^3 + \dfrac{1}{16}(6)^4 = -324$

Now, given $EI = 2 \times 10^9 \text{ Nm}^2$

$$= 2 \times 10^6 \text{ kNm}^2$$

Hence, deflection at the centre can be found by putting $x = 3$ in equation (2).

$$y_c = \frac{1}{2 \times 10^5}\left[15\,(3)^3 - \frac{5}{8}(3)^4 - \frac{1}{16}(3)^3 - 324 \times 3 \right]$$

$$= -0.316 \times 10^{-3}\,m$$

$$= (-)\,0.316\ mm \qquad\qquad (i.e.\ \text{downward}) \downarrow$$

N.B. Deflection should always be expressed in (mm) in Answer.

EXAMPLE 10 *A tube 40 mm outside diameter, 5 mm thick and 1.5 metre long is simply supported at 125 mm from each end and carries a concentrated load of 1 kN at each extreme end.*

Compute the maximum deflection in terms of E and I.

SOLUTION Let us treat the tube like beam to get the deflection subjected to concentrated load as shown in Fig. 10.22.

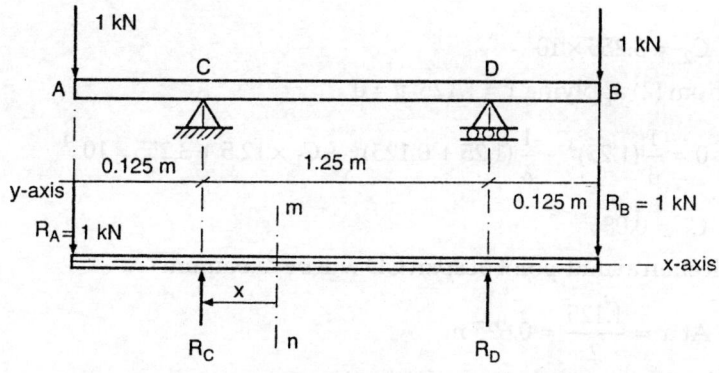

Fig. 10.22

Let us take an imaginary section *mn* to study the case and to get the desired result. Now, taking moment atbout *C*

$$1 \times 0.125 + R_D + 1.25 = 1 \times 1.375$$

$$R_D = \left(\frac{1.375 - 0.125}{1.25} \right)$$

$$= \left(\frac{1.250}{1.25} \right)$$

$$= 1\,kN$$

$$R_C + R_D = 2$$

∴ $$R_C = 1\,kN$$

Now, $$M\,(x) = R_C \cdot x - 1\,(x + 0.125)$$

$$EI \cdot \frac{d^2 y}{dx^2} = x - (x + 0.125)\ kNm$$

Integrating

$$EI \cdot \frac{dy}{dx} = \frac{x^2}{2} - \frac{1}{2}(x + 0.125)^2 + C_1 \qquad \ldots(1)$$

Again, integrating

$$EIy = +\frac{x^3}{6} - \frac{1}{6}(x + 0.125)^3 + C_1 x + C_2 \qquad \ldots(2)$$

B.C. are

At $x = 0, y = 0$	(For C)
At $x = 1.125, y = 0$	(For D)

$$0 = -\frac{1}{6} \times (0.125)^3 + C_2$$

$$C_2 = 3.255 \times 10^4$$

Again, from (2) applying $x = 1.125, y = 0$

$$0 = \frac{1}{6}(1.25)^3 - \frac{1}{6}(1.25 + 0.125)^3 + C_1 \times 12.5 + 3.255 \times 10^{-4}$$

$$C_1 = 0.086$$

The deflection at mid-point of span CD will be maximum *i.e.*

$$\text{At } x = \frac{1.125}{2} = 0.625 \text{ m}$$

$$\therefore \quad y_{max} = \frac{1}{EI} \left[\begin{array}{l} \frac{1}{6}(0.625)^3 - \frac{1}{6} \times 0.625 + 0.125)^3 \\ -0.086 \times 0.625 - 3.255 \times 10^{-4} \end{array} \right]$$

$$= -\left[\frac{0.024414}{EI} \right] \qquad \textbf{Ans.}$$

EXAMPLE 11 *A Simple supported beam carries the triangular load as shown in the figure. Determine the deflection equation and the magnitude of maximum deflection.*

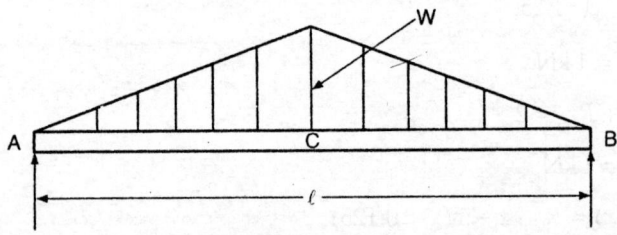

Fig. 10.23

SOLUTION

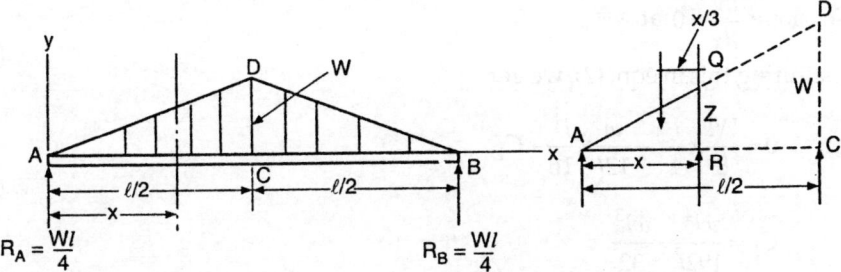

Fig. 10.24

By symmetry $R_A = R_B = \dfrac{wl}{4}$

Since, the beam is symmetrical, so, we will consider half span of the beam for the analysis of deflection.

Further, by taking an imaginary section at a distance x from A we can find at the load intensity (Z). From two similar triangle AQR and ACD, we get

$$\frac{z}{x} = \frac{w}{l/2}$$

$\therefore$ $\qquad Z = \dfrac{2wx}{l}$

Now, total load $= \dfrac{1}{2} \cdot z \cdot x$

$$= \frac{wx^2}{l} \text{ acting at } \left(\frac{x}{3}\right) \text{ from end } Q$$

Now, applying differential equation of elastic curve to part AC we get

$$EI \frac{d^2y}{dx^2} = M_{AC} = \frac{wl}{4}x - \frac{wx^2}{l} \cdot \frac{x}{3} \qquad \qquad ...(1)$$

Integrating

$$EI \frac{dy}{dx} = \frac{wlx^2}{8} - \frac{wx^4}{12l} + C_1 \qquad \qquad ...(2)$$

Again, integrating

$$EIy = \frac{wlx^3}{24} - \frac{wx^5}{60l} + C_1x + C_2 \qquad \qquad ...(3)$$

Here, C_1 and C_2 are constants which can be evaluated by boundary condition BC are, a t $x = 0, y = 0 \Rightarrow C_2 = 0$

Also, slope $\dfrac{dy}{dx} = 0$ at $x = \dfrac{l}{2}$

Substituting this in eqn. (2), we get

$$0 = \frac{Wl}{8} \times \frac{l^2}{4} - \frac{w}{12l} \times \frac{l^4}{16} + C_1$$

$\Rightarrow \qquad C_1 = \dfrac{wl^4}{192l} - \dfrac{wl^3}{32}$

$$= \frac{wl^3}{192} - \frac{wl^3}{32}$$

$$= \frac{wl^3 - 6wl^3}{192}$$

$$= -\frac{5wl^3}{192}$$

Hence, the deflection equation from A to C (also from B to C because of symmetry) becomes

$$EIy = \frac{wlx^3}{24} - \frac{wx^5}{60l} - \frac{5wl^3x}{192}$$

The maximum deflection at mid-point when $x = \dfrac{l}{2}$ is

$$EIy = +\frac{wl}{24} \times \frac{l^3}{8} - \frac{w}{60l} \times \frac{l^5}{32} - \frac{5wl^3}{192} \times \frac{l}{2}$$

$$= +\frac{wl^4}{192} - \frac{wl^4}{1920} - \frac{5wl^4}{384}$$

$$= \frac{wl^4}{120}$$

$\therefore \qquad y_{max} = \dfrac{1}{EI} \cdot \dfrac{wl^4}{120}$ **Ans.**

A simply supported beam subjected to concentrated load, moment and UDL.

EXAMPLE 12 *A simply supported beam shown in Fig. 10.25 has a flexural rigidity $EI = 8 \times 10^6$ Nm^2 find deflection at C and D.*   **(UPTU 2009-10, TME-303)**

SOLUTION **Objective:** To find y_C and y_D

$$R_A + R_E = 40 + 20 \times 2$$

$$= 80$$

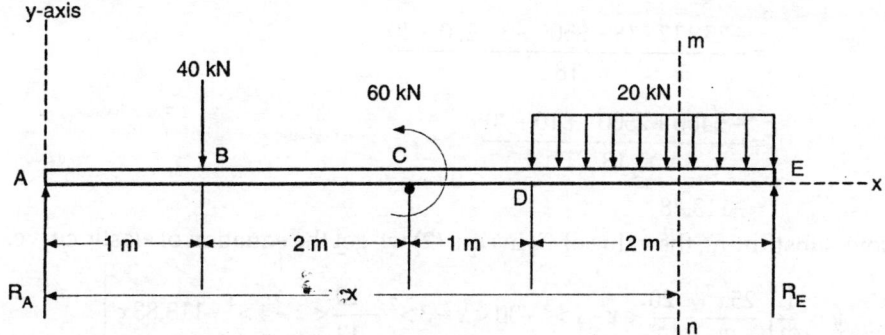

Fig. 10.25

$\Sigma M_E = 0$ gives

$$R_A \times 6 - 40 \times 5 - 60 - 20 \times 2 \times 1 = 0$$

Hence, $R_A = \dfrac{200 + 60 + 40}{6}$

$\qquad\qquad = 50 \text{ kN}$

Taking section mn at a distance x from end A.

Considering beam AE along x-axis then applying Macaulay's method, we get

$$M(x) = R_A \cdot x - 40 < x-1 > -60 < x-3 >^0 - \frac{20}{2} < x-4 >^2 *$$

$$EIy'' = 50x - 40 < x-1 > -60 < x-3 >^0 -10 < x-4 >^2$$

Integrating, we get

$$EIy' = \frac{50x^2}{2} - 20 < x-1 >^2 - 60 < x-3 > - \frac{10}{3} < x-4 >^3 + C_1$$

Again, integrating

$$EIy = 25\frac{x^3}{3} - \frac{20}{3} < x-1 >^3 -30 < x-3 >^2 - \frac{10}{12} < x-4 >^4 + C_1 x + C_2 \qquad \qquad \ldots(2)$$

Now, B.C. are at $x = 0, y = 0 \Rightarrow C_2 = 0$

and   at $x = 6; y = 0 \Rightarrow$

$$0 = 25 \cdot \frac{(6)^3}{3} - \frac{20}{3} < 5 >^3 -30 < 3 >^2 - \frac{10}{12} < 2 >^4 + 6C_1$$

$\Rightarrow \qquad C_1 = -\dfrac{25 \times 6^2}{3} + \dfrac{20}{3 \times 6}(5)^3 + \dfrac{30}{6}(3)^2 + \dfrac{\overset{5}{\cancel{10}}}{\underset{6}{\cancel{12}} \times 6}(2)^4$

$\qquad\qquad = -\dfrac{25 \times 12}{1} + \dfrac{2500}{18} + \dfrac{270}{6} + \dfrac{40}{18}$

*If the moment is clockwise then $M(x)$ will be as

$$M(x) = R_A \cdot x - 40 < x-1 > +60 < x-3 >^0 - \frac{20}{2} < x-4 >^2$$

$$= \frac{-25 \times 12 \times 18 + 2500 + 3 \times 270 + 40}{18}$$

$$= \frac{-5400 + 2500 + 810 + 40}{18}$$

$$= -113.88$$

Now, substituting the value of C_1 in eqn. (2) we get the equation of elastic curve.

$$y = \frac{1}{EI}\left[\frac{25x^3}{3} - \frac{20}{3} <x-1>^3 -30 <x-3>^2 - \frac{10}{12} <x-4>^4 -113.88x \right]$$

Now, find the deflection at C and D we will substitute $x = 3$ and 4 to get y_C and y_D respectively.

$$y_C = \frac{1}{EI}\left[\frac{24}{3}(3)^3 - \frac{20}{3}(2)^3 - 30\,(0)^2 - 113.88 \times 3 \right]$$

(neclecting (–)ve from bracket < >)

$$= \frac{1}{EI}\left[\frac{25 \times 27}{3} - \frac{20 \times 8}{3} - 113.88 \times 3 \right]$$

$$= \frac{1}{8 \times 10^6}\left[225 - 53.33 - 113.88 \times 3 \right] \text{ metre}$$

$$= 21.24 \times 10^{-6} \text{ m}$$

$$= 21.24 \times 10^{-6} \text{ mm}$$

$\therefore \qquad y_C = 0.0214 \text{ mm} \quad$ **Ans.**

Substituting $x = 4$ for deflection at D i.e. y_D

$$y_D = \frac{1}{8 \times 10^6}\left[\frac{25}{3}(4)^3 - \frac{20}{3}(3)^3 - 30\,(1)^2 - 113.88 \times 4 \right]$$

$$= \frac{1}{8 \times 10^6}\left[\frac{25 \times 64}{3} - \frac{20 \times 27}{3} - 30 - 455.52 \right]$$

$$= \frac{1}{8 \times 10^6}\left[533.33 - 180 - 30 - 455.52 \right]$$

$$= 16.52 \times 10^{-6} \text{ m}$$

$y_D = 0.0165 \text{ mm} \qquad$ **Ans.**

EXAMPLE 13   *A beam, simply supported at ends A and B is loaded with two point loads of 60 kN and 50 kN at a distance 1 metre and 3 metre respectively from end A. Determine the position and magnitude of maximum deflection.*

Take $E = 2 \times 10^5 \text{ N/mm}^2$

and $\qquad I = 8500 \text{ cm}^4$ **(UPTU 2009-10, EME-302)**

SOLUTION

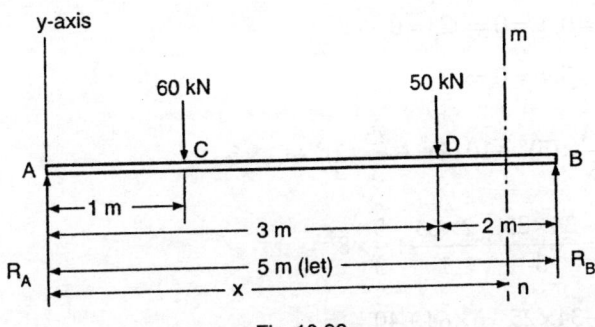

Fig. 10.26

Since, the span AB is not given in the question let us assume $AB = 5$ m

Then $CD = 2$ m

and $DB = 2$ m

Now, taking section mn at a distance 'x' from the end A for the analysis.

Now, let reaction at supports A and B are R_A and R_B respectively.

$$R_A + R_B = 60 + 50$$

$$= 110 \text{ kN}$$

Taking moment about B and equating it to zero

i.e. $\Sigma M_B = 0$

$$R_A \cdot 5 - 60 \times 4 - 50 \times 2 = 0$$

$$R_A = \left(\frac{240 + 100}{5} \right)$$

$$= \frac{340}{5}$$

$$= 68 \text{ kN}$$

Now, $M(x) = R_A \cdot x - 60 < x - 1 > -50 < x - 3 >$

or, $EI \cdot \dfrac{d^2y}{dx^2} = 68x - 60 < x - 1 > -50 < x - 3 >$

Integrating, we get

$$EI \cdot \frac{dy}{dx} = 34x^2 - 30 < x - 1 >^2 -25 < x - 3 >^2 + C_1 \qquad \qquad \text{...(1)}$$

Again, integrating

$$EI \cdot y = \frac{34}{3}x^3 - \frac{30}{3} < x - 1 >^3 - \frac{25}{3} < x - 3 >^3 + C_1 x + C_2 \qquad \text{...(2)}$$

BC are

$$\text{At } x = 0; y = 0 \Rightarrow C_2 = 0$$

$$\text{At } x = 5; y = 0 \Rightarrow$$

$$0 = \frac{34}{3} \times (5)^3 - 10\,(4)^3 - \frac{25}{3}\,(2)^3 + C_1 \times 5$$

$$\Rightarrow \quad C_1 = -\frac{34 \times 25}{3} + \frac{2 \times 64}{1} + \frac{5}{3} \times 8$$

$$= \frac{-34 \times 25 + 6 \times 64 + 40}{3}$$

$$= \frac{-850 + 384 + 40}{3}$$

$$= -142$$

Hence, $\quad Ely = \dfrac{34}{3}x^3 - \dfrac{30}{3} <x-1>^3 - \dfrac{25}{3} <x-3>^3 - 142x$ ...(3)

This is the equations of elastic curve.

Now, to get the maximum deflection we have to equate $\dfrac{dy}{dx} = 0$ in equation (1).

Hence, $\quad 0 = 34x^2 - 30 <x-1>^2 - 25 <x-3>^2 - 142$

$$0 = 34x^2 - 30\,(x^2 - 2x + 1) - 25\,(x^2 - 6x + 9) - 142$$

or, $\quad 34x^2 - 30x^2 + 60x - 30 - 25x^2 + 150x - 225 - 142 = 0$

or, $\quad -21x^2 + 210x - 397 = 0$

or, $\quad 21x^2 - 210x + 397 = 0$

$$x = \frac{210 \pm \sqrt{(210)^2 - 4\,.\,(21)\,(397)}}{2 \times 21}$$

$$= \frac{210 \pm \sqrt{44100 - 33348}}{42}$$

$$= \frac{210 \pm 103.69}{42}$$

$$= 156.84 \quad \text{or} \quad 2.53 \qquad\qquad [\text{As } x \not> \text{span length i.e. } 5\,m\,]$$

So, at $x = 2.53$ m maximum deflection will take place.

Substituting the value of y in equation (3)

$$Ely_{max} = \frac{34}{3} \times (2.53)^3 - \frac{30}{3}(2.53-1)^3 - \frac{25}{3}(2.53-3)^3 - 142 \times 2.53$$

Neglecting the (–)ve value inside the bracket, we get

$$y_{max} = \frac{1}{EI}\left[\frac{34}{3}(2.53)^3 - 10 \times (1.53)^3 - 142 \times 2.53\right]$$

$$= \frac{1}{EI}[183.53 - 3.58 - 359.26]$$

$$= -\frac{179.31}{EI}$$

$$= -\frac{179.31 \times 10^{12}}{EI}$$

$$y_{max} = \frac{-179.31 \times 10^{12}}{2 \times 10^5 \times 8500 \times 10^4} \text{ mm}$$

$$= -\frac{179.3 \times 10}{2 \times 85} \text{ mm}$$

$$= -\frac{1793}{170} \text{ mm}$$

$$= -10.54 \text{ mm} \downarrow \qquad \textbf{Ans.}$$

EXAMPLE 14 *Find the value of Ely at the midway between support and at the overhanging end of the beam*

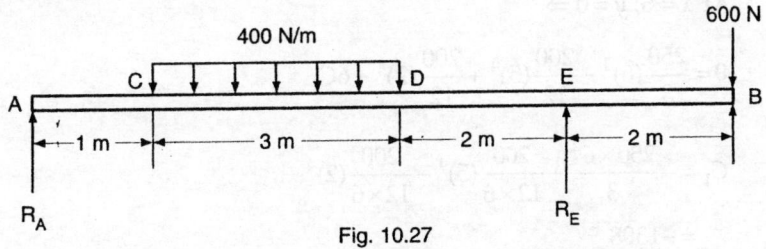

Fig. 10.27

SOLUTION First of all, the U.D.L is extended upto point B. Since extra load has been added so it has to be made zero by applying load from downward of the beam from D to B as shown in figure below.

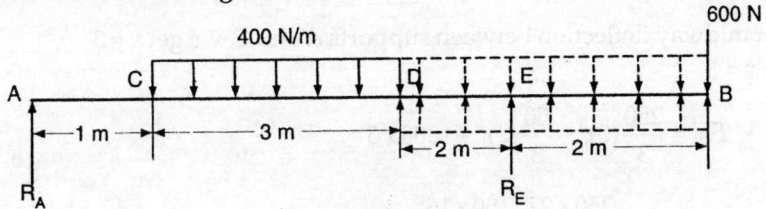

Fig. 10.28

$$R_A \times 6 - 400 \times 3 \times (1.5 + 2) + 600 \times 2 = 0$$

$$R_A = \frac{1200 + 3.5 - 1200}{6}$$

$$= \frac{1200 \times 2.5}{6}$$

$$= 500 \text{ Newton}$$

$\therefore \qquad R_B = 1300 \text{ Newton}$

Applying Macaulay's Method, we have

$$EIy'' = R_A \cdot x - \frac{400}{2} < x - 1 >^2 + \frac{400}{2} < x - 4 >^2 + 1300 < x - 6 >$$

or $\qquad EIy'' = 500x - 200 < x - 1 >^2 + 200 < x - 47 >^2 + 1300 < x - 6 >$

Integrating, we get

$$EIy' = 250x^2 - \frac{200}{3} < x - 1 >^3 + \frac{200}{3} < x - 4 >^3 + 650 < x - 6 >^2 + C_1 \qquad \ldots(1)$$

Again integrating, we get

$$EIy = \frac{250}{3} x^3 - \frac{200}{3 \times 4} < x - 1 >^4 + \frac{200}{3 \times 4} < x - 4 >^4 + \frac{650}{3} < x - 6 >^3 + C_1 x + C_2$$

$$\ldots(2)$$

BC   At $x = 0, y = 0 \Rightarrow C_2 = 0$ (ignoring negative (–ve) value inside bracket)

At $x = 6; y = 0 \Rightarrow$

$$0 = \frac{250}{3} (6)^3 - \frac{200}{12} (5)^4 + \frac{200}{12} (2)^4 + 6C_1$$

$$\Rightarrow \qquad C_1 = -\frac{250 \times 6^2}{3} + \frac{200}{12 \times 6} (5)^4 - \frac{200}{12 \times 6} (2)^4$$

$$= -1308$$

$\therefore$ Eqn. (2) which is a equation of elastic curve reduces to

$$EIy = \frac{250}{3} x^3 - \frac{50}{3} < x - 1 >^4 + \frac{50}{3} < x - 4 >^4 + \frac{650}{3} < x - 6 >^3 - 1308x$$

To get midway deflection between supports A and E, we get $x = 3$

So, at $x = 3$,

$$EIy = \frac{250}{3} (3)^3 - \frac{50}{3} (2)^4 - 1308 \times 3$$

$$= \frac{250 \times 27}{3} - \frac{50 \times 16}{3} - 1308 \times 3$$

$$= \frac{250 \times 27 - 50 \times 16 - 1308 \times 3 \times 3}{3}$$

$$= \frac{6750 - 800 - 11772}{3}$$

$$= -1940.66 \text{ Nm}^3$$

$$\approx -1941 \text{ Nm}^3 \qquad \textbf{Ans.}$$

At the overhang end $x = 8$

So, at $x = 8$, $EIy = \frac{250}{3}(8)^3 - \frac{50}{3}(7)^4 + \frac{50}{3}(4)^4 + \frac{650}{3}(2)^3 - 1308 \times 8$

$$= 42666.66 - 40016.66 + 4266.66 + 1733.33 - 10464$$

$$= -1814.01 \text{ Nm}^3$$

$\therefore \qquad EIy = -1814 \text{ Nm}^3 \qquad \textbf{Ans.}$

EXAMPLE 15 *A beam of uniform section, 10 metre long is simply supported at the ends. It carries a point loads of 150 kN and 65 kN at a distance of 2.5 m and 5.5 m respectively from the left end.*
Calculate:
(a) the deflection under each load,
(b) the maximum deflection.
Take $E = 200 \text{ GN/m}^2$

$$= 200 \times 10^6 \text{ kN/m}^2$$

$$I = 118 \times 10^{-4} \text{ m}^4 \qquad\qquad\qquad \textbf{(UPTU 2006-07)}$$

SOLUTION

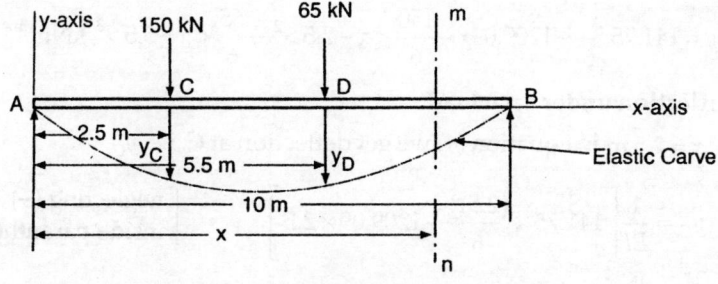

Fig. 10.29

Taking imaginary section mn at a distance x from A.

$$\Sigma F_y = 0 \Rightarrow R_A + R_B = 150 + 65 = 215 \text{ kN}$$

$$\Sigma M_B = 0 \text{ gives}$$

$$R_A \times 10 - 150 \times 7.5 - 65 \times 4.5 = 0$$

$\Rightarrow$ $R_A = 141.75$ kN

and $R_B = 73.25$ kN

Now, $M(x) = R_A \cdot x - 150 <x - 2.5> - 65 <x - 5.5>$

or, $EIy'' = R_A \cdot x - 150 <x - 2.5> - 65 <x - 5.5>$ kNm

Integraing both side

$$EIy' = R_A \cdot \frac{x^2}{2} - \frac{150}{2} <x - 2.5>^2 - \frac{65}{2} <x - 5.5>^2 + C_1 \text{ kNm}^2 \qquad \ldots(1)$$

Again integrating equation (1)

$$EIy = R_A \cdot \frac{x^3}{6} - \frac{150}{2 \times 3} <x - 2.5>^3 - \frac{65}{2 \times 3} <x - 5.5>^3 + C_1 x + C_2 \text{ kNm}^3$$

$$\ldots(2)$$

BC are

At $x = 0$; $y = 0 \Rightarrow C_2 = 0$

At $x = 10$ m; $y = 0 \Rightarrow$

$$0 = 141.75 \times \frac{(10)^3}{6} - \frac{150}{6} \times 7.5^3 - \frac{65}{6} \times 4.5^3 + C_1 \times 10$$

$\Rightarrow$ $C_1 = 1209.09$

Hence, slope and deflection equation are

$$EI \cdot \left(\frac{dy}{dx} \right) = 141.75 \frac{x^2}{2} - 1209.09 - 150 \frac{<x - 2.5>^2}{2} - 65 \frac{<x - 5.5>^2}{2} \text{ kNm}^2 \quad \ldots(3)$$

and $EIy = 141.75 \frac{x^3}{6} - 1209.09x - \frac{150}{6} <x - 2.5>^2 - \frac{65}{6} <x - 5.5>^3 \text{ kNm}^3 \qquad \ldots(4)$

Now, deflection under each load

Putting $x = 2.5$ m in equation (4) we get deflection at C, i.e. y_C

Hence, $y_C = \dfrac{1}{EI} \left[141.75 \times \dfrac{(2.5)^3}{6} - 1209.09 \times 2.5 \right]$ $\left[\begin{array}{l} \text{neglecting (--)ve term} \\ \text{inside parantheses} \end{array} \right]$

$$= \frac{1}{200 \times 10^6 \times 118 \times 10^{-4}} \left[141.75 \times \frac{(2.5)^3}{3} - 1209.09 \times 2.5 \right]$$

$$= 1.1244 \times 10^{-3} \text{ metre}$$

$$= 1.124. \text{ mm} \qquad \textbf{Ans.}$$

Similarly, by substituting $x = 5.5$ m we get deflection at D i.e.

$y_D = 1.438$ mm **Ans.**

Max^m deflection: Maximum deflection will take place between C and D.
Equating slope equation equal to zero, we get

$$0 = 141.75 \times \frac{x^2}{2} - 1209.09 - \frac{150}{2} \times (x^2 + 6.25 - 5x)$$

(Neglecting last term of equation 3 as x less than 5.5 for the maximum deflection, bracket becomes –ve.)

$\Rightarrow \qquad x = 4.72$ m

Now, substituting $x = 4.72$ m in the eqn (4), we get

$$200 \times 16^6 \times 118 \times 10^{-4} \times y_{max} = 141.75 \times \frac{(4.72)^3}{6} - 1209.09 \times 4.72 - \frac{150}{2} \times (2.22)^3$$

$\therefore \qquad y_{max} = 1.481$ mm $\qquad$ **Ans.**

10.7 DEFLECTION OF BEAM BY MOMENT AREA METHOD

Let us consider an arbitrary loading of a simply supported beam AB.

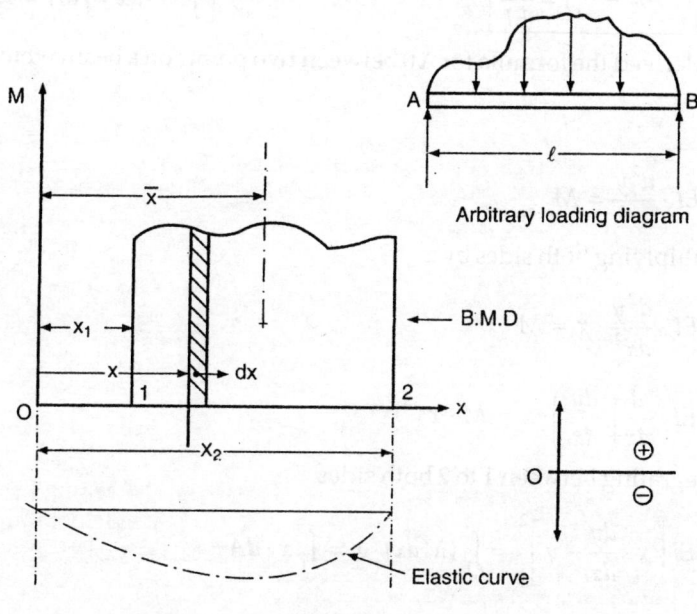

Fig. 10.30

Let $\qquad A$ = Area of B.M.D.

and $\qquad \bar{x}$ = C.G. of the B.M.D. area

Let us consider a small portion of the beam of dx at a distance x from origin.

Area of the hatched part $= \int_1^2 M \cdot dx$

By the beam deflection relation

$$EI \cdot \frac{d^2 y}{dx^2} = M$$

$$\left(\frac{d^2 y}{dx^2}\right) = \frac{M}{EI} \text{ or, } \frac{d}{dx}\left(\frac{dy}{dx}\right) = \frac{M}{EI}$$

Integrating between limit 1 and 2

$$\left[\left(\frac{dy}{dx}\right)\right]_1^2 = \int_1^2 \frac{M\,dx}{EI}$$

Now, $\left(\dfrac{dy}{dx}\right) = \theta$ and θ at $1 \Rightarrow \theta_1$

$$\theta \text{ at } 2 \Rightarrow \theta_2$$

$\therefore$ $[\theta_2 - \theta_1] = \dfrac{1}{EI} \int_1^2 M \cdot dx$

$\boxed{\therefore \ (\theta_2 - \theta_1) = \dfrac{A}{EI}}$ $\left[\int M \cdot dx = \int dA = A\right]$ ...(1)

We have derived the formula for $\Delta\theta$ between two points on a beam which is equal to $\dfrac{A}{EI}$

$\because$ $EI \cdot \dfrac{d^2 y}{dx^2} = M$

Now, multiplying both sides by x

$$EI \cdot \frac{d^2 y}{dx^2} \cdot x = M \cdot x$$

$$EI \cdot \frac{d}{dx}\left(\frac{dy}{dx}\right) \cdot x = M \cdot x$$

Now, integrating between 1 to 2 both sides

$$EI\left[x \cdot \frac{dy}{dx} - y\right]_1^2 = \int_1^2 (M\,dx) \cdot x = \int_1^2 x \cdot dA$$

$$EI\left[x\theta - y\right]_1^2 = A \cdot \bar{x} \qquad\qquad \left[\because \bar{x} = \frac{\int x \cdot dA}{\int dA} = \frac{\int x \cdot dA}{A}\right]$$

$$x_2\,\theta_2 - x_1\,\theta_1 - y_2 + y_1 = \frac{A \cdot \bar{x}}{EI}$$

$$(y_1 - y_2) + (x_2\,\theta_2 - x_1\,\theta_1) = \frac{A \cdot \bar{x}}{EI}$$

If 1 shifts to origin *i.e.* $x_1 = 0$ and θ_2 having zero slope then

$$y_1 - y_2 = \frac{A \cdot \bar{x}}{EI}$$

...(2)

Equation (1) and (2) are known as Mohr's Theorem or Moment Area theorem.

N.B. Before solving the problem based on moment area method one should be acquainted with the C.G. for various type of geometrical shape.

Let the general equation of curve is $y = ax^n$

C.G. $(\bar{x}) = \dfrac{n+1}{n+2} \cdot b$

Area $(A) = \dfrac{b \cdot h}{n+1}$

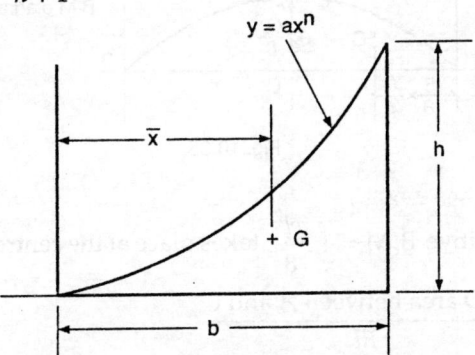

Fig. 10.31

For second degree curve $y = ax^2$

$$\bar{x} = \left(\frac{3}{4}\right) b$$

$$A = \frac{b \cdot h}{3}$$

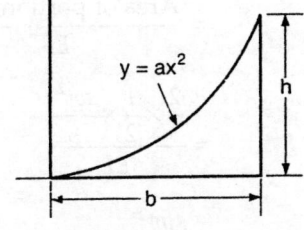

Fig. 10.32

For third degree curve $y = ax^3$

$$\bar{x} = \frac{4}{5} b$$

$$A = \frac{bh}{4}$$

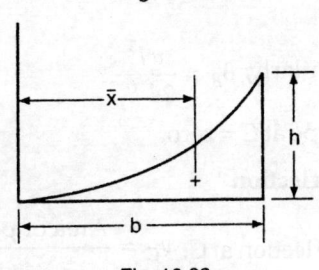

Fig. 10.33

Trapozoidal Area

$$\bar{x} = \frac{h_1 + 2h_2}{3(h_1 + h_2)}$$

$$A = \frac{1}{2} \cdot b \cdot (h_1 + h_2)$$

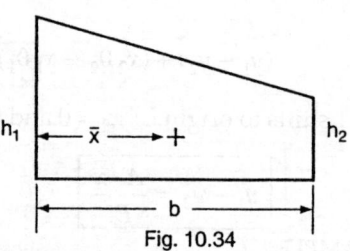

Fig. 10.34

EXAMPLE 1 *Derive slope and deflection expression for a beam subjected to u.d.l. w.*

The span of the beam is l. EI is constant throughout.

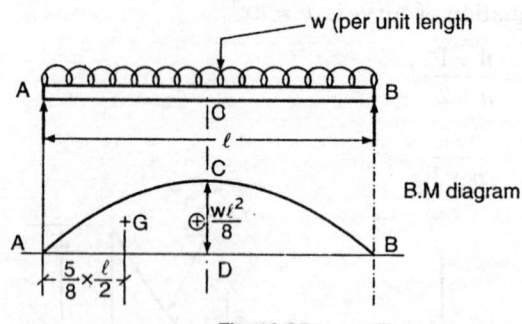

Fig. 10.35

Slope

The maximum positive B.M $= +\dfrac{wl^2}{8}$ takes place at the centre of the beam

$$\theta_A = \frac{\text{BMD area between } A \text{ and } C}{EI}$$

$$= \frac{\text{Area of portion } ACD}{EI}$$

$$= \frac{\dfrac{2}{3} \times \dfrac{l}{2} \times \dfrac{wl^2}{8}}{EI}$$

$$\therefore \quad \theta_A = \frac{wl^3}{24\,EI}$$

$$\boxed{\theta_A = \theta_B = \frac{wl^3}{24\,EI}}$$

Similarly; $\theta_B = \dfrac{wl^3}{24\,EI}$

Slope at C = zero.

Deflection

Deflection at C, $y_C = \dfrac{\text{Area of portion } ACD \times \bar{x}}{EI}$

$$= \frac{\dfrac{\cancel{2}}{3} \times \dfrac{l}{\cancel{2}} \times \dfrac{wl^2}{8} \times \dfrac{5}{8} \times \dfrac{l}{2}}{EI}$$

$$\therefore y_C = y_{max} = \frac{5}{384} \cdot \frac{wl^4}{EI} \qquad \textbf{Ans.}$$

EXAMPLE 2 *Derive the expression for slope and deflection by moment area method for a simply supported beam carrying load W at its centre. The span of beam is l.*
The flexure rigidity (EI) is constant throughout the span.

SOLUTION

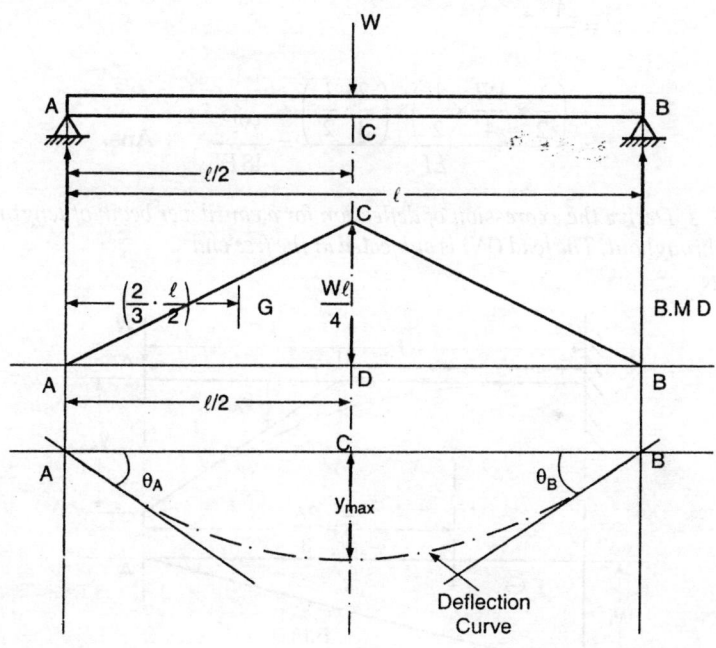

Fig. 10.36

Slope

Slope at $A = \theta_A$

$$= \frac{\text{BMD area between } A \text{ and } C}{EI}$$

$$= \frac{\dfrac{1}{2} \times \dfrac{Wl}{4} \times \dfrac{l}{2}}{EI}$$

$$= \frac{Wl^2}{16\,EI}$$

Owing to symmetry, $\theta_A = \theta_B = \dfrac{Wl^2}{16EI}$

Slope at $C\ (\theta_C) = 0$

Deflection

Deflection at A = deflection at $B = 0$ i.e. $y_A = y_B = 0$

$y_C = y_{max}$, as the load is acting centrally on the beam.

$\therefore \qquad y_C = y_{max} = \dfrac{\text{Moment of BMD area between } A \text{ and } C \text{ about } A}{EI}$

$$= \dfrac{A \cdot \bar{x}}{EI}$$

$$= \dfrac{\left(\dfrac{1}{2} \times \dfrac{Wl}{4} \times \dfrac{l}{2}\right) \times \left(\dfrac{2}{3} \cdot \dfrac{l}{2}\right)}{EI} = \dfrac{Wl^3}{48EI} \qquad \textbf{Ans.}$$

EXAMPLE 3 *Derive the expression of deflection for a cantilever beam of length 'l'. EI is constant throughout. The load (W) is subjected at the free end.*

SOLUTION

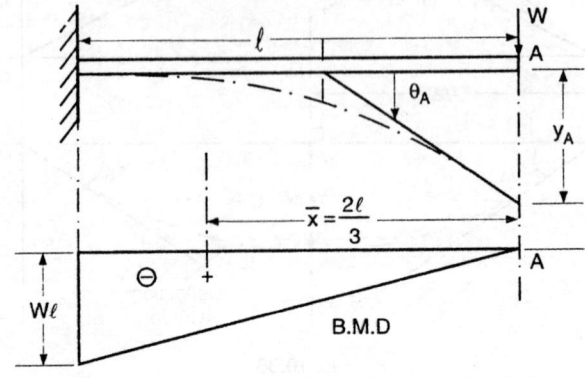

Fig. 10.37

$$\theta_A = -\left[\dfrac{A}{EI}\right]$$

$$= -\left[\dfrac{\dfrac{1}{2} \cdot l \cdot Wl}{EI}\right]$$

$$= -\dfrac{Wl^2}{2EI} \qquad \textbf{Ans.}$$

$$y_A = \left[\frac{A \cdot \bar{x}}{EI} \right]$$

$$= -\left[\frac{\frac{1}{2} \times l \times Wl \times \frac{2l}{3}}{EI} \right]$$

$$= -\left[\frac{Wl^3}{3EI} \right] \quad \textbf{Ans.}$$

EXAMPLE 4 *Find θ and deflection for a cantilever subjected to u.d.l w at the free end.*

SOLUTION

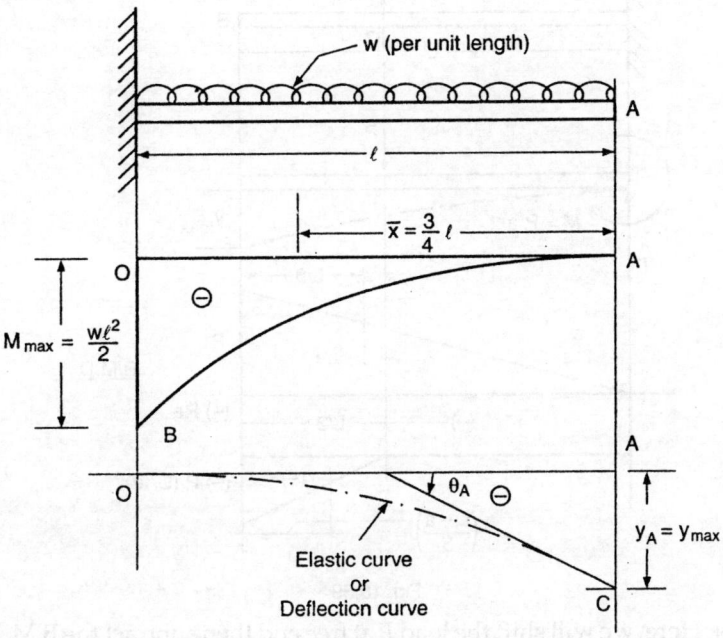

Fig. 10.38

The slope at A, $\theta_A = \dfrac{A}{EI}$

$$= -\frac{\frac{1}{3} \times l \times \frac{wl^2}{2}}{EI}$$

$$= -\frac{wl^3}{6EI}$$

Deflection at A, $y_A = y_{max} = \dfrac{A \cdot \bar{x}}{EI}$

$$= \dfrac{\left[-\dfrac{1}{3} \times l \times \dfrac{wl^2}{2} \right] \left[\dfrac{3}{4} l \right]}{EI}$$

$$= (-) \dfrac{wl^4}{8EI} \qquad \textbf{Ans.}$$

EXAMPLE 5 *Determine δ_{max} for the loaded beam shown in Fig. 10.39.*

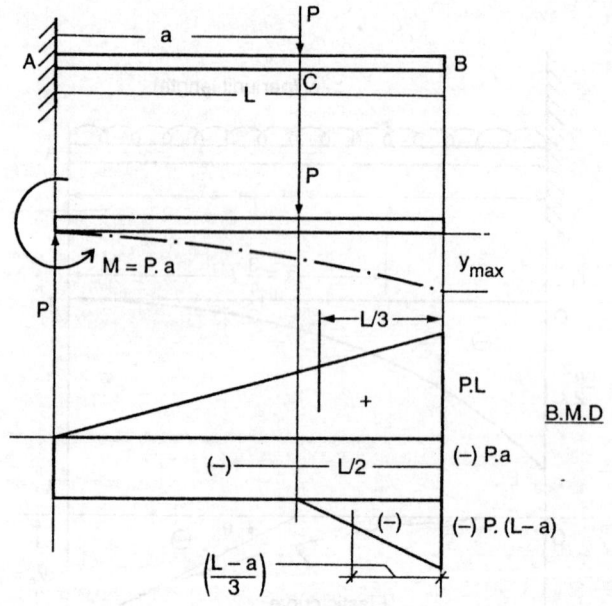

Fig. 10.39

SOLUTION Here, we will shift the load P at free end then subtract the B.M. area of extra portion *i.e.*, for CB to get the objective.

By formula, we have

$$EI \cdot y_{B/A} = (\text{Area of B.M.D. between } B \text{ and } A) \times \bar{x}$$

$$= \left[\left(\dfrac{1}{2} \times L \times PL \right) \cdot \dfrac{L}{3} - (P \cdot a \cdot L) \cdot \dfrac{L}{2} - \dfrac{1}{2} (L - a) \cdot P (L - a) \cdot \left(\dfrac{L - a}{3} \right) \right]$$

$$= \dfrac{1}{6} PL^3 - \dfrac{1}{2} PaL^2 - \dfrac{1}{6} P (L - a)^3$$

$$= \dfrac{1}{6} PL^3 - \dfrac{1}{2} PaL^2 - \dfrac{1}{6} PL^3 + \dfrac{PL^2 a}{2} - \dfrac{PLa^2}{2} + \dfrac{Pa^3}{6}$$

$$= -\frac{PLa^2}{2} + \frac{Pa^3}{6}$$

$$= -\frac{Pa^2}{6}(3L - a)$$

Hence, δ_{max} or $y_B = \dfrac{-Pa^2\,(3L - a)}{6EI} \downarrow$ **Ans.**

EXAMPLE 6 *A cantilever of length 2a carries a load W at free end and a load W at its centre. Determine slope and deflection at free end.*

SOLUTION

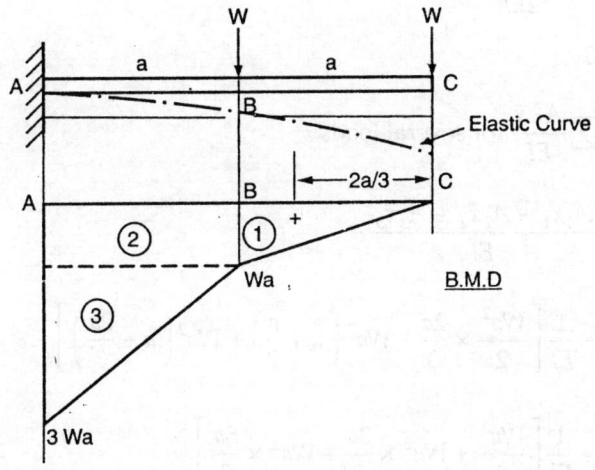

Fig. 10.40

B.M. calculation for cantilever

$$M_C = 0$$

$$M_B = W \cdot a$$

$$M_A = -W \cdot a - W \cdot 2a = -3Wa$$

Slope and deflection both are zero at A.

Hence, slope at free end *i.e.*, at C,

$$\theta_C = -\frac{A}{EI}$$

$$= -\frac{\text{Area of B.M.D. between } C \text{ and } A}{EI}$$

$$= -\left[\frac{A_1 + A_2 + A_3}{EI}\right]$$

$$= -\left[\frac{\left(\frac{1}{2} \times a \times Wa\right) + (Wa \times a) + \left(\frac{1}{2} \times a \times 2Wa\right)}{EI}\right]$$

$$= -\frac{1}{EI}\left[\frac{Wa^2}{2} + Wa^2 + Wa^2\right]$$

$$= (-)\frac{5Wa^2}{2EI} \text{ is the slope at } C.$$

Deflection at C

$$y_C = \sum \frac{A \cdot \bar{x}}{EI} \text{ for several loads}$$

$$= \frac{A_1\bar{x}_1 + A_2\bar{x}_2 + A_3\bar{x}_3}{EI}$$

$$= -\frac{1}{EI}\left[\frac{Wa^2}{2} \times \frac{2a}{3} + Wa^2\left(a + \frac{a}{2}\right) + Wa^2\left(a + \frac{2a}{3}\right)\right]$$

$$= -\frac{1}{EI}\left[\frac{Wa^3}{3} + Wa^2 \times \frac{3a}{2} + Wa^2 \times \frac{5a}{3}\right]$$

$$= -\frac{1}{EI}\left[\frac{Wa^3}{3} + \frac{3Wa^3}{2} + \frac{5Wa^2}{3}\right]$$

$$= -\frac{1}{EI}\left[\frac{2Wa^3 + 9Wa^3 + 10Wa^3}{6}\right]$$

$$= -\frac{1}{EI} \times \frac{21Wa^3}{6}$$

Hence, $\quad y_C = (-)\dfrac{7Wa^3}{2EI} \downarrow$

N.B.: We can draw B.M.D. for load at C, B, and A separately as given in Fig. 10.41 for calculation.

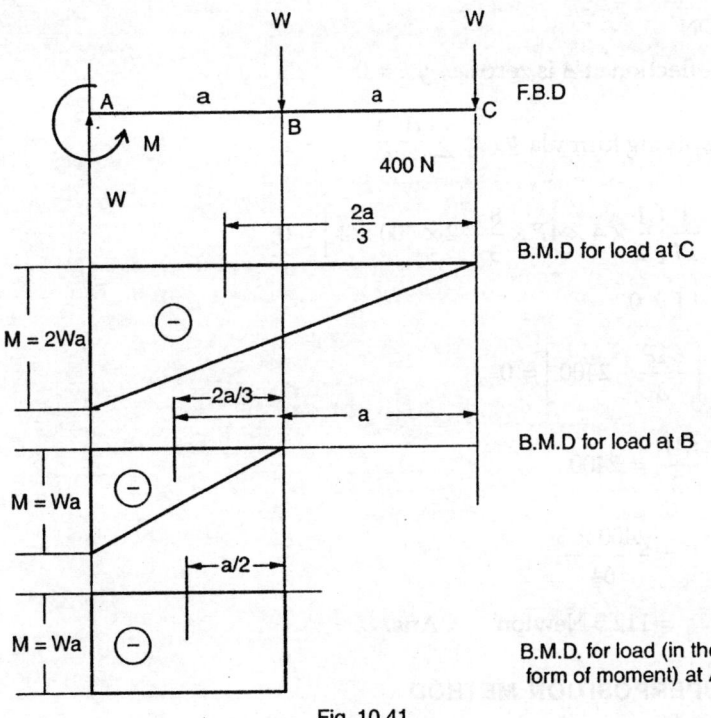

Fig. 10.41

EXAMPLE 7 *Compute P for the loaded cantilever as shown in Fig. 10.42.*

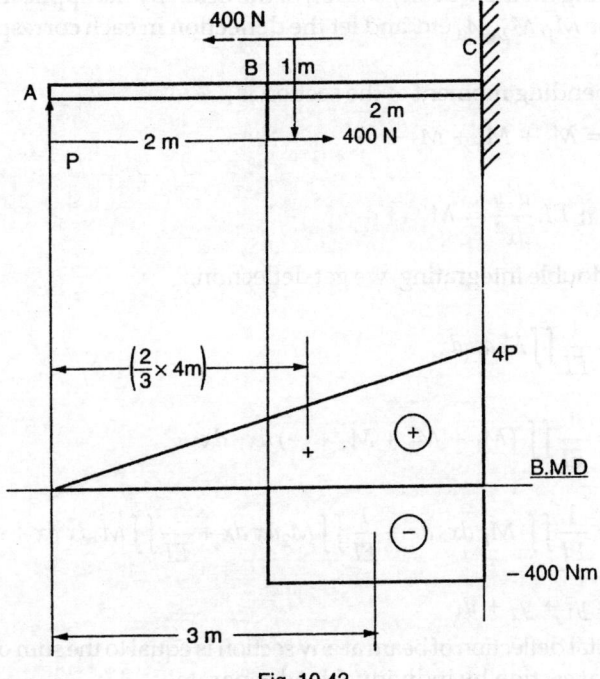

Fig. 10.42

SOLUTION

Since, deflection at A is zero *i.e.*, $y_A = 0$

Now, applying formula $y_A = \sum \dfrac{A \cdot \bar{x}}{EI}$

or, $\dfrac{1}{EI} \left[\dfrac{1}{2} \times 4 \times 4P \times \dfrac{8}{3} - 2 \times 400 \times 3 \right] = 0$

$EI \neq 0$

So, $\left[\dfrac{64P}{3} - 2400 \right] = 0$

or, $\dfrac{64P}{3} = 2400$

$\therefore$ $P = \dfrac{2400 \times 3}{64}$

$= 112.5 \text{ Newton}$ **Ans.**

10.8 SUPERPOSITION METHOD

Let us consider a beam subjected to a number of concentrated loads W_1, W_2, W_3.... etc.

Let the bending moment at any section of the beam by the application of each load separately be M_1, M_2, M_3 etc. and let the deflection in each corresponding case be y_1 ; y_2 ; y_3 etc.

Then, total bending moment at the section is

$M = M_1 + M_2 + M_3 + \cdots\cdots$

We know that $EI \cdot \dfrac{d^2y}{dx^2} = M$

$\therefore$ By double integrating, we get deflection,

i.e., $y = \dfrac{1}{EI} \iint M \, dx \, dx$

$= \dfrac{1}{EI} \iint (M_1 + M_2 + M_3 + \cdots) \, dx \cdot dx$

$= \dfrac{1}{EI} \iint M_1 \, dx \, dx + \dfrac{1}{EI} \iint M_2 dx \, dx + \dfrac{1}{EI} \iint M_3 dx \, dx + \cdots$

$= y_1 + y_2 + y_3$

Hence, the total deflection of beam at any section is equal to the sum of the deflections caused at that section by individual load separately.

EXAMPLE 1 *Use method of superposition to find the slope at end A and the deflection at the centre D for the beam loaded as shown in Fig. 10.43.*

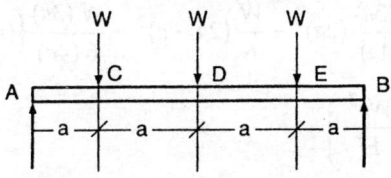

Fig. 10.43

SOLUTION Let θ_C, θ_D and θ_E be the slope at A due to loads W at C, D and E respectively.

Further, let y_C, y_D and y_E be the deflection at point C, D, E due to loads at C, D and E respectively.

Thus, using superposition theorem

$$\theta_C = \frac{W \cdot a \times 3a \, (4a + 3a)}{6 \, EI \, (4a)}$$

Here, $a = a, b = 3a$ and $L = 4a$

$$= \frac{7}{8} \cdot \frac{Wa^2}{EI}$$

$$\theta_D = \frac{W \, (4a)^2}{16 \, EI}$$

$$= \frac{Wa^2}{EI}$$

$$\theta_E = \frac{W \, (3a) \, (a) \, (4a + a)}{6 \, EI \, (4a)} \qquad [\text{Here } a = 3a, b = a \text{ and } L = 4a]$$

$$= \frac{5}{8} \cdot \frac{Wa^2}{EI}$$

Hence, slope at $A = \theta_C + \theta_D + \theta_E$

$$= \left(\frac{7}{8} + 1 + \frac{5}{8}\right) \frac{Wa^2}{EI}$$

$$= \frac{2.5 \, Wa^2}{EI}$$

Now, we have already evaluated deflection (y) at distance x simply supported beam with eccentric load (W) and having span length l (in Macaulay's method) *i.e.*

$$y = \frac{1}{EI} \left\{ \frac{Wb}{6l} x^3 - \frac{W}{6} \langle x - a \rangle^3 - \frac{Wb}{6l} \langle l^2 - b^2 \rangle x \right\}$$

where, x is the arbitrary distance from left end.

Now, for load W at C, $a = a$, $b = 3a$, and $L = 4a$.

$$\therefore \qquad y_C = \frac{1}{EI}\left[\frac{W(3a)}{6(4a)}(2a)^3 - \frac{W}{6}(2a-a)^3 - \frac{W(3a)}{6(4a)}\left\{(4a)^2 - (3a)^2\right\}2a\right]$$

$$= -\left(\frac{11}{12}\cdot\frac{Wa^3}{EI}\right)$$

By symmetry $y_E = y_C = -\dfrac{11}{12}\cdot\dfrac{Wa^3}{EI}$

and $\qquad y_D = -\dfrac{WL^3}{48\,EI}$

$$= -\frac{W(4a)^3}{48\,EI}$$

$$= -\frac{4}{3}\cdot\frac{Wa^3}{EI}$$

$\therefore \qquad$ Deflection at point $D = -y_C + y_D + y_E$

$$= \left(-\frac{11}{12} - \frac{4}{3} - \frac{11}{12}\right)\frac{Wa^3}{EI}$$

$$= -\left(\frac{19}{6}\right)\frac{Wa^3}{EI}$$

N.B: This problem can be easily solved by Macaulay's method by taking imaginary section mn at a distance 'x' from A, leaving only support B.

The equation will be

$$M(x) = R_A \cdot x - W\langle x - a\rangle - W\langle x - 2a\rangle - W\langle x - 3a\rangle$$

By integrating twice and applying boundary condition, we can evaluate slope and deflection at any point of beam.

EXAMPLE 2 *Using superpostion method, determine the slope and deflection at the free end of the cantilever beam shown in Fig. 10.44.*

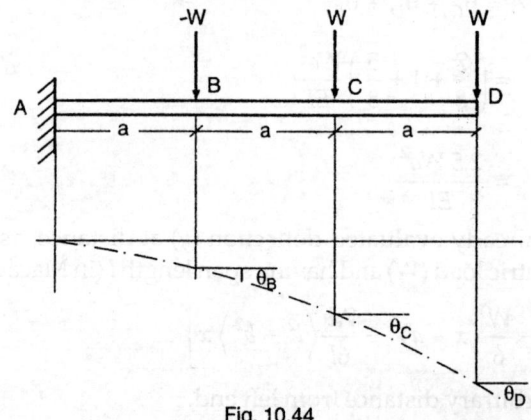

Fig. 10.44

SOLUTION

Now, $\theta_B = \dfrac{Wa^2}{2\,EI}$

$\theta_C = \dfrac{W\,(2a)^2}{2\,EI}$

$= \dfrac{2\,Wa^2}{EI}$

$\theta_D = \dfrac{W\,(3a)^2}{2\,EI}$

$= \dfrac{9\,Wa^2}{2\,EI}$

$\therefore$ Slope at free end $= \theta_B + \theta_C + \theta_D$

$$= \dfrac{Wa^2}{EI}\left[\dfrac{1}{2} + 2 + \dfrac{9}{2}\right]$$

$$= \dfrac{7\,Wa^2}{EI}$$

Deflection $(y_B) = -\left\{\dfrac{Wa^3}{3\,EI} + \theta_B \times 2a\right\}$

$$= -\left\{\dfrac{Wa^3}{3\,EI} + \dfrac{Wa^2}{2\,EI} \times 2a\right\}$$

$$= -\dfrac{4\,Wa^3}{3\,EI}$$

$y_C = -\left\{\dfrac{W\,(2a)^3}{3\,EI} + \theta_C \times a\right\}$

$$= -\left\{\dfrac{8\,Wa^3}{3\,EI} + \dfrac{2\,Wa^2}{EI} \times a\right\}$$

$$= -\dfrac{14\,Wa^3}{3\,EI}$$

$y_D = -\dfrac{W\,(3a)^3}{3\,EI} - -\dfrac{9\,Wa^3}{EI}$

∴ Deflection at free end = $(y_B + y_C + y_D)$

$$= -\frac{4Wa^3}{3EI} - \frac{14Wa^3}{3EI} - \frac{9Wa^3}{EI} = \frac{(-)15Wa^3}{EI} (\downarrow) \quad \textbf{Ans.}$$

PROBLEMS FOR PRACTICE

1. For the beam shown below, find the value of EIy at the point of application of the couple.

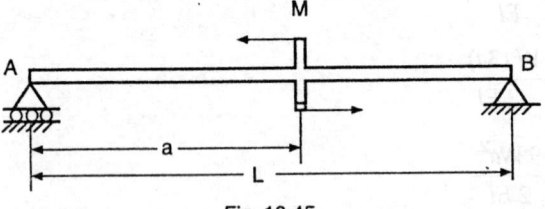

Fig. 10.45

2. Find the value of EIy at the point of application of the 200 N.m couple in the figure.

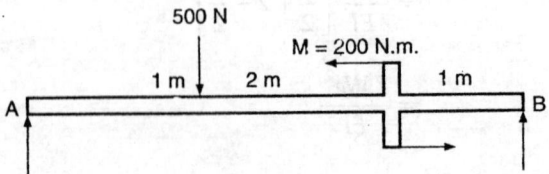

Fig. 10.46

3. A simple supported beam supports a concentrated load placed any where on the span as shown in figure. Measuring x from A, show that the maximum deflection occurs at $x = \sqrt{(L^2 - b^2)/3}$. Find maximum deflection.

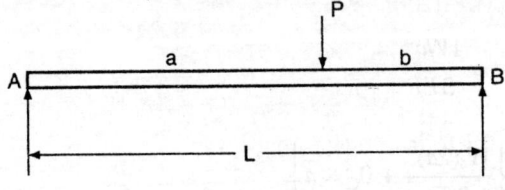

Fig. 10.47

4. A simply supported beam is loaded with a couple M at its right end as shown in figure. Show that the maximum deflection occurs at $x = 0.577 L$.

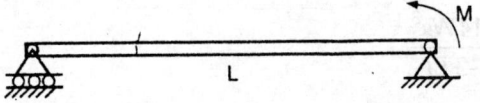

Fig. 10.48

5. Determine the mid-span deflection for the simply supported beam loaded with the couple.

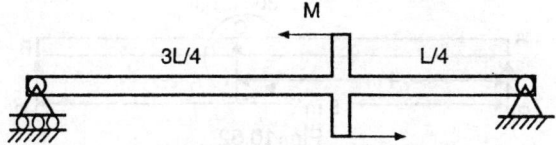

Fig. 10.49

6. The frame shown in figure is of constant cross-section and is perfectly restrained at its lower end. Compute the vertical deflection caused by the couple M.

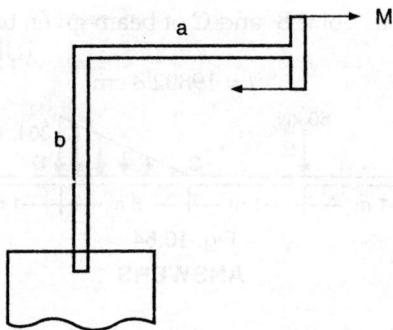

Fig. 10.50

7. In the above figure, if the couple is replaced by vertical downward load P then the vertical deflection will be

$$y = \frac{Pa^2(3b + a)}{3EI}$$

8. Find y_c for the following beam.

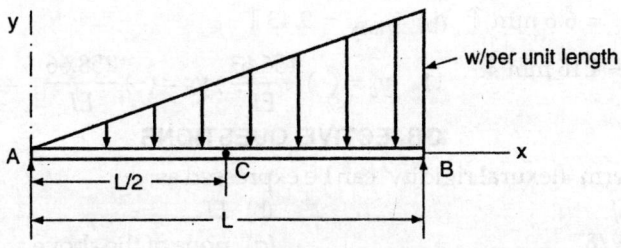

Fig. 10.51

9. If $E = 2 \times 10^5$ N/mm^2 and $I = 2 \times 10^8$ mm^4, determine
   (a) deflection at C,
   (b) the maximum deflection in the following beam:

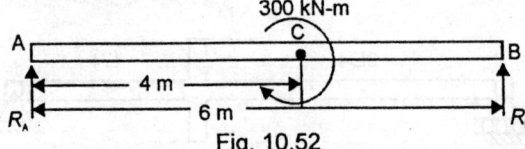

Fig. 10.52

10. An overhanging beam ABC is loaded as shown in Fig. 10.53. Determine deflection at C. Assume $E = 2 \times 10^5$ N/mm^2 and $I = 5 \times 10^8$ mm^4.

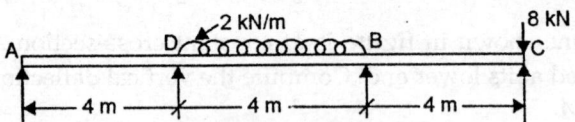

Fig. 10.53

11. Find deflection at point B and C of beam given below.

(UPTU, 3rd Sem 2013-14)

$E = 200$ GPa; $\qquad$ $I = 19802.8$ cm^4

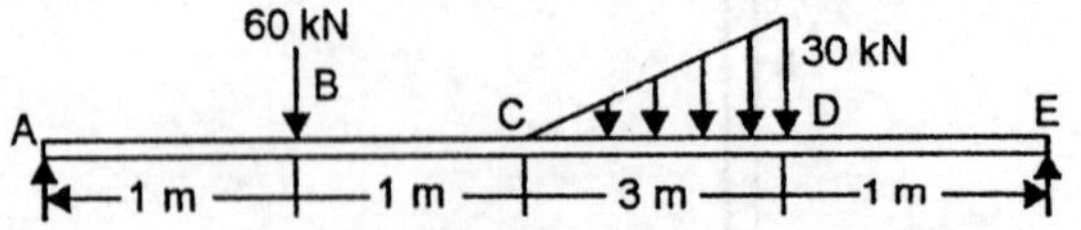

60 kN
B
30 kN
A
C
D
E
1 m — 1 m — 3 m — 1 m

Fig. 10.54

ANSWERS

1. $EIy = \dfrac{Ma}{3L}(L^2 - 3La + 2a^2)$

2. $EIy = 392$ Nm^3

3. $y_{max} = \dfrac{Pb}{48\,EI}(3L^2 - 4b^2)$

5. $y = \dfrac{3ML^2}{64\,EI}$

6. $y = \dfrac{M \cdot a\,(2b + a)}{2\,EI}$

7. $y = \dfrac{Pa^2\,(3b + a)}{3\,EI}$

8. $y_c = (-)\dfrac{5}{768} \cdot \dfrac{wL^4}{EI} \downarrow$

9. (a) $y_c = 6.6$ mm $\uparrow$ (b) $y_{max} = 9.43 \uparrow$

10. $y_c = -4.16$ mm $\downarrow$

11. $y_B = (-)\dfrac{156.63}{EI}$; $y_C = (-)\dfrac{258.66}{EI}$

OBJECTIVE QUESTIONS

1. The term 'flexural rigidity' can be expressed as:
   (a) GJ
   (b) EI
   (c) W/δ
   (d) none of the above

2. The slope and deflection at a section in a loaded beam can be found out by:
   (a) double Integration method
   (b) moment area method
   (c) Macaulay's method
   (d) any of the above

3. Which of the following statements is/are true for the deflection of a beam:
   (a) the beam is subjected to pure bending and the deflections produced are very small.
   (b) bending takes place within elastic limit and modulus of elasticity, intension and compression are equal.
   (c) the beam material is isotropic.
   (d) all the above

4. A higher value of flexural rigidity is an indication of:
   (a) higher stiffness and lower deflection
   (b) lower stiffness and lower deflection
   (c) lower hardness and higher deflection
   (d) none of the above

5. Which of the following statement is true?
   (a) load deflection relationship is linear
   (b) load deflection relationship is parabolic
   (c) load deflection relationship is cubic curve
   (d) none of the above

6. A simply supported rectangular beam of span 'l' and depth 'd' carries a central load W. The ratio of maximum deflection to maximum bending stress is:

   (a) $\dfrac{l^2}{6\,Ed}$ (b) $\dfrac{l^2}{8\,Ed}$ (c) $\dfrac{l^2}{48\,Ed}$ (d) $\dfrac{l^2}{12\,Ed}$

7. The deflection at the free end of a cantilever of length 'l' carrying a point load W at its free end is given as:

   (a) $\dfrac{Wl}{2\,EI}$ (b) $\dfrac{Wl^2}{2\,EI}$ (c) $\dfrac{Wl^3}{2\,EI}$ (d) $\dfrac{Wl^3}{3\,EI}$

8. A cantilever of length l is carrying a uniformly distributed load of w per unit run over the whole span. The deflection at the free end is given by:

   (a) $\dfrac{Wl^3}{4\,EI}$ (b) $\dfrac{Wl^2}{4\,EI}$ (c) $\dfrac{Wl^4}{8\,EI}$ (d) $\dfrac{Wl^4}{16\,EI}$

9. A cantilever of length 'l' is carrying a uniformly distributed load of W per unit run for a distance 'a' from fixed end. The slope at the free end is given as:

   (a) $\dfrac{W a^3}{6\,EI}$ (b) $\dfrac{W a^3}{8\,EI}$ (c) $\dfrac{W a^3}{12\,EI}$ (d) $\dfrac{W a^3}{24\,EI}$

10. A cantilever AB of length 'l' has a moment M applied at free end. The deflection at the free end B is given by:

   (a) $\dfrac{M^2 l}{EI}$ (b) $\dfrac{M^2 l}{2\,EI}$ (c) $\dfrac{Ml}{2\,EI}$ (d) $\dfrac{Ml^3}{2\,EI}$

11. A cantilever AB of length 'l' is carrying a distributed load whose intensity varies uniformly from zero at the free end to w per unit at the fixed end. The deflection at the free end is given by:

(a) $\dfrac{wl^2}{30\,EI}$ (b) $\dfrac{wl^3}{30\,EI}$ (c) $\dfrac{wl^4}{30\,EI}$ (d) $\dfrac{wl^5}{30\,EI}$

12. A cantilever AB of length 'l' is carrying a distributed load whose intensity varies uniformly from zero at the fixed end to 'w' per unit run at the free end. The deflection at free end is given as:

(a) $\dfrac{wl^3}{48\,EI}$

(b) $\dfrac{wl^4}{30\,EI}$

(c) $\dfrac{6}{124}\cdot\dfrac{wl^4}{EI}$

(d) $\dfrac{11}{120}\cdot\dfrac{wl^4}{EI}$

13. A simply supported beam of span 'l' is carrying point load 'w' at the mid span. What is the deflection at the centre of the beam?

(a) $\dfrac{wl^2}{48\,EI}$

(b) $\dfrac{wl^3}{48\,EI}$

(c) $\dfrac{5\,wl^3}{348\,EI}$

(d) $\dfrac{11}{120}\cdot\dfrac{wl^3}{348\,EI}$

14. y_{max} in the following loaded beam will be

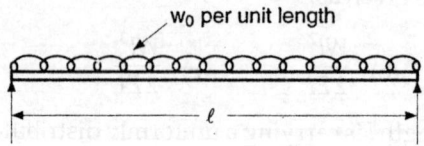

w₀ per unit length

ℓ

Fig. 10.54

(a) $\dfrac{w_0\,l^3}{48\,EI}$ (b) $\dfrac{5\,w_0\,l^4}{348\,EI}$ (c) $\dfrac{11}{121}\dfrac{wl^3}{EI}$ (d) $\dfrac{5\,w_0\,l^4}{384\,EI}$

15. The step function to express couple while using Macaulay's method is:

(a) $\langle x - a\rangle^0$

(b) $\langle x - a\rangle^1$

(c) $\langle x - a\rangle^2$

(d) none of the above

ANSWERS

1. (b)	2. (d)	3. (d)	4. (a)	5. (a)	6. (a)
7. (d)	8. (c)	9. (a)	10. (c)	11. (c)	12. (d)
13. (b)	14. (d)	15. (a)			

— ❖❖ —

INDETERMINATE BEAM
(Fixed, Propped and Continuous Beams)

11.1 INTRODUCTION

Beams in which the equation of static equilibrium (i.e. $\Sigma F_x = 0, \Sigma F_y = 0$ and $\Sigma M = 0$) alone are not sufficient to determine the internal forces and reactions are called statically **indeterminate beams.**

Examples of indeterminate beams are the fixed or encastre or built-in beams; the propped beams or cantilever and the continuous beam as shown in Fig. 11.1 (a), (b), (c) respectively.

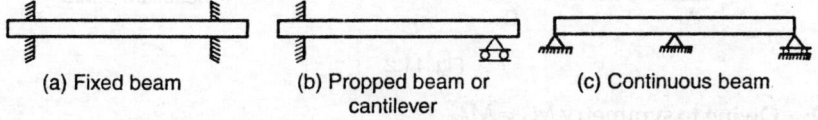

(a) Fixed beam   (b) Propped beam or   (c) Continuous beam
                         cantilever

Fig. 11.1

The unknown reaction in such beams are determined by writing the equation for compatibility of deformations in addition to the equilibrium equation. These compatibility equations are written from the slope and deflection characteristics of beam.

When the unknown reactions are known, the shear force and bending moment distribution can be known, from which we can analyse the 'slope' and 'deflection' as we have evaluated in deflection of beam.

Fixed Beam: *For fixed beam $\Sigma A = 0$ and $\Sigma A \cdot \bar{x} = 0$*

11.2 EXPRESSION FOR SLOPE AND DEFLECTION FOR A FIXED BEAM CARRYING A POINT LOAD AT THE CENTRE

Figure 11.2 shows a fixed beam AB of length L, carrying a point load W at the centre C of the beam.

Let M_A = fixed end moment at A
           M_B = fixed end moment at B
           R_A = reaction at A
and R_B = reaction at B

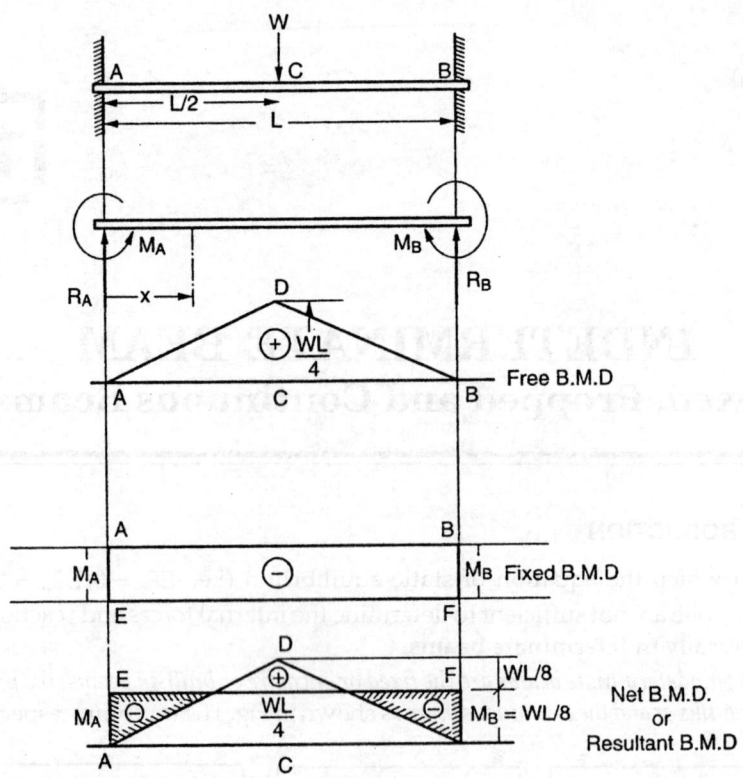

Fig. 11.2

BMD: Owing to symmetry $M_A = M_B$.

Further, for a simply supported beam carrying a point load at the centre the BMD

will be triangle with max B.M. at the centre equal to $\left(\dfrac{W \cdot L}{4} \right)$.

Equating the areas of the two B.M.D.

Area of triangle ADC = Area of rectangle $AEFB$

$$\frac{1}{2} \times AB \times CD = AB \times AE$$

$$\frac{1}{2} \times L \times \frac{WL}{4} = L \times M_A$$

$\therefore$ $M_A = \dfrac{WL}{8}$

Also $M_B = M_A = \dfrac{WL}{8}$

Reaction force R_A and R_B

For this, we will equate clockwise moments and anticlockwise moments about A or B.

Let us take point A

$$\therefore \qquad R_B \times L + M_A = M_B + W \cdot \frac{L}{2}$$

$$R_B \times L + M_B = M_B + \frac{WL}{2} \qquad\qquad [\because M_A = M_B]$$

$$\therefore \qquad R_B = \frac{W}{2}$$

Due to symmetry, $R_A = \dfrac{W}{2}$

Slope and Deflection

The B.M. at any point between AC at a distance x from A is given by

$$M(x) = EI \cdot \frac{d^2 y}{dx^2} = R_A \cdot x - M_A$$

or, $\qquad EI \cdot \dfrac{d^2 y}{dx^2} = R_A \cdot x - M_A$

or, $\qquad EI \cdot \dfrac{d^2 y}{dx^2} = \dfrac{Wx}{2} - \dfrac{WL}{8}$

Integrating both sides, we get

$$EI \cdot \frac{dy}{dx} = \frac{W}{2} \cdot \frac{x^2}{2} - \frac{WL}{8} \cdot x + C_1$$

where, C_1 = constant of integration.

At $x = 0, \dfrac{dy}{dx} = 0$

Hence, $C_1 = 0$

The equation reduces to

$$EI \cdot \frac{dy}{dx} = \frac{wx^2}{4} - \frac{WL}{8} x \qquad\qquad …(1)$$

Equation (1) gives the slope of the beam at any point.

Integrating (1) again, we get

$$EI \cdot y = \frac{W}{4} \cdot \frac{x^3}{3} - \frac{WL}{8} \cdot \frac{x^2}{2} + C_2$$

where, C_2 is another constant of integration.

At $x = 0, y = 0$. Hence, $C_2 = 0$.

The above equation reduces to

$$EIy = \frac{Wx^3}{12} - \frac{WLx^2}{16} \qquad \qquad \dots(2)$$

Equation (2) gives the deflection of the beam at any arbitrary point along the span.

The deflection is maximum at the centre of the beam *i.e.* at $x = \dfrac{L}{2}$.

Therefore, substituting $x = \dfrac{L}{2}$ in eqn. (2).

$$EI\,y_{max} = \frac{W}{12}\left(\frac{L}{2}\right)^3 - \frac{WL}{16}\left(\frac{L}{2}\right)^2$$

$$= \left(\frac{WL^3}{96} - \frac{WL^3}{64}\right)$$

$$= \left(\frac{2WL^3 - 3WL^3}{192}\right)$$

$$= -\left(\frac{WL^3}{192}\right)$$

$$\therefore \qquad y_{max} = (-)\frac{WL^3}{192\,EI} \downarrow \qquad \text{(downward deflection)}$$

N.B: If we compare the max deflection (y_{max}) with the beam having simply supported and loaded at the mid-point, we find that in the case of fixed beam, max deflection (y_{max}) is 4 times less than that of simply supported beam.

$$y_{max} \text{ (for simply supported beam)} = \frac{WL^3}{48\,EI}$$

$$y_{max} \text{ (for fixed beam)} = \left(\frac{WL^3}{192\,EI}\right)$$

$$= \frac{1}{4} \times \left(\frac{WL^3}{48\,EI}\right)$$

$$= \frac{1}{4} \times \text{deflection in simply supported beam}$$

This shows that fixed beams are more stronger and stiffer.

Expression for deflection for a fixed beam with concentrated load anywhere on the span

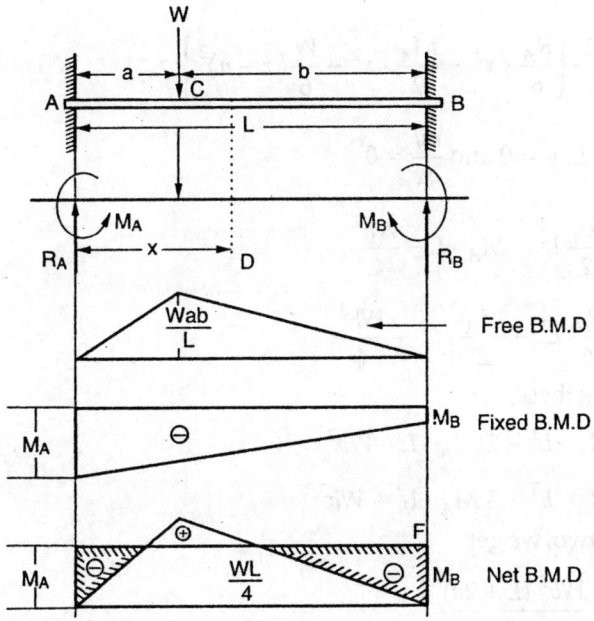

Fig. 11.3

Here, we will adopt Macaulay's Method to find the deflection, reaction at support and moment at fixed end.

At any section at distance x from A

$$M(x) = R_A \cdot x - M_A - W \langle x - a \rangle$$

$$\therefore \quad EI \cdot \frac{d^2y}{dx^2} = R_A x - M_A - W \langle x - a \rangle$$

Integrating both sides

$$EI \cdot \left(\frac{dy}{dx} \right) = R_A \cdot \frac{x^2}{2} - M_A \cdot x - \frac{W}{2} \langle x - a \rangle^2 + A$$

and

$$EI y = R_A \cdot \frac{x^3}{6} - M_A \cdot \frac{x^2}{2} - \frac{W}{6} \langle x - a \rangle^3 + A_x + B$$

Boundary condition are

at $\quad x = 0, y = 0$ and $\dfrac{dy}{dx} = 0$

Therefore, $A = B = 0$.

$$\therefore \qquad \left(\frac{dy}{dx}\right) = \frac{1}{EI}\left\{\frac{R_A}{2}\cdot x^2 - M_A \cdot x - \frac{W}{2}\langle x-a\rangle^2\right\}$$

and, $\qquad y = \frac{1}{EI}\left\{\frac{R_A}{6}\cdot x^3 - \frac{M_A}{2}\cdot x^2 - \frac{W}{6}\langle x-a\rangle^3\right\}$ ...(1)

Again, at $x = L$, $y = 0$ and $\dfrac{dy}{dx} = 0$

$$\therefore \qquad 0 = \frac{R_A}{2}L^2 - M_A \cdot L - \frac{Wb^2}{2}$$

and $\qquad 0 = \dfrac{R_A}{6}L^3 - \dfrac{M_A}{2}\cdot L^2 - \dfrac{Wb^3}{6}$

On simplifying these,

$$0 = R_A \cdot L^2 - 2M_A \cdot L - Wb^2$$

and $\qquad 0 = R_A \cdot L^3 - 3M_A \cdot L^2 - Wb^3$

Solving these two, we get

$$R_A = \frac{Wb^2(L+2a)}{L^3}$$ ...(2)

and $\qquad M_A = \dfrac{Wab^2}{L^2}$ ...(3)

Further, the equations of static equilibrium are

$$R_A + R_B - W = 0$$ ...(4)

and $\qquad R_A L - W(L-a) - M_A + M_B = 0$ ...(5)

From (3) and (5)

$$M_B = \left[\frac{Wa^2b}{L^2}\right]$$

From the eqn. (1), deflection at $x = a$ is

$$y_c = \frac{1}{EI}\left\{\frac{R_A}{6}a^3 - \frac{M_A}{2}a^2\right\}$$ ...(6)

Substituting the value of R_a and M_A from eqns. (2) and (3) in eqn. (6), we get

$$y_c = -\frac{Wa^3b^3}{3\,EIL^3}$$

N.B: For the particular case when load is in the middle, the deflection in the middle can be found by putting $a = b = \dfrac{L}{2}$.

$$R_A = R_B = \frac{W}{2}$$

$$M_A = M_B = \frac{WL}{8}$$

Hence, when load is in the middle

Then $\qquad y_{max} = -\dfrac{WL^3}{192\,EI}$

Alternative Method: *Moment area Method*

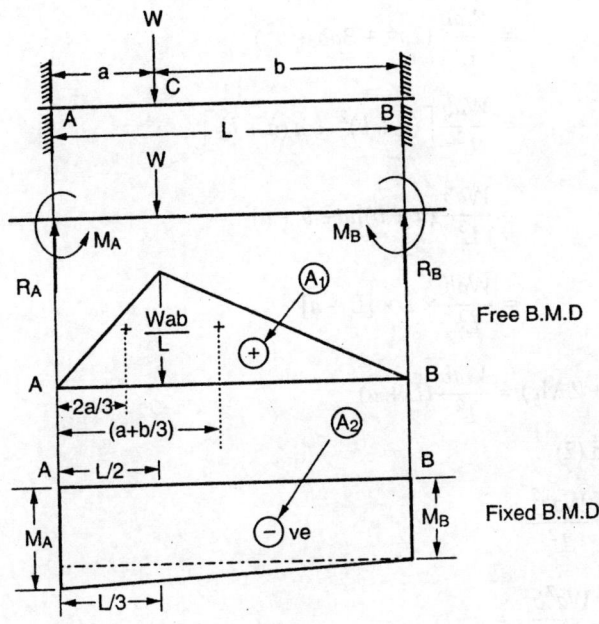

Fig. 11.4

Taking into consideration the sign of A_1 and A_2

i.e., $\qquad A_1 + A_2 = 0$

$$\left[\frac{1}{2} \cdot \frac{W \cdot a \cdot b}{L} \cdot L \right] - \left[\frac{M_A + M_B}{2} \times L \right] = 0$$

or, $\qquad M_A + M_B = \dfrac{Wab}{L}$ ...(1)

$$A_1 \overline{x_1} + A_2 \overline{x_2} = 0$$

$$\left\{ \left(\frac{1}{2} \cdot \frac{Wab}{L} \cdot a \right) \cdot \frac{2a}{3} + \left(\frac{1}{2} \cdot \frac{Wab}{L} \cdot b \right) \left(a + \frac{b}{3} \right) \right\}$$

$$- \left[(M_B \cdot L) \cdot \frac{L}{2} \right] - \left[(M_A - M_B) \cdot \frac{L}{2} \right] \times \frac{L}{3} = 0$$

or, $$\left\{ \frac{Wa^3 b}{3L} + \frac{Wa^2 b^2}{2L} + \frac{Wab^3}{6L} - M_B \cdot \frac{L^2}{2} - M_A \cdot \frac{L^2}{6} + M_B \cdot \frac{L^2}{6} \right\} = 0$$

or, $$\left\{ 2Wa^3 b + 3Wa^2 b^2 + Wab^3 - 2M_B L^3 - M_A L^3 \right\} = 0$$

or, $$M_A + 2M_b = \frac{1}{L^3} \left(2Wa^3 b + 3Wa^2 b^2 + Wab^3 \right)$$

$$= \frac{Wab}{L^3} (2a^2 + 3ab + b^2)$$

$$= \frac{Wab}{L^3} \left[(a+b)^2 + a(a+b) \right]$$

$$= \frac{Wab}{L^3} (a+b)[a+b+a]$$

$$= \frac{Wab}{L^3} \times L \times [L+a]$$

∴ $$(M_A + 2M_b) = \frac{Wab}{L^2} (L+a)$$ …(2)

Solving (1) and (2)

$$M_A = \frac{Wab^2}{L^2}$$

and $$M_B = \frac{Wa^2 b}{L^2}$$

Advantages of Fixed Beam

(i) In a fixed beam, the fixing ends of a beam makes it stronger than when the same is simply supported.

(ii) In a fixed beam the maximum bending moment occurs at the end points.

For this reason the beam needs to be strengthened at the ends only to take up the maximum bending moment.

In the case of a simply supported beam the maximum bending moment occurs not at the ends but in the middle.

Hence, a fixed beam to take up the same maximum bending moment as a simply supported beam will be lighter.

11.3 SLOPE AND DEFLECTION FOR A FIXED BEAM CARRYING A UNIFORMLY DISTRIBUTED LOAD OVER THE ENTIRE LENGTH

(U.P.T.U. 2008-09)

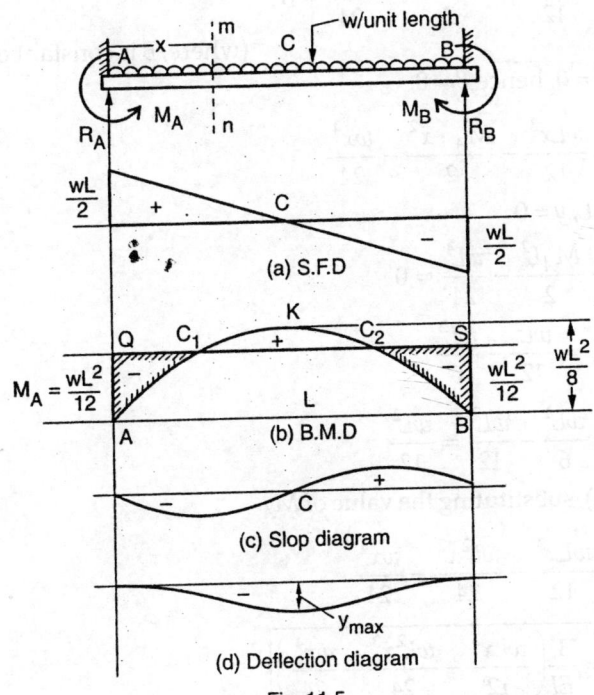

(a) S.F.D

(b) B.M.D

(c) Slop diagram

(d) Deflection diagram

Fig. 11.5

Due to symmetry $R_A = \dfrac{wL}{2}$ and $M_A = M_B$

The BMD for a simply supported beam carrying a uniformly distributed load w will be a parabola having central ordinate $\dfrac{wL^2}{8}$. So, $KL = \dfrac{wL^2}{8}$.

Now, $\qquad M(x) = R_A \cdot x - M_A \cdot x^0 - \dfrac{wx^2}{2}$

or, $\qquad EIy'' = \dfrac{wLx}{2} - M_A - x^0 - \dfrac{wx^2}{2}$

Integrating both sides

$$EIy' = \frac{wLx^2}{4} - M_A \cdot x - \frac{wx^3}{6} + A$$

(where, A = constant of integration)

B.C. is at $x = 0$, $\dfrac{dy}{dx} = 0$ i.e., $y' = 0 \Rightarrow A = 0$

$\therefore \qquad EIy' = \dfrac{wLx^2}{4} - M_A \cdot x - \dfrac{wx^3}{6}$ ...(I)

Again, integrating (I), we get

$$EIy = \frac{wLx^3}{12} - \frac{M_A \cdot x^2}{2} - \frac{wx^4}{24} + B \qquad \qquad ...(II)$$

(where, B is constant of integration)

B.C. at $x = 0$, $y = 0$, hence $B = 0$.

Hence, $EIy = \dfrac{wLx^3}{12} - \dfrac{M_A \cdot x^2}{2} - \dfrac{wx^4}{24}$

Further, at $x = L$, $y = 0$

$$\frac{wL^4}{12} - \frac{M_A L^2}{2} - \frac{wL^4}{24} = 0$$

$$(-)M_A = \frac{wL^2}{12} - \frac{wL^2}{6}$$

$$\therefore \qquad M_A = \frac{wL^2}{6} - \frac{wL^2}{12} = \frac{wL^2}{12}$$

Hence, from (II), substituting the value of M_A

$$EIy = \frac{wLx^3}{12} - \frac{wL^2 x^2}{24} - \frac{wx^4}{24}$$

$$\boxed{\therefore \quad y = \frac{1}{EI}\left(\frac{wLx^3}{12} - \frac{wL^2 x^3}{24} - \frac{wx^4}{24} \right)}$$

For $y_{\max}$, putting $x = \dfrac{1}{2}$, we get

$$y_{\max} = \frac{1}{EI}\left[\frac{wL}{12} \times \left(\frac{L}{2}\right)^3 - \frac{wL^2}{24} \times \left(\frac{L}{2}\right)^2 - \frac{w}{24} \times \left(\frac{L}{2}\right)^4 \right]$$

$$= \frac{1}{EI}\left[\frac{wL^4}{96} - \frac{wL^4}{96} - \frac{wL^4}{384} \right]$$

$$\boxed{\therefore \quad y_{\max} = (-)\frac{wl^4}{384\ EI} \quad \downarrow}$$

*If we compare the result of $y_{\max}$ of a simply supported beam having u.d.l. w over the entire length then we find that the **central deflection for a fixed beam having u.d.l. w is one fifth of the central deflection of the simply supported beam.**

Alternative method: *Moment Area Method*
We have,

$$A_1 + A_2 = 0$$

$y_{\max}$ of a simply supported beam having u.d.l. w over entire length is $(-)\dfrac{5}{384} \cdot \dfrac{wl^4}{EI}$.

$$\frac{2}{3} \times \frac{wL^2}{8} \times L + M \cdot L = 0$$

$$\Rightarrow \quad M = \frac{wL^2}{12}$$

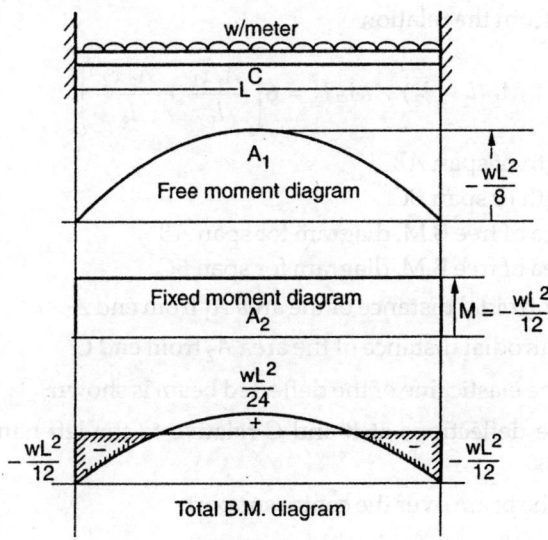

Fig. 11.6

Deflection at centre C,

$$y_C = y_{max} = \frac{1}{EI} \left[A_1 \bar{x}_1 + a_2 \bar{x}_2 \right]$$

$$= \frac{1}{EI} \left[\left(\frac{2}{3} \times \frac{wL^2}{8} \times \frac{L}{2} \right) \left(\frac{3}{8} \times \frac{L}{2} \right) + \left(\frac{ML}{2} \times \frac{L}{4} \right) \right]$$

$$= \frac{1}{EI} \left[\frac{3wL^4}{384} + \frac{ML^2}{8} \right]$$

$$= \frac{1}{EI} \left[\frac{3wL^4}{384} - \frac{wL^4}{96} \right]$$

$$= (-) \frac{wL^4}{384\,EI} \downarrow$$

11.4 CONTINUOUS BEAM

A beam resting on more than two supports is called a continuous beam.

A long beam is generally provided with many supports to prevent excessive deflection. One of the supports is usually an immovable hinge while the other are hinges or roller.

11.5 CLAPEYRON'S EQUATION

If AB and BC are two consecutive spans of a continuous beam subjected to some external loading, the support moments M_A, M_B and M_C at the supports A, B and C can be obtained from the relation

$$M_A l_1 + 2 M_B (l_1 + l_2) + M_C l_2 = 6 \left(\frac{A_1 \bar{x}_1}{l_1} + \frac{A_2 \bar{x}_2}{l_2} \right)$$

where, l_1 = length of span AB

l_2 = length of span BC

A_1 = Area of free B.M. diagram for span AB

A_2 = Area of free B.M. diagram for span BC

$\bar{x}_1$ = Centroidal distance of the area A_1 from end A

$\bar{x}_2$ = centrodial distance of the area A_2 from end C.

In Fig. 11.7 (d), the elastic line of the deflected beam is shown.

δ_1 and δ_2 are the deflections at B and C relative to the left hand support and positive upwards.

θ is the slope of the beam over the centre support.

z_1 and z_2 are the intercepts for l_1 and l_2.

Hence, $\quad \theta = \dfrac{Z_1 + \delta_1}{l_1} = \dfrac{Z_2 + \delta_2 - \delta_1}{l_2} \qquad$ (Slopes are small every where)

i.e. $\quad \dfrac{Z_1}{l_1} + \dfrac{\delta_1}{l_1} = \dfrac{Z_2}{l_2} + \dfrac{\delta_2 - \delta_1}{l_2}$

or, $\quad \dfrac{A_1 \bar{x}_1 - \left(\dfrac{M_A \cdot l_1}{2} \right) \cdot \left(\dfrac{l_1}{3} \right) - \left(\dfrac{M_B \cdot l_1}{2} \right) \cdot \left(\dfrac{2 l_1}{3} \right)}{E I_1 l_1} + \dfrac{\delta_1}{l_1}$

$= (-) \dfrac{A_2 \bar{x}_2 - \left(\dfrac{M_C l_2}{2} \right) \left(\dfrac{l_2}{3} \right) - \left(M_B l_2 \right) \left(\dfrac{2 l_3}{3} \right)}{E I_2 l_2} + \dfrac{\delta_2 - \delta_1}{l_2}$

$$\hspace{6cm} (Z_2 \text{ is negative intercept})$$

or, $\quad \dfrac{M_A \cdot l_1}{I_1} + 2 M_B \left(\dfrac{l_1}{I_1} + \dfrac{l_2}{I_2} \right) + \dfrac{M_C l_2}{I_2}$

$$= 6 \left(\frac{A_1 \bar{x}_1}{I_1 l_1} + \frac{A_2 \bar{x}_2}{I_2 l_2} \right) + 6 E \left[\frac{\delta_1}{l_1} + \frac{\delta_1 - \delta_2}{l_2} \right] \qquad \dots (1)$$

where, I_1 and I_2 are the M.I. of span l_1 and l_2 respectively.

If $\qquad I_1 = I_2$

Then, $\quad M_A l_1 + 2 M_B (l_1 + l_2) + M_C l_2$

$$= 6\left(\frac{A_1 \bar{x}_1}{l_1} + \frac{A_2 \bar{x}_2}{l_2} \right) + 6EI\left(\frac{\delta_1}{l_1} + \frac{\delta_1 - \delta_2}{l_2} \right) \qquad \text{...(2)}$$

If the support are at the same level.

Then, $\quad M_A l_1 + 2 M_B (l_1 + l_2) + M_C \cdot l_2 = 6\left(\frac{A_1 \bar{x}_1}{l_1} + \frac{A_2 \bar{x}_2}{l_2} \right) \qquad \text{...(3)}$

If the ends are simply supported, then,

$$M_A = M_C = 0$$

$\therefore \qquad M_B (l_1 + l_2) = 3\left(\frac{A_1 \bar{x}_1}{l_1} + \frac{A_2 \bar{x}_2}{l_2} \right)$

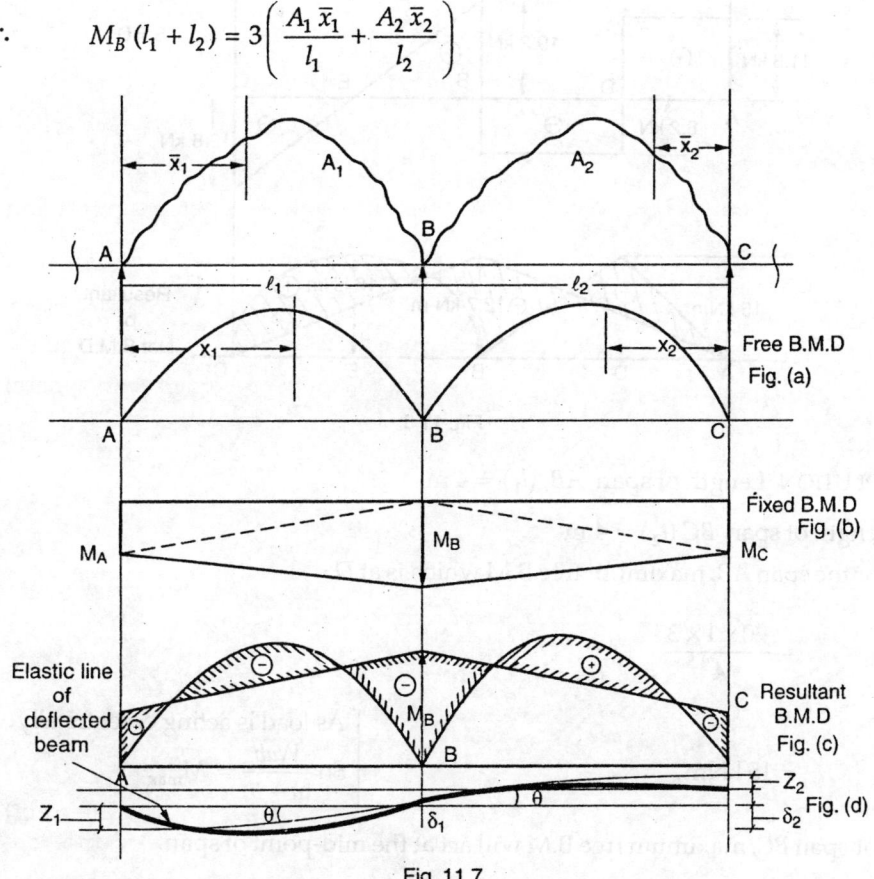

Fig. 11.7

Equation (1) is the general form of Clapeyron's equation.

Equation (2) and (3) are special cases of Clapeyron's equation.

N.B: While solving the problem of continuous beam, we must see if there are more than two supports *i.e.* there are two span length l_1 and l_2, if not, we have to add one span of zero length so that problem may be solved by Three Moment Method *i.e.* by Clapeyron's equation.

EXAMPLE 1 *Draw the S.F.D. and B.M.D. of a continuous beam ABC when span length AB = 4 m and BC = 4 m.*

The span AB carries a point load of 20 kN at a distance of 1 m from support A and the span BC carries a u.d.l. having intensity of 8 kN/m.

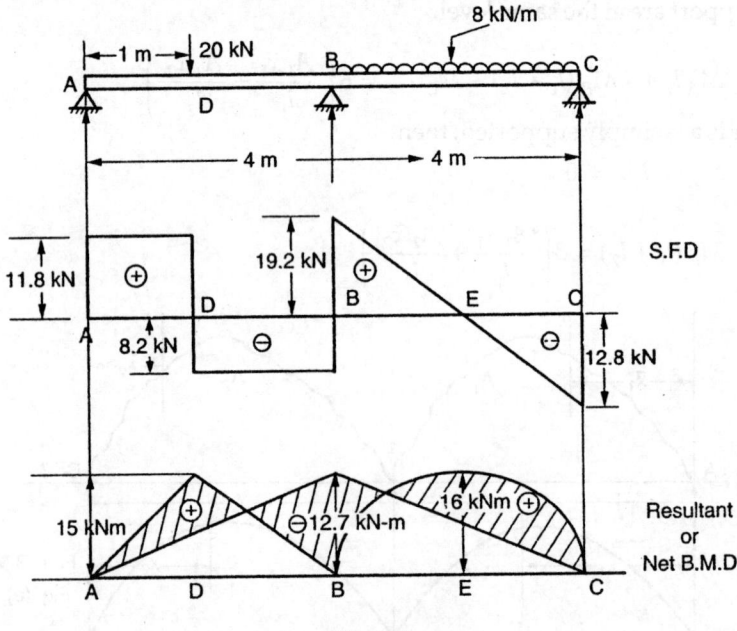

Fig. 11.8

SOLUTION Length of span AB, (l_1) = 4 m

Length of span BC (l_2) = 4 m

For the span AB, maximum free B.M which is at D

$$= \frac{\overset{5}{\cancel{20}} \times 1 \times 3}{\cancel{4}}$$

$$= 15 \text{ kNm.}$$

$$\left[\begin{array}{l} \text{As load is acting eccentrically.} \\ \text{So } \dfrac{Wab}{(a+b)} = M_{max} \end{array} \right]$$

For span BC, maximum free B.M will act at the mid-point of span.

$$\therefore \qquad M_{max} = \frac{Wl^2}{8}$$

$$= \frac{\cancel{8} \times 4}{\cancel{8}} = 16 \text{ kNm}$$

Now, the area of the B.M diagram for span AB

$$A_1 = \frac{1}{\cancel{2}} \times \cancel{4}^2 \times 15$$

$$= 30 \text{ kNm}^2$$

Centroid $\bar{x}_1$ for this area A_1 from end A

$$\bar{x}_1 = \frac{1+4}{3}$$

$$= \left(\frac{5}{3}\right) \text{m}$$

Similarly, area of the free B.M diagram for span BC,

$$A_2 = \frac{2}{3} \times 4 \times 16$$

$$= 42.7 \text{ kNm}^2$$

Centroidal distance of area A_2 from end C

$$\bar{x}_2 = \frac{4}{2} = 2 \text{ m}$$

If M_A, M_B and M_C are the support moments at A, B and C respectively, then applying Claypeyron's theorem of three moments (when the supports are at same level)

$$M_A \cdot l_1 + 2 M_B (l_1 + l_2) + M_C l_2 = \frac{6 A_1 x_1}{l_1} + \frac{6 A_2 x_2}{l_2}$$

Now, since A and C are simply supported. So, $M_A = 0$ and $M_C = 0$.

$$\therefore \qquad 0 + 2 M_B (4 + 4) + 0 = \frac{6 \times 30 \times \left(\dfrac{5}{3}\right)}{4} + \frac{6 \times 42.7 \times 2}{4}$$

$$\boxed{M_B = 12.7 \text{ kNm}} \qquad \textbf{Ans.}$$

Reaction
Let R_A, R_B and R_C are the reaction at supports A, B and C respectively.
Considering span AB,

B.M at $B = -12.7 = R_A \times 4 - 20 (4 - 1)$

$$\therefore \qquad \boxed{R_A = 11.8 \text{ kN}}$$

Similarly, considering span BC,

$$\boxed{R_C = 12.8 \text{ kN}}$$

$$\therefore \qquad R_B = \text{Total load} - R_A - R_C$$

$$= 20 + (8 \times 4) - 11.8 - 12.8$$

$$\boxed{R_B = 27.4 \text{ kN}}$$

HIGHLIGHTS

1. A beam whose both ends are fixed is known as fixed beam and a beam which is supported on more than two supports is known as a continuous beam.
2. The B.M. diagram of a fixed beam is obtained by superimposing its free and the fixed B.M. diagram.
3. *In fixed Beam:* Area of fixing moment = Area of free moments.
   Moment area of fixing diagram = Moment area of free diagram.
4. For single concentrated load:

$$M_a = \frac{Wab^2}{l^2}\,; M_b = \frac{Wa^2 l}{l^2}$$

If $\qquad a = b = \dfrac{l}{2}$ then $M = \dfrac{Wl}{8}$ $\qquad\qquad [wl = W]$

and $\quad y = \dfrac{Wl^3}{192\,EI}$ $\qquad\qquad\qquad [W = wl]$

For distributed load, $M = \dfrac{wl^2}{12}$

and $\quad y = \dfrac{wl^4}{384\,EI}$

5. Continuous Beam:

$$M_1 l_1 + 2 M_2 (l_2 + l_1) + M_3 l_2 = 6\left(\frac{A_1 \bar{x}_1}{l_1} + \frac{A_2 \bar{x}_2}{l_2} \right)$$

6. To apply three moment equation sometimes span of zero length is added and then the above equation is applied.

OBJECTIVE QUESTIONS

1. Which is the odd term of the following:
   - (a) simply supported beam
   - (b) fixed beam
   - (c) continuous beam
   - (d) encastre beam
2. The number of points of contraflexure occuring in a fixed beam subjected to a uniformly distributed load throughout its span is:
   - (a) one
   - (b) two
   - (c) three
   - (d) none of the above

3. Out of the fixed beam and the simply supported beam, both designed for the same loading:
   - (a) fixed beam is heavier
   - (b) fixed beam is lighter
   - (c) both have the same weight
   - (d) none of the above

4. Using fixed beam (in practice) is avoided because of:
   - (a) uncertainty of stress
   - (b) lesser stiffness
   - (b) higher stresses
   - (d) none of the above

5. Clapeyron's equation is used for analysis of:
   - (a) continuous beams
   - (b) fixed beam
   - (b) simple supported beam
   - (d) none of the above

ANSWERS

1. (a)   2. (b)   3. (b)   4. (a)   5. (a)

— ❖❖ —

TORSION

12.1 INTRODUCTION

The machine members, besides axial force, shear force and bending moment, are subjected to twisting moment about it's longitudinal axis resulting in twisting of the machine member. Such kind of loading mode is called torsion.

Examples of torsion in engineering are found in springs; shaft transmitting power of turbine, engine, electric generator, automobiles etc.

12.2 WHAT IS SHAFT?

Shaft is a rotating machine element used to transmit power from driver to driven. In order to transmit power from one shaft to another the various members such as pulley, gears etc are mounted on it. A shaft rotating with constant angular velocity ω radian per second is being acted on by a twisting moment T and hence transmit power, $P = T \cdot \omega$.

The shaft is made up of mild steel, alloy steel etc.

The shafts are normally cylindrical in shape but may be square or elliptical also in section.

In most cases, shafts are cylindrical in shape (solid or hollow).

Due to 'torque' and 'Bending Moment 'shear stress and bending stress is induced in the shaft due to the forces acting on gears, pulley etc. *In other words we can say that shaft is under compound stress due to compound type of loading.*

12.3 TORSION EQUATION FOR A SHAFT

Let us consider a solid shaft of length 'l' diameter 'd' fixed at one end and subjected to torque T at right hand side of the shaft.

To keep the shaft under equilibrium condition, opposite direction torque T has to be shown at left hand side.

As a result of application of torque T the free end will rotate by some angle.

Let it be θ. In the diagram point A is shifted to A' by making an angle θ.

Morever, line BA on the surface of shaft makes an angle ϕ with original position BA. [Fig. 12.1 (a)]

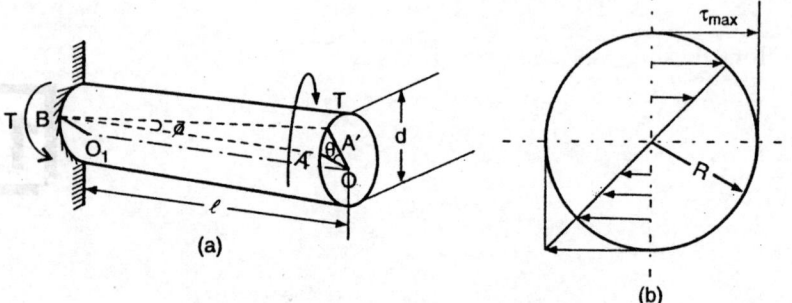

Fig. 12.1

Now, shear strain $= \tan\phi = \phi = \dfrac{AA'}{AB}$ [Since ϕ is small so $\tan\phi = \phi$]

$$= \frac{R\theta}{l}$$ [R is the radius of the shaft]

Also, $\dfrac{\text{Shear stress}}{\text{Shear strain}} = \text{modulus of rigidity}$

$$\frac{\tau}{\phi} = G$$

$$\tau = \phi G$$

$$= \frac{R\theta}{l} \times G$$

$\therefore$ $\dfrac{\tau}{R} = \dfrac{G\theta}{l}$ ...(1)

τ is maximum when R is maximum, i.e. shear stress is maximum on the outside surface and variation of shear stress with radius is linear as shown in Fig. 12.1 (b). Let us now consider transverse section of the shaft of Radius R_o. For any concentric tube of thickness dR at radius R from the centre, let us consider shear stress τ (Fig. 12.2).

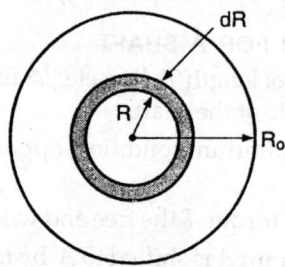

Fig. 12.2

$\therefore$ Total twisting moment $(T) = \int_0^{R_0} \tau\,(2\pi R \cdot dR)\,R$

$$= \int_0^{R_0} \frac{G\theta R}{l} \times 2\pi R^2 dR \qquad \left[\begin{array}{l}\text{From eqn. 1}\\ \tau = \dfrac{G\theta R}{l}\end{array}\right]$$

$$= \frac{2\pi G\theta}{l} \times \frac{R_o^{\,4}}{4}$$

$$= \frac{G\theta}{l} \times \frac{\pi R_o^{\,4}}{2}$$

$$= \frac{G\theta}{l} \times J$$

where,   J = polar moment of inertia of the shaft section.

$\therefore$ $\dfrac{T}{J} = \dfrac{G\theta}{l}$ ...(2)

From equation (1) and (2), we get

$$\boxed{\dfrac{T}{J} = \dfrac{G\theta}{l} = \dfrac{\tau}{R}}$$ **Proved.**

The above derivation is based on the following assumptions:
  (i) The shaft is straight and of uniform cross-section along its length.
 (ii) The torque (T) is constant throughout the shaft length.
(iii) The material of the shaft is homogenous, isotropic and follows hook's law.
(iv) Cross-sections of the shaft which are plane before twist remain plain after twist.
 (v) All radii which are straight before twist remain straight after twist.

12.4 POLAR MODULUS

The polar modulus (Z_p) is defined as the ratio of the polar moment of inertia to the radius of the shaft.

It is also called torsional sectional modulus and denoted by (Z_p).

Mathematically $(Z_p) = \dfrac{J}{R}$

For a solid Shaft

$$J = \frac{\pi}{32} D^4$$

$$\therefore \quad Z_p = \frac{\dfrac{\pi}{32}D^4}{\dfrac{D}{2}}$$

$$= \frac{\pi}{16}D^3$$

For a hollow shaft

$$J = \frac{\pi}{32}\left[D_o^{\;4} - D_i^{\;}\right].$$

$$\therefore \quad Z_p = \frac{\dfrac{\pi}{32}[D_o^{\;4} - D_i^4]}{R_o}$$

$$= \frac{\dfrac{\pi}{32}[D_o^{\;4} - D_i^4]}{\dfrac{D_o}{2}}$$

$$= \frac{\pi}{16\,D_o}[D_o^{\;4} - D_i^4]$$

12.5 STRENGTH OF A SHAFT
Strength of a shaft is the maximum torque 'or' power, the shaft can transmit.

12.6 TORSIONAL RIGIDITY
Torsional rigidity 'or' stiffness of the shaft is defined as the product of modulus of rigidity (G) and the polar moment of inertia (J) of the shaft.

So,   Torsional rigidity = $G \times J$.

In other words, torsional rigidity is also defined as the torque required to produce a twist of one radian per unit length of the shaft. Members made up of long thin section which do not form a closed tube like shape are very weak and are flexible in torsion. The various shape that are weak in torsion are $\text{I}\text{C}\text{ }\text{L}\text{T}$. Pipe, solid bar and rectangular tubes are torsionally stiff.

The torsional stiffness increases from (a) to (d) gradually as the section is formed towards a close section.

$$\text{I}\quad\text{L}\quad\text{L}\quad\text{U}$$
(a)   (b)   (c)   (d)

Let twisting moment T produces a twist of θ radian in a shaft of length l.
Then, by the equation, we get

$$\frac{T}{J} = \frac{G\theta}{l}$$

or, $G \times J = \dfrac{T \times l}{\theta}$

But, $G \times J$ = Torsional rigidity

$\therefore$ Torsional rigidity $= \left(\dfrac{T \times l}{\theta} \right)$

If $l = 1$ metre

and $\theta = 1$ radian

Then torsional rigidity = Torque applied.

Maximum Torque transmitted by a Circular Solid Shaft

$$T \text{ or } T_{max} = \frac{\pi}{16} \cdot \tau_{max} \cdot D^3$$

where τ_{max} = maximum shear stress

D = diameter of shaft.

Torque transmitted by a hollow circular shaft

$$T = \frac{\pi}{16} \cdot \tau_{max} \left[\frac{D_0^{\,4} - D_i^{\,4}}{D_0} \right]$$

Power transmitted by a shaft

Let T_{mean} = mean torque transmitted in Nm.

ω = Angular speed of shaft

N = r.p. m of the shaft

$$\text{Power} = \frac{2\pi N T_{mean}}{60} \text{ watt}$$

$$= \omega \times T \qquad\qquad \left[\because \omega = \frac{2\pi N}{60} \right]$$

12.7 SHAFT IN SERIES

In practice, shafts are having stepping and common axis of rotation. Such an arrangement is called shaft in series.

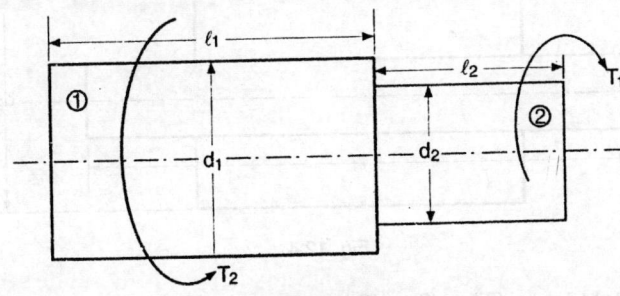

Fig. 12.3

The steppings are provided as per the requirement of attachment *i.e.* fly wheel; gear, bearings etc. Each attachments have different ID and steppings. Different diameters are provided in the shaft.

When shafts are in series, then $T_1 = T_2 = T$.

Now, applying torsion formula for portion (1)

$$\frac{T_1}{J_1} = \frac{\tau}{R} = \frac{G\theta}{l}$$

or, $\dfrac{T_1}{J_1} = \dfrac{\tau_1}{d_1/2} = \dfrac{G_1\,\theta_1}{l_1}$

and $\dfrac{T_2}{J_2} = \dfrac{\tau_2}{d_2/2} = \dfrac{G_2\,\theta_2}{l_2}$

$\therefore$ $T_1 = \dfrac{G_1\,J_1\,\theta_1}{l_1}$ and $T_2 = \dfrac{G_2\,J_2\,\theta_2}{l_2}$

Similarly, $\tau_1 = \dfrac{2\,T_1\,d_1}{J_1}$

$\tau_1 = \dfrac{2\,T_2\,d_2}{J_2}$

$\therefore$ $\dfrac{\tau_1}{\tau_2} = \dfrac{\pi d_2{}^4/32 \times d_1}{\pi d_1{}^4/32 \times d_2} = \dfrac{d_2{}^3}{d_1{}^3}$

and $\theta_1 = \dfrac{T_1\,l_1}{G_1\,J_1}$ and $\theta_2 = \dfrac{T_2\,l_2}{G_2\,J_2}$

12.8 SHAFT IN PARALLEL

When one shaft is shrunk fit into the other in such a way that there is no relative movement between the two shafts then such combination of shafts are in parallel.

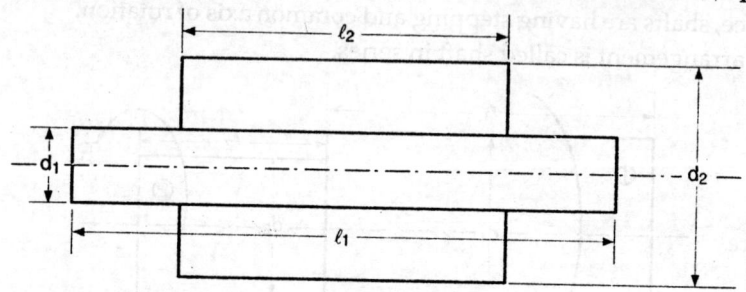

Fig. 12.4

In this case Total torque $(T) = (T_1 + T_2)$.

where, T_1 and T_2 are the individual torque transmission of shaft 1 and 2 respectively.

Now, by formula, $T_1 = \dfrac{G_1\,J_1\,\theta_1}{l_1}$

and $T_2 = \dfrac{G_2\,J_2\,\theta_2}{l_2}$

$$\therefore \quad T = \left(\frac{G_1 J_1 \theta_1}{l_1} + \frac{G_2 J_2 \theta_2}{l_2} \right)$$

If both the shafts have the same length and same angle of twist, then

$$l_1 = l_2 = l$$

and $\quad \theta_1 = \theta_2 = \theta$

$$\therefore \quad T = \frac{\theta}{l}(G_1 J_1 + G_2 J_2)$$

$$\therefore \quad \theta = \left(\frac{T \cdot l}{G_1 J_1 + G_2 J_2} \right)$$

EXAMPLE 1 *A shaft is transmitting 100 kW at 160 rpm. Find a suitable diameter for the shaft if the maximum torque transmitted exceeds the mean by 25%. Take maximum allowable shear stress 70 N/mm².*

SOLUTION Power transmitted by shaft $(P) = \dfrac{2 \pi N T_{mean}}{60}$

$$100 \times 10^3 = \frac{2\pi \times 160 \times T_{mean}}{60}$$

$$\therefore \quad T_{mean} = \left(\frac{10^5 \times 60}{2\pi \times 160} \right)$$

$$= 5965.9 \text{ Nm}$$
$$\approx 5965.9 \text{ Nm}$$

Given, $\quad T_{max} = 1.25 \, T_{mean}$

$$= 1.25 \times 5966$$

$$= 7457.5 \text{ Nm}$$

Shear stress $(\tau) = \dfrac{16 \, T_{max}}{\pi d^3}$

$$70 = \frac{16 \times 7457.5 \times 7}{22 \times d^3}$$

$$d = \left(\frac{16 \times 7 \times 7457.5}{70 \times 22} \right)^{1/3} \times (10^3)^{1/3}$$

$$= (542.36)^{1/3} \times 10$$

$$= 10 \times 7.985 \text{ mm}$$

$$= 79.85 \text{ mm}$$

$$\approx 80 \text{ mm}$$

EXAMPLE 2 *Find the maximum torque that can be applied safely to shaft of 300 mm diameter. The permissible angle of twist is 1.5 in a length of 7.5 metre. The shearing stress should not exceed 42 N/mm². Take G = 84.4 kN/mm².*

SOLUTION Given $\theta = 1.5° = 0.02618$ radian

Polar moment of inertia of the shaft $(J) = \dfrac{\pi}{32} d^4$

$$= \frac{\pi}{32} \times 300^4$$

$$= 7.952 \times 10^8 \text{ mm}^4$$

From torsion equation, $\dfrac{T}{J} = \dfrac{\tau_{max}}{\left(\dfrac{d}{2}\right)}$

$\therefore \qquad T = \dfrac{2 \times \tau_{max} \times J}{d}$

$$= \frac{2 \times 42 \times 7.952 \times 10^8}{300} \times \frac{1}{10^6} \text{ kNm}$$

$$= 222.65 \text{ kNm}$$

Again, from torsion equation, we have

$$\frac{T}{J} = \frac{G\theta}{l}$$

$$T = \frac{G\theta}{l} \times J$$

$$= \frac{84.4 \times 0.02618 \times 7.952 \times 10^8}{7.5 \times 1000} \times \frac{1}{10^3} \text{ kNm}$$

$$= 234.27 \text{ kNm}$$

Selecting smaller of the two values, we have

$$T = 222.65 \text{ kNm} \qquad \textbf{Ans.}$$

EXAMPLE 3 *A solid steel shaft of 2 m length is to transmit 50 kW at 150 rpm. If the shear stress in the shaft material is not to exceed 50 MPa and maximum allowable twist in the shaft is 1°. Calculate the shaft diameter G = 80 GPa.*

SOLUTION Let d = shaft diameter in mm.

and $\qquad T$ = Torque transmitted in Nm

Hence, Power $(P) = \dfrac{2\pi NT}{60}$

$$50 \times 10^3 = \frac{2 \times \pi \times 150 \times T}{60}$$

$$T = 3183 \text{ Nm}$$

$$= \left[3.183 \times 10^6 \right] \text{Nmm}$$

Now, considering stress as the basis,

We have, $\dfrac{T}{J} = \dfrac{\tau_{max}}{d/2}$

$$\dfrac{3.183 \times 10^6}{\dfrac{\pi}{32} d^4} = \dfrac{50}{d/2} \Rightarrow d = 68.7 \text{ mm}$$

Again, considering twist as the basis

$$\dfrac{T}{J} = \dfrac{G\theta}{l}$$

$$\dfrac{3.183 \times 10^6}{\dfrac{\pi}{32} d^4} = \dfrac{(80 \times 10^3) \times \left(\dfrac{\pi}{180} \times 1 \right)}{2000}$$

$$d = 82.55 \text{ mm}$$

The desired shaft dia. will be the larger of the two values

i.e. Shaft diameter = 82.55 mm **Ans.**

EXAMPLE 4 *Two shafts of the same material and same length are subjected to the same torque. If the first shaft is solid circular section and the second is of a hollow circular section, whose internal dia is 2/3 of the outside dia and the maximum shear stress developed in each shaft is same, compare the weight of the two shafts.*

SOLUTION Given

$$T_{\text{hollow}} = T_{\text{solid}} = T$$

$$\tau_h = \tau_s = \tau$$

$$l_h = l_s = l$$

$$\dfrac{di}{do} = \dfrac{2}{3}$$

ρ = demerit of shaft material

$\because$ $\qquad T_s = \dfrac{\pi}{16} \tau_s \cdot di^3$ ...(1)

$$T_h = \dfrac{\pi}{16} \tau_h \cdot (do^3 - di^3)$$

$$= \dfrac{\pi}{16} \tau_h \, do^3 \left\{ 1 - \left(\dfrac{di}{do} \right)^3 \right\}$$

$$= \frac{\pi}{16} \times \tau \times do^3 \left\{ 1 - \left(\frac{2}{3}\right)^3 \right\}$$

$$= \frac{\pi}{16} \times \tau \times do^3 \left\{ 1 - \frac{8}{27} \right\}$$

Now, $T_h = T_s$

$$\frac{\pi}{16} \times \tau \times do^3 \times \left\{ 1 - \frac{8}{27} \right\} = \frac{\pi}{16} \times \tau \, d^3$$

$$d = 0.929 \, do$$

Again, $\dfrac{W_s}{W_h} = \dfrac{V_s \times \rho}{V_h \times \rho} = \dfrac{V_s}{V_h} = \dfrac{\dfrac{\pi}{4} d^2 \times \ell}{\dfrac{\pi}{4} (do^2 - di^2) \times \ell}$

$$= \frac{d^2}{(do^2 - di^2)}$$

$$= \frac{(0.929 \, do)^2}{do^2 \left(1 - \dfrac{di^2}{do^2} \right)}$$

$$= \frac{(0.929) \, do^2}{do^2 \left(1 - \dfrac{4}{9} \right)}$$

$$= \frac{0.929 \times 9}{5} = 1.55$$

$$\boxed{\frac{W_s}{W_h} = 1.55}$$

EXAMPLE 5 *Calculate the ratios of torques transmitted by the hollow and the solid circular shafts of the same material, length and weight.*
SOLUTION

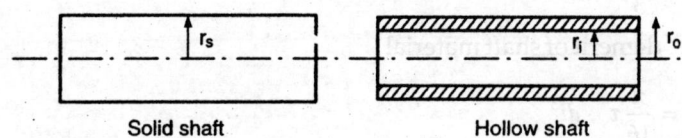

Fig. 12.5

Let r_s = radius of solid shaft
      r_o = external radius of hollow shaft
      r_i = internal radius of hollow shaft
We will use Suffix 'h' for hollow shaft and 'S' for solid shaft.

As the shafts given are made up of the same material, therefore, maximum allowable shear stress τ will be same for both.

$\therefore$ By torsion formula for hollow shaft $\dfrac{T_h}{J} = \dfrac{\tau}{r_o}$

and $\dfrac{T_s}{J} = \dfrac{\tau}{r_s}$

Now, putting the formula of J for hollow and solid shaft

$$\frac{T_h}{\frac{\pi}{2}(r_o^4 - r_i^4)} = \frac{\tau}{r_o} \qquad \qquad \text{...(1)}$$

and

$$\frac{T_s}{\frac{\pi}{2} r_s^4} = \frac{\tau}{r_s} \qquad \qquad \text{...(2)}$$

From eqn. (1) and eqn. (2)

$$\frac{T_h}{T_s} = \frac{r_o^4 - r_i^4}{r_o \cdot r_s^3} \qquad \qquad \text{...(3)}$$

Again, given, the weights, lengths and materials of the two shaft are same.

$\therefore \qquad \rho \pi (r_o^2 - r_i^2) \cdot l = \rho \cdot \pi \cdot r_s^2 \cdot l$

$\therefore \qquad (r_o^2 - r_i^2) = r_s^2 \qquad \qquad \text{...(4)}$

From eqn. (3) and eqn. (4)

$$\frac{T_h}{T_s} = \frac{(r_o^2 + r_i^2)(r_o^2 - r_i^2)}{r_o \cdot r_s^3}$$

$$= \frac{(r_o^2 + r_i^2) \times r_s^2}{r_o \cdot r_s^3}$$

$$= \frac{r_o^2 + r_i^2}{r_o \cdot r_s}$$

$$= \frac{r_o}{r_s}\left[1 + \frac{1}{n^2}\right] \qquad \qquad \text{...(5)}$$

where $\dfrac{r_o}{r_i} = n$

Again from eqn. (4)

$$1 - \left(\frac{r_i}{r_o}\right)^2 = \left(\frac{r_s}{r_o}\right)^2$$

$$1 - \frac{1}{n^2} = \left(\frac{r_s}{r_o}\right)^2$$

or,
$$\left(\frac{r_s}{r_o}\right)^2 = \frac{n^2 - 1}{n^2}$$

or,
$$\frac{r_o}{r_s} = \frac{n}{\sqrt{n^2 - 1}}$$

Substituting the value of $\left(\dfrac{r_o}{r_s}\right)$ in eqn. (5), we get

$$\frac{T_h}{T_s} = \frac{n}{\sqrt{n^2 - 1}} \left[\frac{n^2 + 1}{n^2}\right]$$

i.e.
$$\frac{T_h}{T_s} = \frac{n^2 + 1}{n\sqrt{n^2 - 1}}$$

Taking $n = 2$

$$\left(\frac{T_h}{T_s}\right) = \frac{2^2 + 1}{2\sqrt{2^2 - 1}}$$

$$= \frac{5}{2\sqrt{3}}$$

$$= \frac{5}{2 \times 1.732}$$

$$= \frac{5}{3.464}$$

$$= 1.44$$

$$\boxed{\therefore T_h = 1.44 \times T_s}$$

The above relation reveals that hollow shaft can transmit 44% more torque than the solid shaft of the same material, length and weight.

EXAMPLE 6 *Determine the diameter of the solid shaft which will transmit 300 kW at 250 rpm. The maximum shear stress should not exceed 30 N/mm² and twist should not be more than 1° on a shaft length of 2 m. Take modulus of rigidity = 1 × 10⁶ N/mm².*

SOLUTION

$$\text{Power } (P) = \frac{2\pi NT}{60}$$

$$300 \times 10^3 = \frac{2\pi \times 250 \times T}{60}$$

$$T = \frac{300 \times 10^3 \times 60}{2\pi \times 250}$$

$$= 11459.1 \, \text{Nm}$$

$$= 11459.1 \times 10^3 \, \text{Nmm}$$

$$= 11459100 \, \text{Nmm}$$

(a) Diameter of the shaft when $\tau_{max} = 30 \, \text{N/mm}^2$

By Torsion equation

$$\frac{T}{J} = \frac{\tau_{max}}{(d/2)}$$

$$\frac{T}{\frac{\pi}{32} d^4} = \frac{\tau_{max} \times 2}{d}$$

$$\frac{32T}{\pi d^3} = \frac{2\tau_{max}}{1}$$

$$\therefore \qquad T = \frac{\pi}{16} \times \tau_{max} \times d^3$$

$$\therefore \qquad d = \left(\frac{16T}{\pi \times \tau_{max}} \right)^{1/3} = \left(\frac{16 \times 11459100}{3.14 \times 30} \right)^{0.33} = 118.97 \, \text{mm}$$

(b) Diameter of the shaft when twist should not be more than 1°

Torsion formula considering twist as basis

$$\frac{T}{J} = \frac{G\theta}{l}$$

$$\frac{T}{\frac{\pi}{32} d^4} = \frac{G\theta}{l} \qquad\qquad \left[\begin{array}{l} \because 180° = \pi \, \text{radian} \\ \therefore 1° = \dfrac{\pi}{180} \, \text{radian} \end{array} \right]$$

$$\frac{32T}{\pi d^4} = \frac{G \times \pi}{180 l}$$

$$\therefore \qquad d = \left(\frac{32 \times 180 \times T \times l}{\pi^2 \times G} \right)^{1/4}$$

$$= \left(\frac{32 \times 180 \times 11459100 \times 2}{3.14^2 \times 1 \times 10^5 \times 10^{-3}} \right)^{1/4}$$

$$d = 107.56 \, \text{mm}$$

Therefore, from (a) and (b) suitable diameter of the shaft is greater of the two

i.e.   118.97 mm

            $\approx$ 119 mm   **Ans.**

N.B: For placing order for shaft one should see the standard size from manufacturer's catalogue.

EXAMPLE 7 *The compound shaft shown in figure is built in at the two ends. It is subjected to a twisting moment T in the middle. What is the ratio of the reaction torques T_1 and T_2 at the ends?*

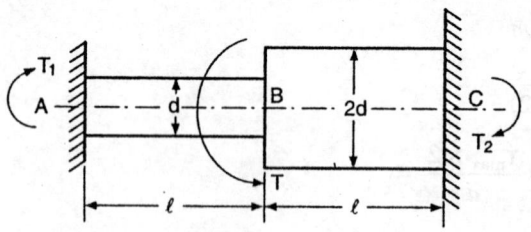

Fig. 12.6

SOLUTION Given that twisting moment T is applied in the middle.

$\therefore$ $T_1 + T_2 = T$

Further, the ends of the shaft are fixed hence they cannot rotate *i.e.* $\theta_{AB} = \theta_{BC}$

$$\frac{T_1 \times l_{AB}}{J_{AB} \times G_{AB}} = \frac{T_2 \times l_{BC}}{J_{BC} \times G_{BC}}$$

$$\frac{T_1}{\frac{\pi}{32} d^4} = \frac{T_2}{\frac{\pi}{32} (2d)^4}$$

or, $$\frac{T_1}{T_2} = \frac{\frac{\pi}{32} d^4}{\frac{\pi}{32} \times 16 \times d^4}$$

$\therefore$ $$\frac{T_1}{T_2} = \left(\frac{1}{16}\right)$$ **Ans.**

EXAMPLE 8 *A shaft 700 mm long consists of two circular portions length wise. One portion is made up of steel is 300 mm long and 30 mm diameter. The other portion of brass is 400 mm long and 60 mm diameter. The shaft is fixed at the ends and a torque is applied at the junction of the two portions.*

Calculate the maximum torque that can be applied to shaft if the safe working shear stress for steel is 50 MPa.

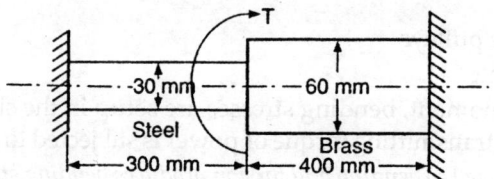

Fig. 12.7

SOLUTION From the given, we have

$$T = (T_s + T_b)$$

Now, torque transmitted by steel shaft,

$$T_s = J \cdot \frac{\tau_s}{r_s}$$

$$= \frac{\pi}{32}(30)^4 \times \frac{50 \times 2}{30}$$

$$= \frac{\pi}{32} \times (2 \times 15)^4 \times \frac{10}{3}$$

$$= \frac{\pi}{2} \times \frac{15^4 \times 10}{3}$$

$$= 265 \times 10^3 \text{ Nmm}$$

At the junction of shaft

$$\theta_s = \theta_b$$

$$\therefore \quad \frac{T_s \cdot L_s}{G_s \cdot J_s} = \frac{T_b \cdot L_b}{G_b \cdot J_b}$$

$$\therefore \quad \frac{(265 \times 10^3) \times 300}{(80 \times 10^3) \times \left(\frac{\pi}{2} \times 15^4\right)} = \frac{T_b \times 400}{(40 \times 10^3) \times \left(\frac{\pi}{2} \times 30^4\right)}$$

$$\therefore \quad T_b = 1590 \times 10^3 \text{ N mm}$$

$$\therefore \quad \text{Total torque at the joint}$$

$$T = (265 + 1590) \times 10^3$$

$$= 1855 \times 10^3 \text{ N mm}$$

$$= 1855 \text{ N m} \qquad \textbf{Ans.}$$

12.9 COMBINED BENDING AND TORSION

So far, we studied the effect of pure twisting on a shaft. However, it is observed that the shafts transmitting power are also subjected to bending moment due to:

(i) self weight

(ii) weight of the pulleys

(iii) belt tension etc.

Due to bending moment, bending stresses are setup in the shaft. We have seen earlier that a shaft transmitting torque or power is subjected to shear stresses also. *Hence, a shaft subjected to bending and torsion produces bending stress and shear stress respectively.*

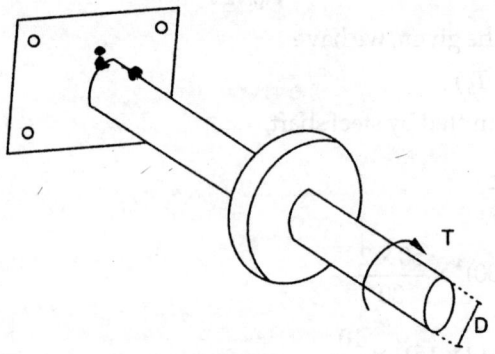

Fig. 12.8

Let us consider any point on the cross-section of the shaft.

Let T = Torque at the section

            D = Diameter of the shaft

            M = B.M. at the section.

The torque (T) will produce shear stress at the point and bending moment (M) will produce bending stress.

Let τ = shear stress at the point produced by torque T.

and σ_b = bending stress at the point produced by B.M. (M).

Now, the shear stress at a point due to torque T is given by

$$\tau = \frac{T}{J} \times r = \left(\frac{16T}{\pi D^3} \right) \qquad \left[\because \frac{T}{J} = \frac{\tau}{r} = \frac{G\theta}{l} \text{ and } J = \frac{\pi}{32} D^3 \right]$$

Similarly, the bending stress at a point due to bending moment (M) is given by

$$\sigma_b = \left[\frac{M}{I} \times y \right]$$

$$\because \qquad y = \frac{D}{2}$$

$$\therefore \qquad \sigma_b = \frac{M}{I} \times \frac{D}{2}$$

$$= \left(\frac{M}{\frac{\pi}{64} D^4} \times \frac{D}{2} \right)$$

$$\therefore \qquad \sigma_b = \left(\frac{32\,M}{\pi D^3}\right)$$

The principal stresses are

$$\sigma_{1,2} = \frac{\sigma_b}{2} \pm \sqrt{\left(\frac{\sigma_b}{2}\right)^2 + \tau^2_{max}}$$

$$= \frac{32\,M}{2\pi D^3} \pm \sqrt{\left(\frac{32\,M}{2\times\pi D^3}\right)^2 + \left(\frac{16\,T}{\pi D^3}\right)^2}$$

$$= \frac{16}{\pi D^3}\left[M + \sqrt{M^2 + T^2}\right]$$

∴ Major principal stress

$$\sigma_1 = \frac{16}{\pi D^3}\left[M + \sqrt{M^2 + T^2}\right]$$

and Minor principal stress

$$\sigma_2 = \frac{16}{\pi D^3}\left[M - \sqrt{M^2 + T^2}\right]$$

Maximum shear stress $(\tau_{max}) = \left(\frac{\sigma_1 - \sigma_2}{2}\right)$

$$\therefore \qquad \tau_{max} = \frac{16}{\pi D^3}\sqrt{M^2 + T^2}$$

For Hollow shaft

Major principal stress $(\sigma_1) = \dfrac{16 D_0}{\pi\,[D_0{}^4 - D_i{}^4]}\left(M + \sqrt{M^2 + T^2}\right)$

and Minor principal stress $(\sigma_2) = \dfrac{16 D_0}{\pi\,[D_0{}^4 - D_i{}^4]}\left(M - \sqrt{M^2 + T^2}\right)$

Maximum shear stress $(\tau_{max}) = \dfrac{16 D_0}{\pi\,[D_0{}^4 - D_i{}^4]}\left(\sqrt{M^2 + T^2}\right)$

12.10 EFFECT OF END THRUST ON SHAFT

So far, we studied that when a shaft is subjected to torsion (T) and B.M (M) due to gear, pulley or due to the weight of shaft itself, then shear stress (τ) and bending stress (σ_b) are developed in the shaft.

Besides these two stresses, sometimes shafts are also subjected to **end thrust**. For example, in a propeller shaft, end thrust is developed which causes a compressive stress in the shaft.

Under such circumstances, total direct stress in the shaft

= Stresses due to B.M. (M) + Stress due to end thrust (P)

But since end thrust is compressive in nature so negative (–) sign will be used while evaluating the total stress.

Thus, at the ends of vertical diameter total direct stress

$$(\sigma_{\text{direct}}) = \left(\pm \sigma_b - \frac{P}{A} \right)$$

EXAMPLE 9 *A propeller shaft of a ship has 180 mm diameter, transmits 1000 kW at 120 rpm. The shaft is subjected to a bending moment of 10^4 Nm and an end thrust of 100 kN. Calculate principal stresses.*

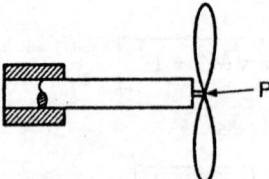

Fig. 12.9

SOLUTION Let T newton metre be the torque transmitted.

$$\because \qquad P = \frac{2 \pi NT}{60}$$

$$\therefore \qquad T = \left(\frac{P \times 60}{2 \pi N} \right)$$

$$= \left[\frac{1000 \times 10^3 \times 60}{2 \pi \times 120} \right] \text{Nm} = 79545.45 \text{ Nm}$$

Given $M = 10^4$ Nm

End thrust $P = -10^5$ N   (Since thrust is compressive in nature)

Direct stress due to end thrust $= \dfrac{P}{A}$

$$= \frac{-10^5}{\dfrac{\pi}{4}(180)^2}$$

$$= -3.928 \text{ N/mm}^2$$

$$= -3.93 \text{ N/mm}^2$$

Bending stress $(\sigma_b) = \pm \dfrac{M}{I} \cdot y$

$$= \pm \frac{M}{(I/y)}$$

$$= \pm \frac{M}{Z} \qquad\qquad \left[\because Z = \frac{I}{y} \right]$$

$$= \pm \frac{(10^4 \times 10^3)}{\frac{\pi}{32}(180)^3}$$

$$= \pm 17.458 \text{ N/mm}^2$$

$$= \pm 17.46 \text{ N/mm}^2$$

Shear stress $(\tau) = \dfrac{T \cdot r}{J}$

$$= \frac{T}{(J/r)}$$

$$= \frac{T}{Z_t} \qquad\qquad [Z_t = \text{section modulus in torsion}]$$

$$= \frac{79545.45 \times 10^3}{\frac{\pi}{16} \times (180)^3}$$

$$= 69.43 \text{ N/mm}^2$$

$\therefore$ Total direct net stress $(\sigma_d) = \left(\pm \sigma_b - \dfrac{P}{A} \right)$

$$= \pm 17.46 - 3.93$$

$$= 13.53 \text{ N/mm}^2$$

or

$$= -21.39 \text{ N/mm}^2$$

Principal stresses on tension side,

$$\sigma_{1,2} = \frac{13.53}{2} \pm \sqrt{\left(\frac{13.53}{2} \right)^2 + (69.49)^2}$$

$$= 6.76 \pm 69.82$$

$$= 76.58 \text{ MPa or} -63.06 \text{ MPa} \qquad \textbf{Ans.}$$

Principal stresses on compression sides,

$$\sigma_{1,2} = \frac{-21.39}{2} \pm \sqrt{\left(\frac{-21.39}{2}\right)^2 + (69.49)^2}$$

$$= -10.7 \pm 70.3$$

$$= 59.6 \, \text{MPa} \quad \text{or} \quad -81 \, \text{MPa} \qquad \textbf{Ans.}$$

EXAMPLE 10 *In a hollow circular shaft, the external diameter is 100 mm and internal diameter is 60 mm. The allowable shear stress in the shaft material is 55 N/mm². Determine the angle of twist in a length of twenty times the external diameter of the shaft. (Take $G = 8.5 \times 10^4 \, \text{N/mm}^2$)* **[UPTU 2006-07]**

SOLUTION Given $d_o = 100$ mm

$$d_i = 60 \, \text{mm}$$

$$\tau = 55 \, \text{N/mm}^2$$

$$\theta = ?$$

$$l = 20 \, d_o = 20 \times 100 = 2000 \, \text{mm}$$

$$G = 8.5 \times 10^4 \, \text{N/mm}^2$$

We have,

$$\frac{\tau}{R} = \frac{G\theta}{l}$$

Hence, $\quad \theta = \dfrac{\tau \times l}{R \times G}$

$$= \left(\frac{55 \times 2000}{50 \times 8.5 \times 10^4}\right)$$

$$= 0.02588 \, \text{radian}$$

$$= 1.483 \, \text{degree} \qquad \textbf{Ans.}$$

HIGHLIGHTS

1. A shaft is in torsion, when equal and opposite torques are applied at the two ends of a shaft.
2. The shear stress is maximum on the surface of the shaft and zero at the axis of shaft.
3. The torsion formula for shaft is

$$\frac{T}{J} = \frac{\tau}{r} = \frac{G\theta}{l}$$

where T - torque

J = polar moment of inertia

$$= \frac{\pi D^4}{32} \text{ for solid shaft}$$

$$= \frac{\pi}{32} [D^4 - d^4] \text{ for hollow shaft}$$

$$\tau_{max} = \frac{16T}{\pi D^3}$$

$$r = \frac{D}{2}$$

l = Length of shaft.

G = Modulus of rigidity.

θ = Angle of twist.

4. Torsional stiffness (K) = Torque per radian twist

$$= \frac{T}{\theta} = \frac{GJ}{l}$$

5. (a) Torque transmitted by a solid shaft

$$T = \frac{\pi}{16} \tau_{max} D^3$$

(b) Torque transmitted by a hollow circular shaft

$$T = \frac{\pi}{16} \times \tau_{max} \left(\frac{D_0^{\,4} - D_i^{\,4}}{D_0} \right)$$

6. Polar modulus (Z_p) $= \dfrac{J}{R}$

$$= \frac{\pi}{16} D^3 \text{ for solid shaft}$$

$$= \frac{\pi}{16 D_0} [D_0^{\,4} - D_i^{\,4}] \text{ for a hollow shaft.}$$

7. The power transmitted by a shaft

$$P = \frac{2\pi NT}{60} \text{ watt}$$

where, N = rpm of the shaft

T = applied torque in Nm

8. Strength of a shaft means the maximum torque or maximum power the shaft can transmit.

9. The strain energy stored in a shaft due to torsion is given by

$$U = \frac{\tau^2}{4G} \times V \text{ for a solid shaft}$$

$$= \frac{\tau^2}{4G}\left[1 + \left(\frac{d}{D}\right)^2\right] \times \text{Volume of shaft}$$

where, τ = Shear stress on the surface of the shaft

D = External diameter of shaft

d = Internal diameter of shaft

10. A shaft when subjected to combined bending and twisting:

Maximum principal stress $(\sigma) = \frac{16}{\pi D^3}\left[M + \sqrt{M^2 + T^2}\right]$

Maximum shear stress $(\tau) = \frac{16}{\pi D^3}\sqrt{M^2 + T^2}$ for solid shaft.

PROBLEMS FOR PRACTICE
(THEORETICAL)

1. Derive the relation $\frac{T}{J} = \frac{\tau}{R} = \frac{G \cdot \theta}{L}$.

2. Define the term : Torsion; Torsional Rigidity; Polar Moment of inertia.

3. Prove that strain energy stored in a body due to shear stress is given by

$$U = \frac{\tau^2}{2G} \times V$$

4. What do you mean by strength of shaft?

5. Prove strain energy due to torsion, $U = \frac{\tau^2}{4G} \times V$.

6. Why hollow shaft is preferred to solid shaft?

(NUMERICAL)

1. A solid steel shaft transmitts 560 kW at 300 rev/min with a maximum shear stress of 60 N/mm².
   (a) What is the shaft diameter?
   (b) What would be the diameter of a hollow shaft of the same material (diameter ratio 2) to transmit the same power at the same speed and stress?
   (c) Compare the stiffness of equal lengths of these shafts.

2. A shaft 3 m long stores 300 Nm of energy when transmitting 1500 kW at 3600 rpm.
   What is the shaft diameter and maximum shear stresss? G = 80,000 N/mm².

3. The dimensions of an angle section are 75 mm × 50 mm × 3.2 mm. Calculate the maximum shear stress and twist per metre length if a torque of 10 Nm is applied. G = 83 × 10³ N/mm².

4. Find the maximum shear stress induced in the shaft as shown in figure.

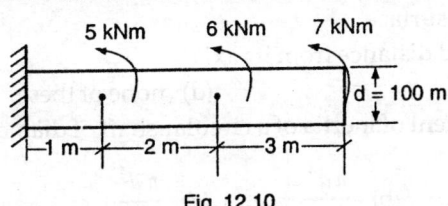

Fig. 12.10

5. What must be the diameter of a solid shaft to transmit a twisting moment of 600 kNm and a bending moment of 150 kNm, the maximum direct stress being limited to 80 MPa?

   What should be the external diameter of a hollow shaft to perform this, if the internal diameter is 0.6 of the external diameter?

6. A torque transmitting solid steel shaft of 100 mm diameter is replaced by a hollow one of the same material having its outside diameter twice its inside diameter.

   Maximum shear stress in the hollow shaft remains same as that in the solid one.

   Compare torsional rigidity (JG) for the two shafts.

7. The compound shaft shown in figure is built-in at the two ends. It is subjected to a twisting moment T at the middle.

   What is the ratio of reaction torques T_1 and T_2 at the ends?

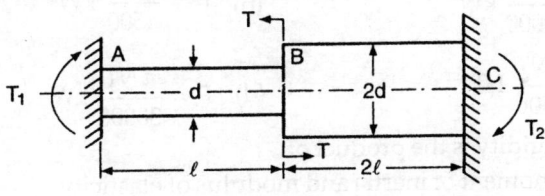

Fig. 12.11

ANSWERS

1. 115 mm; 117 mm; 58.5 mm; 0.98
2. 178 mm; 35.9 N/mm²
3. 23.5 N/mm²; 5.1°
4. 92 N/mm²
5. $d = 366$ mm; $d_0 = 383$ mm
6. $J_s : J_h = 0.98 : 1$
7. $T_1 : T_2 = 1 : 8$

OBJECTIVE QUESTIONS

1. Torsional member are subjected to:
   (a) bending moments
   (b) twisting moments
   (c) combined moments
   (d) none of the above
2. Shafts are made up of:
   (a) mild steel
   (b) alloy steel
   (c) copper alloy
   (d) any of the above

3. The shear stress in a circular shaft is zero at its following location:
   (a) at its outer surface
   (b) at two third distance from its axis
   (c) at its axis
   (d) none of these

4. The polar moment of inertia of a circular shaft of diameter 'd' is:

   (a) $\dfrac{\pi d^4}{8}$
   (b) $\dfrac{\pi d^4}{16}$
   (c) $\dfrac{\pi d^4}{32}$
   (d) $\dfrac{\pi d^4}{64}$

5. The polar moment of inertia of a hollow circular shaft of outside diameter d_o and wide diameter d_i is given by:

   (a) $\dfrac{\pi}{8}(d_o^4 - d_i^4)$
   (b) $\dfrac{\pi}{16}(d_o^4 - d_i^4)$

   (c) $\dfrac{\pi}{64}(d_o^4 - d_i^4)$
   (d) $\dfrac{\pi}{32}(d_o^4 - d_i^4)$

6. The variation of shear stress with respect to radius in a circular shaft is shown by a:
   (a) parabola
   (b) cubic curve
   (c) line
   (d) none of these

7. The power transmitted by a shaft is expressed as:

   (a) $P = \dfrac{\pi NT}{60000}$ kW
   (b) $P = \dfrac{\pi NT}{4500}$ kW

   (c) $P = \dfrac{\pi NT}{4500}$ HP
   (d) $P = \dfrac{\pi NT}{30000}$ kW

8. Torsional rigidity is the product of:
   (a) polar moment of inertia and modulus of elasticity
   (b) modulus of rigidity and modulus of elasticity
   (c) polar moment of inertia and modulus of rigidity
   (d) none of the above

9. The polar modulus for a circular shaft of diameter 'd' is:

   (a) $\dfrac{\pi}{16}d^3$
   (b) $\dfrac{\pi}{32}d^3$
   (c) $\dfrac{\pi}{64}d^3$
   (d) $\dfrac{\pi}{128}d^3$

10. The following assumptions is/are made in torsion equation:
    (a) stresses induced are within elastic limit
    (b) shaft material is homogenous and isotropic
    (c) shaft is of uniform cross-section throughout
    (d) all of the above

11. A hollow shaft made up of steel has external diameter 100 mm and internal diameter 50 mm is to be replaced by a solid alloy shaft. Assuming the same value of polar modulus for both, the diameter of the solid alloy shaft will be:

(a) $10\sqrt[3]{9375}$ mm

(b) $10 \times \sqrt[3]{9375 \times 10}$ mm

(c) $10 \times \sqrt[3]{\dfrac{9375}{10}}$ mm

(d) $\sqrt[3]{9375}$ mm

12. A shaft of diameter 'd' is subjected to bending moment M and twisting moment T. The developed principal stress will be:

(a) $\pm \dfrac{16}{\pi d^3}\sqrt{M^2 + T^2}$

(b) $\pm \dfrac{16}{\pi d^3}\left[M \pm \sqrt{M^2 + T^2} \right]$

(c) $\pm \dfrac{16}{\pi d^3}\left[T \pm \sqrt{M^2 + T^2} \right]$

(d) $\dfrac{16}{\pi d^3}\sqrt{M^2 + T^2} \pm M$

13. If the diameter of a shaft subjected to torque is doubled then horse power P can be increased to:

(a) $16\,P$ (b) $8\,P$ (c) $4\,P$ (d) $2\,P$

14. If a circular shaft is subjected to a torque T and a bending moment M then the ratio of the maximum shear stress to the maximum bending stress is given by:

(a) $\dfrac{2M}{T}$

(b) $\dfrac{T}{2M}$

(c) $\dfrac{2T}{M}$

(d) $\dfrac{M}{2T}$

15. A circular shaft is subjected to a twisting moment T and a bending moment M. The ratio of maximum bending stress to maximum shear stress is given by:

(a) $\dfrac{2M}{T}$

(b) $\dfrac{M}{T}$

(c) $\dfrac{2T}{M}$

(d) $\dfrac{M}{2T}$

16. A circular shaft with diameter D is subjected to bending moment M and torque T. The expression for the maximum principal stress at the section is:

(a) $\dfrac{16}{\pi D^3}\sqrt{M^2 + T^2}$

(b) $\dfrac{2M + T}{\pi D^3}$

(c) $\dfrac{16\pi}{D^3}\left(M + \sqrt{M^2 + T^2} \right)$

(d) $\dfrac{16}{\pi D^3}\left(M + \sqrt{M^2 + T^2} \right)$

17. Arrange the following sections in increasing torsional stiffness.

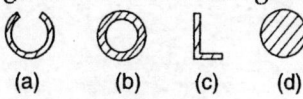

(a)   (b)   (c)   (d)

ANSWERS

1. (b)	2. (d)	3. (c)	4. (c)	5. (d)	6. (c)
7. (d)	8. (c)	9. (a)	10. (d)	11. (c)	12. (b)
13. (b)	14. (b)	15. (a)	16. (d)	17. (c), (a) (b) (d)	

— ❖❖ —

STRAIN ENERGY AND ITS APPLICATION

13.1 INTRODUCTION

We studied in chapter "Simple Stresses and Strains" that external load acting on a elastic body causes deformation. In the process of deformation, their point of application undergo displacement. Therefore, work is done on the body by the external force.

All the work performed during elastic deformation is stored and is recovered on the release of load. This recoverable stored energy in an elastic body is called the elastic *Strain Energy or Resilience.*

Within elastic limit it is equal to the work done in straining the elastic body (may be rod; prismatic bar; wire etc) but if the material is loaded beyond its elastic limit, only a part of the work done in straining can be recovered and the remaining is used in producing the material slip and reappears in the form of heat.

The maximum amount of strain energy which can be stored in the material per unit of its volume, within its elastic limit is called 'Proof Resilience' and is equal to the work done is straining the material upto its elastic limit.

Figure 13.1 shows load extension diagram of a elastic body under tensile test upto elastic limit. The tensile load P increases gradually from zero to the value of P and the extension of the elastic body increases from zero to the value of δ.

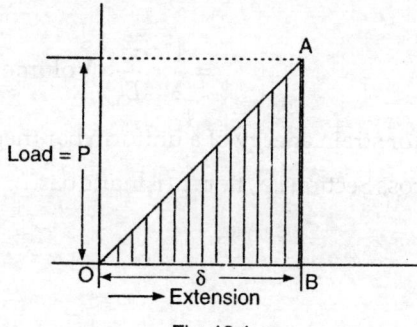

Fig. 13.1

Work done by the load P = Area of triangle OAB

$$= \frac{1}{2}P \times \delta$$

$$= \text{Average load} \times \text{Extension}$$

Strain energy is denoted by letter U.

Strain energy per unit volume of the material is called strain energy density (u).

Strain energy density (u) = $\dfrac{\sigma^2}{2E}$.

13.1.1 Strain Energy in a Bar under Different Cases of Loading

Let us consider a prismatic bar subjected to tensile load P applied gradually as shown in figure. The bar on application of load undergoes an extension (δ).

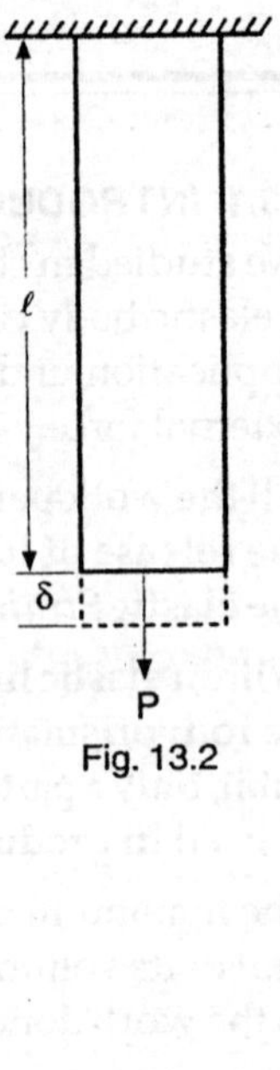

Since, the point of application of the load P has moved through δ. Hence, work done in straining the prismatic bar

$$= \text{Average load} \times \text{deflection}$$

$$= \frac{1}{2} \times P \times \delta$$

$$= \frac{1}{2} \times P \times \frac{PL}{AE}$$

Fig. 13.2

i.e.   Word done in Uniaxial loading $= \dfrac{1}{2} \cdot \dfrac{P^2 L}{AE}$

$$= \frac{1}{2} \cdot \frac{P^2}{A^2} \times \frac{AL}{E}$$

$$= \frac{1}{2} \times \frac{\sigma^2}{E} \times AL$$

$$= \frac{1}{2} \times \frac{\sigma^2}{E} \times \text{Volume of bar}.$$

This is the expression for strain energy of a uniform bar (neglecting its weight).

For a bar of varying Cross Section *i.e.*, non-prismatic bar.

$$U = \int \frac{P^2 \cdot dx}{2A \cdot E}$$

13.2 STRAIN ENERGY OF A BAR (INCLUDING ITS WEIGHT)

Consider a bar of length l mounted vertically. At any section AB, the total load on the section will he the external load P together with the weight of the bar material below AB.

Assuming a uniform cross section of area A with density P load on section

$$AB = P \pm \rho g AS$$

(The positive sign is used when P is tensile and negative sign is used when P is compressive).

For a tensile force P, the extension of the element dS is given by the following expression

$$\delta = \frac{\sigma \cdot dS}{E}$$

$$= \frac{(P + \rho g AS)\, dS}{AE}$$

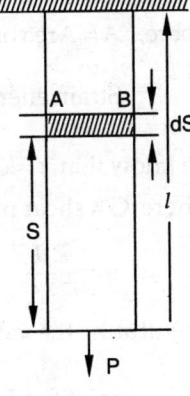

Fig. 13.3

∴   Work done $= \dfrac{1}{2} \times$ load $\times$ extension

$$= \frac{1}{2}(P + \rho g AS)\frac{(P + \rho g AS)}{AE}\,dS$$

$$= \frac{P^2}{2AE}\,dS + \frac{P\rho g}{E}\,S\,dS + \frac{(\rho g)^2 A}{2E}\,S^2\,dS$$

∴   Total strain energy or work done

$$= \int_0^l \frac{P^2}{2AE}\,dS + \int_0^l \frac{P\rho g}{E}\,S\,dS + \int_0^l \frac{(\rho g)^2 A}{2E}\,S^2 dS$$

$$= \frac{P^2 l}{2AE} + \frac{P\rho g l^2}{2E} + \frac{(\rho g)^2 A l^3}{6E}$$

13.3 A RECTANGULAR BLOCK IN SHEAR

In the given figure a rectangular block is subjected to a shear load P, as a result the face AB moves through distance 'S' relative to the Fixed face CD.

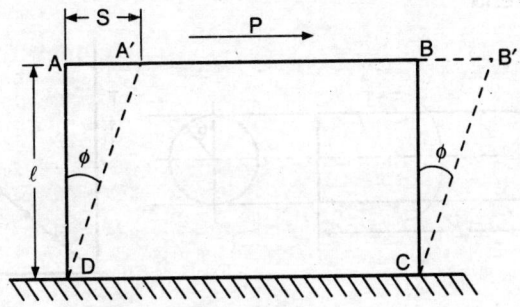

Fig. 13.4

For the linear elastic material, shear strain $(\phi) = \dfrac{s}{l}$

is proportional to the sheer stress $(\tau) = \dfrac{P}{A}$

where, A = Area of the top face.

$\therefore$ Strain energy (U) of the block $= \dfrac{1}{2} \cdot P.S$ ...(i)

We know that $\tau = G\phi$

Where, G = shear modulus.

$\therefore$ $S = \dfrac{F \cdot l}{G \cdot A}$

Substituting the value of S is equation (i), we get

$$U = \dfrac{P^2 l}{2\,GA}$$

$$= \dfrac{1}{2} \cdot \left(\dfrac{P}{A}\right)^2 \times \dfrac{Al}{G}$$

$$= \dfrac{1}{2} \times \dfrac{\tau^2}{G} \times V$$

$$U_{\text{shear loading}} = \dfrac{\tau^2}{2G} \times V$$

$$\boxed{U \text{ (due to shear)} = \dfrac{\tau^2}{2\,G} \times V}$$

13.4 STRAIN ENERGY WHEN THE SHAFT IN TORSIONAL LOADING

Let the Shaft of length l is subjected to torsional loading T and let 'θ' is the angle of twist at the free end.

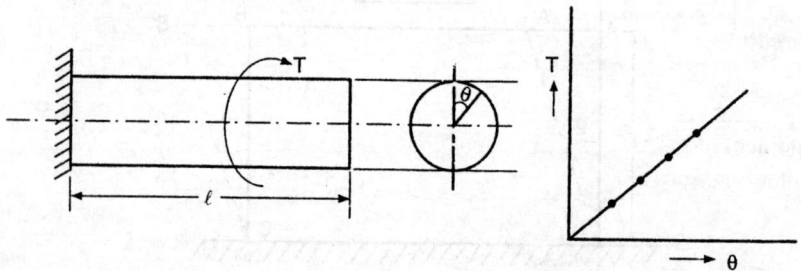

Fig. 13.5

From Torsion Formula, $\dfrac{T}{I_p} = \dfrac{G\theta}{l}$

where, $I_p =$ *Polar $M \cdot I$ of the Shaft.

$G =$ Shear modulus of the material.

Now, $U = \dfrac{1}{2} \cdot T \cdot \theta$

$$= \dfrac{1}{2} \times T \times \dfrac{Tl}{G \times I_p}$$

$$= \dfrac{1}{2} \times \dfrac{T^2 l}{G \times I_p} \quad \text{when torque } T \text{ is constant}$$

13.5 STRAIN ENERGY FOR HOLLOW SHAFT

We observed in section 13.4 that strain energy due to torsional loading of solid shaft is

$$U = \dfrac{T^2 l}{2GI_p} \quad \text{or} \quad \dfrac{T^2 l}{2GJ} \qquad\qquad \text{where, } J = \text{Polar moment of inertia*}$$

For hollow shaft,

$$J \text{ or } \overset{**}{I_p} = \dfrac{\pi}{2}(R^4 - r^4) \qquad\qquad \text{where, } R \text{ is the outer radius}$$

Now, by torsion formula,

$$\dfrac{T}{J} = \dfrac{\tau_{max}}{R}$$

$\therefore \qquad T = \dfrac{\tau_{max}}{R} \cdot J$

$$= \dfrac{\tau_{max}}{R} \cdot \dfrac{\pi}{2}(R^4 - r^4)$$

$$= \dfrac{\pi}{2R}\, \tau_{max}\, (R^4 - r^4)$$

Substituting the value of T in the equation of strain energy

$$U = \dfrac{\left[\dfrac{\pi \tau_{max}}{2R}(R^4 - r^4)\right]^2 l}{2G \cdot \dfrac{\pi}{2}(R^4 - r^4)}$$

---

*Polar moment of Inertia is either denoted by I_p or J.

**For hollow shaft J or $I_p = \dfrac{\pi}{32}[D^4 - d^4]$

$$= \dfrac{\pi}{32}[16R^4 - 16r^4]$$

$$= \dfrac{\pi}{2}[R^4 - r^4]$$

$$= \frac{\tau_{max}^2}{4G} \cdot \frac{\pi (R^4 - r^4) l}{R^2}$$

$$\therefore \quad U_{\text{hollow shaft}} = \frac{\tau_{max}^2}{4G} \cdot \frac{(R^2 + r^2)}{R^2} \times \text{Volume of shaft}$$

Hence, strain energy per unit volume of a hollow shaft $= \dfrac{\tau_{max}^2}{4G} \cdot \dfrac{(R^2 + r^2)}{R^2}$.

13.6 STRAIN ENERGY DUE TO PURE BENDING OF BAR

Let a prismatic bar of length 'l' is subjected to gradually applied end couple M.

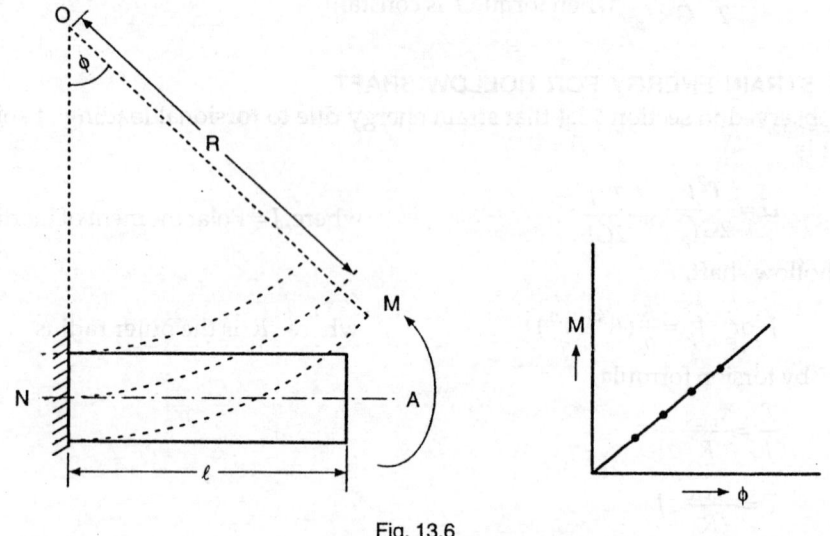

Fig. 13.6

As a result of couple M, the bar bends in the form of arc and subtends an angle ϕ at the centre of curvature.

Let R = Radius of Curvature of the neutral surface, then $\phi = \dfrac{l}{R}$

From bending formula,

$$\frac{M}{I} = \frac{E}{R}$$

where, $I = M \cdot I$ of the cross-section about N.A

$E = $ Young's Modulus

$$\therefore \quad \phi = \frac{Ml}{EI}$$

$\therefore \qquad U = \dfrac{1}{2} \times M \times \dfrac{Ml}{EI}$

$\qquad\qquad = \dfrac{M^2 l}{2EI}$ when M is constant

When M varies then

$$U = \int_0^l \dfrac{M^2 dx}{2EI}$$

N.B.: It should be noted that in the four types of loading case (13.1, 13.4, 13.5 and 13.6) mentioned so far the strain energy expressions are all identical in the following form

i.e. $\qquad$ Strain Energy $(U) = \dfrac{(\text{Applied load})^2 \times l}{2 \times \text{Product of two related constants}}$

The constants being related to the type of loading considered. In bending it is E and I while for torsion G and J.

13.7 STRESS DUE TO IMPACT LOAD

Let us consider a rigid vertical bar with a rigid collar attached to the end of bar.

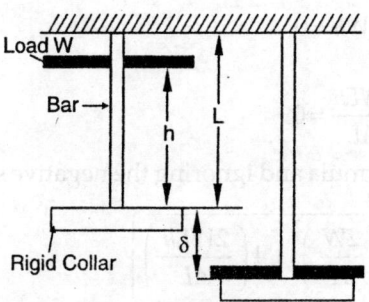

Fig. 13.7

The load W is free to slide vertically and is suspended by some means at a distance 'h' above the collar.

When the load is dropped, it will produce a maximum instantaneous extension δ of the bar.

Since, there is displacement of the bar owing to impact load, so work done will be

$\qquad$ = force $\times$ distance

$\qquad$ = $W (h + \delta)$

This work done will be stored as strain energy and is given by $U = \dfrac{\sigma^2 Al}{2E}$

where, σ = instantaneous stress set up.

Now, $\dfrac{\sigma^2 Al}{2E} = W(h + \delta)$ ...(1)

If the extension δ is small compared with h it may be ignored, then

$$\sigma^2 = \frac{2WEh}{AL}$$

i.e. $\sigma = \sqrt{\dfrac{2WEh}{AL}}$

If, however, δ is not small compared with h it must be expressed in terms of σ thus

$$E = \frac{\text{Stress}}{\text{Strain}}$$

$$= \frac{\sigma L}{\delta}$$

and $\delta = \dfrac{\sigma L}{E}$

Substituting in eqn. (1)

$$\frac{\sigma^2 AL}{2E} = Wh + \frac{W\sigma L}{E}$$

$$\frac{\sigma^2 AL}{2E} - \sigma \frac{WL}{E} - Wh = 0$$

$$\sigma^2 - \frac{2W}{A} \cdot \sigma - \frac{2WEh}{AL} = 0$$

Solving by quadratic formula and ignoring the negative sign

$$\sigma = \frac{1}{2} \left\{ \frac{2W}{A} + \sqrt{\left(\frac{2W}{A}\right)^2 + 4\left(\frac{2WEh}{AL}\right)} \right\}$$

i.e. $\boxed{\sigma = \dfrac{W}{A} + \sqrt{\left(\dfrac{W}{A}\right)^2 + \dfrac{2WEh}{AL}}}$

This is the equation for the maximum stress setup due to impact loading.
If the load is not dropped but *suddenly applied* from effectively zero height $h = 0$, then the above equation reduces to

$$\sigma = \frac{W}{A} + \frac{W}{A}$$

$\boxed{\therefore \ \sigma = \dfrac{2W}{A}}$ (when the load is applied suddenly)

EXAMPLE 1 *An unknown weight falls through 10 mm on a collar rigidly attached to the lower end of a vertical bar 3 m long and 600 mm² in section. If the extension is 2 mm, what is the corresponding stress and the value of the unknown weight?*

$\quad$ *Assume $E = 2 \times 10^5 \, N/mm^2$*

SOLUTION $\;$ Given, $h = 10$ mm; $E = 2 \times 10^5 \, \text{N/mm}^2$

$$l = 3 \, \text{m} = 3000 \, \text{mm}$$

$$A = 600 \, \text{mm}^2$$

$$\delta l = 2 \, \text{mm}$$

$$\sigma = ?$$

$$W = ?$$

By formula, Maximum stress $= E \times$ Maximum strain

$$= 2 \times 10^5 \times \frac{2}{3000}$$

$$= \frac{4}{3} \times 10^2 \, \text{N/mm}^2$$

$$= 1.333 \times 10^2 \, \text{N/mm}^2$$

$$\sigma = 133.3 \, \text{N/mm}^2$$

Let W is the unknown weight then

$\quad$ Loss of Potential Energy $=$ Strain energy stored by the rod

So, $\qquad W(h + \delta l) = \dfrac{\sigma^2}{2E} Al$

$$W(10 + 2) = \frac{(133.33)^2}{2 \times 2 \times 10^5} \times 600 \times 3000$$

$\therefore \qquad W = \left[\dfrac{(133.33)^2 \times 18 \times 10^5}{4 \times 12 \times 10^5} \right]$

$$= 6666.33 \, \text{Newton} \qquad \textbf{Ans.}$$

EXAMPLE 2 *A load of 500 N falls freely through a height of 150 mm on to a collar attached to the end of a vertical rod of 50 mm diameter and 2 metre long, the upper end of the rod being fixed to the ceiling. Calculate the maximum instantaneous extension of the bar. Also calculate the maximum stress in the bar.*

Assume $E = 2 \times 10^5 \, N/mm^2$

SOLUTION $\;$ Given load $(W) = 500 \, \text{N}$

$h = 150$ mm

$d = 150$ mm

$L = 2000$ mm

$E = 2 \times 10^5$ N/mm^2

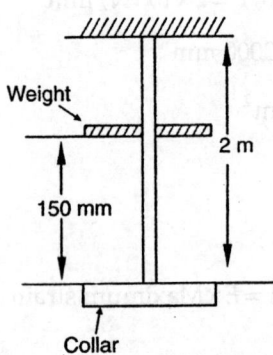

Fig. 13.8

Cross-Sectional Area of vertical rod $(A) = \dfrac{\pi}{4} \times d^2$

$$= \dfrac{\pi}{4} \times (50)^2$$

$$= 1964.28 \text{ mm}^2$$

$$\left(\dfrac{W}{A}\right) = \dfrac{500}{1964.28}$$

$$= 0.254$$

$$\left(\dfrac{W}{A}\right)^2 = (0.254)^2$$

$$= 0.0645$$

(a) Now, instantaneous stress $(\sigma) = \dfrac{W}{A} + \sqrt{\left(\dfrac{W}{A}\right)^2 + \dfrac{2WEh}{AL}}$

$$= 0.254 + \sqrt{0.0645 + \dfrac{2 \times 500 \times 2 \times 10^5 \times 150}{1964.28 \times 2000}}$$

$$= 0.254 + \sqrt{0.0645 + 7636.3858}$$

$$= 0.254 + 87.386$$

$$= 87.64 \text{ N/mm}^2 \qquad \textbf{Ans.}$$

(b) Instantaneous extension $(\delta) = \dfrac{\sigma}{E} \times l$

$$= \dfrac{87.64}{2 \times 10^5} \times 200$$

$$= 0.876 \text{ mm} \quad \textbf{Ans.}$$

EXAMPLE 3 *A wire 600 mm long and cross sectional area 10 mm^2 disc attached at bottom. Calculate the height h from which the load of 2 Newton can be permitted, to fall on the disc, so that the maximum stress in the wire does not exceed 150 N/mm^2.*

Take E for the material of the wire as $2 \times 10^5 N/mm^2$

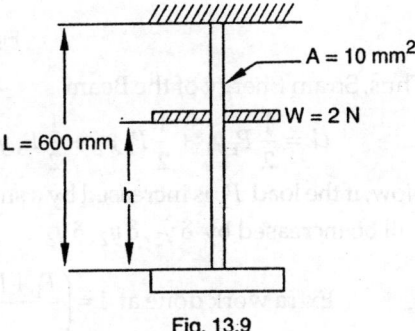

Fig. 13.9

SOLUTION Given $W = 2 \text{ N}$

$$l = 600 \text{ mm}$$
$$A = 10 \text{ mm}^2$$
$$\sigma = 150 \text{ N/mm}^2$$
$$E = 2 \times 10^5 \text{ N/mm}^2$$

Now, by formula, instantaneous stress

$$\sigma = \frac{W}{A} + \sqrt{\left(\frac{W}{A}\right)^2 + \frac{2WEh}{AL}}$$

$$150 = \frac{2}{10} + \sqrt{\left(\frac{2}{10}\right)^2 + \frac{2 \times 2 \times 2 \times 10^5 \times h}{10 \times 600}}$$

or, $150 = 0.2 + \sqrt{\times 0.04 + 133.33\, h}$

or, $149.8 = \sqrt{0.04 + 133.33h}$

or, $h = \left[\dfrac{(149.8)^2 - 0.04}{133.33}\right]$

∴ $h = 168.30 \text{ mm}$

13.8 CASTIGLIANO'S THEOREM

If an elastic body is subjected to external load(s) then the deflection at any point is equal to the partial derivative of the strain energy with respect to that load.

$$\left(i.e.,\ \delta_i = \frac{\delta U}{\delta P_i}\ \text{and}\ \theta_i = \frac{\delta U}{\delta M_i}\right)$$

Proof

Let us consider a portion of beam AB which is under the action of load $P_1, P_2, P_3 \dots P_n$ at point $1, 2, 3 \dots n$ respectively and let $y_1, y_2, y_3 \dots$ be the corresponding deflection at $1, 2, 3, \dots$ respectively.

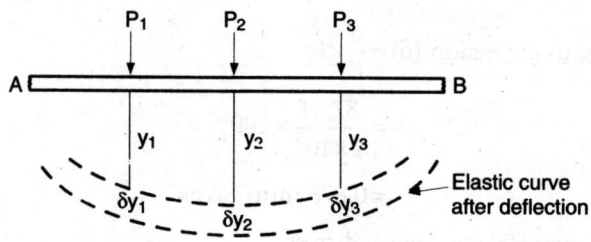

Fig. 13.10

Thus, Strain Energy of the Beam

$$U = \frac{1}{2} P_1 y_1 + \frac{1}{2} P_2 y_2 + \frac{1}{2} P_3 y_3 \qquad \text{...(1)}$$

Now, if the load P_1 is increased by a small amount δP_1 then the deflection at 1, 2, 3 will be increased by $\delta y_1, \delta y_2, \delta y_3 \dots$

∴   Extra work done at $1 = \left(\dfrac{P_1 + P_1 + \delta P_1}{2} \right) \cdot \delta y_1 = \left(P_1 + \dfrac{1}{2} \delta P_1 \right) \cdot \delta y_1$

$$= P_1 \cdot \delta y_1 \qquad \text{(Neglecting smaller quantity)}$$

Extra work done at $2 = P_2 \cdot \delta y_2$

Extra work done at $3 = P_3 \cdot \delta y_3$

∴   Increase in strain energy $\delta U = $ Total extra work done

on $\delta U = P_1 \, \delta y_1 + P_2 \, \delta y_2 + P_3 \, \delta y_3 \qquad \text{...(2)}$

If the external loads $(P_1 + \delta P_1)$; P_2 and P_3 were applied gradually, the total strain energy would be

$$U + \delta U = \Sigma \left(\frac{1}{2} \times \text{load} \times \text{deflection} \right)$$

$$= \frac{1}{2}(P_1 + \delta P_1)(y_1 + \delta y_1) + \frac{1}{2} P_2 (y_2 + \delta y_2) + \frac{1}{2} P_3 (y_3 + \delta y_3) + \dots$$

$$= \left(\frac{1}{2} P_1 y_1 + \frac{1}{2} P_1 \delta y_1 + \frac{1}{2} \delta P_1 \cdot y_1 \right) + \left(\frac{1}{2} P_2 y_2 + \frac{1}{2} P_2 \delta y_2 \right)$$

$$+ \left(\frac{1}{2} P_3 y_3 + \frac{1}{2} P_2 \delta y_3 \right) \qquad \text{(Neglecting small quantities)}$$

$$= \left(\frac{1}{2} P_1 y_1 + \frac{1}{2} P_2 y_2 + \frac{1}{2} P_3 y_3 \right) + \left(\frac{1}{2} P_1 \delta y_1 + \frac{1}{2} P_2 \delta y_2 + \frac{1}{2} P_3 \delta y_3 \right)$$

$$+ \frac{1}{2} \delta P_1 \cdot y_1$$

$$= U + \frac{1}{2} \delta U + \frac{1}{2} \delta P_1 \, y_1 \qquad \text{[from equation (1) and (2)]}$$

Hence, $U + \delta U = U + \dfrac{1}{2} \delta U + \dfrac{1}{2} \delta P_1 \, y_1$ ...(2)

or, $\dfrac{1}{2} \delta U = \dfrac{1}{2} \delta P_1 \, y_1$

or, $\delta U = \delta P_1 \cdot y_1$

$\therefore \qquad y_1 = \left(\dfrac{\delta U}{\delta P_1} \right)$

In the limit if $\delta P_1 \to 0$

$$\frac{\partial U}{\partial P_1} = y_1$$

Similarly, $\dfrac{\partial U}{\partial P_2} = y_2$

In general $\dfrac{\partial U}{\partial P_i} = y_i$ which is the Castigliano's Theorem.

Castigliano's Theorem can also be applied to determine angular rotation (θ) under the action of bending moment or torque.

Like above we can show that

$$\frac{\partial U}{\partial M_i} = \theta_i$$

13.9 DEFLECTION AND ROTATION OF ELASTIC BODIES UNDER VARIOUS TYPE OF LOADING

(a) Deflection under axial load

Strain Energy under axial load P

$$U = \frac{1}{2} \int \frac{P^2 dx}{AE}$$

$\therefore \qquad \delta = \left(\dfrac{\partial U}{\partial P} \right) = \dfrac{\partial}{\partial P} (U) = \displaystyle\int \dfrac{P \cdot dx}{A \cdot E}$

(b) Deflection under bending

Strain Energy under bending moment M

$$U = \int \frac{M^2 dx}{2EI}$$

$\therefore \qquad \delta = \dfrac{\partial U}{\partial P}$

$$\delta = \frac{\partial U}{\partial M} \times \frac{\partial M}{\partial P}$$

$$= \int \frac{M}{EI} dx \times \frac{\partial M}{\partial P}$$

$$= \int \frac{M}{EI} \cdot \frac{\partial M}{\partial P} \cdot dx$$

(c) Rotation under torsion

Strain energy under torque T

$$U = \int \frac{T^2 dx}{2GJ}$$

$$\therefore \qquad \theta = \left(\frac{\partial U}{\partial T} \right)$$

$$= \int \frac{T dx}{GJ}$$

(d) Rotation under bending

$$U = \int \frac{M^2 dx}{2EI}$$

$$\therefore \qquad \phi = \frac{\partial U}{\partial M}$$

$$= \int \frac{M dx}{2EI}$$

(e) Deflection under torsion

$$U = \int \frac{T^2 dx}{2GJ}$$

$$\therefore \qquad \delta = \frac{\partial U}{\partial P}$$

$$= \frac{\partial U}{\partial T} \times \frac{\partial T}{\partial P}$$

$$= \int \frac{T dx}{GJ} \cdot \frac{\partial T}{\partial P}$$

$$= \int \frac{T}{GJ} \cdot \frac{\partial T}{\partial P} \cdot dx$$

(f) Deflection under shear

Strain Energy under Shear Force F

$$U = \int \frac{F^2 dx}{2AG}$$

$$\therefore \quad \delta = \frac{\partial U}{\partial F}$$

$$= \int \frac{F dx}{A \cdot G}$$

EXAMPLE 1 *Find the deflection at the Free end of a Cantilever of Span L, carrying u.d.l of intensity w per unit run over the entire span using strain energy method.*
SOLUTION Let us consider an imaginary load P at the Free end B.

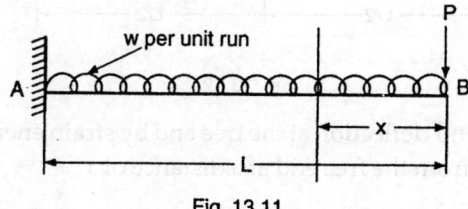

Fig. 13.11

Then, $B.M$ at a distance x from free end

$$M(x) = -\left(\frac{wx^2}{2} + P \cdot x \right)$$

$$\therefore \quad \frac{\partial M_x}{\partial P} = -x$$

Now, applying Castigliano's Theorem
Deflection at free end of the Cantilever

$$y_B = \frac{1}{EI} \int_0^L M_x \cdot \frac{\partial M_x}{\partial P} \cdot dx$$

$$= \frac{1}{EI} \int_0^L \left(-\frac{wx^2}{2} - P \cdot x \right) \cdot (-x) \, dx$$

$$= \frac{1}{EI} \int_0^L \left(\frac{wx^3}{2} + Px \right) dx$$

$$= \frac{1}{EI} \left[\frac{wx^4}{8} + \frac{P \cdot x^2}{2} \right]_0^L$$

$$= \frac{1}{EI} \left[\frac{wL^4}{8} + \frac{P \cdot L^2}{2} \right]$$

As the load is fictitions (Imaginary) so putting $P = 0$

$$y_B = \frac{1}{EI}\left[\frac{wL^4}{8}\right]$$

EXAMPLE 2 *A Cantilever of length L carries a point load W at its free end. The member is circular section having diameter D for a distance* $\left(\dfrac{L}{2}\right)$ *from the fixed end and a diameter* $\dfrac{D}{2}$ *for the remaining length. Find the deflection at the free end.*

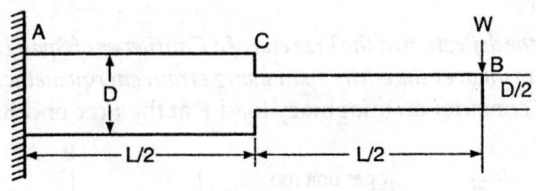

Fig. 13.12

SOLUTION We will find deflection at the free end by strain energy method.
Let us take a section from the free end at a distance of x.

Then, $U = \int_0^L \dfrac{M^2 dx}{2EI}$ where x is measured from B.

For BC Portion, $I_{BC} = \dfrac{\pi}{64}\left(\dfrac{D}{2}\right)^4$

$$= \frac{\pi D^4}{64 \times 16}$$

For CA Portion, $I_{CA} = \dfrac{\pi}{64} \times D^4$

Now if $I_{BC} = I$

$\quad I_{CA} = 16I$

$\therefore\quad U = \int_0^{L/2} \dfrac{M_x^2 \cdot dx}{2\,EI} + \int_{L/2}^{L} \dfrac{M_x^2 \cdot dx}{2\,E\cdot(16I)}$

Now, $U_{BC} = \int_0^{L/2} \dfrac{(-W \cdot x)^2\, dx}{2\,EI}$

$$= \frac{W^2}{2\,EI}\left[\frac{x^3}{3}\right]_0^{L/2}$$

$$= \frac{W^2 L^3}{48\,EI}$$

$$U_{CA} = \int_{L/2}^{L} \frac{(-W \cdot x)^2\, dx}{2E(16I)}$$

$$= \frac{W^2}{32EI}\left[\frac{x^3}{3}\right]_{L/2}^{L}$$

$$= \frac{7W^2L^3}{96 \times 8EI}$$

$$\therefore \quad U = U_{BC} + U_{CA}$$

$$= \frac{W^2L^3}{48EI} + \frac{7W^2L^3}{96 \times 8EI}$$

$$= \frac{23}{768} \cdot \frac{W^2L^3}{EI}$$

Now, work done by load $W = \dfrac{1}{2} \times W \times Y_B$

By equating these two

$$\frac{1}{2}W \cdot Y_B = \frac{23}{768} \cdot \frac{W^2L^3}{EI}$$

$$\therefore \qquad Y_B = \frac{23}{384} \cdot \frac{WL^3}{EI} \quad \textbf{Ans.}$$

EXAMPLE 3 *Derive the expression for deflection of the beam at the free end. The beam is uniform having flexural rigidity EI.*

SOLUTION

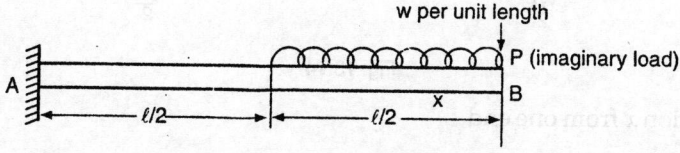

Fig. 13..13

Applying an imaginary load at free end, we have

$$M(x) = P \cdot x + w \cdot \frac{x^2}{2}$$

Applying Castigliano's Theorem

$$\frac{\partial M}{\partial P} = x$$

Deflection at free end of the cantilever

$$y_B = \frac{1}{EI} \int_0^{l/2} \left(Px + \frac{wx^2}{2} \right) x \, dx$$

$$= \frac{1}{EI} \int_0^{l/2} \left(P \cdot x^2 + \frac{wx^3}{2} \right) dx$$

$$= \frac{1}{EI} \left[\frac{Px^2}{3} + \frac{wx^4}{8} \right]_0^{l/2}$$

Since, we have applied imaginary load at free end which is not given in the question so making $P = 0$, we have

$$y_B = \frac{1}{EI} \times \frac{W}{8} \left(\frac{l}{2} \right)^4$$

$$= \frac{1}{EI} \times \frac{Wl^4}{8 \times 16}$$

$$= \frac{1}{EI} \frac{Wl^4}{128} \qquad \textbf{Ans.}$$

EXAMPLE 4 *Derive the expression for strain energy of a simply supported beam with U.D.L w per unit length by Castigliano's Theorem.*
SOLUTION

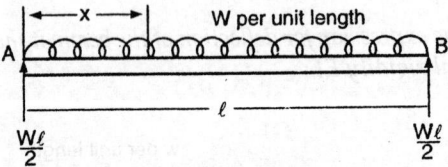

Fig. 13.14

At any section x from one end

$$M(x) = \left(\frac{wl}{2} x - \frac{wx^2}{2} \right)$$

Hence, strain energy $(U) = \int_0^l \frac{M^2 dx}{2EI}$

$$= \int_0^l \left(\frac{wl}{2} x - \frac{wx^2}{2} \right)^2 \cdot \frac{1}{2EI} dx$$

$$= \frac{w^2}{8EI} \int_0^l (lx - x^2)^2 \, dx$$

$$= \frac{w^2}{8EI} \int_0^l \left[l^2 x^2 + x^4 - 2lx^3 \right] dx$$

$$= \frac{w^2}{8EI} \left[\frac{l^5}{3} + \frac{l^5}{5} - \frac{2l^5}{4} \right]$$

$$= \frac{w^2 l^5}{8EI} \left[\frac{20 + 12 - 30}{60} \right]$$

$$= \frac{w^2 l^5}{240 \, EI} \qquad \textbf{Ans.}$$

EXAMPLE 5 *Derive the expression for strain energy when a beam is simply supported with concentrated load or point load any where on the span.*

SOLUTION

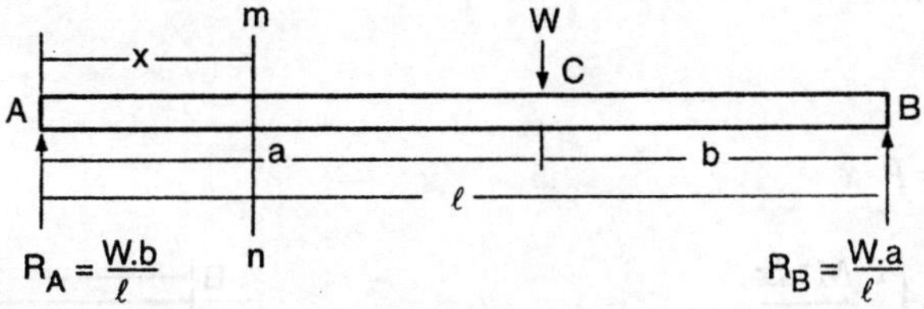

Fig. 13.15

Let us consider a section mn at a distance $'x'$ from end A.

$$M(x) = \left(\frac{w.b}{l} \right) \cdot x$$

and for portion CB of the beam $M(x) = \frac{wa}{l}(l - x)$

Total strain energy $(U) = U_{AC} + U_{CB}$

$$= \int_0^a \left(\frac{Wbx}{l} \right)^2 \cdot \frac{1}{2EI} \, dx + \int_a^l \left\{ \frac{Wa(l - x)}{l} \right\}^2 \cdot \frac{1}{2EI} \, dx$$

$$= \frac{W^2 b^2}{2EI \, l^2} \int_0^a x^2 dx + \frac{W^2 a^2}{2EI \, l^2} \int_a^l (l - x)^2 \, dx$$

$$= \frac{W^2 b^2}{2EI \, l^2} \left[\frac{x^3}{3} \right]_0^a + \frac{W^2 a^2}{2EI \, l^2} \left[\frac{(l - x)^3}{-3} \right]_a^l$$

$$= \frac{W^2 b^2 a^3}{6EI\, l^2} + \frac{W^2 a^2}{6EI\, l^2}(l-a)^3$$

$$= \frac{W^2 b^2 a^3}{6EI l^2} + \frac{W^2 a^2 b^3}{6EI\, l^2} \qquad [\because l-a=b]$$

$$= \frac{W^2 b^2 a^2}{6EI l^2}\,(a+b)$$

$$= \frac{W^2 b^2 a^2}{6EI l} \qquad \textbf{Ans.} \qquad [a+b=l]$$

N.B: When the load is at the centre then $a = b = \dfrac{l}{2}$

and
$$U = \frac{w^2 \left(\dfrac{l}{2}\right)^2 \left(\dfrac{l}{2}\right)^2}{6EI l} = \frac{w^2 l^3}{96EI}$$

EXAMPLE 6 *Find the strain energy stored by the structure shown in the figure and hence determine the vertical deflection of end A. Assume that the member is of uniform cross section throughout.*

SOLUTION

For section AB,

$$M(x) = P \cdot x$$

$\therefore \qquad U_{AB} = \int_0^l \frac{M^2 dx}{2EI}$

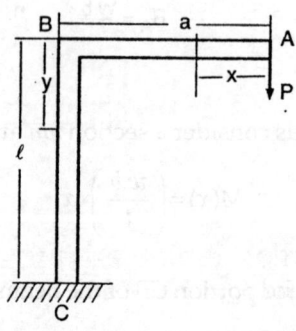

Fig. 13.16

$$= \int_0^a \frac{P^2 x^2 dx}{2EI}$$

$$= \frac{P^2}{2EI}\left[\frac{x^3}{3}\right]_0^a$$

$$= \frac{P^2 a^3}{6EI}$$

For section BC

$$U_{BC} = \int_0^l \frac{M^2 dy}{2EI}$$

$$= \int_0^a \frac{P^2 a^2 dy}{2EI}$$

$$= \frac{P^2 a^2 l}{2EI}$$

$\therefore$ Total strain energy $(U) = U_{AB} + U_{BC}$

$$= \frac{P^2 a^2}{6EI} + \frac{P^2 a^2 l}{2EI}$$

$$= \frac{P^2 a^2}{6EI}(a+3l)$$

Let δ_A = deflection at A

Then, WD by P = Total strain energy stored.

$$\frac{1}{2} \cdot P \cdot \delta_A = \frac{P^2 a^2}{6EI}(a+3l)$$

$\therefore$ $\delta A = \dfrac{Pa^2}{3EI}(a+3l)$ **Ans.**

EXAMPLE 7 *A circular bar ABC of diameter 'd' bent at B as shown in figure through a right angle, is held in x-y plane and fixed at end A.*

A vertical load P is applied parallel to z-axis at end C. Length AB = a and BC = b.

Determine the total strain energy and deflection. E and G are Young's Modulus and Shear modulus of the material respectively. Neglect S.F. energy.

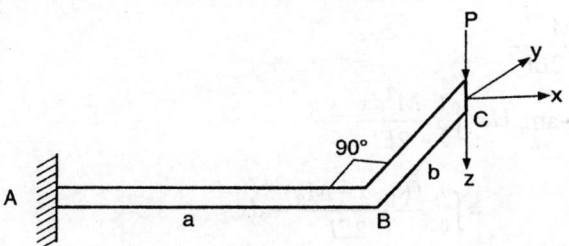

Fig. 13.17

SOLUTION Portion AB of bar is subjected to torsion $P.b$ and a cantilever load P at free end whereas BC acts as a cantilever with load P at free end and fixed at B.

Hence, strain energy $= U_{AB}$ (Cantilever) $+ U_{AB}$ (Torque) $+ U_{BC}$ (Cantilever)

$$U = \frac{P^2 a^3}{6EI} + \frac{T^2 a}{2GI_p} + \frac{P^2 b^3}{6EI}$$

where, $T = P \cdot b$

$\therefore$ $U = \dfrac{P^2 a^3}{6EI} + \dfrac{P^2 b^2 a}{2GI_p} + \dfrac{P^2 b^3}{6EI}$

Now, $I = \dfrac{\pi}{64} d^4 ; I_p = \dfrac{\pi}{32} d^4$

$\therefore$ $U = \dfrac{32P^2}{\pi d^2}\left(\dfrac{a^3}{3E}+\dfrac{ab^2}{2G}+\dfrac{b^3}{3E}\right)$ **Ans.**

Now, $\delta = \left(\dfrac{\partial U}{\partial P}\right)$

$= \dfrac{64P}{\pi d^4}\left(\dfrac{a^3}{3E}+\dfrac{ab^2}{2G}+\dfrac{b^3}{3E}\right)$ **Ans.**

EXAMPLE 8 *Using Castigleano's theorem determine the reaction at the support for the beam shown in Fig. 13.18.*

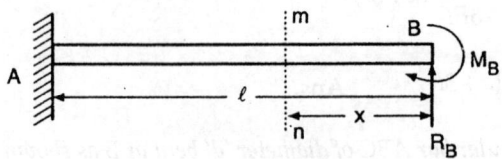

Fig. 13.18

SOLUTION Here $M(x) = R_B \cdot x - M_B$

Strain energy when load is in the form of moment is

$$U = \int \dfrac{M^2 dx}{2EI}$$

For the given beam, $U = \displaystyle\int_0^l \dfrac{M^2 dx}{2EI}$

$$= \int_0^l \dfrac{(R_B \cdot x - M_B)^2}{2EI}\,dx$$

$$= \dfrac{1}{2EI}\int_0^l (R_B^2 \cdot x^2 + M_B^2 - 2R_B \cdot x \cdot M_B)\,dx$$

By Castigliano's theorem, deflection at B, $\delta_B = \dfrac{\partial U}{\partial R_B} = 0$

Also, $\delta_B = \dfrac{\partial U}{\partial M} = 0$

But, since R_B is to be evaluated.

So, omitting the second one

$\therefore$ $\displaystyle\int_0^l (2R_B x^2 - 2x\,M_B)\,dx = 0$

or, $2R_B \dfrac{l^3}{3} - 2M_B \dfrac{l^2}{2} = 0$

$\therefore$ $R_B = \dfrac{3M_B}{2l}\uparrow$ **Ans.**

13.10 MAXWELL'S RECIPROCAL THEOREM

Reciprocal theorem apply only to linear elastic structures i.e., structures for which the principle of superposition is valid.

Two basic conditions must be satisfied:

1. The material must follow Hook's Law.
2. The displacement must be small enough so that all calculations can be based upon the undeformed geometry of the structure.

We will adopt the concepts of work and strain energy to derive the theorem.

Reciprocal displacement theorem — Introduction

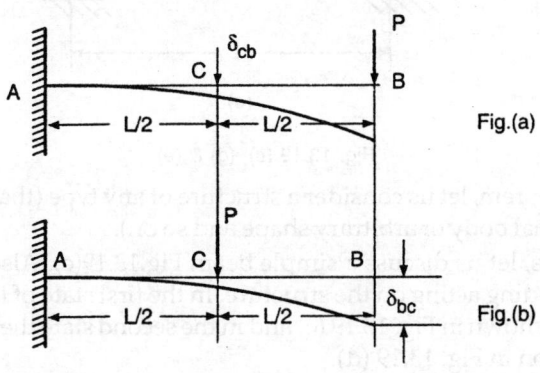

Fig. 13.19 (a) & (b)

Let us take as an example of a cantilever beam AB subjected to a concentrated load P at the free end B as shown in Fig. 13.19 (a). We can obtain the deflection at the mid-point C of this beam.

Thus $\qquad \delta_{cb} = \dfrac{5PL^3}{48EL}$ $\qquad\qquad$ (by deflection of beam formula)

The first subscript notation used with the symbol δ denotes the point at which deflection occurs and the second subscript denotes the point at which load is applied. Thus, the symbol δ_{cb} identifies the deflection of point C caused by a load acting at point B.

Now, let the same cantilever beam subjected to a load P acting at the mid-point C as shown in Fig. 13.19 (b). In this case, we wish to find the deflection at the free end B denoted by symbol δ_{bc}.

Thus $\qquad \delta_{bc} = \dfrac{5PL^3}{48EI}$ $\qquad\qquad$ (by deflection of beam formula)

Thus, we observe that the deflection at C due to load acting at B is equal to the deflection at B due to the load acting at C. This statement is an example of the **Maxwell's reciprocal displacement theorem**.

Proof of Maxwell's Reciprocal-displacement Theorem

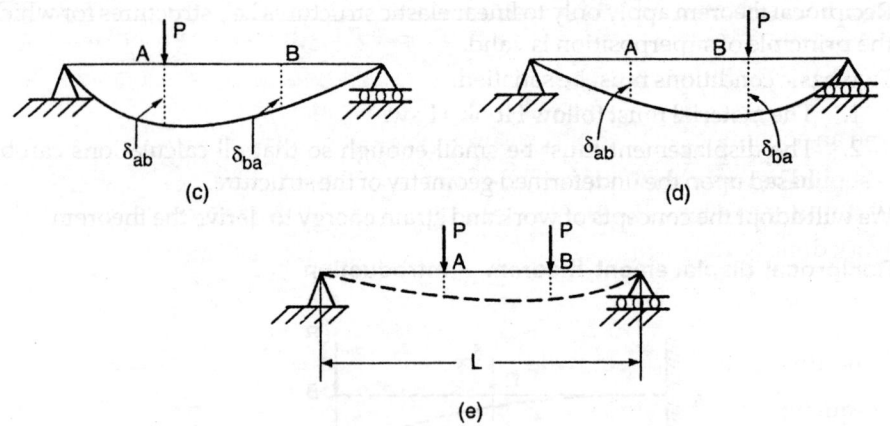

Fig. 13.19 (c), (d) & (e)

To prove the theorem, let us consider a structure of any type (that is a truss beam, three dimensional body of arbitrary shape and so on).

For convenience, let us discuss a simple beam Fig.13.19(c). Also let us consider two states of loading acting on the structure. In the first state of loading, a force P acts at point As shown in Fig. 13.19 (c) and in the second state the same load P acts at point B as shon in Fig. 13.19 (d).

The deflection at A and B for the first state of loading are denoted by δ_{ab} and δ_{ba} respectively in accordance with the subscript notation already discussed. The deflections for the second state of loading are identified as δ_{ab} and δ_{ba}.

Now, let us consider that both loads P acts simultaneously on the beam as shown in Fig. 13.19 (e).

If the material of the beam is linearly elastic and the deflections are small, we can use the principle of superposition to obtain the deflection of the beam.

The deflection corresponding to load P acting at A is $\left(\delta_{aa} + \delta_{ab} \right)$ and the deflection corresponding to the load P acting at B is $\left(\delta_{ba} + \delta_{bb} \right)$.

Knowing these deflections we can calculate the work done by the two loads P as these are slowly and simultaneously applied to the beam.

This work done is equal to the total strain energy U of the beam.

$$U = \frac{1}{2} P \left(\delta_{aa} + \delta_{ab} \right) + \frac{1}{2} P \left(\delta_{ba} + \delta_{bb} \right) \quad ...(a) \quad \text{[By Clapeyron's Theorem]}$$

The total strain energy of the beam subjected to two loads does not depend on the order in which the two loads are applied. Because the beam behaves linearly, the strain energy must be same when the two loads are applied simultaneously.

Let us assume that the load at A is applied first followed by B. Then the strain energy of the beam during the application of the first load is

$$\frac{1}{2} P \, \delta_{aa} \qquad\qquad\qquad\qquad\qquad ...(b)$$

when the second load is applied, an additional deflection results at B equal to δ_{bb}, hence, the second load does work equal to

$$\frac{1}{2} P \cdot \delta_{bb} \qquad \qquad \ldots \text{(c)}$$

and an equal amount of strain energy is developed in the beam.

It should be remembered that while the load at B is being applied, the load acting at A undergoes an additional deflection δ_{ab} and the corresponding amount of work done by that load is

$$P \cdot \delta_{ab} \qquad \qquad \ldots \text{(d)}$$

Thus, this additional strain energy is proceduced. Here, factor $\left(\dfrac{1}{2}\right)$ is not used as in equation (d) because the load P remains constant during the time, the additional deflection δ_{ab} occurs.

Adding (b), (c) and (d) we get the total strain energy for the case when one load is applied before the other.

$$U = \frac{1}{2} P \cdot \delta_{aa} + \frac{1}{2} P \cdot \delta_{bb} + P \cdot \delta_{ab} \qquad \qquad \ldots \text{(e)}$$

This amount of strain energy must be equal to the strain energy produced when the two loads are applied simultaneously, equation (a).

From eqns. (a) and (e), we get

$$\frac{1}{2} P (\delta_{aa} + \delta_{ab}) + \frac{1}{2} P (\delta_{ba} + \delta_{bb}) = \frac{1}{2} P \cdot \delta_{aa} + \frac{1}{2} P \cdot \delta_{bb} + P \cdot \delta_{ab}$$

or, $\delta_{aa} + \delta_{ab} + \delta_{ba} + \delta_{bb} = \delta_{aa} + \delta_{bb} + 2\, \delta_{ab}$

or, $\delta_{ba} = \delta_{ab}$

or, $\delta_{ab} = \delta_{ba}$

This equation represents the **Maxwell's reciprocal displacement theorem** which may he stated, as follows:

The deflection at A due to a load acting at B is equal to the deflection at B due to the same load acting at A.

The reciprocal displacement theorem is also applicable if one load is a force and the other is couple or if both loads are couples.

Consider again a simple beam subjected to two states of loading as shown below in Fig. 13.19 (f).

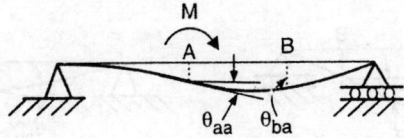

Fig. 13.19 (f)

The first state of loading consists of a couple M acting at point A, as shown in Fig. 13.19 (f).

The displacement corresponding to M is the angle of rotation θ_{aa} and in the second state of loading it is angle θ_{ab}.

In the second loading, the force P acting at B as shown in Fig. 13.19 (g).

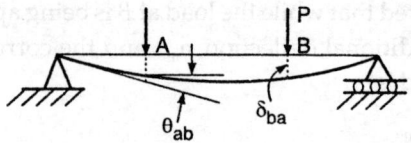

Fig. 13.19 (g)

Repeating the steps like earlier derivation, we get the following expression for the strain energy of the beam when loads M and P are applied simultaneously.

$$U = \frac{1}{2}M(\theta_{aa} + \theta_{ab}) + \frac{1}{2}P(\delta_{ba} + \delta_{bb})$$

When the couple M is applied first, followed by the force P, then the strain energy is

$$U = \frac{1}{2}M\,\theta_{aa} + \frac{1}{2}P\,\delta_{bb} + M\,\theta_{ab}$$

Equating these two expressions for strain energy yields

$$M \cdot \theta_{ab} = P \cdot \delta_{ba}$$

If the load M and P are numerically equal then $\theta_{ab} = \delta_{ba}$, also, the loads will the numerically equal. Therefore, for this case we may state the reciprocal displacement theorem as follows:

The angle of rotation at A due to a force acting at B is equal numerically to the deflection at B due to a couple load acting at A, if force and couples are numerically equal.

If both loads acting on the structure consists of couple M, then, we find

$$\theta_{ab} = \theta_{ba}$$

In this case the theorem is as follows:

The angle of rotation at A due to a couple acting at B is equal to the angle of rotation at B due to the same couple acting at A.

The positive sense of the angles are understood to be the same as the positive sense of the corresponding couples.

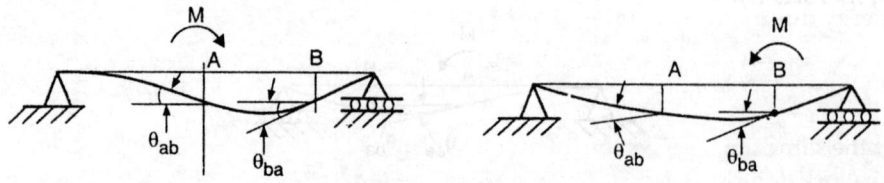

Fig. 13.20

This theorem was first derived by J.C. Maxweil and is often called **Maxwell's Reciprocal theorem.**

Reciprocal Work Theorem

To derive the theorem, let us consider any linear elastic body for which principle of superposition holds as shown in Fig. 13.21.

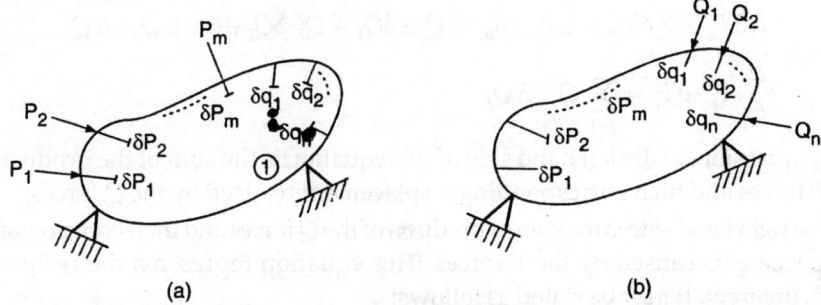

(a)

(b)

Fig. 13.21

The body could represent a beam, truss, frame or other kind of structure. Two states of loading on the structure must be considered.

In the first state as shown in Fig. 13.21 (a) there are m loads $P_1, P_2,...P_m$ and in the second state as in Fig. 13.21 (b) there are n loads $Q_1, Q_2...Q_n$.

To derive the reciprocal work theorem, we use the same ideas about strain energy which we have used in driving the reciprocal displacement theorem. If both load system P and Q are applied simultaneously to the body, the strain energy (equal to the work done by the forces) is

$$U = \frac{1}{2}P_1\left(\delta P_1 + \delta'P_1\right) + \frac{1}{2}P_2\left(\delta P_2 + \delta'P_2\right) + ... + \frac{1}{2}P_m\left(\delta P_m + \delta'P_m\right)$$

$$+\frac{1}{2}Q_1\left(\delta Q_1 + \delta'Q_1\right) + \frac{1}{2}Q_2\left(\delta Q_2 + \delta'Q_2\right) + ... + \frac{1}{2}Q_n\left(\delta Q_n + \delta'Q_n\right) \quad ...(1)$$

This strain energy must be the same as the strain energy obtained when we apply first the entire P-load system and then the entire Q-load system.

When the loads P are applied alone, the strain energy is

$$\frac{1}{2}P_1\,\delta P_1 + \frac{1}{2}P_2\delta P_2 + ... + \frac{1}{2}P_m\cdot\delta P_m \qquad ...(2)$$

When the second set of loads is applied, we get the following amount of strain energy due to the work done by the loads Q,

$$\frac{1}{2}Q_1\cdot\delta'Q_1 + \frac{1}{2}Q_2\cdot\delta'Q_2 + ... + \frac{1}{2}Q_n\cdot\delta'Q_n \qquad ...(3)$$

At the same time, we get the following additional amount of strain energy due to the work done by the loads P.

$$P_1 \cdot \delta' P_1 + P_2 \cdot \delta' P_2 + \dots + P_m \cdot \delta' P_m \qquad \dots(4)$$

Therefore, total strain energy (when the loads P are applied first, followed by the loads Q) is the sum of expressions (2), (3) and (4).

Equating this sum with the strain energy due to simultaneous application of loads (as in equation 1) gives.

$$P_1 \delta' P_1 + P_2 \delta' P_2 + \dots P_m \cdot \delta'_m = Q_1 \cdot \delta Q_1 + Q_2 \, \delta Q_2 + \dots + Q_n \cdot \delta \, Q_n$$

or, $$\sum_{i=1}^{m} P_i \cdot \delta' P_i = \sum_{j=1}^{n} Q_j \cdot \delta \, Q_j$$

The expression on the left hand side of this equation is the sum of the products of the P forces and their corresponding displacements caused by the Q forces.

On the right hand side is the sum of products of the Q forces and their corresponding displacements caused by the P forces. This equation represents the **reciprocal work theorem.** It may be stated as follows:

"The work done by the forces in the first state of loading when they move through their corresponding displacements in the second state of loading is equal to the work done by the forces in the second state of loading when they move through their corresponding displacement in the first state of loading."

The reciprocal work theorem applies to both forces and couples.

The theorem was derived by **E.Betti** and **Lord Rayleigh** hence it is often called — The Betti-Rayleigh reciprocal theorem.

EXAMPLE *For a cantilever beam of length L with a point load at the free end the deflection equation is given as* $y = -\dfrac{P}{6EI}\left(2L^3 - 3L^2 x + x^3\right).$

Using Maxwell reciprocal theorem, determine the deflection at free end of the cantilever when a load N is applied at a distance 'b' from the free end

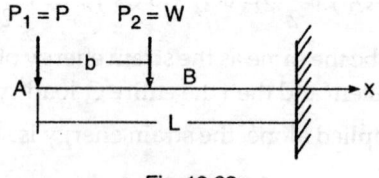

Fig. 13.22

SOLUTION From Maxwell reciprocal work theorem

$$P_1 \cdot \delta A_2 = P_2 \cdot \delta B_1$$

Here, $P_1 = P$

$P_2 = W$

$\delta B_1 = $ deflection at B due to P_1 at A (for point B, $x = b$).

$$= -\frac{P}{6EI}\left(2L^3 - 3L^3\,b + b^3\right)$$

From Maxwell reciprocal work theorem

$$\delta A_1 = \frac{P_2 \cdot \delta B_1}{P_1}$$

$$= \frac{W}{P}\left[-\frac{P}{6EI}\left(2L^3 - 3L^2 b + b^3\right)\right]$$

$$= -\frac{W}{6EI}\left(2L^3 - 3L^2 b + b^3\right).$$

The given problem can be solved by using Maxwell reciprocal displacement theorem as below:

Deflection at $B(x = b)$ due to load W at the free end A is given as

$$\delta B_1 = (-)\frac{W}{6EI}\left(2L^3 - 3L^2 b + b^3\right)$$

From Maxwell reciprocal displacement theorem

$$\delta A_1 = \delta B_1 \text{ when } P_1 = P_2 = W$$

$$\therefore \quad \delta A_1 = -\frac{W}{6EI}\left(2L^3 - 3L^2 b + b^3\right).$$

HIGHLIGHTS

1. All the work performed during elastic deformation is stored and recovered on the release of loads. This recoverable stored energy in an elastic body is called the elastic strain energy.

2. Resilience is the total energy stored in the body. Resilience is also defined as the capacity of a strained body for doing work after the removal of the straining force.

3. Strain energy due to

   (a) Axial loading

   $$U = \frac{1}{2}\cdot\frac{P^2 L}{AE} = \frac{1}{2}\times\frac{\sigma^2}{E}\times \text{Volume of bar}$$

   (b) Shear

   $$U = \frac{\tau^2}{2G}\times V$$

   (c) Torsional loading

   $$U = \frac{T^2 L}{2\cdot G\cdot I_p} \text{ when torque } (T) \text{ is constant.}$$

   when torque (T) varies then $U = \int\frac{T^2\cdot L}{2G\cdot I_p}$

   (d) Pure bending

   $$U = \frac{M^2 L}{2EI} \text{ when } M \text{ is constant}$$

   when bending moment (M) varies then, $U = \int\frac{M^2 L}{2EI}$

PROBLEMS FOR PRACTICE
(THEORETICAL)

1. Define resilience, proof resilience and modulus of resilience.
2. Derive expression for the strain energy stored in a body when:
   (a) load is applied gradually along the axis
   (b) load applied tangentially parallel to the surface.
3. Prove that strain energy stored in a body due to shear stress is given by

$$U = \frac{\tau^2}{2C} \times V$$

4. Prove that when shaft of length l and diameter 'd' is subjected to torque T (variable), then

$$U = \int \frac{T^2 l}{2G \cdot I_p}$$

5. State and prove Maxwell's Reciprocal Theorem.

(NUMERICAL)

1. Using Castigliano's theorem determine the deflection at point C in the beam as shown in figure.

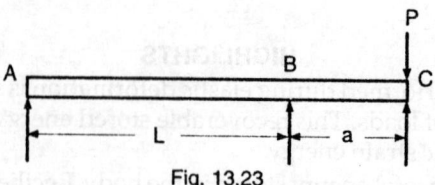

Fig. 13.23

2. Determine the deflection at C of the eleastic frame having flexural rigidity EI throughout.

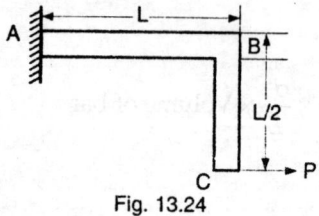

Fig. 13.24

3. A curved member is loaded as shown in figure. Determine the horizontal and vertical displacement of the loaded end.

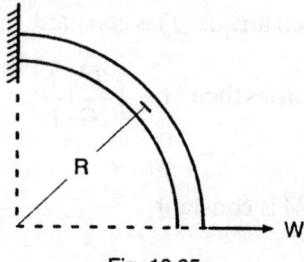

Fig. 13.25

ANSWERS

1. $\delta_C = \dfrac{Pa^2(L+a)}{3\,EI}$ 2. $\dfrac{7}{24} \cdot \dfrac{PL^3}{EI}$ 3. $\delta_h = \dfrac{\pi}{4} \dfrac{WR^3}{EI}$; $\delta_V = \dfrac{WR^3}{2\,EI}$

OBJECTIVE QUESTIONS

1. The strain energy stored in a beam subjected to bending moment M is:

   (a) $\int \dfrac{M^2 dx}{EI}$ (b) $\int \dfrac{M^2 dx}{2\,EI}$ (c) $\int \dfrac{M^2 dx}{3\,EI}$ (d) $\int \dfrac{M^2 dx}{4\,EI}$

2. A material of Young's modulus E and Poisson's ratio v is subjected to two principal stresses σ_1 and σ_2 at a point in a two-dimensional stress-system. The strain energy per unit volume of the material is:

   (a) $\dfrac{1}{2E}\left[\sigma_1^2 + \sigma_2^2 - 2v\,\sigma_1\,\sigma_2\right]$ (b) $\dfrac{1}{2E}\left[\sigma_1^2 + \sigma_2^2 + 2\,\sigma_1\,\sigma_2\,v\right]$

   (c) $\dfrac{1}{2E}\left[\sigma_1^2 - \sigma_2^2 + 2v\sigma_1\,\sigma_2\right]$ (d) $\dfrac{1}{2E}\left[\sigma_1^2 - \sigma_2^2 - 2v\sigma_1\,\sigma_2\right]$

3. Energy stored in a unit volume of the elastic body is called:
   (a) proof resilience   (b) modulus of resilience
   (c) strain energy density   (d) none of the above

4. The area between the load extension curve and extension axis is called:
   (a) strain energy   (b) complementary energy
   (c) proof resilience   (d) none of the above

5. Two shafts of solid circular cross-section are identical except their diameters d_1 and d_2. They are subjected to same torque T. The ratio of strain energies stored U_1/U_2 will be:

   (a) $\left(\dfrac{d_1}{d_2}\right)^4$ (b) $\left(\dfrac{d_1}{d_2}\right)^2$ (c) $\left(\dfrac{d_2}{d_1}\right)^2$ (d) $\left(\dfrac{d_2}{d_1}\right)^4$

6. A simply supported beam of span 'l' and flexural rigidity EI carries a point load at its centre. The strain energy in the beam due to bending is:

   (a) $\dfrac{l^3}{48\,EI}$ (b) $\dfrac{l^3}{192\,EI}$ (c) $\dfrac{l^3}{96\,EI}$ (d) $\dfrac{l^3}{16\,EI}$

7. If σ_p be the proof stress or maximum stress to which the bar is stressed upto the elastic limit, then modulus of resilience is equal to:

   (a) $\dfrac{\sigma_p}{2E}$ (b) $\dfrac{\sigma_p^2}{2E}$ (c) $\dfrac{\sigma_p^2}{4E}$ (d) $\dfrac{\sigma_p}{2E}$

8. The ratio of stress due to suddenly applied load to gradully applied load is equal to:

    (a) two   (b) three   (c) four   (d) five

9. The shearing strain energy for a block of material (per unit volume) subjected to a constant shearing stress throughout is given by:

    (a) $\dfrac{\tau^2}{G}$ (b) $\dfrac{\tau}{G^2}$ (c) $\dfrac{\tau^2}{2G}$ (d) $\dfrac{\tau^2}{G^2}$

10. Strain energy due to torsion is given by:

    (a) $U = \int \dfrac{T^2 dx}{2\,GJ}$ \qquad\qquad (b) $U = \int \dfrac{T\,dx}{2\,GJ}$

    (c) $U = \int \dfrac{T^2\,dx}{3\,GJ}$ \qquad\qquad (d) $U = \int \dfrac{T^2\,dx}{4\,GJ}$

ANSWERS

1. (b)	2. (a)	3. (a)	4. (c)	5. (d)	6. (c)
7. (b)	8. (a)	9. (c)	10. (a)		

— ❖❖ —

SPRINGS

14.1 INTRODUCTION

A spring is a device used to absorb 'or' store energy and release it when required.

— It is used in clock, shock Absorber, automobile etc. The spring in a mechanical clock absorbs energy when the clock is wound and the same energy is released to run the clock.

— The spring wire may be circular 'or' rectangular cross-section but circular section is frequently used.

— Rectangular sections are used in heavy duty springs.

The following types of springs are in use:

  (i) Leaf spring or laminated spring

 (ii) Helical spring

(iii) Flat spiral spring

Leaf Spring: Leaf spring is also known as carriage or bending spring. Leaf spring consist of a number of thin curved plates of uniform thicknesses but different lengths which are placed over each other and clamped together at the centre. This spring is used to absorb shocks in railway wagon, coaches and road vehicles (such as cars, lorries etc).

Helical Spring: The helical springs are formed by winding a wire around a cylindrical mandrel in the form of a helix. Shock absorber and Front axle suspension vehicles are helical springs. **Depending upon the magnitude of helix angle (α), the helical spring is further divided into close coiled and open coiled helical spring. In the case of close coiled spring, helix angle (α) is zero.**

Spiral Spring: Spiral spring consists of a flat strip of rectangular section wound in the form of a spiral and loaded in torsion.

Let us discuss few related terms associated with spring. They are following:

Resilience: Resilience of the spring is the total strain energy absorbed by it per unit volume.

Sprint Index (C): The spring index is defined as the ratio of the mean diameter of the coil to the diameter of the wire.

Mathematically, spring index (C) $= \left(\dfrac{D}{d}\right)$.

Spring Constant or Stiffness (K): It is defined as the load required per unit deflection of the spring.

$$K = \left(\dfrac{W}{\delta}\right), \text{ where } W \text{ load and } \delta = \text{deflection of spring.}$$

Proof Resilience: Proof resilience is the maximum resilience of the spring without the occurence of permanent deformation.

Proof load: Proof load is the maximum load to which the spring can be subjected without undergoing permanent deformation.

Proof Stress: Proof stress is the maximum stress to which the spring can be subjected without occurring permanent deformation.

Since leaf spring is a combination of flat springs so let us discuss first single leaf spring and the behaviour of load on the single leaf spring.

14.2 SINGLE LEAF SPRING

Let us consider a spring of constant width 'b' and thickness 't' and subjected to concentrated (W) load at the spring.

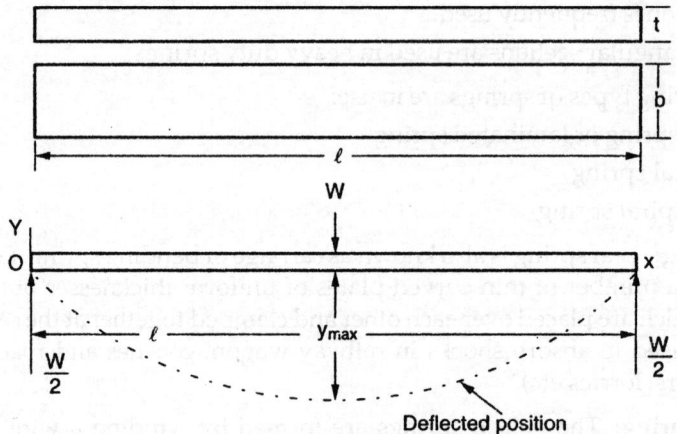

Fig. 14.1

The spring is simply supported.

Now, maximum bending stress $(\sigma_b) = \dfrac{M}{Z}$

$$= \dfrac{\dfrac{WL}{4}}{\dfrac{bt^2}{6}}$$

$$\boxed{\sigma_b = \frac{3}{2} \cdot \frac{Wl}{bt^2}} \qquad \qquad \dots(1)$$

Maximum deflection
(for simply supported beam) $(\delta) = \dfrac{Wl^3}{48EI}$

$$= \frac{Wl^3}{48E} \times \frac{12}{bt^3} \qquad \qquad \left[\because I = \frac{bt^3}{12}\right]$$

$\therefore \qquad \boxed{\delta = \dfrac{Wl^3}{4Ebt^3}}$

So, strain energy stored $(U) = \dfrac{1}{2} \cdot W \cdot \delta$

$$= \frac{1}{2} \times W \times \frac{Wl^3}{4Ebt^3} = \frac{1}{2} \times \frac{W^2 l^2}{4Ebt^3}$$

$$\boxed{U = \frac{W^2 l^3}{8Ebt^3}}$$

Laminated or Leaf spring (Semi-elliptical)

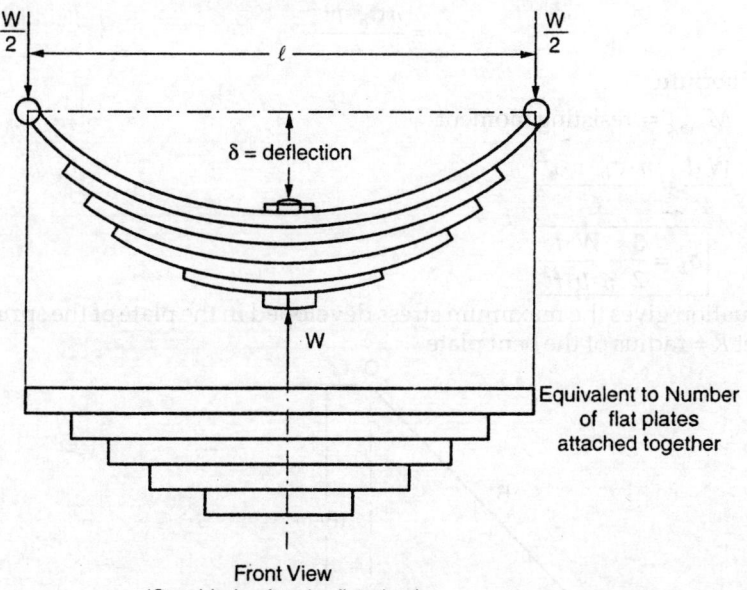

Front View
(Considering it to be flat plate)

Fig. 14.2

Let $\qquad b =$ width of each plate

$n =$ number of plate

$l =$ span of spring

$\sigma_b =$ maximum bending stress developed in the plates

$t =$ thickness of each plates

W = concentrated load acting at the centre of spring
δ = deflection at the top of spring

Now, $M_{max} = \dfrac{Wl}{4}$

MOI of each plate $= \dfrac{bt^3}{12}$

We know $\dfrac{M}{I} = \dfrac{\sigma_b}{y}$

$\therefore$ $M = \dfrac{\sigma_b \cdot I}{y}$

$ = \dfrac{\sigma_b}{y} \cdot I$

$ = \sigma_b \times \dfrac{1}{t/2} \times \dfrac{bt^3}{12}$

$ = \dfrac{\sigma_b \, bt^2}{6}$

Total resisting moment by 'n' plates $= n \times M$

$$= \dfrac{n\,\sigma_b \cdot bt^2}{6}$$

For equilibrium

M_{max} = resisting moment

$$\dfrac{W \cdot l}{4} = \dfrac{n \cdot \sigma_b \cdot b \cdot t^2}{6}$$

$\therefore$ $\boxed{\sigma_b = \dfrac{3}{2} \cdot \dfrac{W \cdot l}{n \cdot b \cdot t^2}}$ ...(2)

This equation gives the maximum stress developed in the plate of the spring.
Now, let R = radius of the bent plate

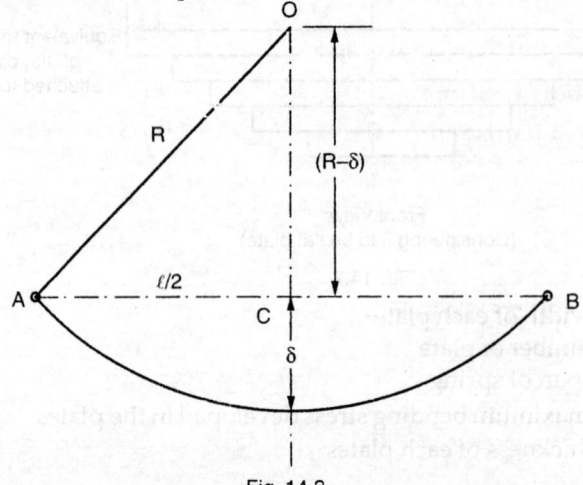

Fig. 14.3

From $\triangle OAC$,

$$AO^2 = AC^2 + CO^2$$

or, $$R^2 = \left(\frac{l}{2}\right)^2 + (R-\delta)^2$$

or, $$R^2 = \frac{l^2}{4} + R^2 + \delta^2 - 2R\delta$$

$\therefore$ $$2R\delta = \frac{l^2}{4}$$ $\left[\begin{array}{l}\text{As } \delta \text{ is small, its square will be}\\ \text{too small and hence neglected}\end{array}\right]$

$\therefore$ $$\delta = \left(\frac{l^2}{8R}\right)$$ ...(3)

From Bending of Beam formula.

$$\frac{\sigma_b}{y} = \frac{E}{R}$$

$\therefore$ $$R = \frac{E \cdot y}{\sigma_b}$$

$$= \left(\frac{E \cdot t}{2\sigma_b}\right)$$ $\left[\because y = \frac{t}{2}\right]$

Putting the value of R in eq. (3)

$$\boxed{\delta = \frac{l^2}{8} \times \frac{2\sigma_b}{E \cdot t} = \frac{\sigma_b \cdot l^2}{4Et}}$$ ... (4)

which is the Central deflection of spring.

Quarter Elliptical Leaf Spring

Let us consider quarter elliptical spring of length l subjected to load W at its free end.

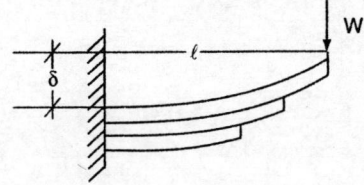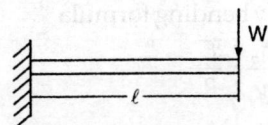

Fig. 14.4

Let l = span of spring

t = thickness of spring

b = width of spring

n = number of plate

σ_b = maximum bending stress induced in the plate

Now, bending moment due to load W

$$M = W \cdot l \qquad \qquad \qquad \dots (1)$$

Further, from bending formula

$$\frac{M}{I} = \frac{\sigma_b}{y}$$

$\therefore$ $$M = \frac{\sigma_b}{y} \times I$$

$$= \frac{\sigma_b}{\dfrac{t}{2}} \times \frac{bt^3}{12}$$

$$= \frac{\sigma_b \cdot t^2 \cdot b}{6}$$

Therefore, total moment of resistance of n number of plate

$$M = \frac{n\, \sigma_b \cdot b \cdot t^2}{6} \qquad \qquad \dots(2)$$

Equating (1) and (2), we get

$$\frac{n\, \sigma_b \cdot b \cdot t^2}{6} = W \cdot l$$

$\therefore$ $$\sigma_b = \frac{6\, W \cdot l}{n \cdot b \cdot t^2} \qquad \dots(3)$$

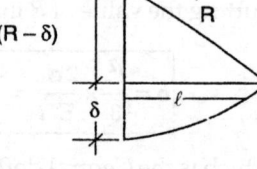

Fig. 14.5

Now, from figure $R^2 = l^2 + (R - \delta)^2$

$$R^2 = l^2 + R^2 - 2R\delta + \delta^2$$

Since δ is small so δ^2 may be neglected.

$\therefore$ $$2R\delta = l^2$$

$$\delta = \frac{l^2}{2R} \qquad \qquad \dots(4)$$

Further, by bending formula

$$\frac{\sigma_b}{y} = \frac{E}{R}$$

$\therefore$ $$\frac{1}{R} = \frac{\sigma_b}{E \cdot y} \qquad \qquad \dots (5)$$

Substituting the value of $\dfrac{1}{R}$ from eqn (5) in equation (4), we get

$$\delta = \frac{l^2}{2} \times \frac{\sigma_b}{E \cdot y}$$

$$= \frac{l^2}{2E \cdot \left(\dfrac{t}{2}\right)} \times \frac{6Wl}{n \cdot b \cdot t^2} \qquad \text{[Substituting the value of } \sigma_b \text{ from eqn (3)]}$$

$$\therefore \ \delta = \frac{6Wl^3}{n \cdot E \cdot b \cdot t^3}$$

14.3 HELICAL SPRING

Helical spring for heavy duty are the thick spring wire coiled in the form of helix.
The helical spring is of two types:

  (i) Closed Coiled helical spring

  (ii) Open Coiled helical spring

Close-Coiled Helical Springs

Close coiled helical springs are springs in which helix angle is very small and therefore the bending effect on the spring is ignored.

That is why close coiled spring is known as torsional spring.

Close-coiled Helical Spring Subjected to Axial Load

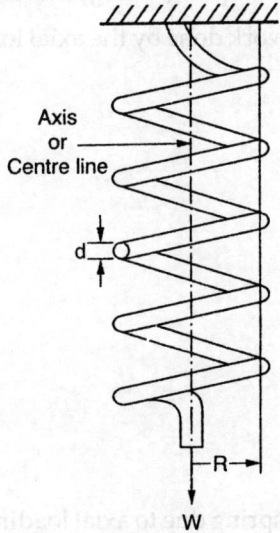

Axis
or
Centre line

Fig. 14.6

Let, l = Total length of the wire

r = Radius of the spring wire = $\left(\dfrac{d}{2}\right)$

R = Mean radius of the coil = $\left(\dfrac{D}{2}\right)$

n = No. of turns, or no. of coils

θ = Wind up angle for the whole length of the spring

Now, from torsion equation

$$\frac{T}{J} = \frac{G\theta}{l}$$

$$\theta = \frac{T \cdot l}{G \cdot J}$$

$$= \frac{(WR) \cdot l}{G \cdot \dfrac{\pi}{32} d^4}$$

$$= \frac{32\, WR \cdot 2\,\pi\, Rn}{G\,\pi\, d^4}$$

$$= \frac{64\, WR^2 n}{Gd^4}$$

When there is a twisting in the spring, energy stored in the spring, $(U) = \dfrac{1}{2} \cdot T \cdot \theta$

This energy is equal to the work done by the axial load W

$$\therefore \qquad \frac{1}{2} \times W \times \delta = \frac{1}{2}\, T\theta$$

$$\therefore \qquad \delta = \frac{T \cdot \theta}{W}$$

$$= \frac{WR\,\theta}{W}$$

$$= R \cdot \frac{64\, WR^2 n}{Gd^4}$$

$$\boxed{\delta = \frac{64\, WR^3 n}{Gd^4}}$$

This gives the deflection of spring due to axial loading W.

Stiffness of spring (k)

Load per unit axial deflection is known as stiffness of spring and denoted by letter k.

$$k = \frac{W}{\delta}$$

$$= \frac{W}{\dfrac{64\,WR^3 n}{Gd^4}}$$

$$= \frac{Gd^4}{64\,R^3 n}$$

Strain Energy (U): $\quad U = \dfrac{1}{2}\,W\delta$

$$= \frac{1}{2}\,T\theta$$

$$= \frac{1}{2} \times WR \times \frac{64\,WR^2 n}{Gd^4}$$

$$= \frac{1}{2} \times \frac{64\,W^2 R^3 n}{Gd^4}$$

Shear Stress (τ): $\quad \tau = \dfrac{T}{Z_t}$
$$\left[\begin{array}{l} Z_t = \text{Sectional Modulus of shaft in torsion} \\[2mm] \qquad = \left(\dfrac{J}{r_{max}}\right) = \dfrac{\pi\,d^3}{16} \end{array}\right]$$

$$= \frac{WR}{\dfrac{\pi}{16}\,d^3}$$

$$= \frac{16\,WR}{\pi d^3} = \frac{8\,WD}{\pi d^3}$$

In order to consider the effects of both direct shear as well as curvature of the wire, **Wahl's stress factor (k_w)** introduced by A.M. Wahl may be used.

Maximum Shear Stress induced in the wire

$$(\tau) = k_w \cdot \frac{16WR}{\pi d^3}$$

where, $\quad k_w = \dfrac{4C-1}{4C-4} + \dfrac{0.615}{C}$

where, $C = \left(\dfrac{P}{d}\right)$. Most machine have spring index (C) more than 3.

Closed-coiled Spring Subjected to Axial Torque T
(a) Maximum stress
In this case, the material of the spring is subjected to pure bending which tends to reduce the radius R of the coil. The bending moment is constant throughout the spring and equal to the applied torque T.

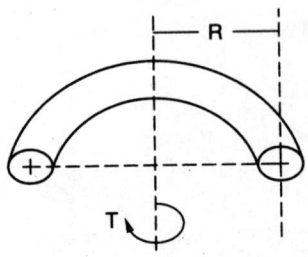

Fig. 14.7

The maximum bending stress $(\sigma_{max}) = \dfrac{M}{I} \cdot y$

$$= \dfrac{T \cdot r}{\dfrac{\pi r^4}{4}}$$

$$= \dfrac{4T}{\pi r^3}$$

$$= \dfrac{4T}{\pi \left(\dfrac{d}{2}\right)^3}$$

$$\boxed{\sigma_{max} = \dfrac{32T}{\pi d^3}}$$

(b) Deflection (Wind up Angle)

Under the action of an axial torque the deflection of the springs becomes the windup angle *i.e.*, the angle through which one end turns relative to the other. This will be equal to the total change of slope along the wire according to Mohr's area moment theorem, is the area of $\dfrac{M}{EI}$ diagram between the ends.

$$\theta = \int_0^L \dfrac{M \cdot dL}{ET} = \dfrac{T \cdot L}{EI}$$

where, L = total length of the wire = $2\pi Rn$

$$\therefore \qquad \theta = \dfrac{T \cdot 2\pi Rn}{E} \times \dfrac{4}{\pi r^4}$$

$$\therefore \qquad \theta = \dfrac{8TRn}{Er^4}$$

EXAMPLE 1 *A leaf spring carries a central load of 6000 Newton. The leaf spring is to be made of 10 steel plates 5 cm wide and 6 mm thick. If the bending stress is limited to 150 N/mm².*

    (i) determine the length of spring

    (ii) deflection at the Centre of spring Take $E = 2 \times 10^5$ N/mm²

SOLUTION

Let $\quad l$ = length of spring

δ = deflection at the centre of spring

$n = 10$, $b = 5$ cm = 50 mm; $t = 6$ mm

$$\sigma_b = \text{Max bending Stress} = \frac{3\,Wl}{2\,nbt^2}$$

$$150 = \frac{3 \times 6000 \times l}{2 \times 10 \times 50 \times (6)^2}$$

$\therefore \quad l = \left[\dfrac{150 \times 2 \times 10 \times 50 \times 36}{3 \times 6000}\right]$

$\qquad = 299.99$ mm

$\qquad \simeq 300$ mm   **Ans.**

Deflection $(\delta) = \dfrac{\sigma_b \cdot l^2}{4\,E \cdot t}$

$$= \frac{150 \times 300^2}{4 \times (2 \times 10^5) \times 6}$$

$$= \frac{15 \times 9 \times 10^5}{48 \times 10^5}$$

$$= \frac{45}{16} = 2.81 \text{ mm} \quad \textbf{Ans.}$$

EXAMPLE 2 *A closely Coiled helical spring of round steel wire 10 mm diameter 10 complete turns with a mean diameter of 12 cm is subjected to an axial load of 200 N. Determine:*
  (i) *The deflection of the spring*
  (ii) *Maximum shear stress in the wire*
 (iii) *Stiffness of the spring (Take $G = 8 \times 10^4$ N/mm^2)*

SOLUTION   Dia. of wire $(d) = 10$ mm

No. of turns $(n) = 10$

Mean dia. of the Coil $(D) = 12$ cm $= 120$ mm

$R = 60$ mm

Axial load $(W) = 200$ N

Modulus of rigidity $(G) = 8 \times 10^4$ N/mm^2

Let δ = deflection of the spring

        τ_{max} = maximum shear stress in the wire

        k = stiffness of the spring

(i) We know that for close Coiled helical spring

$$\text{Deflection } (\delta) = \frac{64WR^3n}{Gd^4}$$

$$= \frac{64 \times 200 \times (60)^3 \times 10}{8 \times 10^4 \times (10)^4}$$

$$= \frac{64 \times 2 \times 216 \times 10^6}{8 \times 10^8}$$

$$= \frac{16 \times 216}{10^2} \text{ mm}$$

$$= 34.56 \text{ mm} \qquad \textbf{Ans.}$$

(ii) By Formula, $\tau_{max} = \left(\dfrac{16WR}{\pi d^3}\right)$

$$= \frac{16 \times 200 \times 60}{3.14 \times (10)^3}$$

$$= \frac{32 \times 10^3 \times 6}{3.14 \times 10^3}$$

$$= 61.146 \text{ N/mm}^2 \qquad \textbf{Ans.}$$

(iii) Stiffness of spring $(k) = \dfrac{W}{\delta}$

$$= \left(\frac{200}{34.56}\right)$$

$$= 5.78 \text{ N/mm} \qquad \textbf{Ans.}$$

EXAMPLE 3 *A closely coiled helical spring of mean diameter 20 cm is made of 3 cm diameter rod and has 16 turns. A weight of 3 kN is dropped on this spring. Find the height by which the weight should be dropped before striking the spring so that the spring may be compressed by 18 cm. [Assume $G = 8 \times 10^4$ N/mm^2].*
SOLUTION

$$\text{Mean radius } (R) \text{ of the Coil} = \left(\frac{200}{2}\right); \ d = 30 \text{ mm}$$

$$= 100 \text{ mm}$$

Let h is the height through which the weight W is dropped.

W = load that produces 180 mm compression of spring.

$\therefore \qquad \delta = \dfrac{64\,WR^3 n}{Gd^4}$

$$180 = \frac{64 \times W \times (100)^3 \times 16}{8 \times 10^4 \times (30)^4}$$

$\therefore \qquad W = \dfrac{180 \times 8 \times 10^4 \times 30^4}{64 \times (100)^3 \times 16}$

$\qquad\qquad = 11390 \ \text{Newton}$

Work done by the falling weight on spring

$\qquad = 3000\,(h + 180)\ \text{N-mm}$

Energy stored in the spring $= \dfrac{1}{2} \times W \times \delta$

$\qquad\qquad\qquad\qquad = \dfrac{1}{2} \times 11390 \times 180$

$\qquad\qquad\qquad\qquad = 1025100\ \text{N/mm}$

Now, we know,

Work done = Energy stored.

$\qquad 3000\,(h + 180) = 1025100$

or, $\qquad h + 180 = \left(\dfrac{1025100}{3000}\right)$

$\therefore \qquad h = (341.7 - 180)$

$\boxed{h = 161.7 \ \text{mm}}$

EXAMPLE 4 *A closely coiled helical spring is to carry a load of 500 Newton. It's mean coil diameter is 10 times that of the wire diameter. Calculate these diameter if the maximum shear stress in the material of the spring is 80 N/mm².*

SOLUTION

Given $W = 500\ \text{N}$

$\qquad \tau_{max} = 80\ \text{N/mm}^2$

If d = diameter of wire and D = mean diameter of coil, then as per given condition,
$D = 10d$

By formula,

$$\tau = \frac{16WR}{\pi d^3}$$

$$80 = \frac{16 \times 500 \times \left(\dfrac{D}{2}\right)}{\pi d^3}$$

$$80\pi d^3 = 8000 \times \left(\frac{10d}{2}\right)$$

or, $80\pi d^3 = 8000 \times 5d$

$$80\pi d^2 = 40,000$$

$$d = \sqrt{\frac{40,000 \times 7}{80 \times 22}} = 12.61 \text{ mm} \quad \textbf{Ans.}$$

∴ $D = 10d$

$$= 10 \times 12.61 = 126.1 \text{ mm} \qquad \textbf{Ans.}$$

EXAMPLE 5 *A close-coiled helical spring a stiffness of 100 N/m in compression with a maximum load of 45 N and a maximum shearing stress is 120 N/mm². The solid length of the spring (i.e. coils touching) is 45 mm, Find:*

(i)   *the wire diameter*
(ii) *the mean coil radius and*
(iii) *the number of coils. (Take G = 0.4 × 10⁵ N/mm²)*

[UPTU, 3rd Sem 2009-10]

SOLUTION

Given, $k = 100 \text{ N/m}$

$$= \frac{100}{1000} \text{ N/mm} = 0.1 \text{ N/mm}$$

$$W = 45 \text{ N}$$

$$\tau_{max} = 120 \text{ N/mm}^2$$

Solid length of spring = $n \cdot d$

where, n = number of spring and d = diameter of spring wire.

By formula

$$k = \frac{G \cdot d^4}{64 R^3 n}$$

$$0.1 = \frac{0.4 \times 10^5 \times d^4}{64 \times R^3 \times n}$$

$$d^4 = \frac{6.4R^3 n}{0.4 \times 10^5}$$

$$= \frac{16R^3 n}{10^5} \qquad \qquad \text{... (1)}$$

Again, shear stress $\tau = \dfrac{16WR}{\pi d^3}$

$$120 = \frac{16 \times 45 \times R}{\pi d^3}$$

$$R = \frac{120\pi d^3}{16 \times 45} = 0.166\, \pi d^3$$

$$= 0.5217 d^3 \qquad \qquad \text{... (2)}$$

Substituting the value of R in eqn. (1), we get

$$d^4 = \frac{16n}{(10)^5} \times (0.5217 d^3)^3$$

or, $\qquad d^4 = \dfrac{16n}{10^5} \times (0.5217)^3 \times d^9$

or, $\qquad \dfrac{1}{d^5} = \dfrac{16n}{10^5} \times (0.5217)^3$

or, $\qquad d^5 n = \dfrac{10^5}{16 \times (0.5217)^3}$

or, $\qquad d^5\left(\dfrac{45}{d}\right) = \dfrac{100000}{16 \times (0.5217)^3}$

or, $\qquad d^4 = \dfrac{100000}{16 \times 45 \times (0.5217)^3}$

$\therefore \qquad d = \left(\dfrac{100000}{16 \times 45 \times (0.5217)^3}\right)^{0.25}$

$\boxed{d = 5.61 \text{ mm}}$ **Ans.**

(ii) From eqn (2), mean radius of the coil $(R) = 0.5217 d^3$

$$= 0.517\,(5.61)^3$$

$\therefore \qquad R = 91.28 \text{ mm}$

(iii) Number of coils $(n) = \left(\dfrac{45}{d}\right)$

$$= \left(\dfrac{45}{5.61}\right)$$

$$= 8.02$$

$$n = 8 \qquad \textbf{Ans.}$$

EXAMPLE 6 *A leaf spring has 12 plates each 50 mm wide and 5 mm thick, the longest plate being 600 mm long. The greatest bending stress is not to exceed 180 N/mm² and the central deflection is 15 mm. Compute the magnitude of the greatest central load that can be applied to the spring. (E = 0.206 × 10⁶ N/mm²)*

[UPTU, 3rd Sem 2009-10, EME-302]

SOLUTION

Given, $n = 12, l = 600$ mm

$$b = 50 \text{ mm}$$

$$t = 5 \text{ mm}$$

Bending stress $\sigma_b \ngtr 180 \text{ N/mm}^2$

Deflection $(\delta) = 15$ mm

Central load $(W) = ?$

$$E = 0.206 \times 10^6 \text{ N/mm}^2$$

By formula,

$$\sigma_b = \frac{3}{2} \cdot \frac{Wl}{nbt^2}$$

$$180 = \frac{3}{2} \cdot \frac{W \times 600}{12 \times 50 \times (5)^2}$$

$$\therefore \qquad W = \left(\frac{180 \times 2 \times 12 \times 50 \times 25}{3 \times 600}\right) \text{Newton}$$

$$= 3000 \text{ Newton}$$

$$= 3 \text{ kN} \qquad \textbf{Ans.}$$

Open-coiled Helical Spring Subjected to Axial Load W

(a) Deflection (δ)

In an open coiled helical spring the helix angled can not be neglected and the spring is subjected to comparable bending and twisting effect.

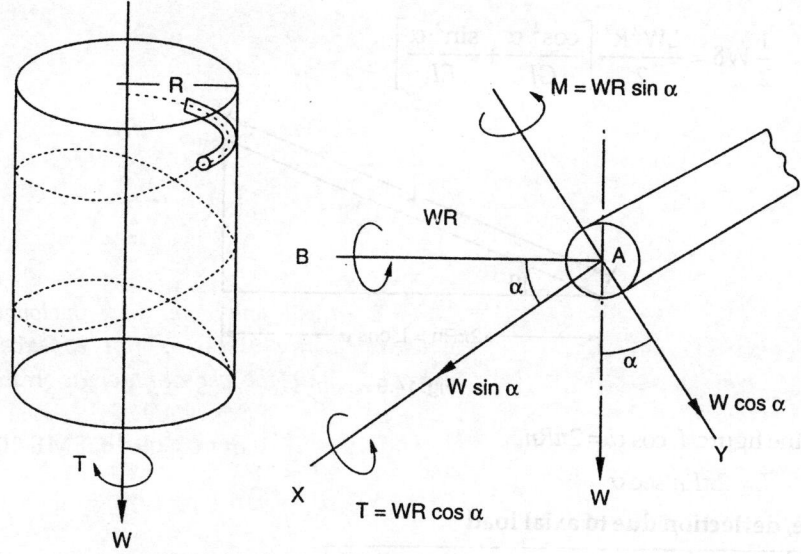

Fig. 14.8

Let W = axial load
       n = number of turn
       d = wire diameter
       D = $2R$ = coil diameter
       α = helix angle
       R = mean coil radius

Here, the open coil is subjected to axial load W together with a couple WR about AB. This couple has component about AX, $WR \cos \alpha$ tending to twist the section and a component about AY of $WR \sin \alpha$ tending to reduce the curvature of the coils.

We are neglecting the shearing effect across the spring being very small in comparison to other.

Thus, $T = WR \cos \alpha$ and $M = WR \sin \alpha$

Now, total strain energy neglecting shear

$$U = \frac{T^2 L}{2GJ} + \frac{M^2 L}{2EI}$$

$$= \frac{L\,(WR \cos \alpha)^2}{2GJ} + \frac{L\,(WR \sin \alpha)^2}{2EI}$$

$$= \frac{LW^2R^2}{2}\left[\frac{\cos^2 \alpha}{GJ} + \frac{\sin^2 \alpha}{EI}\right]$$

Work done by the spring $= \dfrac{1}{2}W\delta$

By strain energy principle, strain energy is equal to the work done by the spring. Therefore,

$$\frac{1}{2} W\delta = \frac{LW^2 R^2}{2}\left[\frac{\cos^2\alpha}{GJ}+\frac{\sin^2\alpha}{EI}\right]$$

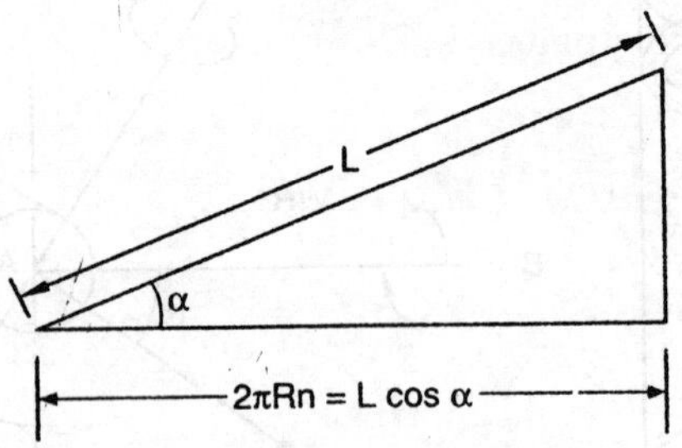

Fig. 14.9

From the figure $L\cos\alpha = 2\pi Rn$

$\therefore \qquad L = 2\pi Rn \sec\alpha$

Hence, deflection due to axial load

$$(\delta) = 2\pi R^3 nW \sec\alpha\left[\frac{\cos^2\alpha}{GJ}+\frac{\sin^2\alpha}{EI}\right] \qquad \text{[Form I]}$$

Alternatively, the deflection (δ) is given by Castigliano's theorem as

$$\delta = \frac{\partial U}{\partial W}$$

$$= \frac{\partial}{\partial W}\left[\frac{LW^2 R^2}{2}\left(\frac{\cos^2\alpha}{GJ}+\frac{\sin^2\alpha}{EI}\right)\right]$$

$$= LWR^2\left[\frac{\cos^2\alpha}{GJ}+\frac{\sin^2\alpha}{EI}\right]$$

$$= 2\pi nWR^3 \sec\alpha\left[\frac{\cos^2\alpha}{GJ}+\frac{\sin^2\alpha}{EI}\right]$$

$$= \frac{2\pi nWR^3}{\cos\alpha}\left[\frac{\cos^2\alpha}{GJ}+\frac{\sin^2\alpha}{EI}\right]$$

$$= \frac{2\pi nWR^3}{\cos\alpha}\left[\frac{\cos^2\alpha}{G\times\dfrac{\pi d^4}{32}}+\frac{\sin^2\alpha}{E\times\dfrac{\pi d^4}{64}}\right]$$

$$= \frac{2\pi nWR^3}{\cos\alpha}\times\frac{32}{\pi d^4}\left[\frac{\cos^2\alpha}{G}+\frac{2\sin^2\alpha}{E}\right]$$

$$\therefore \ \delta = \frac{64\,WR^3 n}{d^4\cos\alpha}\left[\frac{\cos^2\alpha}{G}+\frac{2\sin^2\alpha}{E}\right] \qquad \text{[Form II]}$$

Either form I or form II can be used to compute the deflection (δ) due to axial load (W) in the open coiled helical spring.

(b) Maximum Stress in open coiled helical spring due to axial load

Torque $(T) = WR \cos \alpha$

Bending Moment $(M) = WR \sin \alpha$

Shear Stress $(\tau) = \dfrac{16T}{\pi d^3}$

$$= \frac{16 \, WR \cos \alpha}{\pi d^3}$$

Bending stress $(\sigma) = \dfrac{32M}{\pi d^3}$

$$= \frac{32 \, WR \sin \alpha}{\pi d^3}$$

Principal Stresses are:

$$\sigma_{1,2} = \frac{\sigma}{2} \pm \sqrt{\left(\frac{\sigma}{2}\right)^2 + \tau^2}$$

$$= \frac{\sigma}{2} \pm \frac{1}{2}\sqrt{\sigma^2 + 4\tau^2}$$

$$= \frac{16WR \sin \alpha}{\pi d^3} \pm \frac{1}{2}\sqrt{\left(\frac{32 \, WR \sin \alpha}{\pi d^3}\right)^2 + 4\left(\frac{16WR \cos \alpha}{\pi d^3}\right)^2}$$

$$= \frac{16WR \sin \alpha}{\pi d^3} \pm \frac{16WR}{\pi d^3}\sqrt{\sin^2 \alpha + \cos^2 \alpha}$$

$$= \frac{16WR \sin \alpha}{\pi d^3} \pm \frac{16WR}{\pi d^3}$$

$$= \frac{16WR}{\pi d^3}(\sin \alpha \pm 1)$$

Hence, $\sigma_1 = \dfrac{16 \, WR}{\pi d^3}(\sin \alpha + 1)$, maximum principal stress

and $\sigma_2 = \dfrac{16 \, WR}{\pi d^3}(\sin \alpha - 1)$, minimum principal stress

Maximum Shear Stress $(\tau_{\max}) = \left(\dfrac{\sigma_1 - \sigma_2}{2}\right)$

$$= \frac{16WR}{\pi d^3}\left[\frac{\sin\alpha+1-\sin\alpha+1}{2}\right]$$

$$\therefore \ \tau_{max} = \frac{16WR}{\pi d^3}$$

(c) Angular Rotation (ϕ)

Let us consider an imaginary torque T applied to the spring together with W producing an angular rotation ϕ at one end of the spring relative to the other.

The combined twisting moment on the spring Cross-section is:

$$T = WR\cos\alpha + T\sin\alpha$$

and Combined bending moment $(M) = T\cos\alpha - WR\sin\alpha$

Now, total strain energy $(U) = \dfrac{T^2L}{2GJ} + \dfrac{M^2L}{2EI}$

or, $\quad U = \dfrac{(WR\cos\alpha + T\sin\alpha)^2 \cdot L}{2GJ} + \dfrac{(T\cos\alpha - WR\sin\alpha)^2 \cdot L}{2EI}$

Now, by Castigliano's Theorem $\phi = \dfrac{\partial U}{\partial T}$

Since only W is acting so neglecting term having T.

$$\therefore \qquad \phi = \frac{2WR\cos\alpha \cdot \sin\alpha \cdot L}{2GJ} + \frac{(-2WR\sin\alpha \cdot \cos\alpha) \cdot L}{2EI}$$

$$= LWR\cos\alpha\sin\alpha\left[\frac{1}{GJ} - \frac{1}{EI}\right]$$

Substituting $L = 2\pi RN\sec\alpha$, we get

$$\phi = 2\pi n WR^2 \sin\alpha\left[\frac{1}{GJ} - \frac{1}{EI}\right] \qquad\qquad \text{[Form (I)]}$$

$$= 2\pi n WR^2 \cdot \sin\alpha\left[\frac{1}{G\times\dfrac{\pi d^4}{32}} - \frac{1}{E\times\dfrac{\pi d^4}{64}}\right]$$

$$= \frac{64\pi n WR^2\sin\alpha}{\pi d^4}\left[\frac{1}{G} - \frac{2}{E}\right]$$

$$= \frac{\overset{16}{\cancel{64}}\,\cancel{\pi}nW\times\dfrac{D^2}{\cancel{4}}\sin\alpha}{\cancel{\pi}d^4}\left[\frac{1}{G} - \frac{2}{E}\right]$$

$$\therefore \ \phi \text{ due to axial load} = \frac{16WD^2n\sin\alpha}{d^4}\left[\frac{1}{G} - \frac{2}{E}\right] \qquad \text{[Form (II)]}$$

Open Coiled Helical Spring Subjected to Axial Torque (*T*)
(a) Axial rotation (ϕ)

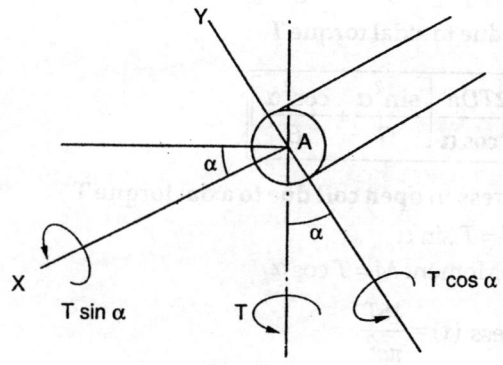

Fig. 14.10

When an axial torque *T* is applied to an open-coiled helical spring, it has a torsional component $T \sin\alpha$ about AX and a bending component $T \cos\alpha$ about AY.

Now, the total strain energy $(U) = \dfrac{T^2 L}{2GJ} + \dfrac{M^2 L}{2EI}$

or,
$$U = \frac{L}{2}\left[\frac{(T\sin\alpha)^2}{GJ} + \frac{(T\cos\alpha)^2}{EI}\right]$$

$$= \frac{T^2 L}{2}\left[\frac{\sin^2\alpha}{GJ} + \frac{\cos^2\alpha}{EI}\right]$$

Work done by torque $(T) = \dfrac{1}{2}\cdot T\cdot\phi$

Now, by strain energy principle, Work done = U

$$\frac{1}{2}T\phi = \frac{T^2 L}{2}\left[\frac{\sin^2\alpha}{GJ} + \frac{\cos^2\alpha}{EI}\right]$$

$\therefore$
$$\phi = T\cdot L\left[\frac{\sin^2\alpha}{GJ} + \frac{\cos^2\alpha}{EI}\right]$$

$$\boxed{\phi = T\cdot 2\pi Rn \sec\alpha\left[\frac{\sin^2\alpha}{GJ} + \frac{\cos^2\alpha}{EI}\right]}$$ [Form (I)]

$$= 2\pi RnT \sec\alpha\left[\frac{\sin^2\alpha}{G\times\dfrac{\pi d^4}{32}} + \frac{\cos^2\alpha}{E\times\dfrac{\pi d^4}{64}}\right]$$

$$= \frac{\pi D n T}{\cos \alpha} \times \frac{32}{\pi d^4} \left[\frac{\sin^2 \alpha}{G} + \frac{\cos^2 \alpha}{E} \right]$$

Angular rotation due to axial torque T

$$\boxed{\therefore \quad \phi = \frac{32 T D n}{d^4 \cos \alpha} \left[\frac{\sin^2 \alpha}{G} + \frac{\cos^2 \alpha}{E} \right]}$$ [Form (II)]

(b) Maximum Stress in open coil due to axial torque T

Torque $T = T \sin \alpha$

and   Bending Moment $M = T \cos \alpha$

$\therefore$ Shear Stress $(\tau) = \dfrac{16T}{\pi d^3}$

$$= \frac{16T \sin \alpha}{\pi d^3}$$

Bending Stress $(\sigma) = \dfrac{32M}{\pi d^3}$

$$= \frac{32T \cos \alpha}{\pi d^3}$$

Principle stresses are:

$$\sigma_{1,2} = \frac{\sigma}{2} \pm \sqrt{\left(\frac{\sigma}{2}\right)^2 + \tau^2}$$

$$= \frac{\sigma}{2} \pm \frac{1}{2}\sqrt{\sigma^2 + 4\tau^2}$$

$$= \frac{16T \cos \alpha}{\pi d^3} \pm \frac{1}{2}\sqrt{\left(\frac{32\, T \cos \alpha}{\pi d^3}\right)^2 + 4\left(\frac{16T \sin \alpha}{\pi d^3}\right)^2}$$

$$= \frac{16T \cos \alpha}{\pi d^3} \pm \frac{16T}{\pi d^3}\sqrt{\cos^2 \alpha + \sin^2 \alpha}$$

$$= \frac{16T \cos \alpha}{\pi d^3} \pm \frac{16T}{\pi d^3}$$

$$= \frac{16T}{\pi d^3}(\cos \alpha \pm 1)$$

$\therefore$ Maximum Stress $(\tau_{max}) = \dfrac{\sigma_1 - \sigma_2}{2}$

$\therefore$ $\tau_{max} = \dfrac{16T}{\pi d^3}$

(c) Axial Deflection due to axial torque (T)

Let us consider that an imaginary axial load W is applied to the spring.
So the total strain energy is given by

$$U = \frac{(WR\cos\alpha + T\sin\alpha)^2 \cdot L}{2GJ} + \frac{(T\cos\alpha - WR\sin\alpha)^2 \cdot L}{2EI}$$

By Castigliano's Theorem, the deflection (δ) in the direction of applied load (W) is given by

$$\delta = \frac{\partial U}{\partial W}$$

$$= TRL\cos\alpha\sin\alpha\left[\frac{1}{GJ} - \frac{1}{EI}\right] \quad \text{when } W = 0$$

$$\therefore \; \delta = 2\pi nTR^2\sin\alpha\left[\frac{1}{GJ} - \frac{1}{EI}\right] \qquad \text{[Form (I)]}$$

$$= 2\pi nTR^2\sin\alpha\left[\frac{1}{G\times\dfrac{\pi d^4}{32}} - \frac{1}{E\times\dfrac{\pi d^4}{64}}\right]$$

$$= \frac{64\pi nTR^2\sin\alpha}{\pi d^4}\cdot\left[\frac{1}{G} - \frac{2}{E}\right]$$

$$\therefore \; \delta = \frac{16TnD^2\sin\alpha}{d^4}\left[\frac{1}{G} - \frac{2}{E}\right] \qquad \text{[Form (II)]}$$

Springs in Series

If two springs of different stiffness are joined together and carry a common load W, they are said to be connected in series and the combined stiffness and deflection are given by the following equations:

$$\text{Deflection }(\delta) = \frac{W}{k} = \delta_1 + \delta_2 = \frac{W}{k_1} + \frac{W}{k_2}$$

$$= W\left(\frac{1}{k_1} + \frac{1}{k_2}\right)$$

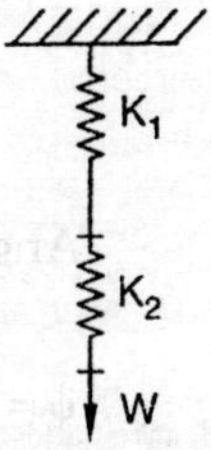

$$\therefore \quad \frac{1}{k} = \frac{1}{k_1} + \frac{1}{k_2}$$

Fig. 14.11

$$\text{Stiffness }(k) = \frac{k_1 k_2}{k_1 + k_2}$$

Springs in Parallel

If the two springs are joined in such a way that they have a common deflection δ then they are said to be connected in parallel. In this case the load carried is shared between the two springs and total load $W = W_1 + W_2$ ...(I)

$$\delta = \frac{W}{k} = \frac{W_1}{k_1} = \frac{W_2}{k_2}$$

So that $W_1 = \dfrac{k_1 W}{k}$ and $W_2 = \dfrac{k_2 W}{k}$

Substituting in equation (I)

$$W = \frac{k_1 W}{k} + \frac{k_2 W}{k}$$

$$= \frac{W}{k}(k_1 + k_2)$$

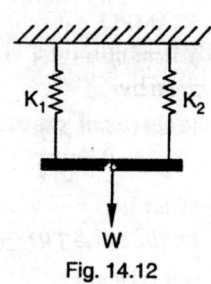

Fig. 14.12

Combined stiffness $(k) = k_1 + k_2$

EXAMPLE 7 *An open-coiled helical spring is made having 10 turns wound to a mean diameter of 120 mm. The wire diameter is 10 mm and the coils make an angle of 30° with a plane perpendicular to the axis of coil.*

Find (a) the axial extension with a load of 100 N. (b) the angle, the free end will turn through with its load if free to rotate.

$$E = 208 \times 10^3 \ N/mm^2; \quad G = 83 \times 10^3 \ N/mm^2$$

SOLUTION

(a)   Axial extension $(\delta) = \dfrac{8WD^3 n}{d^4 \cos \alpha}\left(\dfrac{\cos^2 \alpha}{G} + \dfrac{2 \sin^2 \alpha}{E}\right)$

$$= \frac{8 \times 100 \times 120^3 \times 10}{10^4 \cos 30°}\left(\frac{\cos^2 30°}{83000} + \frac{2 \sin^2 30°}{208000}\right)$$

$$= \frac{800 \times 1728 \times 2}{\sqrt{3} \times 10^4}(0.0905 + 0.024)$$

$$= 18.4 \ mm \quad \textbf{Ans.}$$

(b)   Angle of rotation of free end

$$\phi = \frac{16WD^2 n \sin \alpha}{(d)^4}\left(\frac{1}{G} - \frac{2}{E}\right)$$

$$= \frac{16 \times 100 \times 120^2 \times 10 \sin 30°}{10^4}\left(\frac{1}{83000} - \frac{2}{208000}\right)$$

$$= \frac{16 \times 144 \times 5}{10^4} (0.1205 - 0.098)$$

$$= 0.026 \text{ radian}$$

$$= 1.48°$$

EXAMPLE 8 *Compute the load required to produce an extension of 8 mm on an open coiled helical spring of 10 coils of mean diameter 76 mm with a helix angle of 20° and wire diameter of 6 mm.*

What will be the bending and shear stresses in the surface of the wire?

[*For material of spring E = 210 GN/m² and G = 70 GN/m²*]

What will be the angular twist at the free end of the spring when subjected to an axial torque of 1.5 Nm?

SOLUTION

Given: $\delta = 8$ mm; $n = 10$; $D = 76$ mm; $\alpha = 20°$; $d = 6$ mm

Objective: $\sigma_b = ?$ $\tau = ?$ $\phi = ?$ $W = ?$

By formula, the extension of an open coiled helical spring when subjected to axial load (W) is given by

$$\delta = 2\pi n W R^3 \sec\alpha \left[\frac{\cos^2\alpha}{GJ} + \frac{\sin^2\alpha}{EI} \right]$$

Here, $I = \dfrac{\pi d^4}{64}$

$$= \frac{\pi \times (6 \times 10^{-3})^4}{64}$$

$$= 63.63 \times 10^{-12} \text{ m}^4$$

and $J = \dfrac{\pi d^4}{32}$

$$= \frac{\pi \times (6 \times 10^{-3})^4}{64}$$

$$= 127.26 \times 10^{-12} \text{ m}^4$$

Substituting the known value in the above formula of δ

$$8 \times 10^{-3} = 2\pi \times 10 \times W \times (38 \times 10^{-3}) \cdot \sec 20° \left[\frac{\cos^2 20°}{70 \times 10^9 \times 127.26 \times 10^{-12}} \right.$$

$$\left. + \frac{\sin^2 20°}{210 \times 10^9 \times 63.63 \times 10^{-12}} \right]$$

$$= \frac{20\pi W \times 38^3 \times 10^{-9}}{0.9397} \left[\frac{(0.9397)^2}{8.91} + \frac{(0.342)^2}{13.36} \right]$$

$$= \frac{20\pi W \times 38^3 \times 10^{-9}}{0.9397} [0.1079]$$

$$\therefore \qquad W = \frac{8 \times 10^{-3} \times 0.9397}{20\pi \times 28^3 \times 10^{-9} \times 0.1079}$$

$$= 20 \text{ Newton} \qquad \textbf{Ans.}$$

Bending moment acting on the spring is

$$M = WR \sin \alpha$$

$$= 20 \times 38 \times 10^{-3} \times \sin 20°$$

$$= 20 \times 38 \times 10^{-3} \times 0.342$$

$$= 0.259$$

$$\therefore \qquad M \simeq 0.26 \text{ Nm}$$

Hence, Bending stress $(\sigma_b) = \dfrac{M}{I} \cdot y$

$$y = \left(\frac{d}{2}\right) = 3 \times 10^{-3}$$

$$\therefore \qquad \sigma_b = \frac{0.26}{63.63 \times 10^{-12}} \times 3 \times 10^{-3}$$

$$= 12258368 \text{ N/m}^2$$

$$= 12.26 \text{ MN/m}^2$$

Similarly, Torque on the spring material is

$$T = WR \cos \alpha = 20 \times 38 \times 10^{-3} \times \cos 20°$$

$$= 20 \times 38 \times 10^{-3} \times 0.9397$$

$$\therefore \qquad T = 0.714 \text{ Nm}$$

Shear stress $= \dfrac{T \cdot r}{J}$

$$= \frac{0.714 \times 3 \times 10^{-3}}{127.26 \times 10^{-12}}$$

$$= 16831683 \text{ N/m}^2$$

$$= 16.83 \text{ MN/m}^2$$

Angular twist (ϕ) when subjected to torque 1.5 Nm

$$\phi = 2\pi RnT \sec \alpha \left[\frac{\sin^2 \alpha}{GJ} + \frac{\cos^2 \alpha}{EI} \right]$$

$$= 2\pi \times 38 \times 10^{-3} \times 10 \times 1.5 \times \sec 20° \left[\frac{\sin^2 20°}{70 \times 10^9 \times 127.26 \times 10^{-12}} \right.$$

$$\left. + \frac{\cos^2 20°}{210 \times 10^9 \times 63.63 \times 10^{-12}} \right]$$

$$= 0.302 \text{ radian}$$

$$= 17.3° \qquad \textbf{Ans.}$$

EXAMPLE 9 *A helical spring having 12 coils of mean coil diameter of 20 cm is made of 10 mm diameter steel rod. The helix angle is 25°. Find the angular twist and the axial deflection of one end of spring relative to the other if it is subjected to an axial couple of 14 N-m.*

Calculate the maximum bending and torsional stresses in the wire.

[Take E = 200 GN/m² and G = 80GN/m²]

[UPTU, 3rd Sem. 2006-07]

SOLUTION

Given: $n = 12$

$\qquad\qquad D = 200 \text{ mm}$

$\qquad\qquad R = 100 \text{ mm}$

$\qquad\qquad d = 10 \text{ mm}$

$\qquad\qquad \alpha = 25°$

Axial Couple $= 14 \times 10^3$ Nmm

$$E = \frac{200 \times 10^9}{10^6} \text{ N/mm}^2$$

$$= 2 \times 10^5 \text{ N/mm}^2$$

$$G = 80 \text{ GN/m}^2$$

$$= \frac{80 \times 10^9}{10^6} \text{ N/mm}^2$$

$$= 80 \times 10^3 \text{ N/mm}^2$$

Objective: (i) To compute angular twist *i.e.,* ϕ

$\qquad\qquad$ (ii) To compute deflection *i.e.,* δ

$\qquad\qquad$ (iii) To compute maximum bending stress *i.e.* σ_b maximum

$\qquad\qquad$ (iv) To compute maximum torsional stress *i.e.,* τ_{max}.

Since the coil is subjected to axial couple (T). Hence **angular twist (ϕ)**

$$\phi = \frac{32TDn}{d^4 \cos \alpha} \left(\frac{\sin^2 \alpha}{G} + \frac{2 \cos^2 \alpha}{E} \right)$$

$$= \frac{32 \times 14 \times 10^3 \times 200 \times 12}{(10)^4 \times \cos 25°} \left[\frac{\sin^2 25°}{80 \times 10^3} + \frac{2 \cos^2 25°}{2 \times 10^5} \right]$$

$$= \frac{32 \times 14 \times 2 \times 12 \times 10^5}{10^4 \times 0.906} \left[\frac{(0.423)^2}{80 \times 10^3} + \frac{2 \times (0.906)^2}{2 \times 10^5} \right]$$

$$= 118675.49 \times [2.23661 \times 10^{-6} + 8.20836 \times 10^{-6}]$$

$$= \frac{118675.49}{(10)^6} \times [2.23661 + 8.20836]$$

$$= 1.2395 \text{ radian}$$

$$= \frac{1.2395 \times 180}{\pi} \text{ degree}$$

$$= 71 \text{ degree} \quad \textbf{Ans.}$$

Axial deflection (δ) :

$$\delta = \frac{16 \, TD^2 n \sin \alpha}{d^4} \left(\frac{1}{G} - \frac{2}{E} \right)$$

$$= \frac{16 \times 14 \times 10^3 \times (200)^2 \times 12 \times \sin 25°}{(10)^4} \left(\frac{1}{80 \times 10^3} - \frac{\cancel{2}}{\cancel{2} \times 10^5} \right)$$

$$= \frac{16 \times 14 \times 4 \times 10^7 \times 12 \times 0.423}{(10)^4} \left(\frac{1}{80 \times 10^4} - \frac{1}{10^5} \right)$$

$$= \frac{16 \times 14 \times 4 \times 10^7 \times 12 \times 0.423}{(10)^4} \left(\frac{1}{0.8 \times 10^5} - \frac{1}{10^5} \right)$$

$$= \frac{16 \times 14 \times 4 \times 10^3 \times 12 \times 0.423}{(10)^5} \times 0.2$$

$$= \frac{16 \times 56 \times 12 \times 423 \times 0.2}{(10)^5}$$

$$= 9 \text{ mm} \quad \textbf{Ans.}$$

Maximum bending stress when the coil is subjected to axial couple (T):

By formula bending stress $(\sigma_b) = \dfrac{32M}{\pi d^3}$

when coil is subjected to axial couple (T)

then $\qquad T = T \sin \alpha$

and $\qquad M = T \cos \alpha$

Hence, $\sigma_b = \dfrac{32\, WR \sin \alpha}{\pi d^3}$

$$= \dfrac{32 \times 14 \times \cos 25°}{\left(\dfrac{22}{7}\right) \times \left(\dfrac{10}{1000}\right)^3}$$

$$= 129.146 \times 10^6 \text{ N/m}^2$$

$$\sigma_b = 129.146 \text{MN/m}^2 \qquad \textbf{Ans.}$$

By formula maximum shear stress $(\tau_{max}) = \dfrac{16T}{\pi d^3}$

$$= \dfrac{16\, T \sin 25°}{\dfrac{22}{7} \times \left(\dfrac{10}{10000}\right)^3}$$

$$= \dfrac{16 \times 14 \times 0.423 \times 7}{22 \times \left(\dfrac{1}{10^6}\right)}$$

$$= 30.14 \times 10^6 \text{ N/m}^2$$

$$\tau_{max} = 30.14 \text{MN/m}^2 \qquad \textbf{Ans.}$$

14.4 CONCENTRIC SPRING OR CLUSTER SPRING

Concentric or cluster springs are close-coiled helical springs placed one inside the other as shown in Figure 14.13.

$$\text{Clearance } (\Delta) = \left(\dfrac{D_2 - D_1}{2}\right) - \left(\dfrac{d_1 + d_2}{2}\right)$$

Following conditions have to be satisfied by the spring.

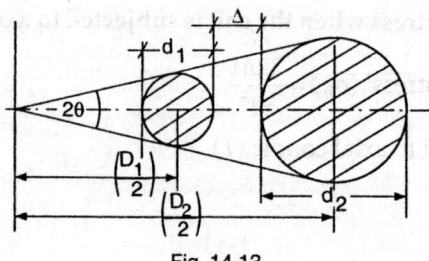

Fig. 14.13

First Condition: When springs are of equal free length and made of the same material then the maximum shear stress in the springs is equal.

$$\therefore \qquad \frac{8W_1 D_1}{\pi d_1^3} = \frac{8W_2 D_2}{\pi d_2^3}$$

$$\Rightarrow \qquad \frac{W_1}{W_2} = \left(\frac{D_2}{D_1}\right) \cdot \left(\frac{d_1}{d_2}\right)^3 \qquad\qquad\qquad \text{...(i)}$$

Second Condition: The deflection is same for both the spring

$$\frac{8W_1 D_1^3 n_1}{G_1 d_1^4} = \frac{8W_2 D_2^3 n_2}{G_2 d_2^4}$$

$$\Rightarrow \qquad \frac{W_1}{W_2} = \left(\frac{D_2}{D_1}\right)^3 \cdot \left(\frac{d_1}{d_2}\right)^4 \cdot \left(\frac{G_1}{G_2}\right) \cdot \left(\frac{n_2}{n_1}\right) \qquad\qquad \text{...(ii)}$$

Third Condition: Both springs have the same solid length *i.e.,*

$$n_1 d_1 = n_2 d_2 \qquad\qquad\qquad\qquad\qquad \text{...(iii)}$$

Comparing equation (i) and (ii), we get

$$1 = \left(\frac{D_2}{D_1}\right)^2 \cdot \left(\frac{d_1}{d_2}\right) \cdot \left(\frac{G_1}{G_2}\right)\left(\frac{n_2}{n_1}\right)$$

Also, $\qquad \dfrac{n_2}{n_1} = \dfrac{d_1}{d_2}$

$$\therefore \qquad 1 = \left(\frac{D_2}{D_1}\right)^2 \cdot \left(\frac{d_1}{d_2}\right)^2 \cdot \left(\frac{G_1}{G_2}\right)$$

If $G_1 = G_2$, then

$$\frac{D_1}{d_1} = \frac{D_2}{d_2}$$

or, $\qquad C_1 = C_2$ *i.e.,* spring indices are equal.

Therefore, equation (i) becomes

$$\frac{W_1}{W_2} = \left(\frac{d_1}{d_2}\right)^2$$

$$\tan \theta = \left(\frac{d_1}{D_1} \right) = \left(\frac{d_2}{D_2} \right)$$

Also, $(W_1 + W_2) = W$

EXAMPLE *Two concentric springs are subjected to an axial load of 6 kN. The maximum allowable deflection of the springs is 40 mm and the solid length is 50 mm. If the springs are made of the same material having G = 84 GPa and maximum allowable shear stress is 850 MPa, Calculate*

  (i) *load shared by the springs*

  (ii) *wire diameters*

Assume inner spring diameter = 80 mm and radial clearance 2.5 mm.

SOLUTION Given $W_1 + W_2 = 6$ kN

$$\delta = 40 \, \text{mm} = 4 \, \text{cm}$$

$$l = 50 \, \text{mm} = 5 \, \text{cm}$$

$$\tau = 850 \, \text{MPa}$$

For the same stress in both the spring

$$\frac{W_1 D_1}{d_1^3} = \frac{W_2 D_2}{d_2^3}$$

For the same deflection in both the spring

$$\frac{W_1 D_1^3 n_1}{d_1^4} = \frac{W_2 D_2^3 n_2}{d_2^4}$$

For solid lengths to be the same

$$n_1 d_1 = n_2 d_2$$

$$\therefore \quad \frac{8 W_1 D_1^3 n_1}{G d_1^4} = 4$$

$$n_1 d_1 = 5$$

$$\frac{8 W_1 D_1}{\pi d_1^3} = 850 \times 10^6$$

$$\frac{\pi D_1^3 n_1}{G_1 d_1} = \frac{4}{850 \times 10^6}$$

$$\frac{\pi D_1^2 5}{G_1 d_1^2} = \frac{4}{850 \times 10^6}$$

$$\therefore \quad \left(\frac{D_1}{d_1} \right)^2 = \frac{4 \times 84 \times 10^9}{\pi \times 5 \times 850 \times 10^6}$$

$$\frac{D_1}{d_1} = c_1 = \sqrt{\frac{4 \times 84 \times 10^9}{\pi \times 5 \times 850 \times 10^6}}$$

$$= 5.016$$

$$\therefore \quad d_1 = \left(\frac{8}{5.016}\right) = 1.595 \text{ cm}$$

Also, $\quad \dfrac{D_2}{d_2} = \dfrac{D_1}{d_1} = 5.016$

$$\therefore \quad D_2 = 5.016 d_2$$

Radial clearance $= \dfrac{1}{2}[(D_1 - D_1) - (d_1 + d_2)]$

$$= \frac{1}{2}[5.016 d_2 - 8 - 1.595 - d_2]$$

$$= 0.25$$

$$\therefore \quad d_2 = 2.514 \text{ cm}$$

$$\frac{W_1}{W_2} = \left(\frac{d_1}{d_2}\right)^2 = \left(\frac{1.595}{2.514}\right)^2 = 0.4025$$

$$W_1 + W_2 = 6$$

$\therefore \quad 1.4025 W_2 = 6$ $\qquad\qquad\qquad (\therefore W_1 = 0.4025 W_2)$

$$W_2 = 4.278 \text{ kN}$$

$$W_1 = 1.722 \text{ kN} \qquad\qquad\qquad\qquad \textbf{Ans.}$$

14.5 FLAT SPIRAL SPRING

Spiral springs are normally constructed from their rectangular section strip wound into a spiral in one plane. They are often used in clockwork mechanism.

The winding torque or moment is applied to the central spindle and the other end firmly anchored to a pin at the outside of the spiral. Under the action of this central moment, all sections of the spring will be subjected to uniform bending which tends to reduce the radius of curvature at all points.

Let us consider the spiral spring as shown in Figure 14.14.

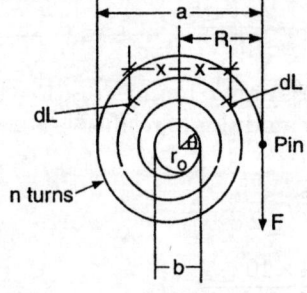

Fig. 14.14

Let M = winding moment applied to the spring spindle
         R = radius of the spring from spindle to pin
         a = maximum dimension of the spring from the pin
         b = breadth of the material of the spring
         t = thickness of the material of the spring
         b = diameter of the spindle

Now, at any instant, $r = r_0 + \left(\dfrac{A}{2\pi}\right)\theta$ where, A = constant when $\theta = 0$, $r = r_0 = \dfrac{b}{2}$

and for the nth turn, $\theta = 2n\pi$ and

$$r = \frac{a}{2} = \frac{b}{2} + \left(\frac{A}{2\pi}\right) \cdot 2n\pi$$

$\therefore$ $A = \left(\dfrac{a-b}{2n}\right)$

i.e., the equation to the spiral is

$$r = \frac{b}{2} + \frac{(a-b)}{4\pi n}\theta$$

When a torque or winding couple M is applied to the spindle, a resistive force F will be set up at the pin such that, winding couple $(M) = F \times R$

Let us consider two small elements in material of length dl at a distance x to each side of the centre line, as shown in Fig. 14.14.

For small deflection, from Mohr's area-moment method, the change in slope between

two points is $\left(\dfrac{M}{EI}\right) \cdot dL$

For the left portion,

$$\text{Change in slope} = d\theta_1 = \frac{F(R+x)\,dL}{EI}$$

Similarly for the right hand portion

$$\text{Change in slope} = d\theta_2 = \frac{F(R-x)\,dL}{EI}$$

The sum of these changes in slope is thus

$$d\theta_1 + d\theta_2 = \frac{F(R+x)\,dL}{EI} + \frac{F(R-x)\,dL}{EI}$$

$$= \frac{2\,FR\,dL}{EI}$$

If this is integrated along the length of the spring, then the result obtained will be twice the total change in slope along the spring i.e., twice the angle of twist.

$$\text{Angle of twist} = \frac{1}{2}\int_0^L \frac{2FR\,dL}{EI}$$

$$= \frac{FRL}{EI}$$

$$= \frac{ML}{EI}$$

where, M = applied winding moment

L = total length of the spring

Now, $$L = \int_0^L dL = \int_0^{2n\pi} r d\theta = \int_0^{2n\pi} \frac{b}{2} + \frac{(a-b)}{4\pi n} \theta \, d\theta$$

$$= \left[\frac{b\theta}{2} + \frac{(a-b)}{4\pi n} \cdot \frac{\theta^2}{2} \right]_0^{2n\pi}$$

$$= \left[\frac{2nb\pi}{2} + \frac{(a-b)}{4\pi n} \cdot \frac{(2n\pi)^2}{2} \right]$$

$$= \pi n = \left[b + \frac{(a-b)}{2} \right]$$

$$= \frac{\pi n}{2} [a+b]$$

Therefore, the wind up angle (θ) of a spiral spring is

$$\boxed{\theta = \frac{M}{EI} \left[\frac{\pi n}{2} (a+b) \right]}$$

Maximum Stress

The maximum bending stress set up in the spring will be at the point of greatest bending moment, since the material of the spring is subjected to pure bending.

Maximum bending moment $= F \times a$

Maximum bending stress $= \dfrac{M}{I} \cdot y$

$$= \frac{F \cdot a \, (t/2)}{I}$$

For rectangular-section spring material of breadth B and thickness t

$$I = \frac{Bt^3}{12}$$

$$\sigma_{max} = \frac{F a t}{2} \times \frac{12}{Bt^3}$$

$$= \frac{6Fa}{Bt^2}$$

Now, the applied moment $(M) = F \times R$

$$\therefore \text{Maximum bending stress } (\sigma_{max}) = \frac{6Ma}{RBt^2}$$

or,   assuming $a = 2R$

$$\sigma_{max} = \frac{12M}{Bt^2}$$

EXAMPLE *A flat spiral spring is pinned at the outer end and a winding cauple is applied to a spindle attached at the inner end as Fig. 14.14 with a = 150 mm; b = 40 mm and R = 75 mm.*

The spring is rectangular in cross-section, 12 mm wide and 2.5 mm thick and there are 5 turns. Determine

   (a) *the angle through which spindle turns.*

   (b) *the maximum bending stress produced in the spring material when a torque of 1.5 Nm is applied to the winding spindle.*
      E of spring material = 210 GN/m².

SOLUTION (a) The angle of twist $= \dfrac{ML}{EI}$

where $L = \dfrac{\pi n}{2}(a + b)$

$$= \frac{\pi \times 5}{2}(150 + 40) \times 10^{-3}$$

$$= 1492.3 + 10^{-3} \text{ m}$$

$$= 1.492 \text{ m}$$

$$\text{Angle of twist} = \frac{1.5 \times 1.492 \times 12}{210 \times 10^9 \times 12 \times 2.5^3 \times 10^{-12}}$$

$$= 0.682 \text{ radian}$$

$$= 39.1°$$

(b) Maximum bending moment $= F \times a$

Where applied moment $= F \times R = 1.5 \text{ Nm}$

i.e., $F = \dfrac{1.5}{75 \times 10^{-3}} = 20 \text{ N}$

Maximum bending moment $= 20 \times 150 \times 10^{-3}$

Maximum bending stress $= \left(\dfrac{M}{I}\right)y = \dfrac{3 \times (t/2)}{I}$

$$= \frac{3 \times 1.25 \times 10^{-3} \times 12}{12 \times 2.5^3 \times 10^{-12}}$$

$$= 240 \times 10^6 = 240 \ \text{MN/m}^2 \qquad\qquad \textbf{Ans.}$$

HIGHLIGHTS

1. Spring is a device used to store energy and release it when required.
2. Springs are of the following types:
    (i) Leaf spring or laminated spring
    (ii) Helical spring
    (iii) Flat spiral spring
3. Laminated springs are used in car; truck etc.
4. Helical springs are the thick spring wires coiled into a helix. They are of two types:
    (i) close coiled helical spring $(\alpha = 0)$
    (ii) open coiled helical spring $(\alpha \neq 0)$
5. The maximum shear stress induced in the wire of the closed coiled helical spring which carries an axial load (W) is given by

$$\tau = \frac{16 \, WR}{\pi d^3}$$

   where W = axil load on the spring
          R = mean radius of spring coil
   and d = diameter of the spring wire
6. For a closed-coiled helical spring which carries an axial load, we have

    (i) strain energy stored $(U) = \dfrac{32 \, W^2 R^3 \eta}{G d^4}$

    (ii) deflection of the spring (δ) at the centre due to axial load is given as

$$\delta = \frac{64 \, W \cdot R^3 \eta}{G d^4}$$

    (iii) stiffness of the spring $(k) = \dfrac{G d^4}{64 \, R^3 \eta}$

7. Open Coiled Helical spring
    (i) When axial load is applied only

   Then (a) Axial deflection $(\delta) = \dfrac{8 \, W D^3 n}{d^4 \cos \alpha} \left(\dfrac{\cos^2 \alpha}{G} + \dfrac{2 \sin^2 \alpha}{E} \right)$

   and (b) Axial rotation $(\phi) = \dfrac{16 W D^2 n \sin \alpha}{d^4} \left(\dfrac{1}{G} - \dfrac{2}{E} \right)$

    (ii) When Axial torque is applied only then

   (c) Axial deflection $(\delta) = \dfrac{16 \, T D^2 n \sin \alpha}{d^4} \left(\dfrac{1}{G} - \dfrac{2}{E} \right)$

and (d) Axial rotation $(\phi) = \dfrac{32\,TDn}{d^4\cos\alpha}\left(\dfrac{\sin^2\alpha}{G} + \dfrac{2\cos^2\alpha}{E}\right)$

8. Leaf spring

   (a) Single: $\delta = \dfrac{Wl^3}{4Ebt^3}$

   where W = concentrated load

   b = width

   t = thickness

   l = span length,

   E = modulus of elasticity

   and $U = \dfrac{W^2 l^3}{8Ebt^3}$ and $\sigma_b = \dfrac{3Wl}{2nbt^2}$

   (b) Laminated: $\delta = \dfrac{\sigma_b \cdot l^2}{4E \cdot t}$

   (c) Quarter elliptical spring

   $\sigma_b = \dfrac{\sigma Wl}{n \cdot b \cdot t^2}$

   $\delta = \dfrac{Wl^3}{n \cdot E \cdot bt^3}$

9. Flat spiral spring

   $\theta = \dfrac{M}{EI}\left[\dfrac{\pi n}{2}(a+b)\right]$

   where M = Winding moment

   n = No. of turns

   a = Maximum dimension of the spring from the pin

   b = diameter of the spindle

   Maximum bending stress $(\sigma_{b\ max}) = \dfrac{6\,M \cdot a}{RBt^2}$

   If $a = 2R$ then $\sigma_{max} = \dfrac{12\,M}{Bt^2}$

10. (a) When springs are in series then stiffness $k = \dfrac{k_1 k_2}{k_1 + k_2}$

    (b) When springs are in parallel then $k = k_1 + k_2$

PROBLEMS FOR PRACTICE
(THEORETICAL)

1. What is spring? Describe the characteristic features of different types of springs. Give an example of the application of each type.

2. Derive expressions for maximum stress, axial deflection; axial rotation and the strain energy stored in the spring.
3. Derive expression for the strain energy stored in a laminated spring.
4. Differentiate between close coiled helical spring and open coiled helical spring.
5. Find what percentage the axial deflection of the coil is neglected for spring in which $\alpha = 2.5°$. Assume n and R remain constant.   **(UPTU 2013-14)**

(NUMERICAL)

1. A leaf spring consists of seven steel plates each 60 mm wide and 6 mm thick. What would be the length of the spring if it is to carry a central load of 3 kN without the stress exceeding 150 MPa? Calculate also the deflection at the centre of the spring.

   Assume E for the spring material = 210 GPa.

2. A close coiled helical spring of circular section extends 25 mm when subjected to an axial load W and there is an angular rotation of 1 (one) radian when a torque T is independently applied about the axis of the spring.

   If Poission's ratio is v and the mean diameter of the coil is D show that

   $$\frac{T}{W} = \frac{D^2(1+v)}{100}$$

3. Two springs one close coiled and the other open coiled are made of the same material and have the same coil radius, the wire diameter and the number of coils. The angle of helix for the open coiled spring is $30°$. Compare the stiffness of the two springs when subjected to an axial load. $E = 2.5 \, G$. What inference do you arrive from this problem.

4. A wagon weighing 200 kN is moving at a speed of 1 m/sec. Find the volume of the buffer spring which should be able to absorb energy of the wagon with the bending and the shearing stresses not exceeding 400 MPa and 300 MPa respectively; if the impact is absorbed by
   (i) compression of the spring
   (ii) twisting of the spring.
   Assume spring to be close coiled $E = 200$ MPa ; $G = 80$ GPa.

ANSWERS

1. Length (l) of spring = 504 mm; deflection (δ) = 7.56 mm

3. $\left[\dfrac{k_0}{k_c} = 0.91\right]$

4. (i) Volume of spring = 72487×10^3 mm^3
   (ii) Volume of spring = 20387×10^4 mm^3

OBJECTIVE QUESTIONS

1. The load deflection graph for a springs is
   (a) parabolic   (b) cubic curve
   (c) linear   (d) none of the above

2. The spring index is the ratio of:
   (a) load and deflection
   (b) load and angle of twist.
   (c) mean coil diameter and spring wire diameter
   (d) mean coil diameter and spring length
3. A load applied at the centre of a carriage spring to straighten all its leaves is known as:
   (a) ultimate load
   (b) safe load
   (c) yield load
   (d) proof load
4. The angle of helix in a practical close coiled spring is:
   (a) nearly zero
   (b) $10 - 15°$
   (c) about $15°$
   (d) none of the above
5. The stress which can always be neglected in the light close coiled spring is:
   (a) direct shear stress
   (b) torsional shear stress
   (c) bending stress
   (d) none of the above
6. Out of the leaf spring, close coiled helical spring and the open coiled helical spring, the maximum energy per unit volume is absorbed in case of:
   (a) leaf spring
   (b) close coiled spring
   (c) open coiled spring
   (d) none of the above
7. The spring used in the mechanical watches is:
   (a) leaf spring
   (b) close coiled spring
   (c) open coiled helical spring
   (d) flat spiral spring
8. Leaf spring is commonly used in case of:
   (a) automobiles
   (b) instruments
   (c) clocks
   (d) none of the above
9. Master leaf in a leaf spring is:
   (a) the shortest spring
   (b) the longest leaf
   (c) the middle leaf
   (d) none of the above
10. The energy stored in a close-coiled helical spring when subjected to an 'axial twist' is given by:

   (a) $\dfrac{\sigma_b^{2}}{6E} \times$ volume of the spring
   (b) $\dfrac{\sigma_b^{2}}{8E} \times$ volume of the spring

   (c) $\dfrac{\sigma_b^{2}}{4E} \times$ volume of the spring
   (d) $\dfrac{\sigma_b^{2}}{2E} \times$ volume of the spring

   (where σ_b = bending stress)
11. Two springs of stiffness k_1 and k_2 are connected in series, the stiffness of the composite spring (K) will be given by:

   (a) $k = k_1 + k_2$
   (b) $k = k_1 \times k_2$

   (c) $k = \dfrac{k_1 k_2}{k_1 + k_2}$
   (d) $k = \dfrac{k_1 + k_2}{k_1 k_2}$

12. The rescilience of a flat spiral spring is given by:

(a) $\dfrac{\sigma_{max}}{24E}$ (b) $\dfrac{\sigma^2_{max}}{24E}$ (c) $\dfrac{\sigma^2_{max}}{12E}$ (d) $\dfrac{\sigma^2_{max}}{8E}$

ANSWERS

1. (c)	2. (c)	3. (d)	4. (b)	5. (a)	6. (c)
7. (d)	8. (a)	9. (b)	10. (b)	11. (c)	12. (b)

— ❖❖ —

THEORIES OF FAILURE

15.1 INTRODUCTION

A material is said to have failed when it is loaded beyond the elastic limit and permanent deformation (non-recoverable) occurs.

Failure of materials represent either separation of a particles from each other (brittle fracture) or slipping of particle (ductile fracture 'or' yielding) accompanied by considerable plastic deformation. Yielding is considered as the most important failure criteria. The onset of plastic deformation is called yielding of material. The criteria for deciding as to which combination of multi axial stresses will cause yielding are called yield criteria.

If the material is subjected to simple stress followed by uniaxial loading then it is easy to predict the failure of material. However, if the material is subjected to complex stresses followed by biaxial or triaxial loading then it is difficult to predict the failure of material.

In order to analyse the theories of failure various theories have been given. In these theories, the complex state of stress has been related to the elastic limit in simple tension or compression.

Let us consider a complex state of stress expressed by three principal stresses $\sigma_1, \sigma_2, \sigma_3$ such that $\sigma_1 > \sigma_2 > \sigma_3$.

We will discuss theory of failure for 2-D stress system.

Five theories have been given and these are:

1. Maximum Principal Stress Theory
2. Maximum Shear Stress Theory
3. Maximum Principal Strain Theory
4. Total Strain Energy Theory
5. Shear Strain Energy Theory or (Distortion Theory).

1. Maximum Principal Stress Theory (Rankine Theory)

According to this theory, failure of material occurs when the maximum principal stress in the complex stress system is equal to the yield stress in simple tension or minimum principal stress is equal to yield stress in simple compression.

Let σ_o be the yield stress then according to this theory, failure of material will occur when

$$\sigma_1 = \pm\, \sigma_o$$

$$\sigma_2 = \pm\, \sigma_o$$

By the experiments it is seen that brittle materials fail due to tensile stress, so this theory can be used to predict the failure for brittle materials and should not be applied for ductile materials.

Further, we know that brittle materials do not have yield point therefore instead of yield stress, ultimate stress (σ_u) is used as the failure criterion. It is general practice to use factor of safety (F.O.S.) to find the permissible stress or working stress.

$$\text{Working stress } (\sigma_1) = \pm \frac{\sigma_u}{\text{F.O.S.}}$$

and

$$(\sigma_2) = \pm \frac{\sigma_u}{\text{F.O.S.}}$$

2. Maximum Shear Stress Theory (Guest or Tresca or Coulomb Theory)

According to this theory, failure of material occurs when the maximum shear stress in the complex system becomes equal to that of the value of maximum shear stress in simple tension or compression.

Since, the maximum shear stress is half the greatest difference between two principal stresses, the criterion of failure becomes

$$\frac{\sigma_1 - \sigma_2}{2} = \pm \frac{\sigma_o}{2}$$

$$\sigma_1 - \sigma_2 = \pm\, \sigma_o$$

This theory is used for ductile materials.

In 3-D stress system $\tau_{max} = \dfrac{\sigma_1 - \sigma_3}{2}$.

3. Maximum Principal Strain Theory or St. Venant's Theory

According to this theory, failure of material occurs when the maximum strain in the complex stress system equals the value of maximum strain at yield point in simple tension or compression test.

Mathematically, failure of material will occur when

$$\varepsilon_{complex} = \varepsilon_{simple}$$

$$\frac{1}{E}\left[\sigma_1 - v \cdot \sigma_2\right] = \pm \frac{\sigma_o}{E}$$

$$\sigma_1 - v \cdot \sigma_2 = \pm\, \sigma_o \qquad\qquad\text{(for tensile test)}$$

and $\qquad \sigma_2 - v \cdot \sigma_1 = \pm\, \sigma_o \qquad\qquad\text{(for compression test)}$

[N.B.: This theory is not used now a days as it does not match with experimental results except for brittle materials].

4. Total Strain Energy Theory (Haigh Theory)

According to this theory, failure of material occurs when the total strain energy*. density in the complex stress system is equal to the strain energy density at yield point in simple tension or compression test.

So, failure will occur when

$$\left[\frac{U}{V}\right]_{\text{in complex system}} = \left[\frac{U}{V}\right]_{\text{in simple tension or compression}}$$

or, $\dfrac{1}{2E}\left[\sigma_1^2 + \sigma_2^2 - 2v\sigma_1\sigma_2\right] = \dfrac{\sigma_o^2}{2E}$

or, $\sigma_1^2 + \sigma_2^2 - 2v\sigma_1\sigma_2 = \sigma_o^2$

5. Shear Strain Energy Theory or (Distortion Theory) or (VON MISES & HENCKY Theory)

According to this theory, failure of material occurs when shear strain energy in the complex stress system equal to the shear strain energy at yield point in simple tension or compression test.

(a) For 3-D Stress System

$$\frac{1}{12G}\left[(\sigma_1 - \sigma_2)^2 + (\sigma_2 - \sigma_3)^2 + (\sigma_3 - \sigma_1)^2\right] = \frac{\sigma_o^2}{6G}$$

or, $(\sigma_1 - \sigma_2)^2 + (\sigma_2 - \sigma_3)^2 + (\sigma_3 - \sigma_1)^2 = 2\sigma_o^2$

(b) For 2-D Stress System, putting $\sigma_3 = 0$ we get

$\sigma_1^2 + \sigma_2^2 - \sigma_1\sigma_2 = \sigma_o^2$

or, $(\sigma_1^2 + \sigma_2^2 - \sigma_1\sigma_2)^{\frac{1}{2}} = \sigma_o$

---

*Strain energy per unit volume is called strain energy density (u).

$$\text{Strain energy density} = \left(\frac{U}{V}\right) = \frac{1}{2} \times P \times \delta \times \frac{1}{V}$$

$$= \frac{1}{2} \times P \times \frac{PL}{AE} \times \frac{1}{V}$$

$$= \frac{1}{2} \cdot \frac{P^2L}{AE} \times \frac{1}{V} = \frac{1}{2} \times \left(\frac{P}{A}\right)^2 \times \frac{AL}{E} \times \frac{1}{V}$$

$$= \frac{1}{2} \times \sigma^2 \times \frac{V}{E} \times \frac{1}{V}$$

$$\therefore \qquad \frac{U}{V} = \left(\frac{\sigma^2}{2E}\right)$$

This is the best theory of the five. It is also known as *OCTAHEDRAL SHEAR STRESS THEORY.

In the above theories, it has been assumed that the properties of material in tension and compression are similar. However, certain materials like concrete; cast iron, soils etc. shows different properties depending on the nature of applied load.

EXAMPLE 1 *The load on a bolt consists of an axial pull of 10 kN together with transverse shear force of 5 kN.*
Estimate the diameter of the bolt using all theories of failure.
Elastic limit in tension = 270 N/mm²
Factor of Safety (F.O.S) = 3
Poisson's Ratio (v) = 0.3   **(Similar problem 3rd semester MTU 2011-12)**

SOLUTION Permissible simple tensile stress $= \left[\dfrac{270}{3}\right]$

$\therefore \qquad \sigma_o = 90 \text{ N/mm}^2$

Let d = diameter of bolt.

Then, normal stress is $= \dfrac{10 \times 10^3}{\dfrac{\pi}{4} d^2}$

$$\sigma = \frac{40,000}{\pi d^2} \text{N/mm}^2$$

and   Shear stress $(\tau) = \dfrac{5000}{\dfrac{\pi d^2}{4}}$

$$= \frac{20,000}{\pi d^2} \text{N/mm}^2$$

Hence, principal stresses are

$$\sigma_1, \sigma_2 = \frac{\sigma_x}{2} \pm \sqrt{\left(\frac{\sigma_x}{2}\right)^2 + \tau^2} \qquad \text{and} \qquad \sigma_3 = 0$$

---

*OCTAHEDRAL Stresses are defined as the normal and shear stress in a cross-section where, normal forms the same angle with all the principal axes.

$$\sigma_{\text{oct}} = \frac{\sigma_1 + \sigma_2 + \sigma_3}{3} ; \tau_{\text{oct}} = \frac{1}{3}\sqrt{(\sigma_1 - \sigma_2)^2 + (\sigma_2 - \sigma_3)^2 + (\sigma_3 - \sigma_1)^2}$$

For uniaxial loading at yield point, $\tau_{\text{oct}} = \dfrac{\sqrt{2}}{3}\sigma_0$ and for biaxial stress system,

$$\tau_{\text{oct}} = \frac{\sqrt{2}}{3}\sqrt{\sigma_1{}^2 + \sigma_2{}^2 - \sigma_1\sigma_2} .$$

$$\sigma_1, \sigma_2 = \frac{40,000}{2} \pm \sqrt{\left(\frac{40,000}{\pi d^2}\right)^2 + \left(\frac{20,000}{\pi d^2}\right)^2}$$

i.e. $\sigma_1 = \dfrac{48290}{\pi d^2}$

and $\sigma_2 = -\dfrac{8290}{\pi d^2}$

$\sigma_3 = 0$

1. Applying Rankine Theory (Principal Stress Theory)

Maximum principal stress in bolt

$$\sigma_1 = \frac{1}{2}\sigma + \frac{1}{2}\sqrt{\sigma^2 + 4\tau^2} \qquad\qquad \text{(Here, } \sigma_x = \sigma; \ \sigma_y = 0\text{)}$$

$$= \frac{1}{2} \times \frac{40,000}{\pi d^2} + \frac{1}{2}\sqrt{\left(\frac{40,000}{\pi d^2}\right) + 4\left(\frac{20,000}{\pi d^2}\right)^2}$$

$\therefore \qquad \sigma_1 = \dfrac{48,290}{\pi d^2}$

Maximum stress in simple tension = 90 N/mm^2 = σ_0

Now, equating the above gives i.e. $\sigma_1 = \sigma_0$

$$\frac{48290}{\pi d^2} = 90$$

$$d = \sqrt{\frac{48290}{90\,\pi}} = 13 \text{ mm}$$

2. Maximum Shear Stress Theory

$$\tau_{max} = \frac{1}{2}\sqrt{\sigma^2 + 4\tau^2}$$

$$= \frac{1}{2}\sqrt{\left(\frac{40,000}{\pi d^2}\right)^2 + 4\left(\frac{20,000}{\pi d^2}\right)^2}$$

$$= \frac{1}{2\pi d^2} \times 100\sqrt{16 + 4 \times 4}$$

$$= \frac{28290}{\pi d^2}$$

Given τ is simple tension = 45 N/mm²

$$\left[\because \tau = \frac{1}{2}(\sigma_2 - \sigma_1) = \frac{1}{2} \times \sigma = \frac{1}{2} \times 90 = 45 \text{ N/mm}^2\right]$$

$\therefore \quad \dfrac{28,290}{\pi d^2} = \dfrac{1}{2}\sigma$

or, $\quad \dfrac{28290}{\pi d^2} = 45$

$$d = \sqrt{\frac{28290}{45\,\pi}} = 14.4 \text{ mm}$$

3. Strain Energy Theory
By this theory

$$\sigma_1^2 + \sigma_2^2 - 2\nu\,\sigma_1\,\sigma_2 = \sigma_o^2$$

$$\left(\frac{48290}{\pi d^2}\right)^2 + \left(-\frac{8290}{\pi d^2}\right)^2 - 2 \times 0.3 \times \left(\frac{48290}{\pi d^2}\right)\left(\frac{-8290}{\pi d^2}\right) = \frac{40000}{\pi d^2}$$

On solving, we get

$$d = 13.5 \text{ mm}$$

4. Shear Strain Theory
$$(\sigma_1 - \sigma_2)^2 + \sigma_2^2 = \sigma_o^2$$

Substituting the value of σ_1, σ_2 and σ_o we get, d = 13.7 mm.

EXAMPLE 2 *A cylindrical shell made up of mild steel plate 1.2 m in diameter is to be subjected to an internal pressure of 1.5 MN/m². If the material yields at 200 MN/m². Calculate the thickness of the plate on the basis of the following three theories, assuming a factor of safety 3 in each case:*

  (i) Maximum principal stress theory

  (ii) Maximum shear stress theory

  (iii) Maximum shear strain theory.

SOLUTION d = 1.2 m

   Internal pressure, p = 1.5 MN/m²
   Yield stress   = 200 MN/m²
   F.O.S.   = 3

$\therefore$ Allowable stress in simple tension $\sigma_o = \left(\dfrac{200}{3}\right)$ MN/m²

Thinckness (t)
Hoop (or circumferential) stress

$$\sigma_h \text{ or } \sigma_c = \frac{pd}{2t}$$

$$= \frac{1.5 \times 1.2}{2t}$$

$$\therefore \qquad \sigma_1 \text{ or } \sigma_h = \left(\frac{0.9}{t}\right) \text{MN/m}^2 \qquad\qquad [\sigma_1 = \text{Max Principal Stress} = \sigma_h]$$

Longitudinal stress $(\sigma_l) = \dfrac{pd}{4t}$

$$= \frac{1.5 \times 1.2}{4 \times t}$$

$$= \frac{0.45}{t} \text{MN/m}^2$$

1. According to maximum principal stress theory $\sigma_1 = \sigma_o$

$$\frac{0.9}{\cdot t} = \frac{200}{3}$$

$$t = 0.0135 \text{ m}$$

$$\boxed{t = 13.5 \text{ mm}} \qquad \textbf{Ans.}$$

2. According to maximum shear stress theory

$$\frac{\sigma_c - \sigma_l}{2} = \frac{\sigma}{2}$$

$$\frac{0.9 - 0.45}{2t} = \frac{200}{6}$$

$$t = \frac{1}{2}\left[\frac{(0.9 - 0.45) \times 6}{200}\right]$$

$$= 0.00675 \text{ m}$$

$$\boxed{t = 6.75 \text{ mm}} \qquad \textbf{Ans.}$$

3. According to shear strain energy theory

$$\sigma_1{}^2 + \sigma_2{}^2 - \sigma_1 \sigma_2 = \sigma_o{}^2$$

$$\therefore \qquad \frac{1}{t^2}\left[(0.9)^2 + (0.45)^2 - 0.9 \times 0.45\right] = \left(\frac{200}{3}\right)^2$$

$$\frac{1}{t^2}\left[0.81 + 0.2025 - 0.405\right] = 4444.4$$

or, $\qquad t^2 = \left(\dfrac{0.6075}{4444.4}\right)$

$$t = 0.0117 \text{ m} = 11.69 \text{ mm} \simeq 11.7 \text{ mm} \qquad \textbf{Ans.}$$

EXAMPLE 3 *At a point on a machine member, it was found that* $\dot{\sigma}_{xx} = 150$ *MPa and* $\sigma_{yy} = -100$ *MPa* .

The yield strength of the material is 300 MPa. Calculate the maximum safe value of τ_{xy} *according to (i) Rankine theory;* (ii) *Guest theory.*

SOLUTION We know that,

$$\sigma_{1,2} = \frac{\sigma_x + \sigma_y}{2} \pm \sqrt{\left(\frac{\sigma_x - \sigma_y}{2}\right)^2 + \tau^2}$$

$$= \left(\frac{150 - 100}{2}\right) \pm \sqrt{\left(\frac{150 + 100}{2}\right)^2 + \tau^2}$$

$$= 25 \pm \sqrt{15625 + \tau^2} \text{ N/mm}^2 \text{ or MPa}$$

(i) Rankine Theory

$$\sigma_1 = \sigma_o$$

$\therefore \qquad 25 + \sqrt{15625 + \tau_{xy}^2} = 300$

$$\tau_{xy} = \sqrt{(300 - 25)^2 - 15625}$$

$$= 245 \text{ MPa}$$

(ii) Guest Theory

$$\sigma_1 - \sigma_2 = \sigma_o$$

$\therefore \qquad 2\sqrt{156 + \tau_{xy}^2} = 300$

$$\tau_{xy} = \sqrt{(150)^2 - 15625}$$

$$= 84.7 \text{ MPa}$$

$$\approx 85 \text{ MPa}$$

EXAMPLE 4 *A mild steel shaft 100 mm diameter is subjected to a maximum torque of 15 kNm and a maximum bending moment of 10 kNm at a particular section. Find the factor of safety according to the maximum shear stress theory of failure if the elastic limit is simple tension is 240 MN/m².* **[UPTU 2006-07]**

SOLUTION Given $d = 100$ mm

$$T_{max} = 15 \text{ kNm} = 15 \times 10^6 \text{ Nmm}$$
$$M_{max} = 10 \text{ kNm} = 10 \times 10^6 \text{ Nmm}$$

$$\tau = \frac{16T}{\pi d^3}$$

$$= \frac{16 \times 15 \times 10^6}{\left(\dfrac{22}{7}\right) \times (100)^3} = \frac{16 \times 15 \times 7}{22 \times 1} = 76.36 \text{ N/mm}^2$$

$$\sigma_b = \frac{M}{I} \cdot y = \frac{10 \times 10^5}{\left(\dfrac{I}{y}\right)}$$

$$= \frac{10 \times 10^6}{Z} = \frac{10 \times 10^6}{\dfrac{\pi}{32}(100)^3}$$

$$= \frac{10^7 \times 32}{\pi \times 10^6} = 101.81 \text{ N/mm}^2$$

$$\sigma_1, \sigma_2 = \frac{\sigma_b}{2} \pm \sqrt{\left(\frac{\sigma_b}{2}\right)^2 + \tau^2}$$

$$= 50.90 \pm \sqrt{(50.90)^2 + (76.36)^2}$$

$$= 50.90 \pm 91.76$$

$$= 142.66 \text{ or } -40.86 \text{ N/mm}^2$$

$$\tau_{max} = \frac{1}{2}(\sigma_{max} - \sigma_{min})$$

$$= \frac{1}{2}(142.66 + 40.86)$$

$$= 91.76 \text{ N/mm}^2$$

$$\tau_{max} \text{ (simple)} = \left[\frac{240 \times 10^6}{2 \times 10^6}\right] \text{N/mm}^2 \qquad \left[\because \tau = \frac{\sigma_t}{2}\right]$$

$$= 120 \text{ N/mm}^2$$

Now, $\qquad 91.76 = \dfrac{120}{\text{fos}}$

$\therefore \qquad F.O.S = \dfrac{120}{91.76} = 1.30$ **Ans.**

15.2 GRAPHICAL REPRESENTATION OF THEORIES OF FAILURE FOR TWO DIMENSIONAL STRESS SYSTEM

The different theories of failure can be represented graphically for two dimensional stress system.

1. Maximum Principal Stress Theory

According to this theory, the failure of a material will occur when the maximum principal tensile stress (σ_1) in the complex system reaches the value of the maximum stress at the elastic limit in simple tension or the minimum principal stress (σ_2) i.e. compressive stress reaches the values of the maximum stress at the elastic limit in simple compression.

So, mathematically, failure will occur if σ_1 or $\sigma_2 = \sigma_{et}$ or σ_{ec}.

If $\sigma_{et} = \sigma_{ec} = {}^{*}\sigma_o$ then these are represented graphically on σ_1, σ_2 coordinate.

Failure will take place if any point having coordinates (σ_1, σ_2) falls outside the square.

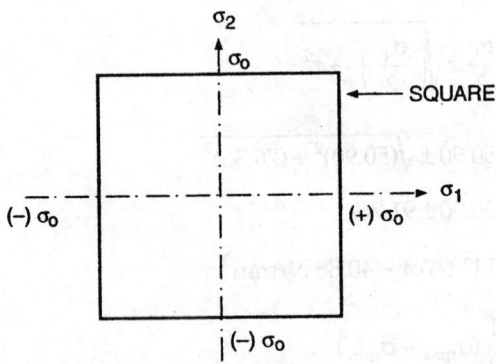

Fig. 15.1 Representation of maximum principal stress theories

2. Maximum Shear Stress Theory

According to this theory failure will occur when τ_{max} in a material reaches the value of maximum shear stress in simple tension at the elastic limit.

$$\tau_{max} \text{ in a material} = \frac{\sigma_{max} - \sigma_{min}}{2}$$

$$= \left(\frac{\sigma_1 - \sigma_2}{2} \right)$$

When σ_1 and σ_2 are of opposite sign, the greater shearing stress is given by $\left(\dfrac{\sigma_1 - \sigma_2}{2} \right)$ and the failure is represented by $(\sigma_1 - \sigma_2) = \sigma_o$ or $(\sigma_2 - \sigma_1) = -\sigma_o$.

The boundaries of these equations are represented by parallel lines AB and ED.

When σ_1 and σ_2 are like (i.e. Ist or IIIrd quadrant) the maximum shear stress is equal to $\left(\dfrac{\sigma_1}{2} \right)$ or $\left(\dfrac{\sigma_2}{2} \right)$ whichever is more.

σ_o = Yield stress in simple tension or compression.

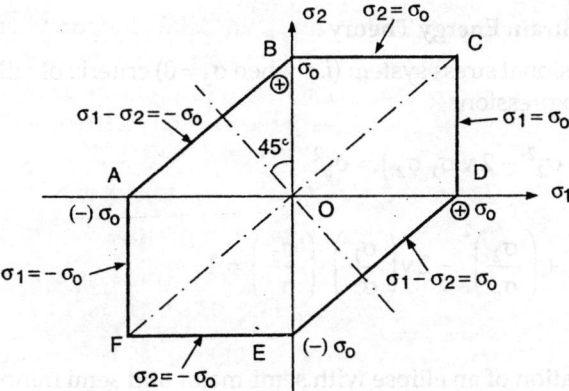

Fig. 15.2 Graphical representation of maximum shear stress theory

Therefore, failure is represented by the following

$$\left.\begin{array}{l} \sigma_1 = \sigma_o \\ \text{or, } \sigma_2 = \sigma_o \end{array}\right\}$$

These are represented by line BC and CD in the Ist quadrant and AF and FE in the third quadrant.

3. Maximum Principal Strain Theory

According to this theory the criteria of failure for two dimensional stress system is

$$(\sigma_1 - \nu\,\sigma_2) = \sigma_t = \sigma_o$$

and $$(\sigma_2 - \nu\,\sigma_1) = \sigma_c = \sigma_o$$

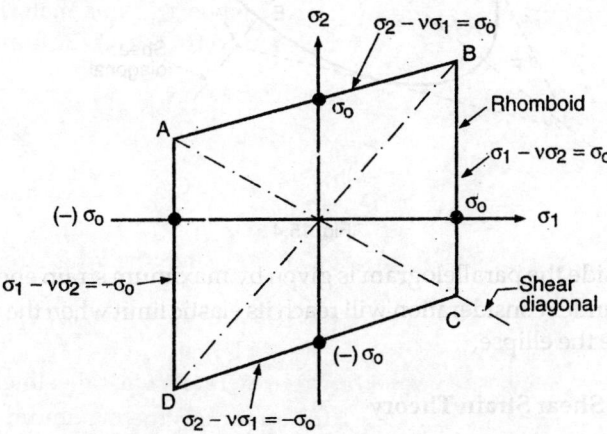

Fig. 15.3 Graphical representation of maximum strain theory

By plotting the above equation, a 'Rhomboid' is obtained.

The failure of the material will occur if any point having coordinates (σ_1, σ_2) falls outside $ABCD$.

4. Maximum Strain Energy Theory

For two dimensional stress system (*i.e.* when $\sigma_3 = 0$) criteria of failure is given by the following expression:

$$\left(\sigma_1^2 + \sigma_2^2 - 2\,v\,\sigma_1\,\sigma_2\right) = \sigma_o^2$$

or,

$$\left(\frac{\sigma_1}{\sigma_o}\right)^2 + \left(\frac{\sigma_2}{\sigma_o}\right)^2 - 2v\left(\frac{\sigma_1}{\sigma_o}\right)\cdot\left(\frac{\sigma_2}{\sigma_o}\right) = 1$$

This is the equation of an ellipse with semi-major and semi minor axes $\dfrac{\sigma_o}{\sqrt{1-v}}$;

$\dfrac{\sigma_o}{\sqrt{1+v}}$ respectively each at 45° to the coordinate axes as shown in figure.

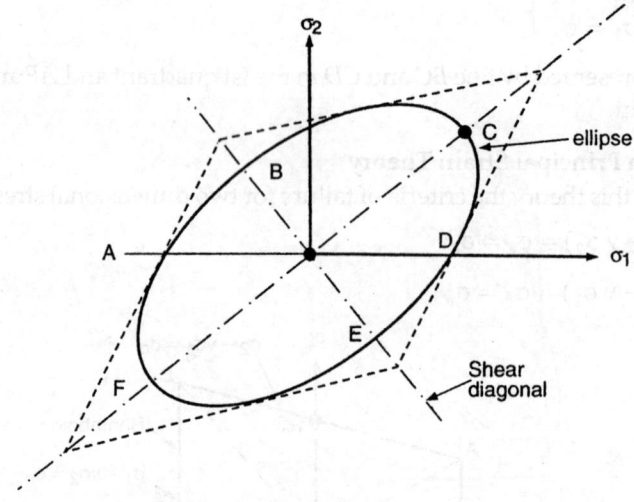

Fig. 15.4

The ellipse inside the parallelogram is given by maximum strain energy theory. The material under consideration will reach its elastic limit when the point (σ_1, σ_2) passes outside the ellipse.

5. Maximum Shear Strain Theory

For two dimensional case (when $\sigma_3 = 0$), the criteria of failure given by this theory is

$$\sigma_1^2 + \sigma_2^2 - \sigma_1\,\sigma_2 = \sigma_o^2$$

This is an equation of ellipse with centre at the origin and axes inclined at 45°.

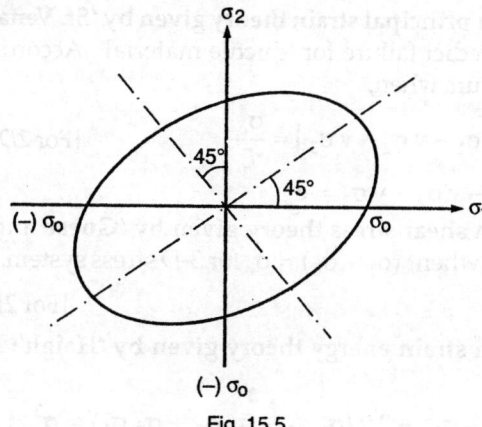

Fig. 15.5

15.3 GRAPHICAL REPRESENTATION OF VARIOUS THEORIES OF FAILURE ON THE SAME DIAGRAM

When $\sigma_t = \sigma_c$ and $\varepsilon_t = \varepsilon_c$.

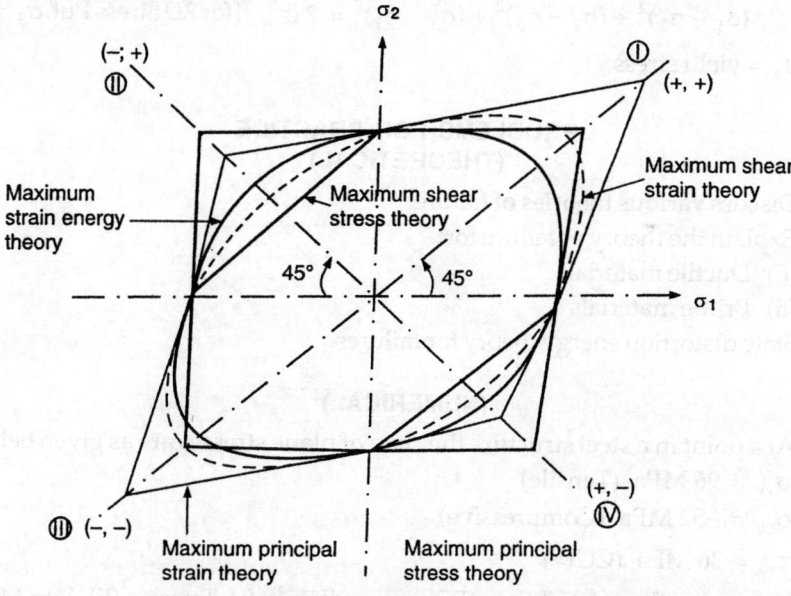

Fig. 15.6 Graphical representation of theories of failure

HIGHLIGHTS

1. A material is said to have failed when permanent deformation occurs.

   If at a point in a strained body σ_1, σ_2 and σ_3 are the principal stresses such that $\sigma_1 > \sigma_2 > \sigma_3$ and σ is the stress in simple tension, then

   The theories of failure are the following:

   (a) **Maximum principal stress theory given by 'Rankine:** According to this theory failure of material under complex stress occurs when $\sigma_1 = \sigma_o$. This theory is used to predict failure of 'brittle material'.

(b) **Maximum principal strain theory given by 'St. Venant':** This theory is used to predict failure for 'ductile material'. According to this theory failure occurs when,

$$\frac{1}{E}[\sigma_1 - v\,\sigma_2 - v\,\sigma_3] = \frac{\sigma_o}{E} \qquad \text{[For 2D Problem } \sigma_3 = 0]$$

or, $\sigma_1 - v\,\sigma_2 - v\,\sigma_3 = \sigma_o$

(c) **Maximum shear stress theory given by 'Guest' and 'Tresca':** Failure will occur when, $(\sigma_1 - \sigma_3) = \sigma_o$ for 3-D stress system.

$$\text{[For 2D } (\sigma_1 - \sigma_2) = \sigma_o]$$

(d) **Maximum strain energy theory given by 'Haigh':** Failure will occur when,

$$\sigma_1^2 + \sigma_2^2 + \sigma_3^2 - 2v\,(\sigma_1\,\sigma_2 + \sigma_2\,\sigma_3 + \sigma_3\,\sigma_1) = \sigma_o^2$$

$$\text{[Put } \sigma_3 = 0 \text{ for 2D Problem]}$$

(e) **Shear strain theory given by v_0 Mises and Hencky: Failure will occur when**

$$(\sigma_1 - \sigma_2)^2 + (\sigma_2 - \sigma_3)^2 + (\sigma_3 - \sigma_1)^2 = 2\sigma_o^2 \quad \text{[for 2D Stress Put } \sigma_3 = 0]$$

NB: σ_o = yield stress

PROBLEMS FOR PRACTICE
(THEORETICAL)

1. Discuss various theories of failure.
2. Explain the theory of failure for:
   (i) Ductile materials
   (ii) Brittle materials
3. State distortion energy theory for failures.

(NUMERICAL)

1. At a point in a steel structure the state of plane stresses are as given below:

   $\sigma_{xx} = 96$ MPa (Tensile)

   $\sigma_{yy} = -52$ MPa (Compressive)

   $\tau_{xy} = 36$ MPa (CCW)

   Determine the safety factor (FOS) according to (i) Tresca (ii) Von Mises. Yield point for steel is 320 MPa.
2. A shaft of uniform circular section is subjected to torsion. Determine the ratio of requisite diameters according to maximum shear stress theory.
3. A bar of mild steel carries an axial pull of 10 kN and a transverse shear force of 5 kN. Taking the elastic limit in tension as 240 MPa, a factor of safety 3 and poisson's ratio is 0.3. Calculate the diameter of the bar if the criterion is:
   (i) Maximum principal stress theory (ii) Maximum strain energy theory.
4. A steel tube has a mean diameter of 120 mm and a thickness of 2 mm. Calculate the torque that can be transmitted by the tube with a factor of safety 3 if the criterion of failure is:

    (a) maximum shear stress

    (b) maximum strain energy

    (c) maximum shear strain energy

    The elastic limit of steel in tension is 220 MPa and Poisson's ratio is 0.3.

5. A circular shaft of 100 mm diameter is subjected to combined bending and twisting moments, the bending moment being three times the twisting moment. If the direct tension yield point of the material is 400 MPa and factor of safety is 4. Calculate the allowable twisting moment according to the following theories of elastic failure:

    (a) Maximum principal stress theory

    (b) Maximum shear stress theory

    (c) Maximum shear strain energy theory

ANSWERS

1. (i) 2 (ii) 2   2. 1.26
3. (i) 13.85 mm   (ii) 14.3 mm
4. (a) 1659 mm   (b) 2346 Nm (c) 1915 Nm
5. (a) 3185 Nm   (b) 3110 Nm (c) 3150 Nm

OBJECTIVE QUESTIONS

1. According to distortion energy theory failure will not occur when:

    (a) $\dfrac{(\sigma_1 - \sigma_2)^2 + (\sigma_2 - \sigma_3)^2 + (\sigma_3 - \sigma_1)^2}{2} \le \sigma_e$

    (b) $\left[(\sigma_1 - \sigma_2)^2 + 4\tau^2 \right]^{1/2} \le \sigma_e$

    (c) $\left[\sigma_1^2 + \sigma_2^2 + \sigma_3^2 - v(\sigma_1 \sigma_2 + \sigma_2 \sigma_3 + \sigma_3 \sigma_1) \right]^{1/2} \le \sigma_t$

    (d) $\dfrac{(\sigma_1 + \sigma_2)^2 + \left[(\sigma_1 - \sigma_2)^2 + 4\tau^2 \right]^{1/2}}{2} \le \sigma_e$

2. In a strained body, three principal stresses at a point are denoted by σ_1, σ_2 and σ_3 such that $\sigma_1 > \sigma_2 > \sigma_3$. If σ_e denotes yield stress then according to the maximum shear stress theory:

    (a) $\sigma_1 - \sigma_2 = \sigma_e$ (b) $\sigma_1 - \sigma_3 = \sigma_e$

    (c) $\sigma_2 - \sigma_3 = 0$ (d) $\dfrac{\sigma_1 + \sigma_2}{2} = \sigma_e$

3. All the failure theories gives nearly the same result:

    (a) when one of the principal stresses at a point is large in comparison to the other

    (b) when shear stresses act

    (c) when both the principal stresses are numerically equal

    (d) for all situation of stress

4. According to maximum shear stress failure theory, yielding in material occurs when:

   (a) maximum shear stress $= \dfrac{1}{2} \times$ yield stress

   (b) maximum shear stress $= \sqrt{2} \times$ yield stress

   (c) maximum shear stress $= \sqrt{\dfrac{2}{3}} \times$ yield stress

   (d) maximum shear stress $= 2 \times$ yield stress

5. As per maximum principal stress theory, when a shaft is subjected to a bending moment M and torque T and if σ is the allowable stress in axial tension then the diameter 'd' of the shaft is given by:

   (a) $d^3 = \dfrac{16}{\pi\sigma}\left[M + \sqrt{M^2 + T^2} \right]$ 　　(b) $d^3 = \dfrac{4}{\pi\sigma}\left[M + \sqrt{M^2 + T^2} \right]$

   (c) $d^3 = \dfrac{32}{\pi\sigma}\left[M + \sqrt{M^2 + T^2} \right]$ 　　(d) $d^3 = \dfrac{8}{\pi\sigma}\left[M + \sqrt{M^2 + T^2} \right]$

6. A cube is subjected to equal tensile stress on all the three faces. If the yield stress of the material is σ_y, then based on strain energy theory, the maximum tensile stress will be:

   (a) $\dfrac{\sigma_y}{\sqrt{3(1 - 2v)}}$ 　　　　　　(b) $\dfrac{\sigma_y}{\sqrt{3(2 - v)}}$

   (c) $\dfrac{\sigma_y}{\sqrt{3(1 - v)}}$ 　　　　　　(d) $\dfrac{\sigma_y}{\sqrt{3(1 + v)}}$

ANSWERS

1. (a)   **2.** (b)   **3.** (c)   **4.** (a)   **5.** (a)   **6.** (a)

— ❖❖ —

THIN CYLINDRICAL VESSELS

16.1 INTRODUCTION

Thin walled shell both 'cylindrical' as well as 'sphericals', are used as container for storage of liquids, and gases under pressure.

If the ratio of thickness to internal diameter of a shell is less than $\dfrac{1}{20}$ *i.e.* if $\left(\dfrac{t}{D_i}\right) < \dfrac{1}{20}$ then it is termed as thin shell.

Owing to internal fluid (*i.e.* liquid or gas) pressure such shells are subjected to:

   (i)   Circumferential stress or Hoop stress (σ_h)

  (ii)   Longitudinal stress (σ_l)

 (iii)   Radial stress (σ_r)

Among these stresses, Radial stress (σ_r) is small and can be neglected.

Whenever a thin Cylinder is subjected to an internal pressure, it is likely to fail either by splitting into two Cylindrical shell (*i.e.* Circumferentially) or by splitting it up into two troughs (*i.e.* longitudinally) as shown in Fig. 16.1 (a) and (b) respectively.

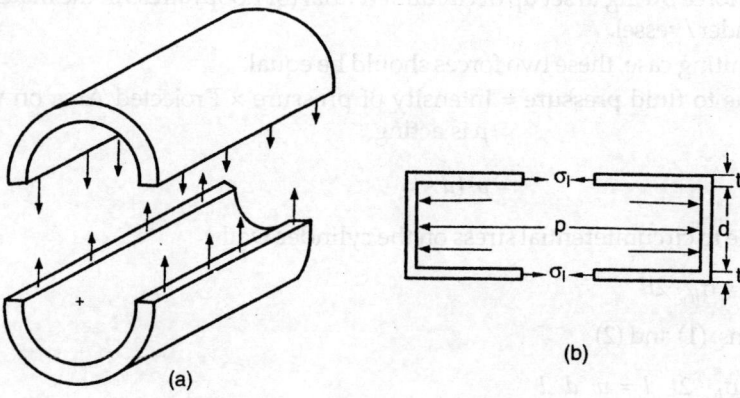

Fig. 16.1

16.2 DERIVATION OF STRESSES IN THIN CYLINDRICAL SHELL

Following assumptions are taken into account
  (i) Radial Stress is negligible
  (ii) Hoop stress is constant along the thickness of the shell.

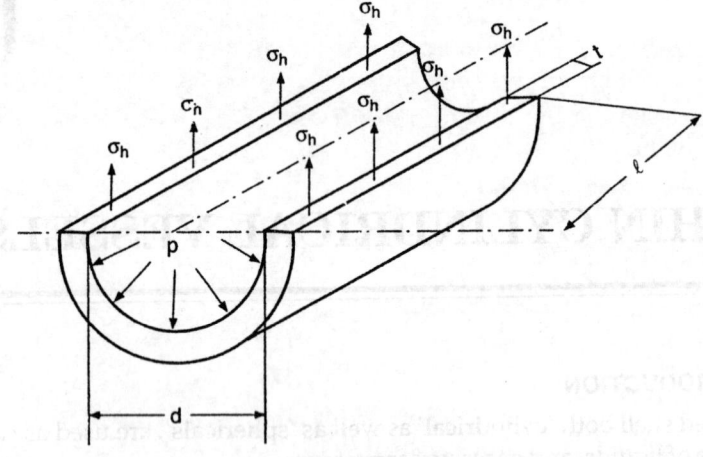

Fig. 16.2

Hoop Stress: When Thin Cylindrical Shell is Subjected to Internal Fluid Pressure

Let us Consider a thin Cylinder/vessel subjected to internal fluid pressure (may be gas or liquid).

Let p = intensity of pressure due to fluid (air/gas/water etc.)

d = dia. of Cylinder

l = length of Cylinder

t = thickness of Cylinder

σ_h = hoop stress or Circumferential stress in the Cylinder/vessel material.

Now, bursting will occur if the force due to fluid pressure 'p' is more than the resisting force owing to set up of circumferential (or hoop) stress in the material of the Cylinder/vessel.

In the limiting case, these two forces should be equal.

Force due to fluid pressure = Intensity of pressure × Projected Area on which
p is acting

$$= p \cdot (d \times l) \qquad \qquad \text{...(1)}$$

Force due to circumferential stress on the cylinder wall

$$= \sigma_h \cdot 2tl \qquad \qquad \text{...(2)}$$

From eqns. (1) and (2)

$$\sigma_h \cdot 2t \cdot l = p \cdot d \cdot l$$

$$\therefore \ \sigma_h = \frac{p \cdot d}{2t}$$

Therefore, Hoop stress $(\sigma_h) = \dfrac{p \cdot d}{2t}$

{N.B.: In constructing large pressure vessels or storage tanks such as boilers, air receiver etc., welding or rivetting may be required for joining the ends of plate.

So, while designing the thickness of pressure vessels, we must consider the efficiency of the joints.

If η_l is the efficiency of longitudinal joint then, hoop stress

$$\sigma_h = \frac{p \cdot d}{2t \cdot \eta_l}$$

If η_h is the efficiency of the circumferential joint then, longitudinal stress

$$\sigma_l = \frac{p \cdot d}{4t \cdot \eta_h}$$

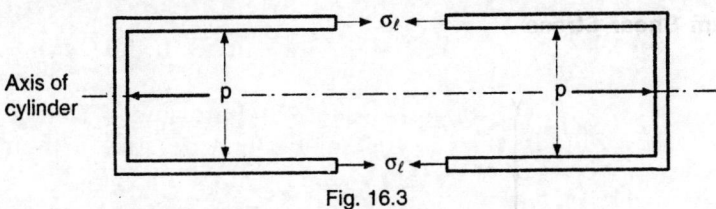

Fig. 16.3 (a)

The thickness of the shell in order that the hoop stress may not exceed the

permissible stress is given by $t = \dfrac{pd}{2\sigma_h \cdot \eta_l} \Bigg].$

Longitudinal Stress (σ_l) When Thin Cylindrical Vessel is Subjected to Internal Fluid Pressure

Let us consider a thin cylindrical vessel which is subjected to internal fluid pressure (p). Longitudinal stress (σ_l) will set-up in the material of the cylinder along the direction of axis of the cylinder.

Axis of cylinder

Fig. 16.3

Let σ_l = longitudinal stress.

The bursting of the vessel will occur if the fluid pressure (due to gas or liquid) kept inside the vessel is more than the resisting force due to longitudinal stress (σ_1) developed in the material.

Force due to fluid pressure = p × Area on which p is acting.

$$= p \times \frac{\pi}{4}d^2 \qquad\qquad ...(1)$$

Resisting force offered by the material

$$= \sigma_l \times \pi \, dt \qquad\qquad ...(2)$$

From eqns. (1) and (2)

$$\sigma_l \times \pi\, d \times t = p \times \frac{\pi}{4} d^2$$

$$\therefore\ \sigma_l = \frac{pd}{4t}$$

Hence, longitudinal stress is half of hoop stress.

"Therefore the design of a pressure vessel must be based on maximum stress
i.e. **hoop stress".**

We can say now that in the case of a thin Cylinder subjected to internal fluid
pressure, the tendency to burst circumferentially is twice that of the longitudinal
direction.

So, in a thin Cylindrical shell, at any point there are two principal stresses:

(i) Circumferential stress $(\sigma_h) = \dfrac{pd}{2t}$ acting circumferentially, this a major stress.

(ii) Longitudinal stress $(\sigma_l) = \dfrac{pd}{4t}$ acting longitudinally and parallel to the axis
of the Cylinder, that is a minor stress.

We also observe that both the stresses (σ_h and σ_l) are tensile in nature and act at
right angle to each other.

Since, these two stresses (σ_h and σ_l) act perpendicular to each other and are
maximum and minimum respectively, we can call them principal stresses also.

Maximum Shear Stress

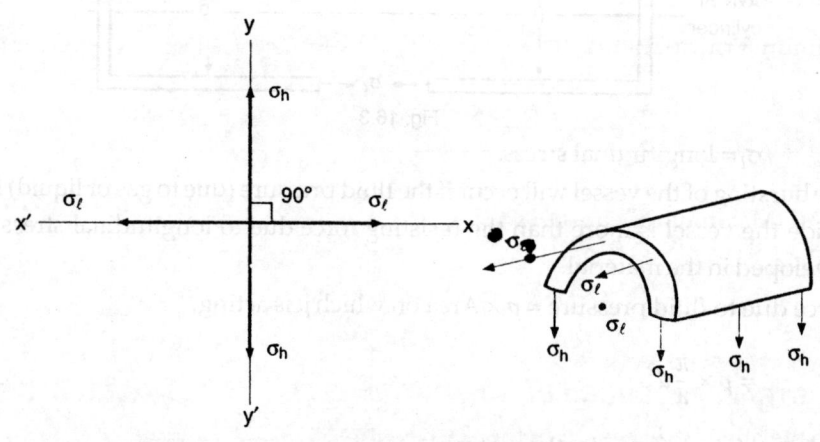

Fig. 16.4

Maximum shear stress $(\tau_{max}) = \left(\dfrac{\sigma_h - \sigma_l}{2} \right)$

$$\therefore \quad \tau_{max} = \left(\dfrac{\dfrac{pd}{2t} - \dfrac{pd}{4t}}{2} \right) \qquad \left[\because \tau_{max} = \dfrac{\sigma_{max} - \sigma_{min}}{2} = \left(\dfrac{\sigma_h - \sigma_l}{2} \right) \right]$$

$$= \left(\dfrac{pd}{8t} \right)$$

Derivation of Stresses When Thin Cylindrical Vessel is Subjected to Internal 'Fluid Pressure' and 'Torque'

So far, we have studied that when a thin cylindrical vessel is subjected to load due to the pressure of fluid (gas or liquid) then hoop stress (σ_h) and longitudinal stresses (σ_l) are set up.

Now, let us study the case when the cylindrical vessel is subjected to fluid pressure and torque. By the theory of torsion we know that torsion produces shear stress (τ) which varies from 0 (zero) at the centre to the maximum at the surface.

So, in this case, shear stress (τ) will also develop in addition to hoop stress (σ_h) and longitudinal stress (σ_l).

Hence, principal stresses due to fluid pressure and torque are

$$\sigma_{1,2} = \frac{\sigma_h + \sigma_l}{2} \pm \sqrt{\left(\frac{\sigma_h - \sigma_l}{2} \right)^2 + \tau^2}$$

Maximum Principal stress (σ_1)

$$= \frac{\sigma_h + \sigma_l}{2} + \sqrt{\left(\frac{\sigma_h - \sigma_l}{2} \right)^2 + \tau^2}$$

Minimum Principal stress (σ_2)

$$= \frac{\sigma_h + \sigma_l}{2} - \sqrt{\left(\frac{\sigma_h - \sigma_l}{2} \right)^2 + \tau^2}$$

and   Maximum Shear stress $(\tau_{max}) = \dfrac{1}{2}(\sigma_1 - \sigma_2)$

$$= \sqrt{\left(\frac{\sigma_h - \sigma_l}{2} \right)^2 + \tau^2}$$

16.3 STRAIN PRODUCED IN A THIN CYLINDRICAL SHELL

We have already discussed in the very beginning that load applied on an elastic body produces stress and deformation (changes in dimensions). Here also owing to internal fluid pressure stresses are developed in the material of the cylinder which ultimately deforms the cylinder, so its dimensions changes.

So at any point in the shell,

Hoop strain $(\varepsilon_h) = \left(\dfrac{\sigma_h}{E} - v \cdot \dfrac{\sigma_l}{E} \right) =$ diametral Strain (ε_d)

where, v is the Poisson's ratio of the material of the shell.

$$\therefore \qquad \varepsilon_h = \frac{pd}{2tE} - v \cdot \frac{pd}{4tE}$$

$$= \frac{pd}{4tE}(2 - v)$$

and Longitudinal strain $(\varepsilon_l) = \dfrac{\sigma_l}{E} - v \cdot \dfrac{\sigma_h}{E}$

$$= \frac{pd}{4tE} - v \cdot \frac{pd}{2tE}$$

$$= \frac{pd}{4tE}(1 - 2v)$$

and Diametral strain $(\varepsilon_d) = \varepsilon_h$

$$= \frac{pd}{4tE}(2 - v)$$

Change in length $(\delta_l) = \varepsilon_l \times l$

$$= \frac{p \cdot d \cdot l}{4tE}(1 - 2v)$$

Change in diameter $(\delta_d) = \varepsilon_h \times d$

$$= \frac{pd^2}{4tE}(2 - v)$$

16.4 VOLUMETRIC STRAIN IN A CYLINDRICAL SHELL

Let $\quad v$ = Volume enclosed by cylindrical shell

$\qquad \delta_d$ = Change in dia. due to stresses setup in the shell material

$\qquad \delta_l$ = Change in length

and, $\quad \delta v$ = Change in volume

$\qquad \varepsilon_h$ = Circumferential strain

$\qquad \varepsilon_l$ = Longitudinal strain

$\qquad \varepsilon_v$ = Volumetric strain

Now, initial volume of shell, $v = \dfrac{\pi}{4}d^2 \cdot l$ $\qquad\qquad$ ...(1)

Taking log both sides

$$\ln v = \ln \pi + 2\ln d + \ln l$$

Differentiating both sides

$$\frac{dv}{v} = 0 + 2 \cdot \frac{d(d)}{d} + \frac{dl}{l}$$

Volumetric strain = 2 × diametral strain + longitudinal strain

∴   Volumetric strain = 2 × hoop strain + longitudinal strain

$$\varepsilon_v = 2 \cdot \varepsilon_h + \varepsilon_l$$

Now, substituting the values of ε_h and ε_l

$$\varepsilon_v = 2\frac{pd}{4tE}(2-v) + \frac{pd}{4tE}(1-2v)$$

$$= \frac{pd}{4tE}\big[2(2-v)+1(1-2v)\big]$$

$$= \frac{pd}{4tE}\big[4-2v+1-2v\big]$$

$$\boxed{\varepsilon_v = \frac{pd}{4\,tE}\big[5-4v\big]}$$

16.5 STRESSES IN THIN SPHERICAL SHELLS

Let us consider a thin spherical shell of diameter 'd' and thickness 't'. The shell is subjected to internal fluid pressure p. Due to internal fluid pressure (p), the spherical shell is likely to split into two parts along yy' or along xx'. Here, let us consider along yy'.

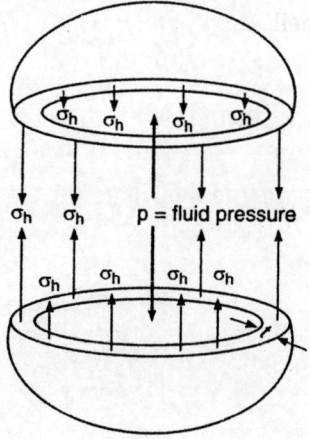 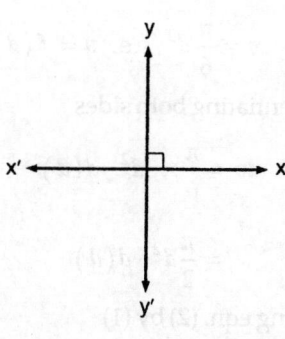

Fig. 16.5

Now, Bursting forces $(P) = p \times$ projected area

$$= p \times \frac{\pi}{4} d^2 \qquad \qquad \text{...(1)}$$

Let the hoop stress (circumferential stress) induced in the material of shell $= \sigma_h$, which will work as a resisting force to prevent from bursting

∴   Resisting force = Stress $(\sigma_h) \times$ area resisting the force P

$$= \sigma_h \times \pi \cdot d \cdot t \qquad \qquad \text{...(2)}$$

Equating eqns. (1) and (2)

$$\sigma_h \times \pi \times d \times t = p \times \frac{\pi}{4} d^2$$

∴ $$\sigma_h = \frac{pd}{4t}$$

It is evident that in the case of thin spherical shell, the two principal stresses σ_h and σ_l (along two axes) at any point is equal.

∴ $$\sigma_h = \sigma_l = \frac{pd}{4t}$$

and $\tau_{max} = \left(\dfrac{\sigma_h - \sigma_l}{2} \right) = 0$ (zero) *i.e.* there in no shear stress developed in the spherical shell.

N.B.: If η_h is the efficiency of the circumferential joint then thickness of the shell

$$(t) = \frac{pd}{4\sigma_l \cdot \eta_h} .$$

16.6 STRAIN PRODUCED IN A THIN SPHERICAL SHELL

Let d = dia. of spherical shell

and, v = volume enclosed by the spherical shell.

∴ $$v = \frac{\pi}{6} d^3 \text{ i.e. } v = f(d) \qquad \qquad \text{...(1)}$$

Differentiating both sides

$$dv = \frac{\pi}{6} \times 3d^2 \cdot d(d)$$

$$= \frac{\pi}{2} d^2 \cdot d(d) \qquad \qquad \text{...(2)}$$

Dividing eqn. (2) by (1)

$$\left(\frac{dv}{v} \right) = 3 \cdot \frac{d(d)}{d}$$

$$\varepsilon_v = 3 \times \text{hoop strain}$$

$$\therefore \qquad \varepsilon_v = 3 \times \varepsilon_h \qquad\qquad \text{...(3)}$$

Now, hoop strain $\left(\varepsilon_h\right) = \dfrac{\sigma_h}{E} - v.\dfrac{\sigma_h}{E}$

$$= \dfrac{\sigma_h}{E}\left(1-v\right)$$

$$= \dfrac{pd}{4tE}\left(1-v\right) = \text{diametral strain } (\varepsilon_d)$$

Substituting the values of ε_h in equation (3) volumetric strain of spherical shell (ε_v)

$$\therefore \qquad \varepsilon_v = 3 \times \dfrac{pd}{4tE}\left(1-v\right)$$

$$\boxed{\varepsilon_v = \dfrac{3pd}{4tE}\left(1-v\right)}$$

where, v is poisson's ratio of the spherical shell.

Increase in diameter of the spherical shell due to internal pressure

$$\delta_d = \varepsilon_d \times d$$

$$\boxed{\delta_d = \dfrac{pd^2}{4tE}(1-v)}$$

Increase in volume $(\delta_v) = \varepsilon_v \times v$

$$= \dfrac{3pd}{4tE}(1-v) \times \dfrac{\pi}{6}d^3$$

$$\boxed{\delta_v = \dfrac{\pi pd^4}{8tE}(1-v)}$$

EXAMPLE 1 *A cylinder 2 m long 0.5 m in dia. and is made up of 10 mm steel is subjected to an internal pressure of 2 MPa. Calculate the cylinder diameter and length under pressure. What will be the maximum shear stress in the cylinder? Assume E = 200 GPa and v = 0.25.*
SOLUTION

$$\tau_{max} = \dfrac{\sigma_1 - \sigma_2}{2} = \left(\dfrac{\sigma_h - \sigma_l}{2}\right)$$

We have to find out $\sigma_1 = $ Maximum principal stress

$$= \text{Hoop stress}$$

$$= \sigma_h$$

$$= \frac{pd}{2t}$$

$$= \frac{2 \times 500}{2 \times 10}$$

$$\sigma_h = 50 \ \text{N/mm}^2$$

and, σ_2 = Minimum principal stress

$\qquad$ = Longitudinal stress

$$= \frac{\sigma_h}{2}$$

$\therefore \qquad \sigma_l = 25 \ \text{N/mm}^2$

$\therefore \qquad$ Change in cylinder diameter $(\delta_d) = \dfrac{D}{E}\left[\sigma_h - v \cdot \sigma_l\right]$

$$= \frac{500}{200 \times 10^3}\left[50 - 0.25 \times 25\right]$$

$$= 0.109 \ \text{mm}$$

Change in cylinder length $(\delta_l) = \dfrac{L}{E}\left[\sigma_l - v \cdot \sigma_h\right]$

$$= \frac{2000}{200 \times 10^3}\left[50 - 0.25 \times 50\right]$$

$$= 0.125 \ \text{mm}$$

$\therefore \qquad$ Final cylinder diameter $(d_f) = 500 + 0.109$

$$= 500.109 \ \text{mm}$$

and,   Final cylinder length $(l_f) = 2000 + 0.125$

$$= 2000 \cdot 125 \ \text{mm}$$

$\therefore \qquad \tau_{max} = \dfrac{\sigma_1 - \sigma_2}{2} = \dfrac{\sigma_h - \sigma_l}{2}$

$$= \frac{50 - 25}{2}$$

$$= 12.5 \ \text{N/mm}^2$$

$$= 12.5 \ \text{MPa.} \qquad \textbf{Ans.}$$

EXAMPLE 2 *A cylinderical steel pressure vessel 400 mm in diameter with a wall thickness of 20 mm is subjected to an internal pressure of 4.5 MN/m².*

(a) Calculate the tangential and longitudinal stresses in the steel.

(b) *To what value may the internal pressure be increased if the stress in the steel is limited to 120 MN/m^2.*

(c) *If the internal pressure were increased until the vessel burst, sketch the type of fracture that would occur.*

SOLUTION

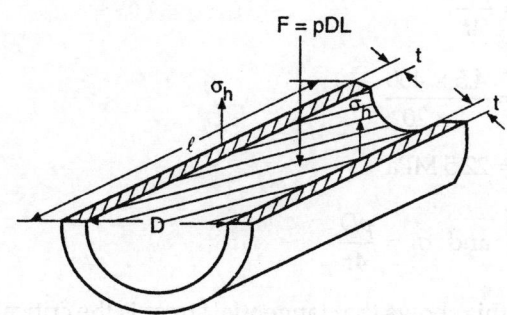

Fig. 16.6

(a) Force due to fluid pressure $(F) = p \cdot D \cdot l$ ...(1)

Force due to circumferential stress on the cylinder wall $= \sigma_h \cdot (2tl)$ ...(2)

where, t = thickness of wall

l = length of the cylinder

σ_h = hoop stress or circumferential stress or tangential stress

Equating (1) and (2), we get

$$\sigma_h \cdot 2tl = p \cdot D \cdot l$$

$$\sigma_h = \frac{p \cdot D}{2t}$$

$$= \frac{4.5 \times 400}{2 \times 20}$$

$$= 45 \text{ MPa} \qquad \textbf{Ans.}$$

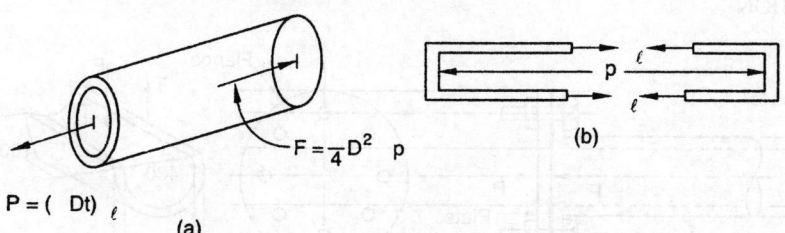

Fig. 16.7

Force due to fluid pressure $= p \times \dfrac{\pi}{4} D^2$ ...(1)

Resisting force offered by the material $= \sigma_l \times \pi D t$ ...(2)

From (1) and (2)

$$\sigma_l \times \pi Dt = p \times \frac{\pi}{4}D^2$$

$$\sigma_l = \frac{pD}{4t}$$

$$= \frac{4.5 \times 400}{4 \times 20}$$

$$= 22.5 \text{ MPa}$$

(b) Since $\sigma_h = \dfrac{pD}{2t}$ and $\sigma_l = \dfrac{pD}{4t}$

Hence, $\sigma_h = 2\sigma_l$, this shows that tangential stress is the critical.

$$\sigma_h = \frac{pD}{2t}$$

$$120 = \frac{p \times 400}{2 \times 20}$$

$$\therefore \qquad p = \frac{120 \times 40}{400} = 12 \text{ MPa} \qquad \textbf{Ans.}$$

(c) The bursting force will cause a stress on the longitudinal section as shown in Fig. 16.7 (b).

EXAMPLE 3 *A pipe carrying steam at 3.5 MPa has an outside diameter of 450 mm and a wall thickness of 10 mm. A gasket is inserted between the flange at one end of the pipe and a flat plate used to cap the end. How many 40 mm diameter bolts must be used to hold the cap on if the allowable stress in the bolts is 80 MPa of which 55 MPa is the initial stress?*

What circumferential stress is developed in the pipe?

SOLUTION

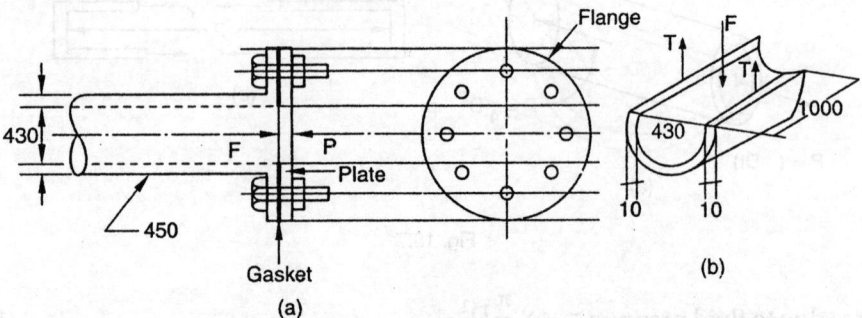

Objective: (a) Number of bolts required (b) Circumferential stress developed in pipe.

Fig. 16.8

Force due to steam is $(F) = \sigma \cdot A$

$$= 3.5 \left[\frac{\pi}{4} (430)^2 \right]$$

$$= 508270.42 \text{ Newton}$$

Now, for equilibrium, $P = F$

$$\sigma_{\text{bolt}} \cdot A \cdot n = 508270.42$$

$$(80 - 55) \left[\frac{1}{4} \pi (40)^2 \right] n = 508270.42$$

∴ $n = 16.19$ say 16 bolts   **Ans.**

Circumferential stress

$$F = p \cdot A$$

$$= 3.5 [430 \times 1000]$$

$$= 1505000 \text{ N}$$

From Fig. 16.8 (b) $2T = F$

$$2 [\sigma_c (1000) (10)] = 1505000$$

⇒ $\sigma_c = 75.25 \text{ MPa}$ **Ans.**

EXAMPLE 4 *A cylindrical pressure vessel is fabricated from steel plating that has a thickness of 20 mm. The diameter of the pressure vessel is 450 mm and its length is 2 metre. Determine the maximum internal pressure that can be applied if the longitudinal stress is limited to 140 MPa and the circumferential stress is limited to 50 MPa.*
SOLUTION

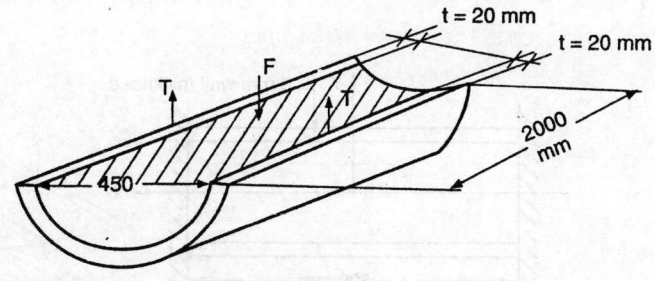

Fig. 16.9

$\Sigma F_v = 0$ gives

$$F = 2T$$

$$p \cdot (DL) = 2 \cdot (\sigma_h \cdot L \cdot t)$$

$$\sigma_h = \frac{p \cdot D}{2t}$$

$$60 = \frac{p \times 450}{2 \times 20}$$

$$\Rightarrow \qquad p = \left(\frac{60 \times 40}{450} \right) = 5.33 \text{ MPa}$$

Based on longitudinal stress

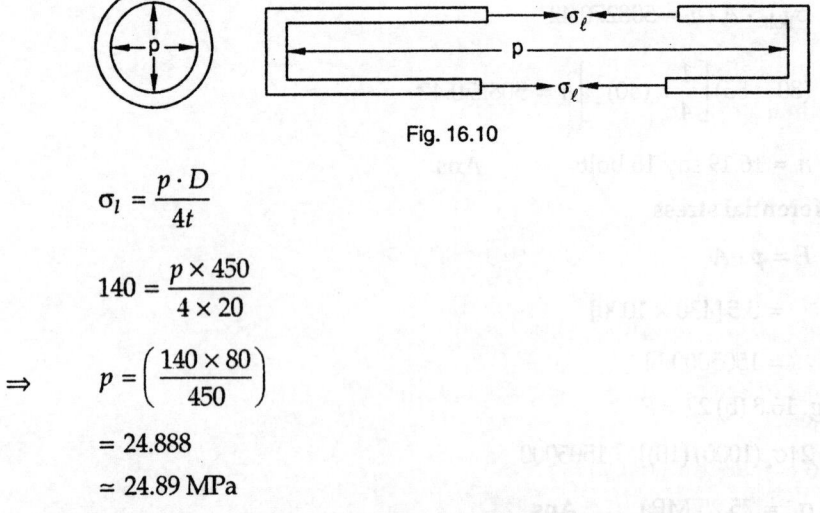

Fig. 16.10

$$\sigma_l = \frac{p \cdot D}{4t}$$

$$140 = \frac{p \times 450}{4 \times 20}$$

$$\Rightarrow \qquad p = \left(\frac{140 \times 80}{450} \right)$$

$$= 24.888$$

$$\simeq 24.89 \text{ MPa}$$

So, the maximum internal pressure for safe working is 5.33 MPa. **Ans.**

EXAMPLE 5 *A 600 mm long bronze tube with its closed ends is 75 mm in diameter with wall thickness of 3 mm. With no internal pressure, the tube just fits between two rigid end walls. Calculate the longitudinal and tangential stresses for an internal pressure of 5 MPa.*

Assume $v = \dfrac{1}{3}$ *and* $E_{br} = 83$ MPa.

SOLUTION

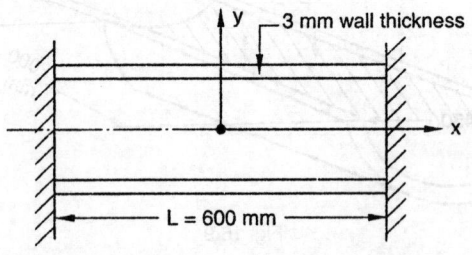

Fig. 16.11

Since the tube is fixed with its ends closed. So, strain along x-axis is zero.

$$\varepsilon_x = \frac{\sigma_x}{E} - v \cdot \frac{\sigma_y}{E} = 0$$

$$\sigma_x = v \cdot \sigma_y$$

Tangential stress or hoop stress $\sigma_h = \sigma_y$

Now, $\quad \sigma_h = \dfrac{pD}{2t}$

$$= \frac{5 \times \cancel{75}^{25}}{2 \times \cancel{3}}$$

$$= 62.5 \text{ MPa}$$

Longitudinal stress (σ_l) or $\sigma_x = \nu \cdot \sigma_y$

$$= \frac{1}{3} \times 62.5$$

$$= 20.83 \text{ MPa} \quad \textbf{Ans.}$$

EXAMPLE 6 *A welded steel cylindrical drum made of 10 mm plate has an internal diameter of 1.20 m. Compute the change in diameter that would be caused by an internal pressure of 1.5 MPa.*
Assume that Poisson's ratio is 0.3 and E = 200 GPa.
SOLUTION

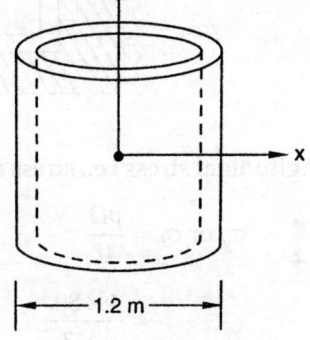

σ_y = longitudinal stress = σ_l

$$= \frac{pD}{4t}$$

$$= \frac{1.5 \times 1200}{4 \times 10}$$

$$= 45 \text{ MPa}$$

σ_x = Tangential stress = σ_h = hoop stress

Fig. 16.12

$$= \frac{pD}{2t}$$

$$= \frac{1.5 \times 1200}{2 \times 10}$$

$$= 90 \text{ MPa}$$

Strain along x-axis $(\varepsilon_x) = \dfrac{\sigma_x}{E} - \nu \cdot \dfrac{\sigma_y}{E}$

$$= \frac{90}{2 \times 10^5} - 0.3 \left(\frac{45}{2 \times 10^5} \right)$$

$$= 38.25 \times 10^{-5}$$

Also, $\quad \varepsilon_x = \dfrac{\Delta D}{D}$

$\therefore \quad \Delta D = \varepsilon_x \cdot D$

$\qquad = 38.25 \times 10^{-5} \times 1200$

$\qquad = 0.459 \text{ mm}$ **Ans.**

EXAMPLE 7 *A 150 mm long bronze tube closed at its ends is 80 mm in diameter and has a wall thickness of 3 mm. It fits without clearance in an 80 mm hole in a rigid block. The tube is then subjected to internal pressure of 4 MPa. Assuming $\nu = \dfrac{1}{3}$ and E = 83 GPa, determine the tangential stress in the tube.*

SOLUTION

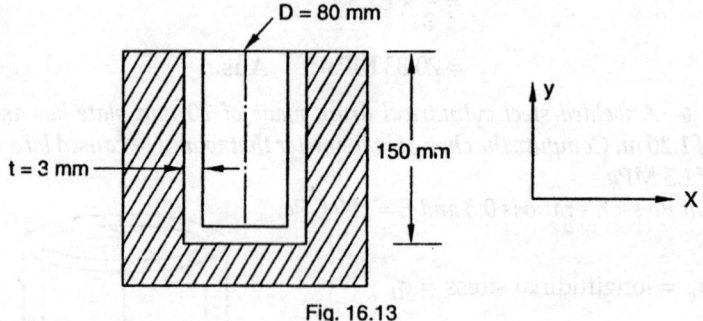

Fig. 16.13

Longitudinal stress i.e., stress along the axis of the cylinder

$$\sigma_y \text{ or } \sigma_l = \frac{pD}{4t}$$

$$= \frac{4 \times 80}{4 \times 3}$$

$$= \left(\frac{80}{3}\right) \text{MPa}$$

Strain in the x-direction

$$\varepsilon_x = \frac{\sigma_x}{E} - \nu \cdot \frac{\sigma_y}{E} = 0 \qquad \text{(Since the tube is fixed in block)}$$

or, $\qquad \sigma_x = \nu \cdot \sigma_y$

$$= \frac{1}{3}\left(\frac{80}{3}\right)$$

$$= 8.89 \text{ MPa} \qquad \textbf{Ans.}$$

EXAMPLE 8 *A boiler shell is to be made of 15 mm thick plate having a limiting value of tensile stress 120 N/mm². If the efficiencies of the longitudinal and circumferential joints are 70% and 30% respectively, determine:*

(i) *the maximum permissible diameter of the shell for the internal pressure of 2N/mm² and*

(ii) *permissible intensity of internal pressure when the shell diameter is 1.5 m.*

SOLUTION

(i) **Given data's are:** t = thickness of shell = 15 mm

$$\sigma_t = 120 \text{ N/mm}^2 = \sigma_h \text{ or } \sigma_c \text{ (let)}$$

$$\eta_l = 70\% = 0.7$$

$$\eta_c = 30\% = 0.3$$

$$p_i = 2 \text{ N/mm}^2$$

Now, applying formula

$$\text{Circumferential stress } (\sigma_c) = \frac{pd}{2\eta_l t}$$

$$120 = \frac{2 \times d}{2 \times 0.7 \times 15}$$

$$\Rightarrow \qquad d = \frac{120 \times \cancel{2} \times 0.7 \times 15}{\cancel{2}}$$

$$= 1260 \text{ mm}$$

Let the limiting tensile stress = longitudinal stress = 120 N/mm²

Now, $\qquad \sigma_l = \dfrac{pd}{4\eta_c t}$

$$120 = \frac{2 \times d}{4 \times 0.3 \times 15}$$

$$\Rightarrow \qquad d = \frac{120 \times \overset{2}{\cancel{4}} \times 0.3 \times 15}{\cancel{2}}$$

$$= 1080 \text{ mm}$$

Hence, maximum dia to meet both condition is 1080 mm. **Ans.**

(ii) **Permissible intensity of internal pressure**

Here, we will also assume limiting tensile stress equal to circumferential stress and longitudinal stress one by one.

Now, $\qquad \sigma_h \text{ or } \sigma_c = \dfrac{pd}{2\eta_l t}$

$$120 = \frac{p \times 1500}{2 \times 0.7 \times 15}$$

$$\Rightarrow \qquad p = \frac{120 \times 2 \times 0.7 \times \overset{}{\cancel{15}}}{\underset{100}{\cancel{1500}}}$$

$$= 1.68 \text{ N/mm}^2$$

Again, $\sigma_l = \dfrac{pd}{4\eta_c t}$

$$120 = \dfrac{p \times 1500}{4 \times 0.30 \times 15}$$

$\Rightarrow$ $d = \dfrac{120 \times 4 \times 0.30 \times 15}{1500}$

          $= 1.44 \text{ N/mm}^2$

To satisfy both the conditions permissible internal pressure $= 1.44 \text{ N/mm}^2$ **Ans.**

(**N.B.:** The chosen internal pressure should be such that calculated stress should not exceed the given limiting stress.

Let us check it:

If we take $p = 1.68 \text{ N/mm}^2$ then

$$\sigma_l = \dfrac{1.68 \times 1500}{4 \times 0.3 \times 15}$$

       $= 139.99$

       $\simeq 140 \text{ N/mm}^2$ which is more than the limiting stress 120N/mm^2.

Hence, not accepted).

EXAMPLE 9 *A thin cylindrical tube of 80 mm internal diameter and 5 mm thick is closed at the ends and is subjected to an internal pressure of 6 N/mm². A torque of 2009600 N/mm is applied to the tube. Find the hoop stress; longitudinal stress; maximum and minimum principal stresses and the maximum shear.*

SOLUTION

Given $d = 80$ mm

       $t = 5$ mm

       $p = 6 \text{ N/mm}^2$

       $T = 2009600$ Nmm

Hoop Stress $(\sigma_h) = \dfrac{pd}{2t}$

          $= \dfrac{6 \times \overset{16}{\cancel{80}}}{\cancel{2} \times \cancel{5}}$

          $= 48 \text{ N/mm}^2$

Longitudinal stress $(\sigma_l) = \dfrac{pd}{4t}$

          $= \dfrac{6 \times 80}{4 \times 5}$

          $= 24 \text{ N/mm}^2$

Maximum and Minimum Principal Stresses:

We know that due to torque, shear stress will be produced in the tube.

Let τ is the shear stress in the wall of the tube

∴   Shear Stress × Area = Shear Force

$$= \tau \times (\pi d \times t)$$

$$= \tau \times \pi \times 80 \times 5$$

$$= 400\,\pi\tau$$

and   Torque (T) = Shear Force $\times \dfrac{d}{2}$

$$= 400\,\pi\tau \times \frac{d}{2}$$

$$= 400\,\pi\tau \times \frac{80}{2}$$

$$= 16000\,\pi \times \tau \; \text{Nmm}$$

But torque applied in the problem is 2009600 Nmm

Equating these two torques, we get

$$16000\,\pi\tau = 2009600$$

∴ $$\tau = \left(\frac{2009600}{16000\pi} \right) = 40 \; \text{N/mm}^2$$

Now, by formula

Maximum Principal Stress $(\sigma_1) = \left(\dfrac{\sigma_h + \sigma_l}{2} \right) + \sqrt{\left(\dfrac{\sigma_h - \sigma_l}{2} \right)^2 + \tau^2}$

$$= \frac{48 + 24}{2} + \sqrt{\left(\frac{48 - 24}{2} \right)^2 + (40)^2}$$

$$= 36 + \sqrt{144 \times 1600}$$

$$= 36 + 41.761$$

∴ $\sigma_1 = 77.761 \; \text{N/mm}^2$ (Tensile) **Ans.**

Minimum Principal Stress $(\sigma_2) = \left(\dfrac{\sigma_h + \sigma_l}{2} \right) - \sqrt{\left(\dfrac{\sigma_h - \sigma_l}{2} \right)^2 + \tau^2}$

$$= \frac{48 + 24}{2} - \sqrt{\left(\frac{48 - 24}{2} \right)^2 + (40)^2}$$

$$= 36 - 41.761$$

∴ $\sigma_2 = -5.761 \; \text{N/mm}^2$ (Compressive)   **Ans.**

We know by formula that,

$$\text{Maximum Shear Stress } (\tau_{max}) = \left(\frac{\sigma_1 - \sigma_2}{2}\right)$$

$$= \left(\frac{77.761 + 5.761}{2}\right)$$

$$= 41.761 \text{ N/mm}^2 \qquad \text{Ans.}$$

EXAMPLE 10 *A cylindrical vessel whose ends are closed by means of rigid flange (plates) of 3 mm thick steel plate. The length and the internal diameter of the vessel are 50 cm and 25 cm respectively.*

Determine the longitudinal and hoop stresses in the cylindrical shell due to internal fluid pressure of 3 N/mm². Also, compute the increase in length, diameter and volume of the vessel. Take E = 2 × 10⁵ N/mm² and v = 0.3.

SOLUTION

Given data's are: $t = 3 \text{ mm} = 0.3 \text{ cm}$

$$l = 50 \text{ cm}$$
$$d = 25 \text{ cm}$$
$$p_i = 3\text{N/mm}^2$$
$$E = 2 \times 10^5 \text{ N/mm}^2$$
$$v = 0.3$$

Hoop Stress $(\sigma_h) = \dfrac{pd}{2t}$

$$= \frac{3 \times 25}{2 \times 0.3}$$

$$= 125 \text{ N/mm}^2 \qquad \text{Ans.}$$

Longitudinal stress $(\sigma_l) = \dfrac{pd}{4t}$

$$= \frac{3 \times 25}{4 \times 0.3}$$

$$= 62.5 \text{ N/mm}^2 \qquad \text{Ans.}$$

Circumferential strain (ε_c) or hoop strain (ε_h)

$$= \left(\frac{\sigma_h}{E} - v \cdot \frac{\sigma_l}{E}\right)$$

$$= \frac{1}{E}(125 - 0.3 \times 62.5)$$

$$= \frac{1}{2 \times 10^5}(125 - 0.3 \times 62.5)$$

$$= \frac{106.25}{2 \times 10^5}$$

$$= 53.125 \times 10^{-5}$$

Also, circumferential strain $(\varepsilon_c) = \dfrac{\delta_d}{d}$

Hence, $\dfrac{\delta_d}{d} = 53.125 \times 10^{-5}$

$\therefore \qquad \delta_d = 53.125 \times 10^{-5} d$

$$= 53.125 \times 10^{-5} \times 25$$

$$= 0.0132812 \text{ cm}$$

$$= 0.0133 \text{ cm}$$

Hence, increase in diameter $(\delta_d) = 0.0133$ cm

Longitudinal Strain $(\varepsilon_l) = \dfrac{\delta_l}{l} = \left(\dfrac{\sigma_l}{E} - \nu \cdot \dfrac{\sigma_h}{E} \right)$

$$= \frac{1}{E} (\sigma_l - \nu \sigma_h)$$

$$= \frac{1}{2 \times 10^5} (62.5 - 0.3 \times 125)$$

$$= \frac{25}{2 \times 10^5}$$

$\therefore \qquad \dfrac{\delta_l}{l} = 12.5 \times 10^{-5}$

Hence, increase in length $(\delta_l) = 12.5 \times 10^{-5} \times l$

$$= 12.5 \times 10^{-5} \times 50$$

$$= 0.00625 \text{ cm} \qquad \qquad \textbf{Ans.}$$

Volumetric Strain of a cylindrical vessel is given by,

$$\varepsilon_v = \left(\frac{\delta V}{V} \right) = \left(2 \cdot \frac{\delta_d}{d} + \frac{\delta_l}{l} \right)$$

$$= 2\varepsilon_c^* + \varepsilon_l$$

$$= 2 \times 53.125 \times 10^{-5} + 12.5 \times 10^{-5}$$

$$= 106.250 \times 10^{-5} + 12.5 \times 10^{-5}$$

$$= 118.75 \times 10^{-5}$$

$*\left(\dfrac{\delta_d}{d} \right) = \varepsilon_c$ circumferential strain or hoop strain (ε_h).

Hence, increase in volume of the cylinder

$$(\delta_V) = 118.75 \times 10^{-5} \times V$$

$$= 118.75 \times 10^{-5} \times \frac{\pi}{4}(25)^2 \times 50$$

$$= 29.145 \text{ cm}^3 \qquad \textbf{Ans.}$$

EXAMPLE 11 *A spherical tank has diameter of 20 meter and wall thickness 15 mm. If the permissible stress in the material is 120 MPa, determine the maximum pressure at which gas can be stored in the tank. Determine the increase in diameter and volume of the tank due to gas pressure. Tak E = 200 GPa and Poisson's ratio (ν) = 0.3.* **(UPTU 2008-09)**

SOLUTION

Given σ_h = 120 MPa

$\qquad d = 20$ m

$\qquad t = 15$ mm

$\qquad \nu = 0.3$

$\qquad E = 200 \times 10^3$ MPa

For spherical tank, Hoop Stress $(\sigma_h) = \dfrac{pd}{4t}$

$$120 = \frac{p \times 20 \times 10^3}{4 \times 15}$$

$\Rightarrow \qquad p = 0.36$ MPa

Increase in diameter of spherical tank (δ_d)

$$= \text{Hoop Strain} \times \text{Diameter}$$

$$= \varepsilon_h \times d = \left\{ \frac{1}{E} (\sigma_h - \nu \cdot \sigma_h) \right\} \times d$$

$$= \frac{pd}{4tE} (1 - \nu) \times d$$

$$= \frac{pd^2}{4tE} (1 - \nu)$$

$$= \frac{0.36 \times (20 \times 10^3)}{4 \times 15 \times 200 \times 10^3} (1 - 0.3)$$

$$= \frac{0.36 \times 400 \times 10^6 \times 0.7}{60 \times 200 \times 10^3}$$

$\therefore \qquad \delta_d = 8.4$ mm $\qquad$ **Ans.**

Increase in volume of spherical tank $(\delta_V) = 3\varepsilon_h \times V$

$$\Rightarrow \qquad \delta_V = 3 \times \frac{pd}{4tE}(1-v) \times \frac{\pi}{6}d^3$$

$$= \frac{\pi pd^4}{8tE}(1-v)$$

$$= \frac{22}{7} \times \frac{(0.36 \times 10^6) \times (20)^4 \times 0.7}{8 \times (15 \times 10^{-3}) \times 200 \times 10^9}$$

$$= \frac{22}{7} \times \frac{0.36 \times (20)^4 \times 0.7 \times \cancel{10^6}}{8 \times 15 \times 200 \times \cancel{10^6}}$$

$$\therefore \qquad \delta_V = 5.275 \text{ m}^3$$

Hence, increase in volume = 5.275 m^3. **Ans.**

EXAMPLE 12 *A thin cylindrical shell is subjected to internal fluid pressure. The ends are closed by*

(a) *Two water tight pistons attached to a common rod.*

(b) *Flanged ends*

Find the increase in internal diameter in each case given that the internal diameter is 20 cm, thickness is 0.5 cm, $v = 0.3$. Young's modulus is 200 GN/m^2, internal pressure is 3.5 MN/m^2.

SOLUTION

In both the cases, the circumferential stress is

$$\sigma_c \text{ or } \sigma_h = \frac{pd}{2t}$$

$$= \frac{\cancel{2}pr}{\cancel{2}t}$$

$$= \frac{3.5 \times 10^6 \times 0.01}{0.005}$$

$$= 70 \times 10^6 \text{ N/m}^2$$

$$= 70 \text{ N/mm}^2$$

(a) In this case there is no longitudinal stress i.e., $\sigma_l = 0$

The circumferential or hoop stress is

$$\varepsilon_h = \frac{\sigma_h}{E}$$

$$= \frac{70 \times 10^6}{200 \times 10^9}$$

$$= 0.35 \times 10^{-3}$$

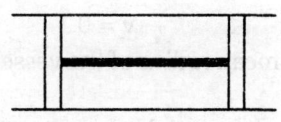

Fig. 16.14

Increase in internal diameter $= 0.2\,(0.35 \times 10^{-3})$
$$= 0.07 \times 10^{-3}\,\text{m}$$
$$= 0.007\,\text{cm} \qquad \textbf{Ans.}$$

(b) In this case, the longitudinal stress

$$\sigma_l = \frac{pd}{4t}$$

$$= \frac{1}{2}(\sigma_h)$$

$$= \frac{1}{2} \times 70$$

$$= 35\,\text{MN/m}^2$$

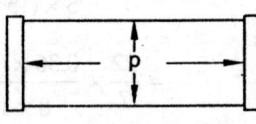

Fig. 16.15

$$\therefore \qquad \varepsilon_h = \frac{1}{E}\,(\sigma_h - v \cdot \sigma_l)$$

$$= \frac{1}{200 \times 10^9}\,(70 \times 10^6 - 0.3 \times 35 \times 10^6)$$

$$= \frac{1}{\underset{10^3}{200 \times 10^9}} \times 10^6\,(70 \times -03 \times 35)$$

$$= \frac{1}{200} \times \frac{35}{10^3}\,(2 - 0.3)$$

$$= \frac{35}{10^3 \times 200} \times 1.7$$

$$= 0.2975$$

Increase in internal diameter $= 0.2 \times 0.2975 \times 10^{-3}\,\text{m}$
$$= 0.2 \times 0.2975 \times 10^{-1}\,\text{cm}$$
$$= 0.00595\,\text{cm} \qquad \textbf{Ans.}$$

EXAMPLE 13 *An air vessel which is made of steel is 2 metre long. It has an external diameter of 45 cm and 1 cm thick. Find the increase in external diameter and increase in length when charged to internal air pressure of 1 MN/m².*
SOLUTION

For steel $E = 200\,\text{GN/m}^2$

$$v = 0.3$$

The mean radius of the vessel $= 0.225\,\text{m}$

Circumferential stress $(\sigma_h \text{ or } \sigma_c) = \frac{pd}{2t}$

$$= \frac{1 \times 10^6 \times 0.225}{0.010}$$

$$= 225 \times 10^5 \text{ N/m}^2$$

$$= 22.5 \text{ MN/m}^2$$

Longitudinal Stress $(\sigma_l) = \dfrac{pd}{4t}$

$$= \frac{1}{2}(\sigma_h)$$

$$= 11.25 \text{ MN/m}^2$$

Circumferential Strain is

$$\varepsilon_h = \frac{1}{E}(\sigma_h - v\sigma_l)$$

$$= \frac{\sigma_h}{E}\left(1 - \frac{v}{2}\right)$$

$$= \frac{22.5 \times 10^6}{200 \times 10^9}\left(1 - \frac{0.3}{2}\right)$$

$$= \frac{22.5 \times -0.85}{200 \times 10^3}$$

$$= 9.56 \times 10^{-5}$$

Longitudinal Strain is

$$\varepsilon_l = \frac{1}{E}(\sigma_l - v\sigma_h)$$

$$= \frac{\sigma_h}{E}\left(\frac{1}{2} - v\right)$$

$$= \frac{22.5 \times 10^6}{200 \times 10^9} \times (0.5 - 0.3)$$

$$= 2.25 \times 10^{-5}$$

The increase in diameter $= D \times \varepsilon_h$

$$= 0.450\,(9.56 \times 10^{-5})$$

$$= 4.302 \times 10^{-5} \text{ m}$$

$$= 4.302 \times 10^{-2} \text{ mm} = 0.0430 \text{ mm}$$

The increase in length $= l \times \varepsilon_l$

$\qquad = 2 \times (2.25 \times 10^{-5})$

$\qquad = 4.50 \times 10^{-5}$ m

$\qquad = 4.50 \times 10^{-2}$ mm

$\qquad = 0.450$ mm

16.7 CYLINDRICAL VESSEL WITH HEMISPHERICAL ENDS

Let us consider the vessel shown in figure in which the wall thickness of the cylindrical and hemispherical portions are different (this is sometimes necessary since the hoop stress in the cylinder is twice that in a sphere of the same radius and wall thickness). For calculation purpose, the internal diameter of both portions is assumed equal.

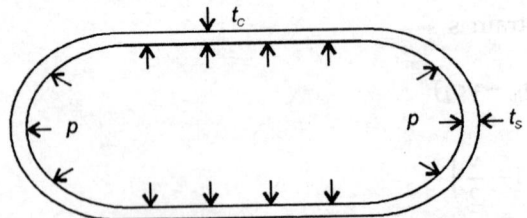

Fig. 16.17 Cross-section of thin cylinder with hemispherical ends

(a) **For the cylindrical portion:**

Hoop or circumferential stress $= \sigma_{h_c} = \dfrac{pd}{2t_C}$

Longitudinal stress $= \sigma_{l_c} = \dfrac{pd}{2t_C}$

Hoop or circumferential strain $= \dfrac{1}{E}[\sigma_{h_c} - v.\sigma_{l_c}]$

$\qquad\qquad = \dfrac{pd}{4t_C \cdot E}[2 - v]$

(b) **For the hemispherical ends:**

Hoop stress $= \sigma_s = \dfrac{pd}{4t_s}$

Hoop strain $= \dfrac{1}{E}[\sigma_{h_s} - v.\sigma_{h_s}]$

$\qquad\qquad = \dfrac{pd}{4t_s \cdot E}[1 - v]$

Now, equating the two strains in order that there shall be no distortion of the junction.

$$\frac{pd}{4t_cE}[2-v] = \frac{pd}{4t_sE}[1-v]$$

or,

$$\frac{t_s}{t_c} = \frac{1-v}{2-v}$$

For steel $v = 0.3$

So,

$$\frac{t_s}{t_c} = \frac{1-0.3}{2-0.3}$$

or,

$$\frac{t_s}{t_c} = \frac{0.7}{1.7}$$

or,

$$\frac{t_c}{t_s} = 2.4$$

or,

$$t_c = 2.4\,t_s$$

i.e. the thickness of the cylinder walls must be approximately 2.4 times that of the hemispherical ends for no distortion of the junction to occur.

Because of the reduced wall thickness of the ends, the maximum stress will occur in the ends. For equal maximum stresses in the two portions, the thickness of the cylinder walls must be twice that in the ends.

16.8 VESSEL SUBJECTED TO FLUID PRESSURE

Let us consider that a cylinder is initially full of fluid at atmospherical pressure. We wish to find out the amount of fluid which must be pumped into the cylinder in order to raise the pressure by a specified amount.

By formula, bulk modulus $(K) = \dfrac{\text{Volumetric stress}}{\text{Volumetric strain}}$

In this case volumetric stress = pressure p

and volumetric strain $= \dfrac{\text{Change in volume}}{\text{Original volume}}$

$$= \frac{\delta V}{V}$$

$\therefore$

$$K = \left(\frac{p}{\dfrac{\delta V}{V}}\right)$$

$$= \frac{p.V}{\delta V}$$

i.e. change in volume of fluid under pressure $= \dfrac{pV}{K}$

Extra fluid pressure to raise cylinder pressure by p

$$= \frac{pd}{4tE}[5-4v]\,V + \frac{pV}{K}$$

Similarly, for spheres, the extra fluid required

$$= \frac{3pd}{4tE}[1-v]\,V + \frac{pV}{K}$$

EXAMPLE   *A thin cylinder of 75 mm diameter, 250 mm long with wall 2.5 mm thick is subjected to an internal pressure of 7 MN/m². Determine the change in internal diameter and the change in length.*

If in addition to the internal pressure, the cylinder is subjected to a torque of 200 Nm, find the magnitude and nature of principal stresses set up in the cylinder.

$$E = 200 \text{ GN}/m^2; \, v = 0.3$$

SOLUTION Given $d = 75$ mm; $l = 250$ mm; $t = 2.5$ mm

$$p = 7 \text{ MN}/m^2$$

$$= 7 \times 10^6 \text{ N}/m^2$$

$$E = 200 \times 10^9 \text{ N}/m^2$$

(a) By formula, change in diameter = hoop strain × d

or circumferential strain × d

$$= \frac{d}{E}\cdot[\sigma_h - v\sigma_l]$$

$$= \frac{pd^2}{4tE}[2-v]$$

$$= \frac{7 \times 10^6 \times 75^2 \times 10^{-6}}{4 \times 2.5 \times 10^{-3} \times 200 \times 10^9}\,(2-0.3)$$

$$= 33.4 \times 10^{-6} \text{ m}$$

(b) Change in length = longitudinal strain × original length

$$= \frac{1}{E}\,(\sigma_l - v\sigma_h) \times l$$

$$= \frac{pd}{4tE}(1-2v)\cdot l$$

$$= \frac{pdl}{4tE}(1-2v)$$

$$= \frac{7\times10^6 \times 75\times10^{-3}\times 250\times10^{-3}}{4\times2.5\times10^{-3}\times 210\times10^9}(1-0.6)$$

$$= 26.2 \times 10^{-6} \text{ m}$$

(c) Hoop stress $(\sigma_h) = \dfrac{pd}{2t}$

$$= \frac{7\times10^6 \times 75\times10^{-3}}{2\times2.5\times10^{-3}} = 105 \text{ MN/m}^2$$

Longitudinal stress $(\sigma_l) = \dfrac{pd}{4t}$

$$= \frac{7\times10^6 \times 75\times10^{-3}}{2\times2.5\times10^{-3}} = 52.5 \text{ MN/m}^2$$

In addition to these stresses, a shear stress τ is also set up.

By Torsion formula, $\dfrac{T}{J} = \dfrac{\tau}{R}$

$\therefore$ $$\tau = \frac{T.R}{J}$$

Now, $$J = \frac{\pi}{32}\frac{(Do^4 - Di^4)}{4}$$

$$= \frac{\pi}{32}\cdot\frac{(80^4 - 75^4)}{10^{12}} = 0.92 \times 10^{-6} \text{ m}^4$$

$\therefore$ Shear stress $\tau = \dfrac{200\times20\times10^{-3}}{0.92\times10^{-6}} = 4.34 \text{ MN/m}^2$

The principal stresses are

$$\sigma_1, \sigma_2 = \frac{\sigma_x + \sigma_y}{2} \pm \frac{1}{2}\sqrt{(\sigma_x - \sigma_y)^2 + 4\tau_{xy}^2}$$

$$= \frac{1}{2}(105 + 52.5) \pm \frac{1}{2}\sqrt{(105 - 52.5)^2 + 4\times(4.34)^2}$$

$$= \frac{1}{2} \times 157.5 \pm \frac{1}{2} \sqrt{2760 + 75.3}$$

$$= 78.75 \pm 26.6$$

Thus, $\sigma_1 = 105.35 \text{ MN/m}^2$ and $\sigma_2 = 52.15 \text{ MN/m}^2$

Therefore, the principal stresses are 105.35 MN/m² and 52.5 MN/m² (both tensile).

EXAMPLE 14 *A boiler drum consists of a cylindrical portion 2 m long, 1 m diameter and 25 mm thick, closed by hemispherical ends.*

In a hydraulic test to 10 N/mm² how much additional water will be pumped in, after initial filling at atmospheric pressure?

Assume the circumferential strain at the junction of the cylinder and hemispherical is same for both.

For drum material E=207000 N/mm² v = 0.3 for water K = 2100 N/mm².

(UPTU 2002-2003)

SOLUTION   **For cylinder**

Since $\frac{t}{D_i} < \frac{1}{20}$ here, so this is a problem of thin cylinder.

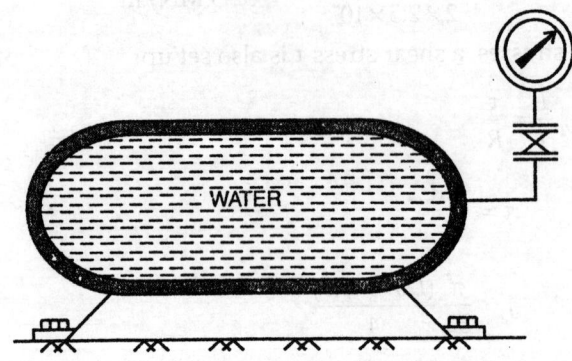

Fig. 16.16

Hoop stress $(\sigma_h) = \frac{pd}{2t}$

$$= \frac{(10 \times 1000)}{2 \times 25}$$

$$= 200 \text{ N/mm}^2$$

Longitudinal stress $(\sigma_l) = \frac{pd}{4t}$

$$= 100 \text{ N/mm}^2$$

Hoop strain $\left(\varepsilon_h\right) = \dfrac{1}{E}\left(\sigma_h - v\sigma_l\right)$

$$= \frac{1}{E}\left(200 - 0.3 \times 100\right)$$

$$= \frac{1}{E} \times 170$$

Longitudinal strain $\left(\varepsilon_l\right) = \dfrac{1}{E}\left(\sigma_l - v\sigma_h\right)$

$$= \frac{1}{E}\left(100 - 0.3 \times 200\right)$$

$$= \frac{1}{E} \times 40$$

Increase in capacity $= \left(2\,\varepsilon_h + \varepsilon_l\right) \times \text{volume}$

$$= \left(2 \times \frac{170}{E} + \frac{40}{E}\right) \times \left[\frac{\pi}{4}\left(1000\right)^2 \times \overset{5}{\cancel{2000}}\right]$$

$$= \frac{1}{E}\left(340 + 40\right) \times \left[3.14 \times 10^6 \times 500\right]$$

$$= \frac{1}{207 \times 10^3} \times 380 \times 314 \times 5 \times 10^6$$

$$= \frac{380 \times 314 \times 5000}{207}$$

$$= 2882125.6 \ \text{mm}^3$$

$$= 2.9 \times 10^6 \ \text{mm}^3 \qquad\qquad \ldots(1)$$

For the two hemispherical ends:

Hoop strain $\varepsilon = \varepsilon_h$ (same as that of cylinder)

Increase in capacity $= 3\,\varepsilon_h \times \text{volume}$

$$= 3 \times \frac{170}{E} \times \frac{\pi \times 1000^3}{6}$$

$$= \frac{3 \times 170}{207000} \times \frac{22}{7} \times \frac{10^3}{6}$$

$$= 1.3 \times 10^6 \ \text{mm}^3 \qquad\qquad \ldots(2)$$

Decrease in volume of water $= \dfrac{p}{k} \times$ volume of cylinder

$$= \dfrac{p}{k} \text{ [Volume of Cylindrical portion + Volume of spherical portion]}$$

$$= \dfrac{10}{2100}\left[\left\{\dfrac{\pi}{4} \times (1000)^2 \times 2000\right\} + \dfrac{\pi \times 1000^3}{6}\right]$$

$$= 10 \times 10^6 \ \ \text{mm}^3 \hspace{3cm} \text{...(3)}$$

Therefore, the additional volume of water required $= (1) + (2) + (3)$

$$= 2.9 \times 10^6 + 1.3 \times 10^6 + 10 \times 10^6$$

$$= 14.25 \times 10^6 \ \ \text{mm}^3 \text{ at atmospheric pressure}$$

16.9 WIRE WOUND CYLINDER

In order to increase the strength of a thin cylinder to withstand high internal pressure without excessive increase in wall thickness, they are sometimes prestressed by winding with steel wire under tension. By winding wire, initial compressive hoop stress is produced in the cylinder. The hoop stress due to fluid pressure is tensile in nature. Therefore, due to wire winding, the final hoop stress in the cylinder shall be reduced.

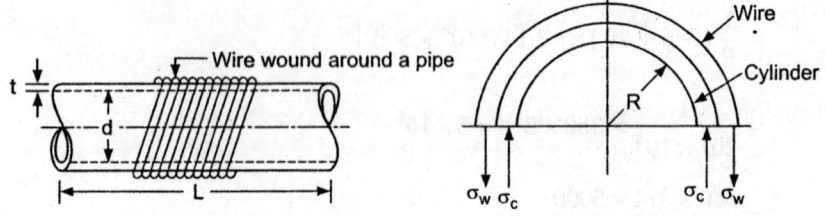

Fig. 16.17

The figure 16.17 shows a cylinder wound with wire.

Let, d = Diameter of the cylinder and L = length of cylinder

        t = Wall thickness of the cylinder

      dw = Diameter of the wire

       n = Number of turns of wire per unit length $= \left(\dfrac{L}{d_w}\right)$

      σ_w = Initial winding stress in wire (tensile)

      σ_c = Compressive circumferential stress developed in the cylinder

Now, when cylinder is subjected to internal pressure p then, let

      σ_c' = Circumferential stress developed in the cylinder

      σ_w' = Stress developed in the wire

      σ_i' = Longitudinal stress developed in the cylinder.

Before admission of fluid into the cylinder

Tensile force exerted by the wire per unit length

$$= 2 \times \frac{\pi}{4} d_w^2 \times \sigma_w \times n$$

Compressive force developed in the cylinder

$$= 2 \times t \times 1 \times \sigma_c$$

$$= 2\sigma_c \cdot t \cdot L$$

For equilibrium $= 2\sigma_c \cdot t = 2 \times \frac{\pi}{4} d_w^2 \times \sigma_w \times n$

But $n = \dfrac{1}{d_w}$

$\therefore \qquad 2\sigma_c \cdot t \cdot L = 2 \times \dfrac{\pi}{4} d_w^2 \times \sigma_w \times \dfrac{L}{d_w}$

$$\boxed{\therefore \ \sigma_c = \frac{\pi d_w}{4t} \cdot \sigma_w} \qquad\qquad \text{...(i)}$$

After the admission of fluid into the cylinder

When the wire wound cylinder is subjected to internal pressure, then, we have

Resisting force of cylinder along longitudinal section $= \sigma_c' \times 2t \times l$

Resisting force of wire per unit length = Number of turns of wire × 2 × Area of Cross-section of wire × Stress in wire due to fluid pressure

$$= n \times 2 \times \frac{\pi}{4} d_w^2 \times \sigma_w'$$

$$= \frac{L}{d_w} \times \frac{\pi}{2} d_w^2 \times \sigma_w' \qquad\qquad \left(n = \frac{L}{d_w} \right)$$

$$= L \times \frac{\pi}{2} d_w \times \sigma_w'$$

Now, bursting force due to fluid pressure

$$= \text{Resisting force of cylinder} + \text{Resisting force of wire}$$

$$p \times d \times L = \sigma_c' \times 2t \times L + L \times \frac{\pi}{4} d_w \times \sigma_w'$$

$$\therefore \qquad p \times d = \sigma_c' \times 2t + \frac{\pi}{2} \times d_w \times \sigma_w' \qquad\qquad \text{...(ii)}$$

Now, since wire and cylinder remain in contact, hence, the circumferential strain in the cylinder = circumferential strains in the wire.

$$\frac{\sigma_c'}{E_c} - v \cdot \frac{\sigma_l'}{E_c} = \frac{\sigma_w'}{E_w}$$

or, $$\frac{\sigma_c'}{E_c} - v \cdot \frac{pd}{4tE_c} = \frac{\sigma_w'}{E_w} \qquad \left(\because \sigma_l' = \frac{pd}{4t} \right)$$

EXAMPLE *A cast iron cylinder of 20 cm inner diameter and 1.25 cm thickness is closely wound with a layer of 4 mm diameter steel wire under a tensile stress of 55 MN/m². Determine the stresses set up in the cylinder and steel wire if water under a pressure of 3 MN/m² is passed in the cylinder. Assume $E_{C.I} = 100$ GN/m²; $E_s = 200$ GN/m² and Poisson's ratio (v) = 0.25.*

SOLUTION Given d_i = 20 cm = 0.2 m

Wall thickness of cylinder (t) = 1.25 cm = 0.0125 m

Diameter of steel wire (d_w) = 4 mm = 0.004

Initial tension of wire (σ_w) = 55 MN/m²

Pressure of water (p) = 3 MN/m²

$E_{C.I} = E_c = 100$ GN/m²

$E_s = E_{\text{wire}} = 200$ GN/m²

Poisson's ratio (v) = 0.25

Stresses setup in the Cylinder and Steel wire

(a) Before the admission of water into the cylinder

Tensile force exerted by wire per unit length

$\quad$ = Compressive force developed in the cylinder

$$2 \times \frac{\pi}{4} d_w^2 \times \sigma_w \times n = 2 \times t \times 1 \times \sigma_c$$

$\therefore \qquad \sigma_c = \frac{\pi d_w}{4t} \times \sigma_w$

$$= \frac{\pi \times 0.004 \times 55}{4 \times 0.0125} = 13.82 \text{ MN/m}^2$$

(b) After the admission of water into the cylinder

Due to internal pressure, longitudinal stress is developed in the cylinder.

$$\sigma_l' = \frac{pd}{4t}$$

$$= \frac{3 \times 0.2}{4 \times 0.0125} = 12 \text{ MN/m}^2$$

Now,

$\qquad$ Total bursting force = Total resisting force

$$p \times d = \sigma_c' \times 2t + \sigma_w' \times 2 \times \frac{\pi}{4} d_w^2 \times n$$

or, $$pd = \sigma_c' \cdot 25 \times \sigma_w' \times \frac{\pi d_w}{2}$$

or $$3 \times 0.2 = \sigma_c' \times 2 \times 0.0125 + \sigma_w' \times \frac{\pi \times 0.004}{2}$$

$$\qquad \dots(i) \qquad \left[\begin{array}{l} n = \dfrac{L}{d_w} \\[2mm] \text{Considering } L = 1 \text{ m and } n = \dfrac{1}{d_w} \end{array} \right]$$

and, Circumferential strain in the cylinder = Circumferential strain in the wire

$$\frac{\sigma_c'}{E_c} - v \frac{\sigma_l'}{E_c} = \frac{\sigma_w'}{E_w}$$

where σ_c' = circumferential stress in the cylinder (MN/m^2)

σ_w' = circumferential stress in the wire, after the water is admitted into the cylinder

Now, substituting the known values, we get

$$\frac{\sigma_c' \times 10^6}{100 \times 10^9} - 0.25 \times \frac{12 \times 10^6}{100 \times 10^9} = \frac{\sigma_w' \times 10^6}{200 \times 10^9}$$

or, $$2\sigma_c' - 6 = \sigma_w' \qquad\qquad \dots(ii)$$

Substituting the value of σ_w' in equation (i) we have

$$3 \times 0.2 = \sigma_c' \times 2 \times 0.0125 + (\sigma_c' - 6) \times \frac{\pi \times 0.004}{2}$$

$$\Rightarrow \qquad \sigma_c' = 17 \text{ MN/m}^2$$

$$\therefore \qquad \sigma_w' = 2 \times 17 - 6$$

$$= 28 \text{ MN/m}^2$$

Resultant stress in the cylinder $= (\sigma_c' - \sigma_c)$

$$= 17 - 13.82$$

$$= 3.18 \text{ MN/m}^2 \text{ (Tensile)} \qquad \textbf{Ans}$$

Resultant stress in the wire $= (\sigma_w - \sigma_w')$

$$= 55 + 28$$

$$= 83 \text{ MN/m}^2 \text{ (Tensile)} \qquad \textbf{Ans}$$

HIGHLIGHTS

1. If $\dfrac{t}{D_i} < \dfrac{1}{20}$ then the cylinder is a thin cylinder.

2. In the case of thin cylinder, the stress distribution is assumed uniform over the thickness of wall.

3. When a thin cylindrical vessel is subjected to internal fluid pressure, the following stresses are setup in the material of a thin cylinder:

   (i) Circumferential or hoop stress (σ_h)

   (ii) Longitudinal stress (σ_l)

   The circumferential stress or hoop stress (σ_h) is given by

   $$\sigma_h = \frac{p \cdot d}{2t} \quad \text{where} \quad p = \text{internal fluid pressure}$$

   $$d = \text{internal diameter of thin cylinder}$$

   and, $\qquad\qquad\qquad t = \text{thickness of wall of cylinder}$

   The longitudinal stress (σ_l) is given by

   $$\sigma_l = \frac{p \cdot d}{4t}$$

   These two formulae are used for the seamless shell i.e., when there is no joints.

   But, when it is not seamless as in the case of rivetted boiler shell, then

   $$\sigma_h = \frac{p \cdot d}{2t\eta_l}$$

   and, $\qquad \sigma_l = \dfrac{p \cdot d}{4 \cdot t \cdot \eta_h}$

   where, η_l = efficiency of the longitudinal joints

   and, $\quad \eta_h$ = efficiency of the circumferential joints.

4. We observed that $\sigma_h = 2 \times \sigma_l$.

5. Maximum shear stress at any point in a thin cylinder subjected to internal fluid pressure is given by

   Maximum shear stress $(\tau_{max}) = \dfrac{\sigma_h - \sigma_l}{2} = \dfrac{p \cdot d}{8t}$

6. If a Cylindrical shell is subjected to an internal fluid pressure p, then Circumferential strain or hoop strain (ε_h).

   $$\therefore \quad \varepsilon_h = \frac{pd}{2tE}\left(1 - \frac{v}{2}\right)$$

   where, v = poisson's ratio;

   Longitudinal strain (ε_l) is given by

   $$\varepsilon_l = \frac{pd}{2tE}\left(\frac{1}{2} - v\right)$$

Change in volume of a cylindrical shell subjected to internal fluid pressure p

$$\delta v = \varepsilon_v \times V$$

$$= (\varepsilon_l + 2\varepsilon_h) \times V$$

$$= \left\{ \frac{pd}{2tE}\left(\frac{1}{2} - v\right) + 2 \cdot \frac{pd}{2tE}\left(1 - \frac{v}{2}\right) \right\} \times V$$

$$= \frac{pd}{2tE}\left[\frac{1}{2} - v + 2 - v\right] \times V$$

$$\therefore \quad \delta v = \frac{pd}{2tE}\left[\frac{5}{2} - 2v\right] \times \frac{\pi}{4}d^2 l = \frac{\pi pd^3 l}{16tE}[5 - 4v]$$

where, ε_v = volumetric strain

E = young's modulus of shell material

v = poisson's ratio

v = volume of shell

t = Thickness of shell

7. When a thin cylindrical shell is subjected to internal fluid pressure (p) and torque then

Major principal stress $(\sigma_1) = \dfrac{\sigma_h + \sigma_l}{2} + \sqrt{\left(\dfrac{\sigma_h - \sigma_l}{2}\right)^2 + \tau^2}$

and Minimum principal stress $(\sigma_2) = \dfrac{\sigma_h - \sigma_l}{2} - \sqrt{\left(\dfrac{\sigma_h - \sigma_l}{2}\right)^2 + \tau^2}$

and $\tau_{max} = \dfrac{(\sigma_1 - \sigma_2)}{2} = \sqrt{\left(\dfrac{\sigma_h - \sigma_l}{2}\right)^2 + \tau^2}$

Thin Sphere:

Hoop stress $(\sigma_h) = \dfrac{pd}{4t}$ = longitudinal stress (σ_l)

Increase in capacity $(\delta_V) = (3 \times \text{hoop strain}) \times \text{Volume}$

$$= 3\varepsilon_h V$$

$$= \frac{3pd}{4tE}(1 - v) \times \frac{\pi}{6}d^3$$

$$= \frac{\pi pd^4}{8tE}(1 - v)$$

Increase in diameter $(\delta_d) = \varepsilon_d \times d = \dfrac{pd^2}{4tE}(1 - v)$

PROBLEMS FOR PRACTICE
(THEORETICAL)

1. What do you mean by thin cylinder? What type of stresses are setup in a thin cylinder when it is subjected to internal fluid pressure?

2. (a) Prove that $(\sigma_h) = \dfrac{pd}{2t}$ and $(\sigma_l) = \dfrac{pd}{4t}$

   (b) Prove that maximum shear stress at any point in a thin cylinder subjected to internal fluid pressure is given by

   $$\tau_{max} = \frac{pd}{8t}$$

   when, p = internal fluid pressure

   d = internal dia. of thin cylinder

   and, t = wall thickness of cylinder.

3. (a) Prove that volumetric strain $(\varepsilon_v) = (2\varepsilon_h + \varepsilon_l)$ when a thin cylinder is subjected to internal fluid pressure.

   (U.P.T.U IIIrd Sem., 2006-2007)

   (b) Prove that when a thin walled Cylindrical vessel of diameter d, length L, and thickness t is subjected to internal pressure p, the change in volume is given by

   $$\frac{\pi pd^3 L}{16 tE}(5 - 4v)$$

4. Prove that when a thin walled spherical vessel of diameter 'd' and thickness 't' is subjected to internal fluid pressure p, the increase in volume is equal to

   $$\frac{\pi pd^4}{8tE}(1 - v)$$

   where, E = Modulus of elasticity

   v = Poisson's ratio

   t = Thickness of wall of sphere

(NUMERICAL)

1. A thin cylinder of internal diameter 2 m contains a fluid at an internal pressure of $3\,N/mm^2$.

   Determine the maximum thickness of the cylinder if (a) longitudinal stress is not to exceed $30\ N/mm^2$ and (b) the circumferential stress is not to exceed $40\,N/mm^2$.

2. A boiler is subjected to internal steam pressure of $3\,N/mm^2$. The thickness of the boiler plate is 2.5 cm and the permissible tensile stress is $125\ N/mm^2$. Find out the maximum diameter, when the efficiency of longitudinal joint is 90% and that of circumferential joint is 35%.

3. A thin spherical copper shell of diameter 0.3 m and thickness 1.6 mm is just full of water at atmospheric pressure.
   Find how much the internal pressure will be increased by pumping in 25,000 mm^3 of water. Given $E = 100,000$ N/mm^2; $v = 0.286$; $K = 2200$ N/mm^2.

4. A thin cylindrical tube of 100 mm internal diameter and 5 mm thick is closed at the ends and is subjected to an internal pressure of 5 N/mm^2. A torque of 2200 NM is also applied to the tube.
   find   (a) hoop stress

              (b) longitudinal stress

              (c) σ_1 and σ_2

              (d) τ_{max}

ANSWERS

3. 1.22 N/mm^2 4. (a) 50 N/mm^2 (b) 25 N/mm^2
(c) 68.16 N/mm^2 ; 6.84 N/mm^2 (d) 30.66 N/mm^2

OBJECTIVE QUESTIONS

1. If $\dfrac{t}{d} < \dfrac{1}{20}$. Then the cylinder is

   (a) thin cylinder   (b) thin shell
   (c) either of the above   (d) none of the above

2. The hoop or circumferential stress in a thin cylindrical shell of diameter D, length L and thickness (t) when subjected to an internal pressure (p) is equal to

   (a) $\dfrac{pD}{4t}$ (b) $\dfrac{pD}{2t}$ (c) $\dfrac{2pD}{t}$ (d) $\dfrac{4pD}{t}$

3. The stress which can be neglected in the case of thin shell compared to other stresses is
   (a) radial stress   (b) hoop stress
   (c) longitudinal stress   (d) tangential stress

4. The hoop stress/longitudinal stress ratio in the case of thin cylindrical shell is
   (a) 1   (b) 2   (c) 3   (d) 4

5. The longitudinal 'or' axial stress in a thin cylindrical shell of diameter (D), length (L) and thickness (t) when subjected to an internal pressure (p) is equal to

   (a) $\dfrac{pD}{4t}$ (b) $\dfrac{pD}{2t}$ (c) $\dfrac{2pD}{t}$ (d) $\dfrac{4pD}{t}$

6. The maximum shear stress in a thin cylindrical shell when subjected to an internal pressure (p) is equal to

   (a) $\dfrac{pD}{4t}$ (b) $\dfrac{pD}{8t}$ (c) $\dfrac{pD}{2t}$ (d) $\dfrac{pD}{t}$

7. The maximum shear stress in a thin spherical shell when subjected to an internal pressure (p) is equal to

   (a) $\dfrac{pD}{4t}$ (b) $\dfrac{pD}{8t}$ (c) $\dfrac{pD}{2t}$ (d) zero

8. The volumetric strain hoop strain ratio in a thin sphere is

   (a) 1   (b) 2   (c) 3   (d) 4

9. The circumferential strain in case of thin cylindrical shell, when subjected to internal pressure (p) is equal to

   (a) $\dfrac{pd}{2tE}\left(\dfrac{1}{2} - v\right)$ (b) $\dfrac{pd}{2tE}\left(1 - \dfrac{1}{2}\cdot v\right)$

   (c) $\dfrac{pd}{4tE}(1 - v)$ (d) $\dfrac{3pd}{4tE}(1 - v)$

10. The longitudinal strain in the case of thin cylindrical shell when subjected to internal pressure (p) is equal to

    (a) $\dfrac{pd}{2tE}\left(\dfrac{1}{2} - v\right)$ (b) $\dfrac{pd}{2tE}\left(1 - \dfrac{v}{2}\right)$

    (c) $\dfrac{pd}{4tE}(1 - v)$ (d) $\dfrac{3pd}{4tE}(1 - v)$

11. The strain in any direction in case of thin spherical shell subjected to internal pressure (p) is equal to

    (a) $\dfrac{pd}{2tE}\cdot\left(\dfrac{1}{2} - v\right)$ (b) $\dfrac{pd}{2tE}\cdot\left(1 - \dfrac{v}{2}\right)$

    (c) $\dfrac{pd}{4tE}\cdot(1 - v)$ (d) $\dfrac{3pd}{4tE}\cdot(1 - v)$

12. The volumetric strain in the case of thin spherical shell, when subjected to internal pressure (p) is equal to

    (a) $\dfrac{pd}{2tE}\left(\dfrac{1}{2} - v\right)$ (b) $\dfrac{pd}{2tE}\left(1 - \dfrac{v}{2}\right)$

    (c) $\dfrac{pd}{4tE}(1 - v)$ (d) $\dfrac{3pd}{4tE}(1 - v)$

13. The hoop or circumferential stress in a rivetted cylindrical shell when subjected to internal pressure (p) is equal to

(a) $\dfrac{pD}{4t\eta_l}$ (b) $\dfrac{pD}{4t\eta_c}$ (c) $\dfrac{pD}{2t\eta_l}$ (d) $\dfrac{pD}{4t\eta_c}$

where η_l = efficiencies of longitudinal joint

η_c = efficiency of circumferential joint

14. The longitudinal stress in a rivetted cylindrical shell when subjected to internal fluid pressure (p) is equal to

(a) $\dfrac{pD}{4t\eta_l}$ (b) $\dfrac{pD}{4t\eta_c}$ (c) $\dfrac{pD}{2t\eta_l}$ (d) $\dfrac{pD}{4t\eta_c}$

ANSWERS

1. (c)	2. (b)	3. (a)	4. (b)	5. (a)	6. (b)
7. (d)	8. (c)	9. (b)	10. (a)	11. (c)	12. (d)
13. (c)	14. (a)				

— ❖❖ —

THICK CYLINDERS AND SPHERES

17.1 INTRODUCTION

It the ratio of thickness to the internal diameter is more than $\frac{1}{20}$, then such cylindrical shell is known as thick cylinder. *i.e.* if $\frac{t}{D_i} > \frac{1}{20}$ then it is thick cylinder.

In thin cylinder, we had assumed that the distribution of circumferential 'or' hoop stress (σ_h) stress over the cross-section is uniform and therefore, radial stress is negligible because thickness of metal is quite less as compared to its internal diameter. These assumptions do not hold good in the case of thick cylinder or tube subjected to pressure.

Circumferential stress (σ_c), as well as radial stress (σ_r) in the case of thick shell varies with thickness 'or' radius.

Uses: *Thick shells are used where fluid is stored or transferred under very high pressure.*

In order to find 'circumferential' and 'radial stresses' in a thick cylinder or tube at any radius following assumptions are made:

   (i) The material of the shell is perfectly homogenous and isotropic.

  (ii) Plane sections perpendicular to the longitudinal axis of the cylinder remain plane after the application of internal pressure.

 (iii) The material is stressed within the elastic limit.

 (iv) Modulus of elasticity for the cylinders' material in tension and compression are equal i.e. $E_t = E_c$.

N.B: We will denote circumferential stress (σ_c) and hoop stress (σ_h). **In fact both are same** but we will use separate notation for each.

17.2 STRESSES IN THICK CYLINDER 'OR' TUBE

Let us consider a thick cylinder having

it's length = l

inner radius = r_i

outer radius = r_o

Let us consider that cylinder is subjected to internal pressure p_i acting on its inner surface and outer pressure p_o acting on its outer surface. We have to evaluate the stress developed due to internal pressure p_i.

Due to internal fluid pressure, following type of stresses will be developed in the cylinder.

   (i) Longitudinal stress (σ_l)

  (ii) Radial stress (σ_r)

 (iii) Circumferential stress (σ_c) or Hoop stress (σ_h)

Note: Circumferential Stress (σ_c) Hoop stress (σ_h) is same, readers are advised to remember both and should not get confused.

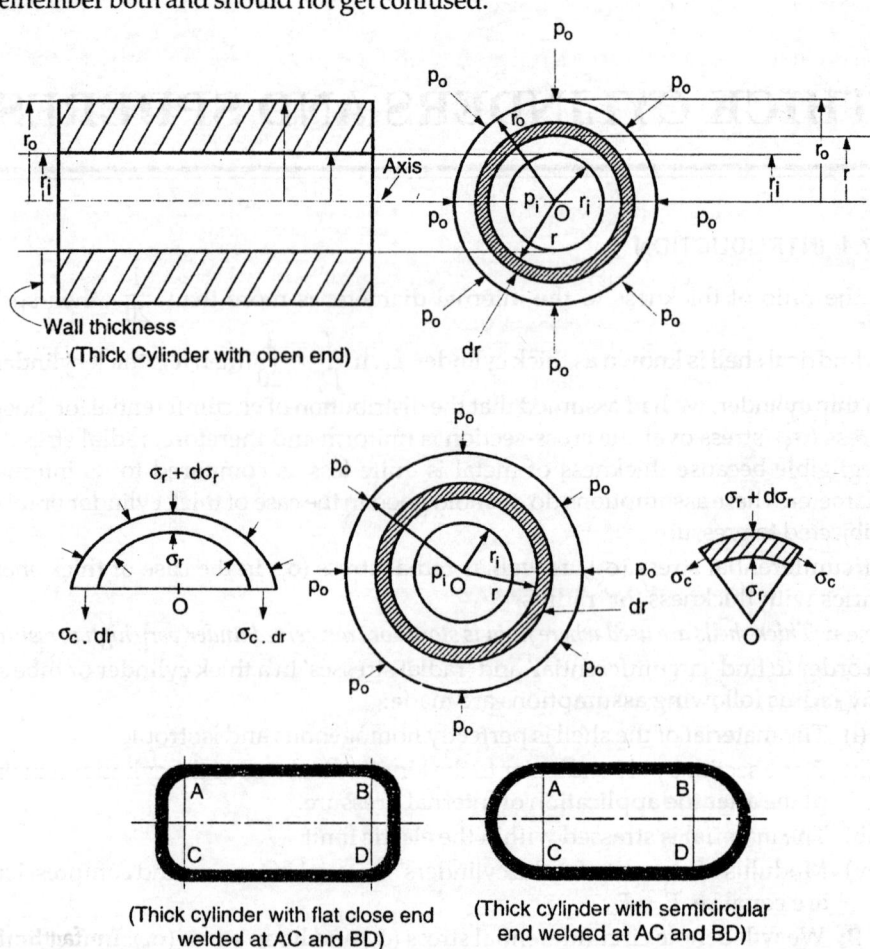

Fig. 17.1

To analyse the above stresses, consider an elementary ring of thickness dr at a distance r from the center as shown in Fig. 17.1.

Considering forces on half the elementary ring of thickness dr and at a distance 'r' from the center O.

         Downword force = Upward force

or, ·   Resisting force = Bursting force

$$2 \cdot \sigma_c \cdot dr \cdot l = l\left[\sigma_r \times 2r - 2(\sigma_r + d\sigma_r)(r + dr)\right]$$

or, $\sigma_c \cdot dr = \sigma_r \cdot r - (\sigma_r \cdot r + \sigma_r \cdot dr + d\sigma_r \cdot r + d\sigma_r \cdot dr)$

or, $\qquad \sigma_c \cdot dr = -\sigma_r \cdot dr - r \cdot d\sigma_r$

$\qquad\qquad\qquad$ (neglecting last term being the product of two small quantities)

Dividing by dr throughout, we get

$$\sigma_c = -\sigma_r - r \cdot \frac{d\sigma_r}{dr}$$

or, $\qquad r \cdot \dfrac{d\sigma_r}{dr} = -\sigma_C - \sigma_r$ $\qquad\qquad\qquad\qquad\qquad\qquad\qquad$ ...(1)

If σ_l = axial longitudinal stress (tensile), then longitudinal strain =

$$(\varepsilon_l) = \frac{\sigma_l}{E} - v \cdot \frac{\sigma_c}{E} + v \cdot \frac{\sigma_r}{E}$$

$$= \frac{1}{E} \left[\sigma_l - v \left(\sigma_c - \sigma_r \right) \right]$$

For ε_l to be constant, $\left(\sigma_C - \sigma_r \right)$ must be constant

Let $\qquad \left(\sigma_C - \sigma_r \right) = 2A$

$\therefore \qquad\quad \sigma_C = 2A + \sigma_r$

Substituting the value of σ_C in eqn. (1).

$$r \cdot \frac{d\sigma_r}{dr} = -\left(2A + \sigma_r \right) - \sigma_r$$

$$r \cdot \frac{d\sigma_r}{dr} = -2\left(\sigma_r + A \right)$$

or, $\qquad \dfrac{d\sigma_r}{\left(\sigma_r + A \right)} = -2 \cdot \dfrac{dr}{r}$

Integrating both sides, we get

$$\log \left(\sigma_r + A \right) = -2 \log r + \text{constant}$$

$$\log \left(\sigma_r + A \right) + 2 \log r = \text{constant}$$

or, $\qquad \log \left(\sigma_r + A \right) + \log r^2 = \text{constant}$

or, $\qquad r^2 \cdot \left(\sigma_r + A \right) = B \text{ (let another constant)}$

or, $\qquad \left(\sigma_r + A \right) = \dfrac{B}{r^2}$

$$\boxed{\therefore \ \sigma_r = \frac{B}{r^2} - A} \qquad\qquad\qquad\qquad\qquad\qquad\qquad ...(2)$$

$$\sigma_c = \sigma_r + 2A$$

$$= \frac{B}{r^2} - A + 2A$$

N.B.: Radial stress (σ_r) is always compressive.

$$\boxed{\sigma_c = \frac{B}{r^2} + A}$$ ...(3)

Equations (2) and (3) are known as **lame's formula 'or' lame's theorem** which give 'radial stress' and circumferential stress, or (hoop stress) between $r = r_i$ and $r = r_o$

At inner radius r_i, $\sigma_r = p_i$

or, $$p_i = \frac{B}{r_i^2} - A$$ ...(4)

where, p_i = internal pressure,

At outer radius $\sigma_r = p_o$

$\therefore$ $$p_o = \frac{B}{r_o^2} - A$$ ...(5)

In most cases $p_o = 0$

Thus, the constants A and B can be evaluated from these equations. Now, circumferential stress (σ_C) can be found out at any radius.

Evaluation of constants 'A' and 'B':

Subtracting (4) from (5)

$$p_i - p_o = \frac{B}{r_i^2} - \frac{B}{r_o^2}$$

$$\boxed{B = \left\{ \frac{\left(p_i - p_o\right)r_i^2 \cdot r_o^2}{\left(r_o^2 - r_i^2\right)} \right\}}$$

and, $$A = \frac{B}{r_i^2} - p_i$$

$$= \frac{\left(p_i - p_o\right)r_i^2 r_o^2}{r_i^2 \cdot \left(r_o^2 - r_i^2\right)} - p_i = \frac{\left(p_i - p_o\right)r_o^2}{r_o^2 - r_i^2} - p_i$$

$$= \frac{p_i r_o^2 - p_o r_o^2 + p_i r_i^2 - p_i r_o^2}{r_o^2 - r_i^2}$$

$$\boxed{A = \frac{\left(p_i r_i^2 - p_o r_o^2\right)}{\left(r_o^2 - r_i^2\right)}}$$

Substituting values of A and B in equation (2) and (3), we get, σ_r and σ_c respectively.

General Case

When the thick cylinder is subjected to internal pressure (p_i) and external pressure (p_o).

Then, radial stress $(\sigma_r) = \dfrac{B}{r^2} - A$

$$= \frac{(p_i - p_o)\, r_i^2 r_o^2}{r^2\,(r_o^2 - r_i^2)} - \frac{(p_i r_i^2 - p_o r_o^2)}{r_o^2 - r_i^2}$$

$$= \frac{1}{(r_o^2 - r_i^2)}\left\{ \frac{(p_i - p_o)\, r_i^2 r_o^2}{r^2} - (p_i r_i^2 - p_o r_o^2) \right\}$$

and, Hoop stress (σ_h) or

Circumferential stress $(\sigma_c) = \dfrac{B}{r^2} + A$

$$= \frac{1}{(r_o^2 - r_i^2)}\left\{ \frac{(p_i - p_o)\, r_i^2\, r_o^2}{r^2} + (p_i r_i^2 - p_o r_o^2) \right\}$$

Special Cases

(a) Thick cylinder subjected to internal pressure only: When the thick cylinder is subjected to internal pressure only, then $p_o = 0$

Now, $\quad \sigma_r = p_i$ at $r = r_i$

and $\quad \sigma_r = 0$ at $r = r_o$

Substituting these value in equation (2).

$$p_i = \frac{B}{r_i^2} - A$$

and $\quad 0 = \dfrac{B}{r_o^2} - A$

$\therefore \quad p_i - 0 = \dfrac{B}{r_i^2} - \dfrac{B}{r_o^2}$

$$= B\left(\frac{r_o^2 - r_i^2}{r_i^2\, r_o^2} \right)$$

$\therefore \quad B = \dfrac{p_i \cdot r_i^2 \cdot r_o^2}{(r_o^2 - r_i^2)}$

and $\quad A = \dfrac{B}{r_o^2}$

$$= \frac{p_i \cdot r_i^2\, \cancel{r_o^2}}{\cancel{r_o^2}\,(r_o^2 - r_i^2)}$$

$$= \frac{p_i \cdot r_i^2}{(r_o^2 - r_i^2)}$$

Now, substituting the value of A and B in equation (2) and (3), we get σ_r and σ_c respectively.

$$\sigma_r = \frac{B}{r^2} - A$$

$$= \frac{p_i \cdot r_i^2 \cdot r_0^2}{r^2 \cdot (r_0^2 - r_i^2)} - \frac{p_i r_i^2}{(r_0^2 - r_i^2)}$$

$$\therefore \quad \boxed{\sigma_r = \frac{p_i r_i^2}{(r_0^2 - r_i^2)} \left(\frac{r_0^2}{r^2} - 1 \right)}$$

and $\quad \sigma_c = \dfrac{B}{r^2} + A$

$$= \frac{p_i \cdot r_i^2 \cdot r_0^2}{r^2 \cdot (r_0^2 - r_i^2)} + \frac{p_i r_i^2}{(r_0^2 - r_i^2)}$$

$$\therefore \quad \boxed{\sigma_c = \frac{p_i r_i^2}{(r_0^2 - r_i^2)} \left(\frac{r_0^2}{r^2} + 1 \right)}$$

From the above expression we observe that σ_c is maximum when r is minimum i.e., when $r = r_i$

$$\therefore \quad \sigma_c \text{ (Maximum)} = \frac{p_i r_i^2}{r_0^2 - r_i^2} \left[\frac{r_0^2}{r_i^2} + 1 \right]$$

$$= p_i \cdot \left(\frac{r_0^2 + r_i^2}{r_0^2 - r_i^2} \right)$$

$$= p_i \cdot \left(\frac{k^2 + 1}{k^2 - 1} \right)$$

where $\quad k = \left(\dfrac{r_0}{r_i} \right)$

At $r = r_0$, σ_c is minimum

$$\sigma_c \text{ (minimum)} = \frac{p_i r_i^2}{r_0^2 - r_i^2} \left[\frac{r_0^2}{r_0^2} + 1 \right]$$

$$= \frac{2 p_i r_i^2}{r_0^2 - r_i^2}$$

$$= p_i \cdot \frac{2}{(k^2 - 1)}$$

Also, σ_r is maximum at $r = r_i$

$\therefore$ $\qquad$ $\sigma_r\,(\text{Maximum}) = p_i$

Hence, at the inner surface,

$$\frac{\sigma_c}{\sigma_r} = \frac{p_i\left(\dfrac{k^2+1}{k^2-1}\right)}{p_i}$$

$$= \left(\frac{k^2+1}{k^2-1}\right)$$

Profile of stress: We observe that maximum stress in thick cylinder is 'Hoop stress'.

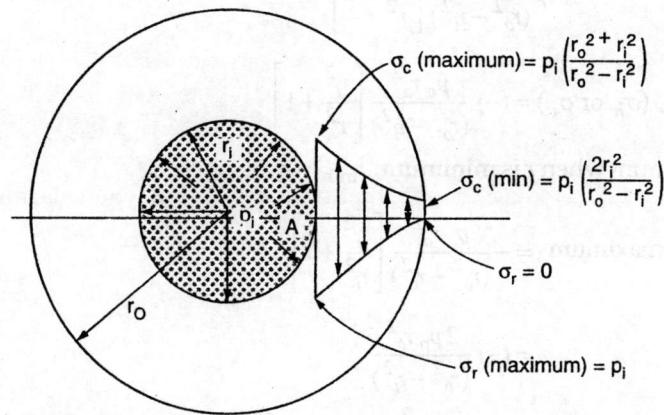

Fig. 17.2

(b) Thick cylinder subjected to external pressure only: When the thick cylinder is subjected to external pressure only, then $p_i = 0$

Now, $\qquad$ $\sigma_r = 0$ when $r = r_i$

and $\qquad$ $\sigma_r = p_o$ when $r = r_o$

Substituting these in Lame's eqn.

$$\sigma_r = 0 = \frac{B}{r_i^2} - A$$

and $\qquad$ $p_o = \dfrac{B}{r_o^2} - A$

$$0 - p_o = B\left\{\frac{1}{r_i^2} - \frac{1}{r_o^2}\right\}$$

$$B = -p_o \cdot \frac{r_i^2\, r_o^2}{r_o^2 - r_i^2}$$

and $A = \dfrac{B}{r_i^2}$

$$= -p_o \cdot \dfrac{r_o^2}{(r_o^2 - r_i^2)}$$

Substituting the value of A and B in Lame's Eqn.

Radial stress $(\sigma_r) = \dfrac{B}{r^2} - A$

$$= -\dfrac{p_o\, r_i\, r_o^2}{(r_o^2 - r_i^2)r^2} + \dfrac{p_o\, r_o^2}{(r_o^2 - r_i^2)}$$

$$= (-)\dfrac{p_o\, r_o^2}{(r_o^2 - r_i^2)}\left[\dfrac{r_i^2}{r^2} - 1\right]$$

Hoop stress $(\sigma_h \text{ or } \sigma_c) = (-)\dfrac{p_o\, r_o^2}{(r_o^2 - r_i^2)}\left[\dfrac{r_i^2}{r^2} + 1\right]$

σ_c is maximum when r is minimum, $r_{min} = r_i$

$\therefore$ σ_c maximum $= -\dfrac{p_o\, r_o^2}{(r_o^2 - r_i^2)}\left[\dfrac{r_i^2}{r_i^2} + 1\right]$

$$= (-)\dfrac{2p_o\, r_o^2}{(r_o^2 - r_i^2)}$$

$$= -p_o \cdot \dfrac{2k^2}{k^2 - 1} \quad \text{where } k = \left(\dfrac{r_o}{r_i}\right)$$

At $r = r_o$, $\sigma_c = -\dfrac{p_o\, r_o^2}{r_o^2 - r_i^2}\left[\dfrac{r_i^2}{r_o^2} + 1\right]$

$$= -p_o \cdot \left(\dfrac{r_o^2 + r_i^2}{r_o^2 - r_i^2}\right)$$

$$= -p_o \cdot \left(\dfrac{k^2 + 1}{k^2 - 1}\right)$$

σ_r is maximum at $r = r_o$ and $\sigma_r \text{ (maximum)} = p_o$

Hence, at the outer surface, $\dfrac{\sigma_c}{\sigma_r} = \left(\dfrac{r_o^2 + r_i^2}{r_o^2 - r_i^2}\right)$

$$= \left(\dfrac{k^2 + 1}{k^2 - 1}\right)$$

Profile of stress: The distribution of hoop stress (σ_c) and radial stress (σ_r) is shown in the figure.

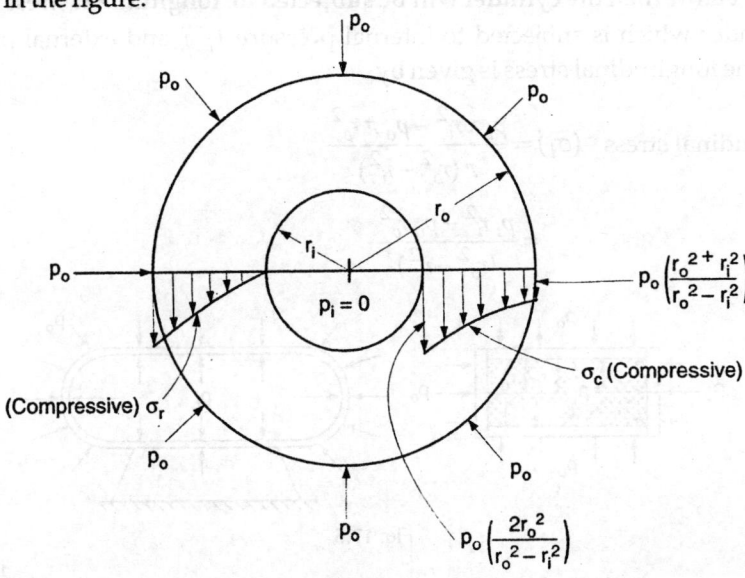

Fig. 17.3

In this case also, Hoop stress is the maximum stress at the inner radius.

(c) Solid circular shaft subjected to external pressure (p_o): We know

$$\sigma_r = \frac{B}{r^2} - A \text{ and } \sigma_c = \frac{B}{r^2} + A$$

Since, σ_r and σ_c are infinite at $r = 0$, so B must be zero so that $\sigma_r = -A$

and $\qquad \sigma_c = A$

$\therefore \qquad (-)\sigma_r = \sigma_c = A$

which follows that both radial and circumferential stress are uniformly distributed and each is equal to the external radial pressure.

17.3 LONGITUDINAL STRESS

If the cylinder is not closed at the ends, for examples, gun barrel or when the pressure is retained by a piston at one or both ends of the cylinder shown below, then the longitudinal (axial) stress is zero. *i.e.* $\sigma_l = 0$

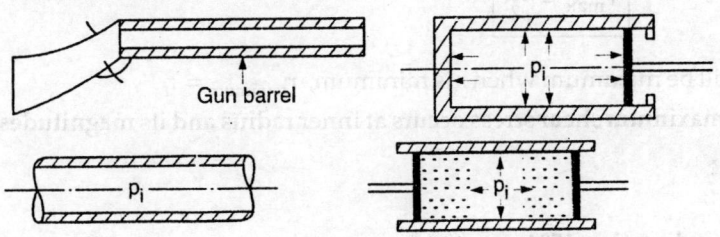

Fig. 17.4

However, if the cylinder is closed at the ends by caps or hemispherical shell as shown below then the cylinder will be subjected to 'longitudinal stress' also.

A cylinder which is subjected to internal pressure (p_i) and external pressure (p_o), the longitudinal stress is given by

$$\text{Longitudinal stress }(\sigma_l) = \frac{p_i \,\pi r_i^2 - p_o\, \pi r_o^2}{\pi(r_o^2 - r_i^2)}$$

$$= \frac{p_i \, r_i^2 - p_o\, r_o^2}{(r_o^2 - r_i^2)}$$

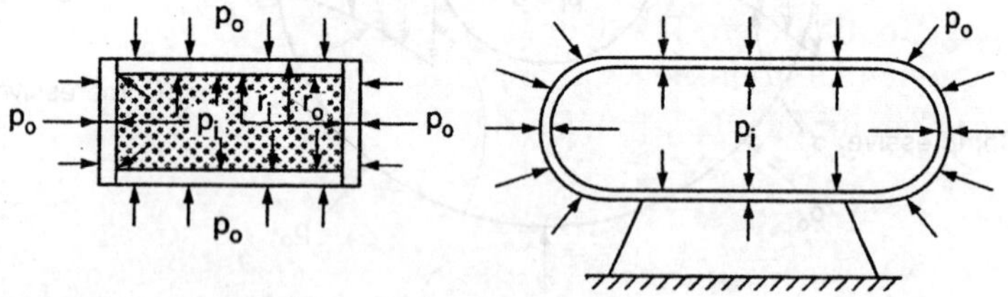

Fig. 17.5

when only internal pressure p_i acts, then, logitudinal stress $(\sigma_l) = \dfrac{p_i \, r_i^2}{(r_o^2 - r_i^2)}$

Principal and shear stresses: Since no torque acts on the cylinder, So, here σ_c, σ_l and σ_r are the principal stresses. σ_r is compressive and σ_c, σ_l are tensile. σ_c is maximum and σ_r is minimum,

Now, we know, $\tau_{max} = \left(\dfrac{\sigma_{max} - \sigma_{min}}{2}\right)$

$$= \frac{\sigma_c - (-\sigma_r)}{2} \quad \text{(as } \sigma_r \text{ is compressive)}$$

$$= \left(\frac{\sigma_c + \sigma_r}{2}\right)$$

$$= \frac{1}{2}\left[\left(\frac{B}{r^2} + A\right) + \left(\frac{B}{r^2} - A\right)\right]$$

$$\boxed{\tau_{max} = \frac{B}{r^2}}$$

τ_{max} will be maximum when r is minimum, $r_{minimum} = r_i$

Hence, maximum shear stress occurs at inner radius and its magnitudes is equal to $\left(\dfrac{B}{r^2}\right)$.

It acts in a direction 45° to σ_r and σ_c

$$\tau_{max} = B \times \frac{1}{r_i^2}$$

$$= \frac{(p_i - p_o) \, r_i^2 r_o^2}{(r_o^2 - r_i^2)} \times \frac{1}{r_i^2}$$

$$= \frac{(p_i - p_o) \, r_o^2}{(r_o^2 - r_i^2)}$$

Change in cylinder dimensions

(a) Change in diameter: The diametral strain of a cylinder is equal to the hoop 'or' circumferential strain, hence, change in diameter = (diametral strain × original diameter) = circumferential strain × original diameter circumferential strain (ε_c), is given by

$$\varepsilon_c = \frac{1}{E} \left[\sigma_c - v \cdot \sigma_r - v \cdot \sigma_l \right]$$

Thus, change is diameter at any radius r of the cylinder is given by

$$\Delta D = \frac{2r}{E} \left[\sigma_c - v \, \sigma_r - v \, \sigma_l \right]$$

(b) Change in length: Similarly, change in length of the cylinder is given by

$$\Delta l = \frac{l}{E} \left[\sigma_l - v\sigma_r - v\sigma_c \right]$$

Effect of Thickness

(i) Let us consider a cylinder having inner radius r_i, thickness t, further, let the cylinder is subjected to internal pressure p_i, then $r_o = (r_i + t)$

$$\sigma_{c_i} = p_i \, \frac{(r_i + t)^2 + r_i^2}{(r_i + t)^2 - r_i^2}$$

$$= p_i \cdot \frac{(r_i + t)^2 + r_i^2}{(2r_i + t) \cdot t}$$

further, $\sigma_{c_0} = p_i \cdot \left(\dfrac{2r_i^2}{r_o^2 - r_i^2} \right)$

$$= p_i \cdot \frac{2r_i^2}{(r_i + t)^2 - r_i^2}$$

$$= p_i \cdot \frac{2r_i^2}{(2r_i + t) \cdot t}$$

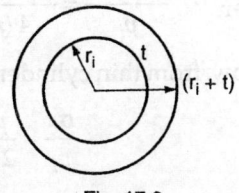

Fig. 17.6

when t is small,

$$\sigma_{c_i} = p_i \cdot \frac{2r_i^2}{2r_i t}$$

$$= \frac{p_i r_i}{t}$$

and $\quad \sigma_{c_0} = p_i \cdot \frac{2r_i^2}{2r_i t}$

$$= \frac{p_i r_i}{t}$$

So, we find that for small value of t, $\sigma_{c_i} = \sigma_{c_0} = \dfrac{p_i r_i}{t}$ which is the same as that of the thin cylinder.

(ii) Let $d = 2r_i$

$\therefore \quad \sigma_{c(\text{max})} = \sigma_{c_i} = p_i \cdot \dfrac{\left(\dfrac{d}{2}+t\right)+\left(\dfrac{d}{2}\right)^2}{(d+t)\cdot t}$

$$= p_i \cdot \frac{(d+2t)+d^2}{4t\,(d+t)}$$

$$= p_i \cdot \frac{\left[\left(\dfrac{d}{t}+2\right)^2+\left(\dfrac{d}{t}\right)^2\right]}{4\left(\dfrac{d}{t}+1\right)}$$

Let $\quad \left(\dfrac{d}{t}\right) = n$

then $\quad \dfrac{\sigma_{c(\text{max})}}{p_i} = \dfrac{(n+2)^2+n^2}{4\,(n+1)}$

Now, from thin cylinder theory where σ_c is assumed uniform,

$$\frac{\sigma_c}{p_i} = \frac{p_i d}{2t\,p_i}$$

$$= \frac{d}{2t}$$

$$= \frac{1}{2}\left(\frac{d}{t}\right) = \frac{n}{2}$$

$\therefore \quad$ Error $= \dfrac{(n+2)^2+n^2}{4(n+1)} - \dfrac{n}{2}$

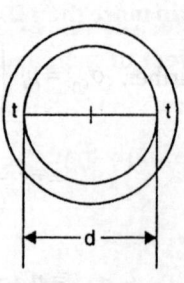

Fig. 17.7

$$= \frac{(n+2)^2 + n^2 - 2n(n+1)}{4(n+1)}$$

$$= \frac{n^2 + 4n + 4 + n^2 - 2n^2 - 2n}{4(n+1)}$$

$$= \frac{2n+4}{4(n+1)}$$

$$= \frac{2(n+2)}{4(n+1)} = \frac{n+2}{2(n+1)}$$

$\therefore$ Percentage error $= \left\{ \dfrac{\dfrac{n+2}{2(n+1)}}{\dfrac{(n+2)^2 + n^2}{4(n+1)}} \times 100 \right\}$

$$= \left\{ \frac{2(n+2)}{(n+2)^2 + n^2} \times 100 \right\}$$

For $n = 20$

$$\text{Percentage error} = \frac{2(20+2)}{(20+2)^2 + (20)^2} \times 100$$

$$= \frac{44}{(22)^2 + (20)^2} \times 100$$

$$= 4.9773\%$$

Thus, it is observed that the error in the value of $\left(\dfrac{\sigma_c}{p_i}\right)$ by assuming it as a thin cylinder is less than 5% when $\left(\dfrac{d}{t}\right)$ ratio is 20. That is why cylinder with $\left(\dfrac{d}{t}\right)$ ratio more than 20 are considered to be thin cylinders.

Effect of Increasing the Cylinder Thickness

We know that $\sigma_r = \dfrac{p_i r_i^2}{r_o^2 - r_i^2} \left(\dfrac{r_o^2}{r^2} - 1 \right)$

and $\sigma_c = \dfrac{p_i r_i^2}{r_o^2 - r_i^2} \left(\dfrac{r_o^2}{r^2} + 1 \right)$

$$\therefore \qquad \sigma_{r_c} = \frac{p_i \, r_i^2}{r_o^2 - r_i^2}\left(\frac{r_o^2}{r^2} \mp 1\right)$$

When $t \to \infty$, then r_i can be neglected in comparison to r_o

$$\equiv \frac{p_i \, r_i^2}{r_o^2}\left(\frac{r_o^2}{r^2}\right)$$

$$\equiv \frac{p_i \, r_i^2}{r^2} \qquad\qquad\qquad (\because r_o^2 \mp r^2 \equiv r_o^2)$$

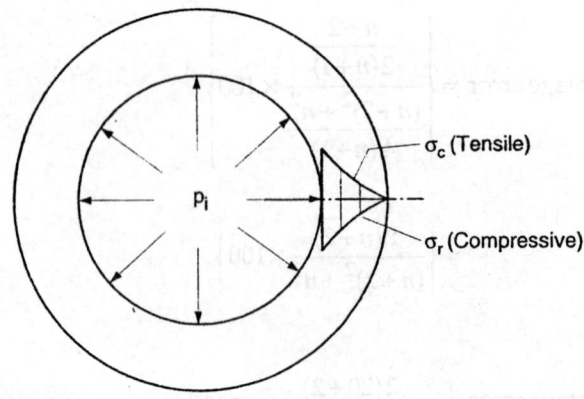

Fig. 17.8

This implies that for a cylinder of very large radius: (Fig. 17.8)

(a) At any point, the radial and the circumferential stresses are equal.

(b) If $\sigma_l = 0$, pure shear exists everywhere is the cylinder.

(c) Both σ_r and σ_c are inversely proportional to r^2, thus, at $r = 4r_i$, stresses are only $\left(\dfrac{1}{16}\right)$ of their maximum value which means that a cylinder of

$k = \dfrac{r_o}{r_i} > 4$ may be reasonably assumed to be a cylinder of infinite thickness.

Strain in Thick Cylinder

1. Circumferential strain $= \dfrac{\pi(d + \delta d) - \pi d}{\pi d}$

$$= \frac{\delta d}{d}$$

= Diametral strain

Diametral strain is always calculated in the direction of σ_c.

Hoop strain $(\varepsilon_c) = \dfrac{\sigma_c}{E} + v \cdot \dfrac{\sigma_r}{E} - v \cdot \dfrac{\sigma_l}{E}$

$$= \frac{1}{E}\left[\sigma_c + v\,(\sigma_r - \sigma_l)\right]$$

Therefore, assuming that the cylinder is closed with caps, then hoop strain

$$\varepsilon_c = \frac{1}{E}\left[\left\{\frac{r_i^2 r_o^2}{r^2} \cdot \frac{p_i - p_o}{r_o^2 - r_i^2} + \frac{p_i r_i^2 - p_o r_o^2}{r_o^2 - r_i^2}\right\}\right.$$

$$\left. + v\left\{\frac{r_i^2 r_o^2}{r^2} \cdot \frac{p_i - p_o}{r_o^2 - r_i^2} - \frac{p_i r_i^2 - p_o r_o^2}{r_o^2 - r_i^2} - \frac{p_i r_i^2 - p_o r_o^2}{r_o^2 - r_i^2}\right\}\right]$$

$$= \left\{\frac{(1+v)}{E} \cdot \frac{r_i^2 r_o^2}{r^2} \cdot \frac{p_i - p_o}{r_o^2 - r_i^2} + \frac{(1-2v)}{E} \cdot \frac{p_i r_i^2 - p_o r_o^2}{r_o^2 - r_i^2}\right\}$$

When, there is no axial or longitudinal stress (*i.e.* cylinder having open ends as that of water pipe) then the above relation reduces to

$$\varepsilon_c = \left(\frac{1+v}{E}\right) \cdot \left(\frac{r_i^2 r_o^2}{r^2}\right) \cdot \left(\frac{p_i - p_o}{r_o^2 - r_i^2}\right)$$

$$\left[\text{As } \sigma_l = \frac{p_i r_i^2 - p_o r_o^2}{r_o^2 - r_i^2} = 0 \text{ when there is no axial or longitudinal stress.}\right]$$

2. The radial strain causing radial shaft at any point is the direction of radial stress (σ_r) is $\varepsilon_r = \dfrac{1}{E}\left[\sigma_r + v\,(\sigma_c + \sigma_l)\right]$

3. Volumetric strain $(\varepsilon_V) = \dfrac{dV}{V}$

$$V = \pi r^2 l$$

$$\therefore \quad dV = \frac{\partial V}{\partial r} \cdot dr + \frac{\partial V}{\partial L} \cdot dl$$

$$= (2\pi r l) \cdot dr + (\pi r^2) \cdot dl$$

$$= \pi r^2 l\left[2 \cdot \frac{dr}{r} + \frac{dl}{l}\right]$$

$$\left(\frac{dV}{V}\right) = 2 \cdot \frac{dr}{r} + \frac{dl}{l}$$

$\therefore$ Volumetric strain = 2 × Diametral (or circumferential) strain
+ Longitudinal strain.

$$\varepsilon_V = (2\varepsilon_c + \varepsilon_l)$$

17.4 THICK CYLINDER FOR HIGH PRESSURE

Following methods are adopted to carry liquid under high pressure.

  (i) By compounding the cylinder

  (ii) By winding steel wire under tension on the cylinder

Compound cylinder 'or' Composite cylinders are formed by shrinking one cylinder on to the other. Due to this, inner cylinder is subjected to initial hoop compression, which enables the compound cylinder to withstand much higher working pressure. The outer cylinder in this case is subjected to initial hoop tension due to shrinkage which results in uniform distribution of pressure.

In addition to withstanding high internal pressure, a compound cylinder results in appreciable saving in weight as compared to thick cylinder.

So, we have studied that in a compound or composite cylinder there are two concentric cylinders, one is shrunk fit on the other end which makes the Cylinder to withstand high pressure of fluid (liquid or gas).

17.5 DERIVATION OF STRESSES IN COMPOUND CYLINDERS (THICK)

Let r_o = outer radius of compound cylinder

  r_i = inner radius

  r_j = radius of the junction of the two cylinder

  p_j = radial pressure at the junction of the two cylinder

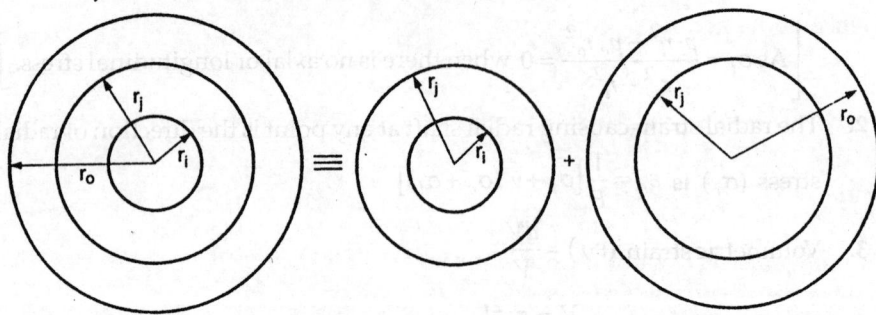

Fig. 17.9

Case I: *Derivation of hoop stress 'or' circumferentials stress when fluid is not admitted in the cylinder.*

(i)   Then **for outer cylinder** Lame's equation at a radius x

$$p_x = \frac{B_1}{x^2} - A_1 \qquad\qquad ...(1)$$

and, $$\sigma_x = \frac{B_1}{x^2} + A_1 \qquad\qquad ...(2)$$

A_1 and B_1 are constant for outer cylinder.

  At $x = r_o$; $p_x = 0 = \sigma_r$

and,   At $x = r_j$; $p_x = p_j$

$$\therefore \qquad 0 = \left(\frac{B_1}{r_i^2} - A_1 \right) \qquad \qquad ...(3)$$

$$\text{and,} \qquad p_j = \left(\frac{B_1}{r_j^2} - A_1 \right) \qquad \qquad ...(4)$$

From eqns. (3) and (4), the constant A_1 and B_1 can be determined and substituted in equation (2) to get hoop stress in the outer cylinder (due to shrinkage) can be obtained.

(ii) For inner cylinder

Lame's equation for inner cylinder at a radius x

$$p_x = \frac{B_2}{x^2} - A_2 \qquad \qquad ...(5)$$

$$\text{and,} \qquad \sigma_x = \frac{B_2}{x^2} + A_2 \qquad \qquad ...(6)$$

where, A_2 and B_2 are other constants

$$\text{At } x = r_i ; \; p_x = 0 \text{ as fluid pressure is not inside the cylinder (inner)}$$

$$\text{and,} \qquad \text{At } x = r_j ; \; p_x = p_j$$

Hence, above equation reduces to

$$0 = \frac{B_2}{r_i^2} - A_2 \qquad \qquad ...(7)$$

$$\text{and,} \qquad p_j = \frac{B_2}{r_j^2} - A_2 \qquad \qquad ...(8)$$

From equations (7) and (8) the constants A_2 and B_2 can be determined. These values are substituted in (6) and the hoop stress is obtained in the inner cylinder.

Case II: *Derivation of hoop stress 'or' Circumferential stress, when fluid is admitted in the Compound Cylinder*

When there is a fluid under pressure inside the cylinder, hoop stress will set-up in the compound cylinder.

In order to find the stresses, the inner cylinder and outer cylinder together will be considered as thick shell.

Let $\qquad p_x =$ internal fluid pressure

Hence, by Lame's theorem

$$p_x = \frac{B}{x^2} - A \qquad \qquad ...(7)$$

$$\sigma_x = \frac{B}{x^2} + A \qquad \qquad ...(8)$$

where, A and B are constants for a single thick shell owing to internal fluid pressure.

At $x = r_0$; $p_x = 0$

Substituting these values in equation (7), we get

$$0 = \frac{B}{r_0^2} - A \qquad \qquad ...(9)$$

At $\qquad x = r_i$; $p_x = p$ $\qquad$ (fluid pressure)

$$p_i = \frac{B}{r_i^2} - A \qquad \qquad ...(10)$$

From equations (9) and (10), the constants A and B can be determined.

The resultant hoop stresses will be the algebraic sum of the hoop stresses caused due to shrinkage and due to internal fluid pressure.

Shrinkage Allowance

In order to get the desired interface pressure p_j at the common surface of the compound cylinder, it is necessary that the inner diameter of the outer cylinder should be slightly smaller then the outer diameter of the inner cylinder.

Practically, outer cylinder is heated as long as the outer cylinder slides over the inner cylinder, on cooling it exerts the required pressure at the common surface.

The initial difference in diameter at this surface is termed as shrinkage allowance.

Let the pressure set-up at the junction of two cylinders due to force or shrink fit be 'p_j'.

Let the hoop stresses set-up at the junction on the inner and outer tubes resulting from the pressure p_j be σ_{h_i} (compressive) and σ_{h_o} (tensile) respectively.

If δ_0 = radial shift of outer cylinder

and δ_i = radial shift of inner cylinder as shown in Fig. 17.10.

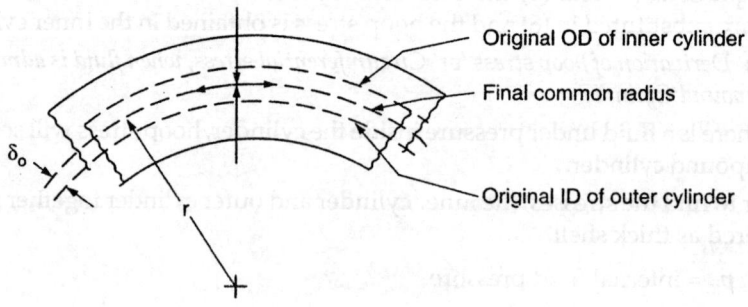

Fig. 17.10

As circumferential strain = diameteral strain

Circumferential strain at radius r on the outer cylinder $= \dfrac{2\delta_0}{2r}$

$$= \frac{\delta_0}{r} = \varepsilon_{h_o}$$

Circumferential strain at radius r on the inner cylinder $= \dfrac{2\delta_i}{2r}$

$$= \dfrac{\delta_i}{r} = -\varepsilon_{h_i}$$

(negative sign, since there is decrease in diameter)

Total interference or shrinkage $= \delta_o + \delta_i$

$$= r\varepsilon_{h_o} + r\left(-\varepsilon_{h_i}\right)$$

$$= \left(\varepsilon_{h_o} - \varepsilon_{h_i}\right) r$$

Assuming the cylinder open ends i.e. $\sigma_l = 0$

$\therefore \qquad \varepsilon_{h_o} = \dfrac{\sigma_{h_o}}{E_1} - \dfrac{v_1}{E_1}\left(-p_j\right)$ $\qquad\qquad \left[\text{As } \varepsilon_{h_o} = -p_j\right]$

and $\qquad \varepsilon_{h_i} = \dfrac{\sigma_{h_i}}{E_2} - \dfrac{v_2}{E_2}\left(-p_j\right)$ $\qquad\qquad \left[\text{As } \varepsilon_{h_i} = -p_j\right]$

where, E_1, E_2, v_1 and v_2 are the elastic modulus and Poisson's ratio of the two tubes respectively.

Hence, total intereference or shrinkage allowance

$$= \left[\dfrac{1}{E_1}\left(\sigma_{h_o} - v_1 p_j\right) - \dfrac{1}{E_2}\left(\sigma_{h_i} + v_2 p_j\right)\right] \cdot r$$

where, r is the initial nominal radius of the mating surfaces.

Generally, the tubes are of the same material.

Hence, $E_1 = E_2 = E$ and $v_1 = v_2 = v$

Therefore, $\boxed{\text{Shrinkage allowance} = \dfrac{r}{E}\left(\sigma_{h_o} - \sigma_{h_i}\right)}$

N.B.: Since hoop stress (σ_h) and circumferential stress (σ_c) are the same, so, we can write σ_c also in the above . Hence, Shrinkage allowance $= \dfrac{r}{E}(\sigma_{c_o} - \sigma_{c_i})$.

17.6 INTERFERENCE

Let there be a shaft of diameter D and a thin hollow sleeve of thickness t and internal diameter 'd' is to be fitted on the shaft of outer dia D. $D > d$.

There is very small difference between D and d.

The difference between two diameter $(D - d)$ is called interference.

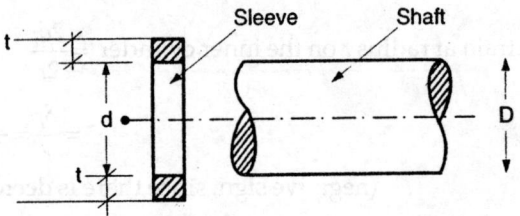

Fig. 17.11

To fit the sleeve over shaft, it is heated and afterward it is made to slide over shaft (D). After the assembly when temperature of both sleeve and shaft becomes normal, sleeve grips the shaft firmly and interference pressure is developed between the surfaces in contact.

This interface *pressure (p_i) tries to compress the shaft and tries to expand the sleeve as shown in Fig. 17.12.

Shrinkage allowance = increase in diameter of outer cylinder + decrease in diameter of inner cylinder.

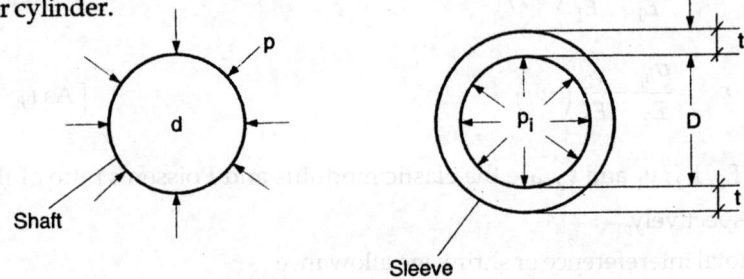

Fig. 17.12

EXAMPLE 1 *A hollow forged boiler drum 1.9 m outside diameter and 130 mm thick, was tested before entering service upto 200 bar. Calculate the maximum and minimum hoop stress under test.*

SOLUTION

At inner surface

$$R_i = \frac{D_i}{2}$$

$$= \frac{D_o - 2 \times t}{2}$$

$$= \frac{1.9 - 2 \times 0.130}{2}$$

$$= \frac{1.9 - 0.260}{2}$$

$$= 0.82 \ m$$

$$= 820 \ mm$$

130 mm → | ← 130 mm

← 1.9 M →

Fig. 17.13

---

*The hoop and radial stresses throughout the solid shaft are everywhere equal to the shrinkage or interference pressure and both are compressive i.e. negative (–). The maximum shear stress $= \frac{1}{2}(\sigma_1 - \sigma_2)$ is thus zero throughout the shaft.

$$\sigma_r = 20 = \frac{B}{(820)^2} - A \qquad \ldots(1)$$

At outer surface

$$R_o = \frac{D_o}{2}$$

$$= \frac{1.9 \times 1000}{2}$$

$$= \frac{1900}{2}$$

$$= 950 \ \text{mm}$$

Now, $\qquad \sigma_r = 0 = \dfrac{B}{(950)^2} - A \qquad \ldots(2)$

$$\therefore \qquad 20 - 0 = \frac{B}{(820)^2} - \frac{B}{(950)^2}$$

$$B = 52.746 \times 10^6$$

$$A = 58.444$$

$$\therefore \qquad \sigma_{C\text{min}} = \frac{B}{R_o^2} + A$$

$$= \frac{52.746 \times 10^6}{(950)^2} + 58.444$$

$$= 116.89 \ \text{N/mm}^2$$

$$\sigma_{C(\text{max})} = \frac{B}{R_2^2} + A$$

$$= \frac{52.746 \times 10^6}{(820)^2} + 58.444$$

$$= 136.89 \ \text{N/mm}^2$$

EXAMPLE 2 *Draw the curves of radial and hoop stress for a tube of 150 mm outside diameter and 70 mm inside diameter when subjected to*

   (a) an internal pressure 600 bar only

   (b) an external pressure 400 bar only

   (c) when subjected to internal pressure and external pressure 600 bar and 400 bar respectively.

SOLUTION

(a)   At internal radius, $R_i = 35$ mm

$$\therefore \qquad \text{Radial stress } (\sigma_r) = \frac{B}{r^2} - A$$

$$*60 = \frac{B}{(35)^2} - A \qquad \qquad \ldots(1)$$

At outer radius, $R_0 = 75$ mm

$$\sigma_r = \frac{B}{75^2} - A$$

$$0 = \frac{B}{(75)^2} - A \qquad \qquad \ldots(2)$$

Substituting (2) from (1)

$$60 = \frac{B}{(35)^2} - \frac{B}{(75)^2}$$

$$\therefore \qquad B = 93.963 \times 10^3$$

and, $A = 16.7$

Since, we have to plot the curve, so, we need some more points to know the shape of the curve. For this purpose r at a interval of 10 mm is taken and then corresponding value of σ_C and σ_r are obtained by calculation and tabulated in the form of table as given below.

r (mm)	$\sigma_C = \left(\dfrac{B}{r^2} + A \right)_{\text{tension}}$	$\sigma_r = \left(\dfrac{B}{r^2} - A \right)_{\text{compression}}$
35	93.4	60
45	63.1	30
55	48	14.3
65	39	6.0
75	33.4	0

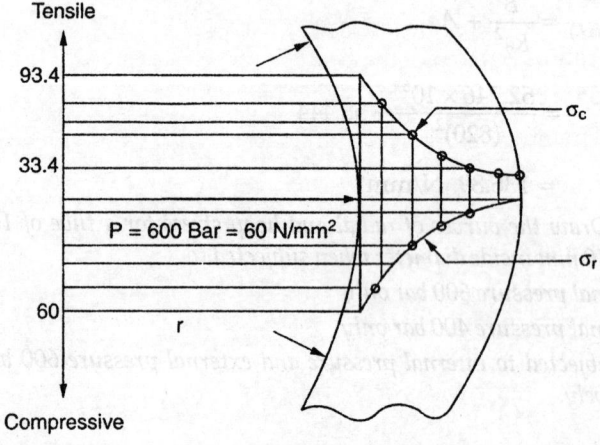

Fig. 17.14

---

*1 bar = 100 kPa = 0.1 MPa = 0.1 N/mm²

Hence, 600 bar = 60 N/mm²

(b) $r_o = 75$ mm

$r_i = 35$ mm

$p_o = 400$ bar

$p_i = 0$

$$0 = \sigma_r = \text{Radial stress} = \frac{B}{(35)^2} - A \qquad \ldots(1)$$

and, $40 = \dfrac{B}{(75)^2} - A$ $\qquad \ldots(2)$

From (2) and (1) gives

$$40 = \frac{B}{(75)^2} - \frac{B}{(35)^2}$$

$$B = -62.642 \times 10^3$$

and, $A = 51.136$

r	$\sigma_C = \left(\dfrac{B}{r^2} + A\right)$	$\sigma_r = \left(\dfrac{B}{r^2} - A\right)$
35	0	− 102.27
45	20.2	− 82.07
55	30.43	− 71.84
65	36.31	− 65.96
75	40.0	− 62.27

Like before, some points at the interval of 10 has been taken between inner radius (r_i) and outer radius (r_o) to plot the curve.

(c) $r_i = 35$ mm

$r_o = 75$ mm

At inner radius, $r_i = 35$ mm

$$\sigma_r = 60 = \frac{B}{(35)^2} - A \qquad \ldots(1)$$

At outer radius $r_o = 75$ mm

$$\sigma_r = 40 = \frac{B}{(75)^2} - A \qquad \ldots(2)$$

∴   (1) and (2) gives

$$20 = \frac{B}{(35)^2} - \frac{B}{(75)^2}$$

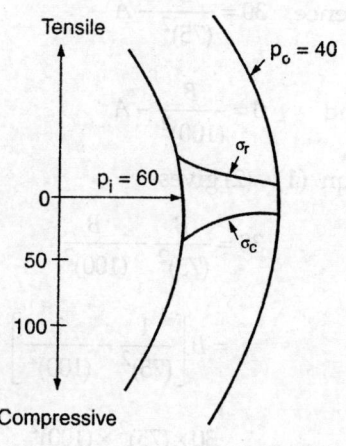

Fig. 17.15

$$B = 31.321 \times 10^2$$

and, $A = -31.43$

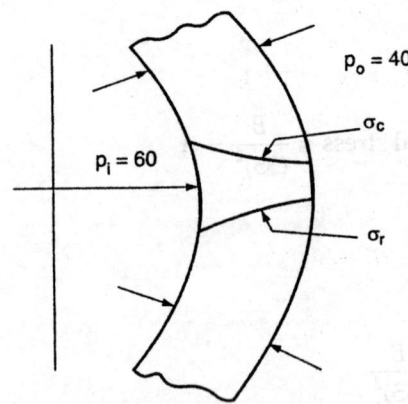

$p_o = 40$

σ_c

$p_i = 60$

σ_r

Fig. 17.16

Like before, some points between the min. and max. radius will be taken and corresponding value of σ_C and σ_r will be evaluated and tabulated in the tabular form, from which graph could be plotted.

EXAMPLE 3 *A hub is shrunk on to a solid shaft and the final dimensions are:*
   Diameter at the junction 150 mm
   External dia. of hub 200 mm
Find the initial difference in the diameters of the hub and the shaft to produce a radial contact pressure of 30MPa; E = 200 GPa.

SOLUTION   **For the hub**

$\sigma_r = 30$ MPa at $r = 75$ mm

and $\sigma_r = 0$ at $r = 100$ mm

Hence, $30 = \dfrac{B}{(75)^2} - A$ ...(1)

and $0 = \dfrac{B}{(100)^2} - A$ ...(2)

Eqn. (1) – (2) gives

$$30 = \frac{B}{(75)^2} - \frac{B}{(100)^2}$$

$$= B\left[\frac{1}{(75)^2} - \frac{1}{(100)^2}\right]$$

$\therefore$ $B = \dfrac{30 \times (75)^2 \times (100)^2}{(100)^2 - (75)^2}$

$$= \frac{30 \times (75)^2 \times 10^4}{175 \times 25}$$

$$= 38.571 \times 10^4$$

$$A = \frac{B}{(100)^2} = 38.571$$

Hence, circumferential stress $(\sigma_c)_{r=75} = \dfrac{B}{r^2} + A$

$$= \frac{38.571 \times 10^4}{(75)^2} + 38.571$$

$$= 68.570 + 38.571$$

$$= 107.141 \text{ MPa}$$

Increase in internal hub diameter $= \dfrac{d}{E}(\sigma_c + v \cdot \sigma_r)$

$$= \frac{150}{200 \times 10^3}(107.141 + v \cdot 30) \qquad \dots(1)$$

For the shaft

$$\sigma_c = -\sigma_r = -30 \text{ MPa}$$

Hence, decrease in shaft diameter

$$= \frac{150}{200 \times 10^3}(30 - v \cdot 30) \qquad \dots(2)$$

Equation (1) + (2) will give initial diffrerence in diameters

Equation (1) + (2) gives $\dfrac{150}{200 \times 10^3}(107.141 + 30)$

$$= \frac{150}{200 \times 10^3} \times 137.141$$

$$= 0.1028 \text{ mm} \quad \textbf{Ans.}$$

EXAMPLE 4 *A cast iron pipe of 400 mm inner diameter and 100 mm thickness carries water under pressure of 80 kg/cm². Determine the maximum and minimum intensities of hoop stress across the section. Also, sketch the radial pressure distribution and hoop stress distribution across the section.*

SOLUTION

$$di = 400 \text{ mm} \qquad\qquad d_o = 600 \text{ mm}$$

$$= 40 \text{ cm.} \qquad\qquad = 60 \text{ cm}$$

$$\therefore \quad r_i = 20 \text{ cm} \qquad\qquad r_o = 30 \text{ cm.}$$

$$p_i = 80 \text{ kg/cm}^2$$

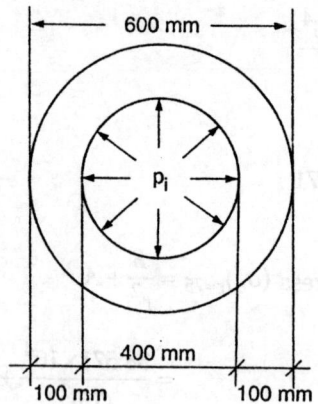

Fig. 17.17

Let us consider an arbitrary radius x of the pipe, then by Lame's Eqn.

$$p_x = \frac{B}{x^2} - A$$

or,

$$80 = \frac{B}{(20)^2} - A$$

$\Rightarrow$

$$A = \frac{B}{400} - 80 \qquad \qquad \dots \text{(I)}$$

Similarly,

$$0 = \frac{B}{(30)^2} - A$$

$\Rightarrow$

$$A = \frac{B}{900} \qquad \qquad \dots \text{(II)}$$

From (I) and (II)

$$\frac{B}{400} - 80 = \frac{B}{900}$$

$$\frac{B - 32,000}{400} = \frac{B}{900}$$

$\Rightarrow$ $9B - 288,000 = 4B$

$\Rightarrow$ $5B = 288000$

$\Rightarrow$ $B = 57600$ and $A = 64$

Hoop stress $(\sigma_h) = \dfrac{B}{x^2} + A$

$$= \frac{57600}{x^2} + 64$$

∴   Hoop stress at radius 20 cm,

$$\sigma_{20} = \frac{57600}{(20)^2} + 64$$

$$= \frac{57600}{400} + 64$$

$$= 144 + 64$$

$$= 208 \text{ kg/cm}^2$$

and, Hoop stress at radius 30 cm,

$$\sigma_{30} = \frac{57600}{(30)^2} + 64$$

$$= \frac{57600}{900} + 64$$

$$= 64 + 64$$

$$= 128 \text{ kg/cm}^2$$

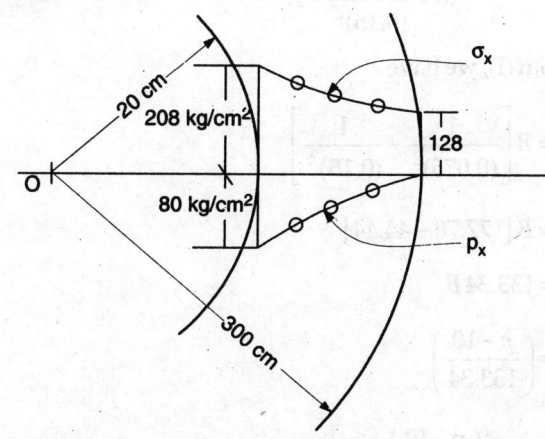

Fig. 17.18 Profile of hoop stress and radial stress

EXAMPLE 5 *An external pressure of 10 MN/m² is applied to a thick cylinder of internal diameter 150 mm. and external diameter 300 mm. If the maximum hoop stress permitted on the inside wall is 35 MN/m², Calculate.* **(MTU 3rd Sem. 2012-13)**

 (i) *The maximum internal pressure that can be applied*
 (ii) *The change in outside diameter if the cylinder has the closed ends. Take*
   $E = 210 \text{ GN/m}^2$ *and* $v = 0.3$

SOLUTION
 (i) Maximum internal pressure (p):
   $r_i = 75 \text{ mm} = 0.075 \text{ m}; r_o = 0.150 \text{ m}$

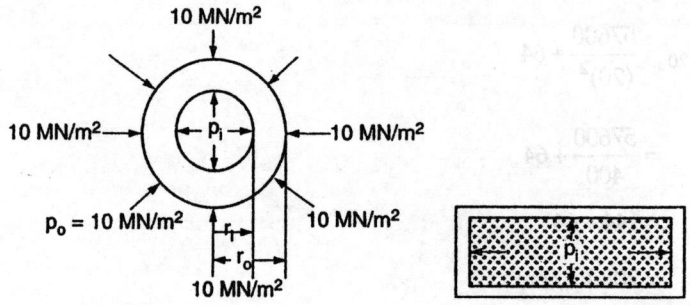

Fig. 17.19

At radius $r_i = 0.075$ m; $p_{r_i} = p$ MN/m^2 (let).

A radius $r_o = 0.15$ m; $p_{r_o} = 10$ MN/m^2

By Lame's Equation,

$$p = \frac{B}{(0.075)^2} - A \qquad \ldots (I)$$

and

$$10 = \frac{B}{(0.15)^2} - A \qquad \ldots (II)$$

Subtracting (II) from (I), we have

$$(p - 10) = B\left[\frac{1}{(0.075)^2} - \frac{1}{(0.15)^2}\right]$$

$$= B[177.78 - 44.44]$$

or, $\quad (p - 10) = 133.34\,B$

$\Rightarrow \qquad B = \left(\dfrac{p - 10}{133.34}\right)$

from equation (II) $A = \left\{\left(\dfrac{p-10}{3}\right) - 10\right\}$

$$= \left\{\frac{p-40}{3}\right\}$$

Now, Hoop stress (σ_h) or $\sigma_c = \dfrac{B}{r^2} + A$

$$\sigma_c \text{ at } r_i = \frac{B}{r_i^2} + A$$

$$35 = \frac{p-10}{133.34} \times \frac{1}{(0.075)^2} + \frac{p-40}{3}$$

or, $$35 = \frac{p-10}{0.75} + \frac{p-40}{3}$$

or, $$3.5 = 1.333\,(p-10) + 0.333\,(p-40)$$

or, $$35 = 1.333\,p - 13.330 + 0.333\,p - 13.32$$

or, $$35 + 13.33 + 13.32 = 1.6666\,p$$

or, $$p = \left(\frac{61.65}{1.666}\right)$$

$$= 37.004 \text{ MN/m}^2$$

$$p \simeq 37 \text{ MN/m}^2 \qquad \textbf{Ans.}$$

(ii) **Change in outside diameter:** Hoop strain or Circumferential strain at outer surface

$$\varepsilon_h \text{ or } \varepsilon_c \text{ at } r = r_o = \left[\frac{\sigma_c}{E} - v \cdot \frac{\sigma_l}{E} - v \cdot \frac{\sigma_r}{E}\right]$$

$$= \frac{1}{E}\left[\sigma_c - v \cdot \sigma_l - v \cdot \sigma_r\right] \qquad \dots \text{(III)}$$

Let us compute σ_c, σ_l at $r = r_o$

From eqs. (III) $B = \left(\dfrac{p-10}{133.34}\right)$ $\qquad$ From (IV) $A = \left(\dfrac{p-40}{3}\right)$

$$= \left(\frac{37-10}{133.34}\right) \qquad\qquad\qquad = \left(\frac{37-40}{3}\right)$$

$$= 0.202 \qquad\qquad\qquad\qquad = (-1)$$

Hoop stress or Circumferential stress σ_h or σ_c at $r = r_0 = \dfrac{B}{r_0^2} + A$

$$= \frac{0.202}{(0.15)^2} + (-1)$$

$$= 7.97 \text{ MN/m}^2$$

Longitudinal stress (σ_c) when cylinder is subjected to internal pressure (p_i) and external pressure (p_0).

Here $p_i = 37$ MN/m^2 and $p_0 = 10$ MN/m^2

Hence, longitudinal stress $(\sigma_l) = \dfrac{p_i r_i^2 - p_0 r_0^2}{r_0^2 - r_i^2}$

$$= \frac{37 \times (0.075)^2 - 10 \times (0.15)^2}{(0.15)^2 - (0.075)^2}$$

$$\sigma_l = (-)\,1\,\text{MN/m}^2 \;\;(\text{Compressive})$$

Given $p_o = \sigma_{r_0} = (-)\,10\,\text{MN/m}^2$

Now, change in diameter $\Delta d = 2r_0 \times \varepsilon_c$ at $r = r_0 = \dfrac{2r_0}{E}\,(\sigma_h - \nu \cdot \sigma_r - \nu \cdot \sigma_l)$

$$= \frac{2 \times 0.15}{210 \times 10^9}\big[7.97 - 0.3 \times (-10) - 0.3\,(-1)\big] \times 10^6$$

$$= \frac{0.3}{210 \times 10^3}\big[7.97 + 3 + 0.3\big]\,\text{metre}$$

$$= \frac{0.3}{210 \times 10^3} \times 11.27\,\text{metre} = 0.0161 \times 10^{-3}\,\text{metre}$$

Hence change in dia $(\Delta d) = 0.0161\,\text{mm}^*$ **Ans.**

EXAMPLE 6 *A thick cylinder has a length of 300 mm and outer and inner diameters 150 mm and 100 mm respectively.*

  (i) *Compute circumferential and longitudinal stresses at inner surface when the cylinder is filled with water under a pressure of 100 bar.*

 (ii) *How much additional water was pumped in above the atmospheric pressure?*

     Take $E = 200\,\text{KN/mm}^2; \nu = 0.3; K_{\text{water}} = 2\text{KN/mm}^2$

SOLUTION

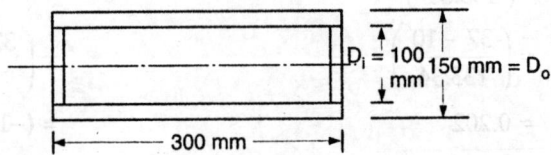

$D_i = 100$ mm   150 mm $= D_o$

$\mid\!\!\longleftarrow\!\!\longrightarrow\!\!\mid$ 300 mm

Fig. 17.20

Given $p = \sigma_r = 100\,\text{bar} = 10\,\text{N/mm}^2$

At inner radius $(r_i) = \dfrac{D_i}{2} = 50\,\text{mm}.$

Radial stress $(\sigma_r) = \dfrac{B}{r_i^2} - A$

Here, $10 = \dfrac{B}{50^2} - A$ ...(I)

---

*Change in dia should be expressed in mm and not in metre.

At outer radius $(r_o) = \dfrac{D_o}{2}$

$$= \frac{150}{2} = 75 \text{ mm}$$

Radial stress $(\sigma_r) = \dfrac{B}{r_0^2} - A$

or, $\qquad\qquad 0 = \dfrac{B}{75^2} - A$ $\qquad\qquad\qquad\qquad\qquad$ ... (II)

(I) – (II) gives

$$10 = \frac{B}{50^2} - \frac{B}{75^2}$$

$\Rightarrow \qquad B = 45000$ and $A = 8$ from (II)

At inner surface $(r_i) = 50$, $\sigma_c = \dfrac{B}{50^2} + A$

$$= \frac{45000}{2500} + 8$$

$$= \frac{450}{25} + 8$$

$$= 26 \text{ N/mm}^2 \text{ (Tensile)}$$

At inner surface Circumferential strain (ε_c)

$$= \frac{\sigma_c - \sigma_l \cdot v - \sigma_r \cdot v}{E} \qquad\qquad \left[\sigma_r = -10 \text{ N/mm}^2 \right]$$

$$= \frac{26 - 8 \times 0.3 + 10 \times 0.3}{2 \times 10^5} = 1.33 \times 10^{-4}$$

Longitudinal strain $(\varepsilon_l) = \dfrac{\sigma_l - v \cdot \sigma_c - v \cdot \sigma_r}{E}$

$$= \frac{8 - 0.3 \times 2.6 + 0.3 \times 10}{2 \times 10^5}$$

$$= 1.6 \times 10^{-5}$$

Total volumetric strain = Volumetric strain of water + Volumetric strain of cylinder.

Now, volumetric strain of water $(\varepsilon_V) = \dfrac{p}{K}$

$$= \dfrac{10}{2 \times 10^3}$$

$$= 5 \times 10^{-3}$$

Volumetric strain of cylinder $(\varepsilon_V) = (\varepsilon_l + 2\varepsilon_c)$

$$= 1.6 \times 10^{-5} + 2 \times 1.33 \times 10^{-4}$$

$$= 2.82 \times 10^{-4}$$

Hence, total volumetric strain $= 5 \times 10^{-3} + 2.82 \times 10^{-4}$

$$= \left(\dfrac{5 + 0.282}{10 + 3} \right)$$

$$= 5.282 \times 10^{-3}$$

∴   Addition volume of water $= 5.282 \times 10^{-3} \times$ Volume of cylinder

$$= 5.282 \times 10^{-3} \times \dfrac{\pi}{4} \left(\dfrac{150}{1000} \right)^2 \times \dfrac{300}{1000}$$

$$= 2.8 \times 10^{-5} \ m^3$$

$$= 2.8 \times 10^{-5} \times 1000 \ \text{litre}$$

$$= 2.8 \times 10^{-2} \ \text{litre}$$

$$= \left(\dfrac{2.8}{100} \right) \text{litre}$$

$$= 0.028 \ \text{litre} \qquad \textbf{Ans.}$$

EXAMPLE 7 *A hollow cylinder of 45 cm internal diameter and 10 cm wall thickness contains the fluid under pressure of 850 N/cm². Find the maximum and minimum hoop stress across the section.*   **(UPTU 2006 - 07)**

SOLUTION   Given $d_i = 45$ cm $\Rightarrow r_i = 22.5$ cm

$t = 10$ cm and $\sigma_r = 850 \ N/cm^2 =$ pressure of fluid inside pipe

Hence, $d_o = 65$ cm $\Rightarrow r_o = 32.5$ cm

By Lame's equation

$$\text{Radial stress } (\sigma_r) = \dfrac{B}{r^2} - A$$

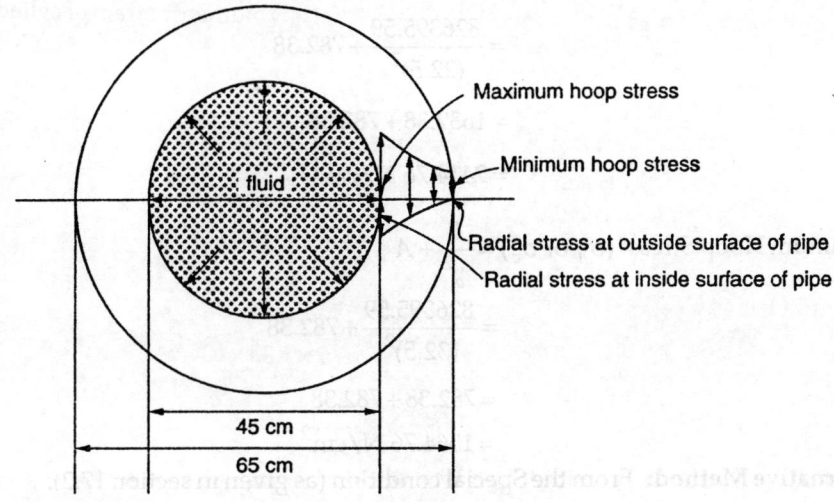

Maximum hoop stress

Minimum hoop stress

Radial stress at outside surface of pipe

Radial stress at inside surface of pipe

fluid

45 cm

65 cm

Fig. 17.21

For inner radius (r_i), $\sigma_r = \dfrac{B}{(22.5)^2} - A$

$$850 = \dfrac{B}{(22.5)^2} - A \qquad \text{... (I)}$$

For outer radius (r_0); $\sigma_r = 0$

Hence, $0 = \dfrac{B}{(32.5)^2} - A \qquad \text{... (II)}$

from (I) and (II), we get

$$850 = \dfrac{B}{(22.5)^2} - \dfrac{B}{(32.5)^2}$$

$\Rightarrow \qquad B = \dfrac{850 \times (22.5)^2 \times (32.5)^2}{(32.5)^2 - (22.5)^2}$

$\qquad = 826395.59$

and, $\qquad A = \dfrac{B}{(32.5)^2}$

$\qquad = \dfrac{826395.59}{(32.5)^2}$

$\qquad = 782.38$

Maximum Hoop Stress $(\sigma_h \text{ or } \sigma_c) = \dfrac{B}{r_i^2} + A$

$$= \frac{826395.59}{(22.5)^2} + 782.38$$

$$= 1632.38 + 782.38$$

$$= 2414.76 \text{ N/cm}^2$$

Minimum Hoop Stress $(\sigma_h \text{ or } \sigma_c) = \dfrac{B}{r_o^2} + A$

$$= \frac{826395.59}{(32.5)^2} + 782.38$$

$$= 782.38 + 782.38$$

$$= 1564.76 \text{ N/cm}^2$$

Alternative Method: From the Special condition (as given in section 17.2).

At inner radius

Hoop stress $\quad (\sigma_h \text{ or } \sigma_c) = \dfrac{p_i r_i^2}{(r_o^2 - r_i^2)}\left[1 + \dfrac{r_o^2}{r_i^2}\right]$

When only internal pressure of fluid (p_i) exist

$$= \frac{850 \times (22.5)^2}{(32.5^2 - 22.5^2)}\left[1 + \frac{(32.5)^2}{(22.5)^2}\right]$$

$$= 782.386 \times 3.086$$

$$= 2414.77 \text{ N/cm}^2$$

At outer radius

Hoop stress $\quad (\sigma_h \text{ or } \sigma_c) = \dfrac{p_i r_i^2}{(r_o^2 - r_i^2)}\left[1 + \dfrac{r_o^2}{r_o^2}\right]$

When only internal pressure (p_i) of fluid exist then σ_h or σ_c

$$= \frac{2p_i \, r_i^2}{(r_o^2 - r_i^2)}$$

$$= \frac{2 \times 850 \times (22.5)^2}{\left\{(32.5)^2 - (22.5)^2\right\}}$$

$$= 1564.77 \text{ N/cm}^2$$

EXAMPLE 8 *A thick cylinder with closed ends has 100 mm internal radius and 150 mm external radius. It is subjected to an internal pressure of 60 MN/m² and external pressure 30 MN/m².*

Determine the hoop and radial stress at the inside and outside cylinder together with longitudinal stress. **(UPTU 3rd Semester 2005-06)**

SOLUTION

Given
$$r_i = 100 \text{ mm} = 0.1 \text{ m}$$
$$r_0 = 150 \text{ mm} = 0.15 \text{ m}$$
$$p_i = 60 \text{ MN/m}^2$$
$$p_0 = 30 \text{ MN/m}^2$$

Following formula exist, when cylinder is subjected to internal pressure (p_i) and external pressure (p_0) then,

Hoop Stress $(\sigma_c) = \dfrac{1}{(r_0^2 - r_i^2)} \left\{ \dfrac{(p_i - p_0)\, r_i^2 r_0^2}{r^2} + (p_i r_i^2 - p_0\, r_0^2) \right\}$

Putting $r = r_i$ and r_0 respectively in the above equation, we can get hoop stress at inner and outer surface of the cylinder.

(σ_c) Hoop stress at inner surface

$$= \dfrac{1}{(0.15)^2 - (0.1)^2} \left\{ \dfrac{(60-30) \times (0.15)^2 \times \cancel{(0.1)^2}}{\cancel{(0.1)^2}} + (60 \times 0.1^2 - 30 \times 0.15^2) \right\}$$

$$= \dfrac{1}{0.0225 - 0.01}\{\cancel{0.675} + 0.6 - \cancel{0.675}\}$$

$$= 48 \text{ MN/m}^2 \text{ (Tensile)} \quad \textbf{Ans.}$$

Similarly, hoop stress at radius $r = r_0$, we have

$$\sigma_c \text{ at } r = r_0 = \dfrac{1}{(0.15)^2 - (0.1)^2}\left[30 \times (0.1)^2 + (60 \times 0.1^2 - 30 \times 0.15^2) \right]$$

$$= \dfrac{1}{0.0225 - 0.01}[0.3 + 0.6 - 0.675]$$

$$= \dfrac{1}{0.0125} \times 0.225$$

$$= 18 \text{ MN/m}^2 \quad \text{(Tensile)} \quad \textbf{Ans.}$$

Radial Stress (σ_r): By formula $\sigma_r = \dfrac{(p_i - p_0)\, r_i^2 r_0^2}{r^2 (r_0^2 - r_i^2)} - \dfrac{p_i r_i^2 - p_0 r_0^2}{(r_0^2 - r_i^2)}$

For inside radius, putting $r = r_i$ in the above, we get

$$\sigma_r = \dfrac{(p_i - p_0)\, r_0^2}{r_0^2 - r_i^2} - \dfrac{p_i r_i^2 - p_0 r_0^2}{r_0^2 - r_i^2}$$

$$= \dfrac{1}{(r_0^2 - r_i^2)}\left\{ (p_i - p_0) r_0^2 - (p_i r_i^2 - p_0 r_0^2) \right\}$$

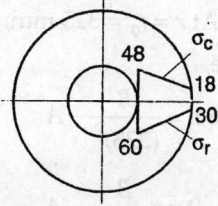

Profile of circumferential (σ_c) and radial stress (σ_s) stresses at inside and outside of the thick cylinder with closed ends:

$$= \frac{1}{(0.15)^2 - (0.1)^2} \left\{ 30 \times 0.15^2 - (60 \times 0.1^2 - 30 \times 0.15^2) \right\}$$

$$= \frac{1}{0.0125} \times \{0.675 - 0.6 + 0.675\}$$

$= 60 \text{ MN/m}^2$ (Compressive) **Ans.**

For outside radius, putting $r = r_0$, we get

$$\sigma_r = \frac{1}{0.0125} \times \{30 \times 0.1^2 - 0.6 + 0.675\}$$

$$= \frac{1}{0.0125} \times \{0.3 - 0.6 + 0.675\}$$

$= 30 \text{ MN/m}^2$ (Compressive)

Longitudinal stress

$$(\sigma_l) = \frac{\pi (p_i r_i^2 - p_o r_o^2)}{\pi (r_o^2 - r_i^2)}$$

$$= \frac{60 \times (0.1)^2 - 30 \times (0.15)^2}{(0.15)^2 - (0.1)^2}$$

$$= \frac{0.6 - 0.675}{0.0125}$$

$= (-) 6 \text{ MN/m}^2$ (Compressive) **Ans.**

Alternative Method:*

$$\sigma_o = \left(\frac{B}{0.1^2} - A \right)$$

$$30 = \left(\frac{B}{0.152} - A \right)$$

Solving $B = 0.54$ $A = (-) 6$

σ_h or σ_c at inner radius at r = 0.5 m

$$\sigma_h = \frac{B}{r^2} + A = \frac{0.54}{(0.1)^2} - 6 = 48 \text{ NM/m}^2$$

σ_h or σ_c at outer radius at r = 0.15 m

$$\sigma_h = \frac{0.54}{(0.15)^2} - 6 = 18 \text{ NM/m}^2$$

σ_h at inner radius

$$\sigma_r = \frac{B}{r_i^2} - A = 54 + 6 = 60 \text{ NM/m}^2$$

σ_r at outer radius

$$\sigma_r = \frac{B}{r_o^2} + A = 23.99 + 6 = 30 \text{ MN/m}^2$$

EXAMPLE 9 *A hollow cylinder of 45 cm internal diameter and 10 cm thickness contains the fluid under pressure of 850 N/cm². Find the maximum and minimum hoop stress across the section.* **(UPTU 2006-07)**

SOLUTION

Given $r_i = 225$ mm; $t = 100$ mm

$r_0 = 325$ mm $p_i = 850 \text{ N/cm}^2 = 8.50 \text{ N/mm}^2$

At $r = r_i = 225$ mm; $\sigma_r = p_i = 8.5 \text{ N/mm}^2$

At $r = r_0 = 325$ mm; $\sigma_r = p_o = 0$

Therefore,

$$8.5 = \frac{B}{(225)^2} - A \qquad \qquad \qquad \text{...(I)}$$

and $$0 = \frac{B}{(325)^2} - A \qquad \qquad \qquad \text{...(II)}$$

*Readers should prefer Alternative method being easier.

Subtracting (II) from (I)

$$8.5 = \frac{B}{(225)^2} - \frac{B}{(325)^2}$$

$\Rightarrow \qquad B = 826.44 \times 10^3$ and $A = 7.824$

Maximum hoop stress will develop at inside surface of the cylinder and minimum hoop stress will develop at the outer cylinder.

So, at $r = r_i = 225$ mm

$$\sigma_c \text{ or } \sigma_h = \frac{b}{r_i^2} + A$$

$$= \frac{826.44 \times 10^3}{(225)^2} + 7.824$$

$\therefore \qquad \sigma_h = 24.14 \text{ N/mm}^2 \qquad \textbf{Ans.}$

At $r = r_o = 325$

$$\sigma_h = \frac{b}{r_o^2} + A$$

$$= \frac{826.44 \times 10^3}{(325)^2} + 7.824$$

Hoop stress $(\sigma_c) = 15.64 \text{ N/mm}^2 \qquad \textbf{Ans.}$

EXAMPLE 10 *For a tube having $E = 2 \times 10^5$ N/mm² and $v = 0.3$, the hoop stress at the inner face is twice the internal pressure. Find the thickness of the wall if internal radius is 60 cm.* **(UPTU 2008-09)**

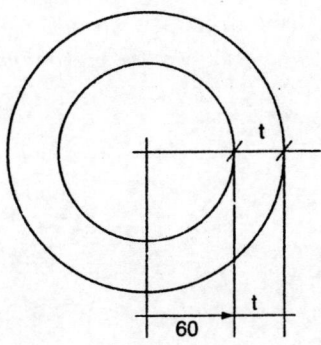

Fig. 17.22

SOLUTION

Given $r_i = 60$ cm; $v = 0.3; E = 2 \times 10^5$ N/mm²

Also, σ_c at inner surface = 2 × Internal Pressure (Given in question).

$$\left(\frac{B}{r_i^2} + A\right) = 2 \cdot \left(\frac{B}{r_i^2} - A\right)$$

or,
$$\left(\frac{\dfrac{B}{r_i^2} + A}{\dfrac{B}{r_i^2} - A}\right) = \frac{2}{1}$$

or,
$$\frac{\dfrac{2B}{r_i^2}}{2A} = \frac{3}{1}$$

or,
$$\frac{2B}{r_i^2} \times \frac{1}{2A} = \frac{3}{1}$$

or,
$$\frac{B}{A} = 3r_i^2$$

or,
$$\frac{B}{A} = 3 \times (60)^2$$

or,
$$\frac{B}{A} = 3 \times 3600$$

$$\therefore \quad \left(\frac{B}{A}\right) = 10800$$

At the outer surface $\sigma_r = 0$

$$\Rightarrow \quad 0 = \frac{B}{(r_i + t)^2} - A$$

$$\Rightarrow \quad A = \frac{B}{(r_i + t)^2}$$

$$\Rightarrow \quad (r_i + t)^2 = \frac{B}{A}$$

$$\Rightarrow \quad (60 + t)^2 = 10800$$

$$\Rightarrow \quad (60 + t) = \sqrt{10800}$$

$$\Rightarrow \quad 60 + t = 103.92$$

$$\Rightarrow \quad t = 43.92 \text{ cm}$$

$$\therefore \quad t = 44 \text{ cm} \quad \textbf{Ans.}$$

EXAMPLE 11 *A compound cylinder is made by shrinking a tube of 160 mm internal diameter and 20 mm thick over another tube of 160 mm external diameter and 20 mm thick. The radial pressure at the common surface after shrinking is 80 kg/cm².*

Find the final stresses set-up across the section, when the compound cylinder is subjected to an internal fluid pressure of 600 kg/cm².

(UPTU 2014-15)

SOLUTION
(Similar Problem)

Outer diameter of outer cylinder $= 16 + 2 + 2$

$$= 20 \text{ cm.}$$

$\therefore$ $r_1 = 10 \text{ cm.}$

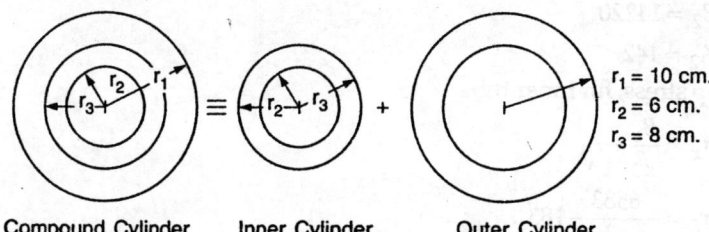

Compound Cylinder	Inner Cylinder	Outer Cylinder

$r_1 = 10$ cm.
$r_2 = 6$ cm.
$r_3 = 8$ cm.

Fig. 17.23

Outer diameter of inner cylinder = 160 mm = 16 cm.

$\therefore$ Radius $r_3 = 8$ cm.

Thickness $= 20$ mm

$$= 2 \text{ cm.}$$

$\therefore$ Inner diameter of inner cylinder $= 16 - 2 - 2 = 12$ cm

Radius (r_2) $= 6$ cm

Let σ_x is the hoop stress at a radius x in the compound cylinder

Now, applying Lame's Eqn. for inner and outer cylinder before fluid pressure is admitted.

$$0 = \frac{B_1}{r_2^2} - A_1$$

$$= \frac{B_1}{(6)^2} - A_1 \qquad \qquad \dots \text{(I)}$$

Similarly, $p = \dfrac{B_1}{r_3^2} - A_1$

$$80 = \frac{B_1}{(8)^2} - A_1 \qquad \qquad \dots \text{(II)}$$

$$p_1 = \frac{B_2}{r_3^2} - A_2$$

$$80 = \frac{B_2}{(8)^2} - A_2 \qquad \text{... (III)}$$

and

$$0 = \frac{B_2}{r_1^2} - A_2 \qquad \text{... (IV)}$$

Solving (I) and (II), we get $B_1 = (-) 6583$

$$A_1 = (-) 183$$

From (III) and (IV), we get

$$B_2 = 14220$$

and $A_2 = 142$

Now, hoop stress, for inner tube

$$\sigma_x = \frac{B_1}{x^2} + A_1$$

$$\sigma_6 = -\frac{6583}{6^2} - 183$$

$$= -365.85 \text{ kg} / \text{cm}^2$$

$$\approx -366 \text{ kg/cm}^2 \qquad \text{... (V)}$$

and $$\sigma_8 = -\frac{6583}{8^2} - 183$$

$$= -286 \text{ kg/cm}^2 \qquad \text{... (VI)}$$

For outer tube,

$$\sigma_8 = \frac{14420}{8^2} + 142$$

$$= 364.187 \text{ kg/cm}^2$$

$$\approx 364. \text{ kg/cm}^2 \qquad \text{... (VII)}$$

and $$\sigma_{10} = \frac{14420}{10^2} + 142$$

$$= 284.2 \text{ kg/cm}^2$$

$$\approx 284. \text{ kg/cm}^2 \qquad \text{... (VIII)}$$

Applying Lame's Equation for inner cylinder only, after the fluid (600 kg/cm^2) is admitted in

$$p_x = \frac{B}{x^2} - A$$

$$600 = \frac{B}{(6)^2} - A \qquad \text{... (IX)}$$

and $\qquad 0 = \dfrac{B}{(10)^2} - A \qquad\qquad\qquad\qquad\qquad$ ... (X)

Equations (IX) − (X) gives

$$600 = \dfrac{B}{36} - \dfrac{B}{100} = \dfrac{4B}{225}$$

∴ $\qquad B = 33750$ and $A = 337.5$

Using Lame's Equation

$$\sigma_x = \dfrac{B}{x^2} + A$$

∴ $\qquad \sigma_6 = \dfrac{33750}{(6)^2} + 337.5$

$$= 1275 \text{ kg/cm}^2$$

$$\sigma_8 = \dfrac{33750}{(8)^2} + 337.5$$

$$= 527.34 + 337.5$$

$$= 864.84 \text{ kg/cm}^2$$

$$\simeq 865 \text{ kg/cm}^2$$

and $\qquad \sigma_{10} = \dfrac{33750}{(10)^2} + 337.5$

$$= 675 \text{ kg/cm}^2$$

Hoop stress (kg/cm²)	Inner Cylinder		Outer Cylinder	
	x = 6 cm	x = 8 cm	x = 8 cm	x = 10 cm
(i) Initial	−366	−286	364	284
(ii) After the fluid is admitted	+1275	+865	+865	+675
Net	+909	+579	+1229	+959

EXAMPLE 12 *A compound tube is composed of a tube of 250 mm internal diameter and 25 mm thick shrunk on a tube of 200 mm internal diameter. The interface radial pressure at the junction is 8 N/mm². The compound tube is subjected to an internal pressure of 60 N/mm². Find the variation of hoop stress over the wall of the compound tube.*

SOLUTION

$\qquad$ Given $\quad p_j = 8 \text{ N/mm}^2$

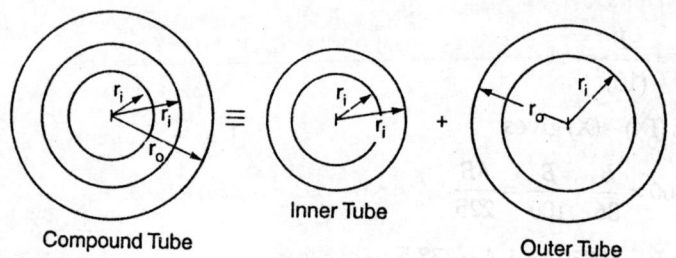

Compound Tube ≡ Inner Tube + Outer Tube

Fig. 17.24

For outer tube

At radius $r_j = 125$ mm

$$\text{Radial stress } (\sigma_r) = \frac{B}{r_o^2} - A$$

$$8 = \frac{B}{(125)^2} - A \qquad \qquad \dots \text{(I)}$$

At radius $r_o = 150$ mm, $\sigma_r = 0$

$$\Rightarrow \quad 0 = \frac{B}{(150)^2} - A \qquad \qquad \dots \text{(II)}$$

From (I) and (II), $8 = \dfrac{B}{(125)^2} - \dfrac{B}{(150)^2}$

$$\Rightarrow \quad B = 409090.9$$

$$\approx 409091$$

and $\quad A = \dfrac{B}{(150)^2}$

$$= \frac{409091}{22500}$$

$$\therefore \quad A = 18.18$$

At radius $r_o = 150$ mm

$$\text{Hoop stress } (\sigma_c) = \frac{409091}{(150)^2} + 18.18$$

$$= 18.18 + 18.18$$

$$= 36.36 \text{ N/mm}^2 \text{ (Tensile)}$$

At radius $r_j = 125$ mm,

$$\text{Hoop stress } (\sigma_c) = \frac{409091}{(125)^2} + 18.18$$

$$= 26.18 + 18.18$$

$$= 44.36 \text{ (Tensile)}$$

For Inner Tube:

At radius $r_j = 125$ mm

Radial stress $(\sigma_r) = \dfrac{B}{r_j^2} - A$

$$8 = \frac{B}{(125)^2} - A$$

at radius $r_i = 100$ mm

$$0 = \frac{B}{(100)^2} - A$$

$$8 = \frac{B}{(125)^2} - \frac{B}{(100)^2}$$

$$B = \frac{8 \times (100)^2 \times (125)^2}{(100)^2 - (125)^2}$$

$$= (-) \, 222222.22$$

$$\simeq (-) \, 222222$$

and $\quad A = \dfrac{B}{(100)^2}$

$$= -22.22$$

At radius $r_j = 125$ mm

Circumferential stress $(\sigma_c) = \dfrac{B}{r_j^2} + A$

$$= \frac{-222222}{(125)^2} - 22.22$$

$$= -14.22 - 22.22$$

$$= -36.44 \text{ N/mm}^2 \text{ (Compressive)}$$

At radius $r_i = 100$ mm Hoop stress or Circumferential stress

$$(\sigma_c) = \frac{-222222}{(100)^2} - 22.22$$

$$= -22.22 - 22.22$$

$$= -44.44 \text{ N/mm}^2 \text{ (Compressive)}$$

Stresses due to internal fluid pressure

At radius $r_j = 100$ mm, $\sigma_r = 60$ N/mm^2

$\Rightarrow \qquad 60 = \dfrac{B}{(100)^2} - A$

At radius $r_0 = 150$, $\sigma_r = 0$

$\Rightarrow \qquad 0 = \dfrac{B}{(150)^2} - A$

$\therefore \qquad 60 = \dfrac{B}{(100)^2} - \dfrac{B}{(150)^2}$

$\qquad B = \dfrac{60 \times (100)^2 \times (150)^2}{(150)^2 - (100)^2}$

$\qquad = 1080000$

$A = \dfrac{B}{(150)^2}$

$\qquad = 47.99$

$\qquad = 47.99$

$\qquad \simeq 48$

Hence, at radius $r_0 = 150$, mm

Hoop stress, $\sigma_c = \dfrac{B}{r_0^2} + A$

$\qquad = \dfrac{1080000}{(150)^2} + 48$

$\qquad = 47.99 + 48$

$\qquad = 48 + 48$

$\qquad = 96$ N/mm^2 (Tensile)

At radius $r_j = 125$ mm

$\qquad \sigma_c = \dfrac{1080000}{(125)^2} + 48$

$\qquad = 69.12 + 48$

$\qquad = 117.12$ N/mm^2 (Tensile)

At radius $r_i = 100$ mm

$$\sigma_c = \frac{1080000}{(100)^2} + 48$$

$$= 108 + 48$$

$$= 156 \, \text{N/mm}^2 \text{ (Tensile)}.$$

Hoop stress (N/mm²)	Inner tube		Outer tube	
	100 mm	125 mm	150 mm	125 mm
Hoop stress (σ_h or σ_c) due to shrinkage	– 44.44	– 36.44	+ 36.36	44.36
Hoop stress (σ_h or σ_c) when subjected to internal pressure 60 N/mm²	+ 156.0	+ 117.12	+ 96	+ 117.12
Net	+ 111.56	80.68	132.36	161.48

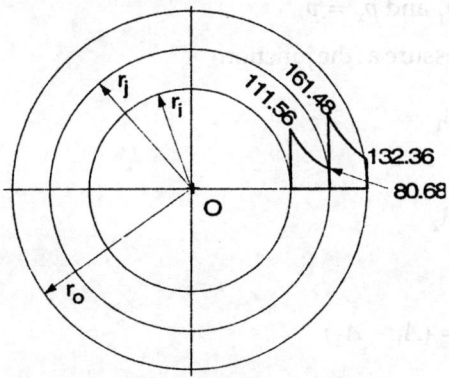

Fig. 17.25

17.7 INITIAL DIFFERENCE IN RADII AT THE JUNCTION OF COMPOUND CYLINDER FOR SHRINKAGE

In order to shrink the outer cylinder over the inner cylinder, the inner diameter of the outer cylinder should be slightly less than the outer diameter of the inner cylinder.

The outer cylinder is heated and inner cylinder is inserted into it. After cooling, the outer cylinder shrinks over the inner cylinder. Therefore, inner cylinder is put into compression and outer cylinder is put into tension.

Due to shrinkage, the outer radius of inner cylinder decreases, whereas, the inner radius of outer cylinder increases from the initial value.

As an engineer, we will evalute σ_x and p_x at the junction and, also, we will evaluate the original difference of radii at the junction.

Let r_o = outer radius of the outer cylinder

r_i = inner radius of the inner cylinder

r_j = radius of junction after shrinking or common radius after shrinking

p_j = radial pressure at the junction after shrinking.

Before shrinking the outer radius of the inner cylinder is little more than r_j and inner radius of the outer cylinder is little less than r_j.

The Lame's equation for outer and inner cylinder are:

$$p_x = \frac{B}{x^2} - A$$

and $$\sigma_x = \frac{B}{x^2} + A$$

The values of constant A and B will be different for each cylinder.

Let the constants for inner cylinder are A_2, B_2 and for outer cylinder A_1, B_1.

The radial pressure at the junction i.e. p_j is the same for outer cylinder and inner cylinder.

At the junction $x = r_j$ and $p_x = p_j$

Therefore, radial pressure at the junction

$$p_j = \frac{B_1}{r_j^2} - A_1 \qquad \qquad \text{...(1)}$$

$$= \frac{B_2}{r_j^2} - A_2 \qquad \qquad \text{...(2)}$$

or, $$\left(\frac{B_2 - B_1}{r_j^2} \right) = (A_1 - A_2) \qquad \qquad \text{...(3)}$$

or, $(B_2 - B_1) = r_j^2 \, (A_1 - A_2)$

Now, hoop strain (circumferential strain) in the cylinder at any point.

$$= \left(\frac{\sigma_x}{E} + v \cdot \frac{p_x}{E} \right) \qquad \qquad \text{...(4)}$$

Circumferential strain $= \dfrac{2\pi \, (r + dr) - 2\pi r}{2\pi r}$

$$= \frac{dr}{r}$$

$$= \text{Radial strain} \qquad \qquad \text{...(5)}$$

Hence, equating circumferential strain given by eqn. (4) and (5), we have

$$\frac{dr}{r} = \frac{\sigma_x}{E} + v \cdot \frac{p_x}{E} \qquad \qquad \text{...(6)}$$

After shrinking at the junction, there is extension in the inner radius of the outer cylinder and compression in the outer radius of the inner cylinder.

At the junction $x = r_{j,}$, increase in the inner radius of the outer cylinder

$$= r_j \left(\frac{\sigma_x}{E} + v \frac{p_x}{E} \right) \qquad \qquad ...(7)$$

For outer cylinder at the junction, we have

$$\sigma_x = \frac{B_1}{r_j^2} + A_1$$

and, $$p_x = \frac{B_1}{r_j^2} - A_1$$

where, A_1 and B_1 are constants for outer cylinder. Substituting the values of σ_x and p_x in equation (7).

We get, increase in the inner radius of the outer cylinder

$$= r_j \times \left[\frac{1}{E} \left(\sigma_x + \frac{p_x}{E} \right) \right]$$

$$= r_j \times \left[\frac{1}{E} \left(\frac{B_1}{r_j^2} + A \right) + \frac{v}{E} \left(\frac{B_1}{r_j^2} - A \right) \right]$$

In the same manner, decrease in the outer radius of the inner cylinder is obtained from equation (6) as

$$= (-) r_j \times \left[\frac{\sigma_x}{E} + v \frac{p_x}{E} \right] \qquad \qquad ...(8)$$

$$(- \text{ve sign is due to decrease in the outer radius})$$

For inner cylinder at the junction, we have

$$\sigma_x = \frac{B_2}{r_j^2} + A_2$$

and, $$p_x = \frac{B_2}{r_j^2} - A_2$$

Substituting these values in equation (8), we have, decrease in the outer radius of the inner cylinder

$$= -r_j \cdot \left[\frac{1}{E} \left(\frac{B_2}{r_j^2} + A_2 \right) + \frac{v}{E} \left(\frac{B_2}{r_j^2} - A_2 \right) \right] \qquad \qquad ...(9)$$

Original difference in the outer radius of the inner cylinder and inner radius of the outer cylinder

 = Increase in inner radius of outer cylinder

 + Decrease in the outer radius of inner cylinder

$$= r_j \left[\frac{1}{E}\left(\frac{B_1}{r_j^2} + A_1 \right) + \frac{v}{E}\left(\frac{B_1}{r_j^2} - A_1 \right) \right] - r_j \left[\frac{1}{E}\left(\frac{B_2}{r_j^2} + A_2 \right) + \frac{v}{E}\left(\frac{B_2}{r_j^2} - A_2 \right) \right]$$

$$= \frac{r_j}{E}\left[\left(\frac{B_1}{r_j^2} + A_1 \right) - \left(\frac{B_2}{r_j^2} + A_2 \right) \right] + v\frac{r_j}{E}\left[\left(\frac{B_1}{r_j^2} - A_1 \right) - \left(\frac{B_2}{r_j^2} - A_2 \right) \right]$$

Now, from equation (1) and (2)

$$\frac{B_1}{r_j^2} - A_1 = \frac{B_2}{r_j^2} - A_2$$

Therefore, the second part of the above equation is zero.

The above equation reduces to as the original difference of radii at the junction

$$= \frac{r_j}{E}\left[\left(\frac{B_1}{r_j} + A_1 \right) - \left(\frac{B_2}{r_j^2} + A_2 \right) \right]$$

$$= \frac{r_j}{E}\left[\frac{B_1 - B_2}{r_j^2} + (A_1 - A_2) \right]$$

$$= \frac{r_j}{E}\left[(A_1 - A_2) + (A_1 - A_2) \right] \qquad \left[\text{From eqn. (3) } \frac{B_1 - B_2}{r_j^2} = (A_1 - A_2) \right]$$

$$= \frac{2r_j}{E}(A_1 - A_2)$$

The values of A_1 and A_2 are obtained from the given condition.

17.8 THICK SPHERICAL SHELL

In figure 17.26, the spherical shell is shown.

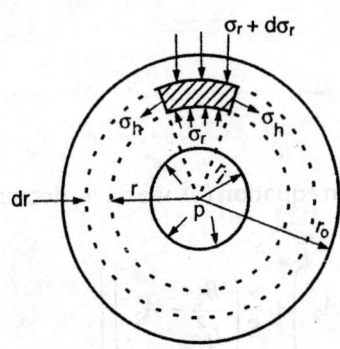

Fig. 17.26

Let r_i = Inner radius
r_o = Outer radius
p = Internal pressure
σ_r = Radial compressive stress at any radius r
$\sigma + d\sigma_r$ = Radial compressive stress at radius $(r + dr)$
σ_h = Circumferential tensile stress 'or' hoop stress in all direction perpendicular to the radius.

Let us consider the forces on elementary spherical shell of radius r and thickness dr.

The bursting force on the section of elemental shell

$$= \sigma_r \cdot \pi r^2 - (\sigma_r + d\sigma_r) \cdot \pi (r + dr)^2$$

Resisting force $= \sigma_h \times 2\pi r\, dr$

Equating the resisting force and bursting force, we have,

$$\sigma_h \times 2\pi r\, dr = \sigma_r \cdot \pi r^2 - (\sigma_r + d\sigma_r) \cdot \pi (r + dr)^2$$

Neglecting squares and products of small quantities, we have

$$2\sigma_h = -2\sigma_r - \frac{r}{2} \cdot \frac{d\sigma_r}{dr}$$

or, $$\sigma_h = -\sigma_r - \frac{r}{2} \cdot \frac{d\sigma_r}{dr} \qquad \qquad ...(1)$$

Differentiating the above relation, we get

$$\frac{d\sigma_h}{dr} = -\frac{d\sigma_r}{dr} - \frac{1}{2}\left[r \cdot \frac{d^2\sigma_r}{dr^2} + \frac{d\sigma_r}{dr} \right] \qquad ...(2)$$

The three principal stresses at any point in the elementary spherical shell at a radius r are:

(i) The radial pressure σ_r (compressive).
(ii) The circumferential 'or' hoop stress σ_h (tensile).
(iii) The circumferential or hoop stress $\sigma_h' = \sigma_h$ (tensile) on a plane perpendicular to the radius.

The radial strain at any point is given by

$$\varepsilon_r = \frac{\sigma_r}{E} + v\frac{2\sigma_h}{E} \qquad \text{(Compressive)}$$

$$= -\frac{1}{E}(\sigma_r + 2v\,\sigma_h) \qquad \text{(Tensile)} \qquad ...(3)$$

The circumferential 'or' hoop strain at any point is given by

$$\varepsilon_h = \left(\frac{\sigma_h}{E} - v \cdot \frac{\sigma_h}{E} + v\frac{\sigma_r}{E} \right) \qquad ...(4)$$

$$= -\frac{1}{E}\{(1 - v) \cdot \sigma_h + v \cdot \sigma_r\} \qquad \text{(Tensile)}$$

Due to internal pressure, let the radius increases from r to $(r + u)$.

$\therefore$ Radial strain $(\varepsilon_r) = \dfrac{d(r + u) - dr}{dr}$

$$= \dfrac{du}{dr} \qquad \qquad \dots(5)$$

and   Circumferential strain $(\varepsilon_h) = \dfrac{(r + u)\, d\theta - r\, d\theta}{r\, d\theta}$

$$= \dfrac{u}{r} \qquad \qquad \dots(6)$$

Now, $\varepsilon_r = \dfrac{du}{dr}$

$$= \dfrac{d}{dr}(u)$$

$$= \dfrac{d}{dr}(r \cdot \varepsilon_h)$$

$$= \varepsilon_h + r \cdot \dfrac{d\varepsilon_h}{dr} \qquad \qquad \dots(7)$$

Substituting the values of ε_r and ε_h from eqn. (3) and (4), we get

$$-\dfrac{1}{E}\left[\sigma_r + 2v \cdot \sigma_h\right] = \dfrac{1}{E}\left[(1-v)\,\sigma_h + v \cdot \sigma_r\right] + \dfrac{r}{E}\left[(1-v)\dfrac{d\sigma_h}{dr} + v \cdot \dfrac{d\sigma_r}{dr}\right]$$

Simplifying and rearranging, we get

$$(1 + v) \cdot (\sigma_r + \sigma_h) + (1 - v) \cdot r \cdot \dfrac{d\sigma_h}{dr} + r \cdot \dfrac{d\sigma_r}{dr} = 0$$

Substituting the value of σ_h and $\dfrac{d\sigma_h}{dr}$ from eqn. (1) and (2), we get

$$(1 + v)\left[\sigma_r - \sigma_r - \dfrac{r}{2} \cdot \dfrac{d\sigma_r}{dr}\right]$$

$$+ (1 - v)\,r\left[(-)\dfrac{d\sigma_r}{dr} - \dfrac{1}{2}\left(r \cdot \dfrac{d^2\sigma_r}{dr^2} + \dfrac{d\sigma_r}{dr}\right)\right] + r \cdot \dfrac{d\sigma_r}{dr} = 0$$

After simplication, we get

$$\dfrac{d^2\sigma_r}{dr^2} + \dfrac{4}{r} \cdot \dfrac{d\sigma_r}{dr} = 0$$

Let $\dfrac{d\sigma_r}{dr} = Z$

Hence, $r \cdot \dfrac{dz}{dr} + 4z = 0$

$$\frac{dz}{z} = -4 \cdot \frac{dr}{r}$$

Integrating both sides, we get

$$\log_e z = -4 \cdot \log_e r + \log_e C_1$$

(where, C_1 = constant of integration)

$$\log_e z = \log_e \left[\frac{C_1}{r^4} \right]$$

$\therefore \qquad Z = \dfrac{C_1}{r^4}$

$\therefore \qquad \left(\dfrac{d\sigma_r}{dr} \right) = \dfrac{C_1}{r^4}$

or, $\qquad d\sigma_r = C_1 \cdot \left(\dfrac{dr}{r^4} \right)$

Integrating both sides, we get

$$\sigma_r = -\frac{C_1}{3r^3} + C_2 \qquad\qquad ...(8)$$

where, C_2 is constant of integration.

From equation (1) $\sigma_h = -\sigma_r - \dfrac{r}{2} \cdot \dfrac{d\sigma_r}{dr}$

$$= -\left[-\frac{C_1}{3r^3} + C_2 \right] - \frac{r}{2} \cdot \frac{d\sigma_r}{dr}$$

$$= \frac{C_1}{3\,r^3} - C_2 - \frac{r}{2} \times \frac{C_1}{r^4}$$

$$= \frac{C_1}{3r^3} - C_2 - \frac{C_1}{2r^3}$$

$$= -\frac{C_1}{6r^3} - C_2 \qquad\qquad ...(9)$$

From (8), $\sigma_r = -\dfrac{C_1}{3\,r^3} + C_2$

and From (9), $\sigma_h = -\dfrac{C_1}{6r^3} - C_2$

Substituting $C_1 = -6B$ and $C_2 = -A$ we get

Radial stress $(\sigma_r) = \dfrac{2B}{r^3} - A$ ...(10)

and Hoop stress $(\sigma_h) = \dfrac{B}{r^3} + A$ ...(11)

Now, the boundary condition will be applied to find the constant A and B.

B.C. are, At $r = r_i$; $\sigma_r = p$

and At $r = r_o$; $\sigma_r = 0$

$\therefore$ $p = \dfrac{2B}{r_i^3} - A$ ...(12)

and $0 = \dfrac{2B}{r_o^3} - A$ ...(13)

Solving (12) and (13), we get

$$B = \frac{p \cdot r_i^3 \, r_o^3}{2\,(r_o^3 - r_i^3)} \text{ and } A = \frac{p\, r_i^3}{r_o^3 - r_i^3}$$

Substituting A and B, we get σ_r and σ_h for spherical shell.

EXAMPLE 1 *A spherical shell of 120 mm internal diameter has to withstand an internal pressure of 30 MN/m². If the permissible tensile stress is 80 MN/m². Calculate thickness of the shell.*

SOLUTION Internal radius (r_i) of the shell

$= \dfrac{120}{2}$

$= 60 \text{ mm}$

$= 0.06 \text{ m}$

Internal fluid pressure $(p) = 30 \text{ MN/m}^2$

Permissible tensile stress $(\sigma_h) = 80 \text{ MN/m}^2$

or
hoop stress

Thickness of shell

By formula, we know that in thick spherical shell

$\sigma_r = \dfrac{2B}{r^3} - A$ ...(1)

and $\sigma_h = \dfrac{B}{r^3} + A$ ...(2)

At $r = 0.06$ m; $\sigma_r = 30$ MN/m^2

$\therefore \qquad \dfrac{2B}{(0.06)^2} - A = 30$

or, $\qquad$ 9259.26 B $- A = 30$ $\hspace{5cm}$ ...(3)

At $r = 0.06$ m; σ_h or $\sigma_c = 80$ MN/m^2

$\therefore \qquad \dfrac{B}{(0.06)^3} + A = 80$

or, $\qquad$ 4629.63 B $+ A = 80$

or, $\qquad$ 4629.63 B $+ A = 80$ $\hspace{5cm}$ ...(4)

Solving (3) and (4) we get

$\qquad B = 0.00792$ and $A = 43.33$

Let the external radius be r_0 then at $r = r_0$; $\sigma_r = 0$

$\therefore \qquad \dfrac{2 \times 0.00792}{(r_o)^3} - 43.33 = 0$

or, $\qquad r_o = \left(\dfrac{2 \times 0.00792}{43.33} \right)^{1/3}$

$\qquad\qquad = 0.0715$ m

$\qquad\qquad = 71.5$ mm

Therefore, thickness of shell $= (r_o - r_i)$

$\qquad\qquad\qquad\qquad\qquad = (71.5 - 60)$

$\qquad\qquad\qquad\qquad\qquad = 11.5$ mm

EXAMPLE 2 *Two thick cylinders A and B of the same size have external diameter twice the internal diameter. Cylinder A is subjected to internal pressure only, while cylinder B is subjected to external pressure only. Calculate the ratio of these pressure when:*

    (i) the largest hoop stresses in the two cases are equal in magnitude.

    (ii) the largest circumferential strains in the two cases are numerically equal. Take poisson's ratio as 0.3.

SOLUTION

(i) Cylinder A

$\qquad \sigma_r = p_i$ at $r = r_i$

$\qquad \sigma_r = 0$ at $r = r_o$

$\therefore \qquad p_i = \dfrac{B}{r_i^2} - A$

and $\qquad 0 = \dfrac{B}{r_o^2} - A$

which gives, $\quad B = p_i \cdot \left(\dfrac{r_i^2 r_o^2}{r_o^2 - r_i^2} \right)$

and $\quad\quad\quad A = p_i \cdot \left(\dfrac{r_i^2}{r_o^2 - r_i^2} \right)$

$\therefore\quad \sigma_{c\,max}$ at $r = r_2 ; = \dfrac{B}{r_i^2} + A$

$$= p_i \cdot \left(\dfrac{r_o^2}{r_o^2 - r_i^2} \right) + p_i \left(\dfrac{r_i^2}{r_o^2 - r_i^2} \right)$$

$$= p_i \cdot \left(\dfrac{r_o^2 + r_i^2}{r_o^2 - r_i^2} \right)$$

$$= p_i \cdot \left(\dfrac{k^2 + 1}{k^2 - 1} \right) \quad\quad\quad\quad\quad …(I)$$

where $\quad k = \left(\dfrac{r_o}{r_i} \right) = 2$

Cylinder B:

$\quad\quad \sigma_i = 0$ at $r = r_i$

$\quad\quad \sigma_r = p_o$ at $r = r_o$

Hence, $\quad 0 = \dfrac{B}{r_i^2} - A$

and $\quad\quad p_o = \dfrac{B}{r_o^2} - A$

which gives, $\quad B = 0 - p_o \cdot \dfrac{r_i^2 r_o^2}{r_o^2 - r_i^2}$

and $\quad\quad\quad A = -p_o \cdot \dfrac{r_o^2}{r_o^2 - r_i^2}$

$\therefore\quad \sigma_{c\,max}$ at $r = r_i ; = \dfrac{B}{r_i^2} + A$

$$= (-) p_o \cdot \left(\dfrac{r_o^2}{r_o^2 - r_i^2} \right) - p_o \left(\dfrac{r_o^2}{r_o^2 - r_i^2} \right)$$

$$= (-) \, p_o \cdot \left(\frac{2r_c^2}{r_o^2 - r_i^2} \right)$$

$$= (-) \, p_o \cdot \left(\frac{2k^2}{k^2 - 1} \right) \qquad \qquad ...(\text{II})$$

Equating (I) and (II)

$$p_i \left(\frac{k^2 + 1}{k^2 - 1} \right) = p_o \cdot \left(\frac{2k^2}{k^2 - 1} \right)$$

$$\left(\frac{p_i}{p_o} \right) = \left(\frac{2k^2}{k^2 - 1} \right)$$

$$= \frac{2(2)^2}{(2)^2 + 1} = \left(\frac{8}{5} \right)$$

$$\therefore \qquad \left(\frac{p_i}{p_o} \right) = 1.6 \qquad \textbf{Ans.}$$

(II) For Cylinder A,

$$\varepsilon_{c \, \max} = \varepsilon_c \text{ at } r = r_i$$

$$= \left[\frac{\sigma_c}{E} + v \cdot \frac{\sigma_r}{E} \right]$$

$$= \frac{1}{E} \left[p_i \frac{k^2 + 1}{k^2 - 1} + v \cdot p_i \right] \qquad \qquad ...(\text{III})$$

For cylinder B,

$$\varepsilon_{c \, \max} = \varepsilon_c \text{ at } r = r_i$$

$$= \left[\frac{\sigma_c}{E} \right]$$

$$= \frac{1}{E} \left[-p_o \frac{2k^2}{k^2 - 1} \right] \qquad \qquad ...(\text{IV})$$

Equating (III) and (IV)

$$p_i \left[\frac{k^2 + 1}{k^2 - 1} + v \right] = p_o \left[\frac{2k^2}{k^2 - 1} \right]$$

$$\Rightarrow \qquad \frac{p_i}{p_o} = \frac{2k^2}{k^2 - 1} \bigg/ \left(\frac{k^2 + 1}{k^2 - 1} + v \right)$$

$$= \frac{2 \times (2)^2}{(2)^2 - 1} \bigg/ \left(\frac{2^2 + 1}{2^2 - 1} + 0.3 \right)$$

$$= \frac{8}{3} \bigg/ \left(\frac{5}{3} + 0.3 \right)$$

$$= \frac{8}{\cancel{3}} \times \frac{\cancel{3}}{5.9} = 1.33 \qquad \textbf{Ans.}$$

EXAMPLE 3 *A cylindrical pressure vessel of external and internal radii 0.3 m and 0.2 m respectively, is subjected to an internal hydraulic pressure of 20 N/mm². If $E = 2 \times 10^5$ N/mm² and $\mu = 0.3$, find the stresses at the internal and external surfaces and calculate the change in the internal and external diameters.*

(UPTU 3rd Sem 2009-10)

SOLUTION

Given $r_o = 0.3$ m $= 300$ mm

$r_i = 0.2$ m $= 200$ mm

$p_i = 20$ N/mm²

$E = 2 \times 10^5$ N/mm²

$\sigma_i = ?$ $\qquad\qquad\qquad$ $\sigma_o = ?$

$\Delta d_i = ?$ $\qquad\qquad\qquad$ $\Delta d_o = ?$

At outer radius $p_o = 0$

So, $\qquad 0 = \dfrac{B}{(300)^2} - A$ $\qquad\qquad\qquad\qquad\qquad$ ...(I)

At inner radius $p_i = 20$ N/mm²

$\therefore \qquad 20 = \dfrac{B}{(200)^2} - A$ $\qquad\qquad\qquad\qquad\qquad$ ...(II)

Now, $\quad 20 = \dfrac{B}{(200)^2} - \dfrac{B}{(300)^2}$

$\therefore \qquad B = \dfrac{20 \times (200)^2 \times (300)^2}{(300 + 200)\,(300 - 200)}$

$\qquad\quad = 144 \times 10^4$

$\qquad A = \dfrac{B}{(300)^2}$

$\qquad\quad = \dfrac{144 \times 10^4}{(300)^2} = 16$

Now, substituting the value of A and B in Lame's eqn.

$$\sigma_c = \left(\frac{B}{r^2} + A \right) \quad \text{at inner surface}$$

$$= \frac{144 \times 10^4}{(200)^2} + 16$$

$$= \frac{\overset{36}{\cancel{144} \times \cancel{10^4}}}{\cancel{4} \times \cancel{10^4}} + 16$$

$$= 52 \text{ N/mm}^2 \qquad \textbf{Ans.}$$

$$\sigma_c = \frac{144 \times 10^4}{(300)^2} + 16 \qquad \text{at outer surface}$$

$$= \frac{\overset{16}{\cancel{144} \times \cancel{10^4}}}{\cancel{9} \times \cancel{10^4}} + 16$$

$$= 32 \text{ N/mm}^2$$

$$\sigma_r = \frac{B}{r^2} - A \qquad \text{at inner surface}$$

$$= \frac{144 \times 10^4}{(200)^2} - 16$$

$$= \frac{\overset{36}{\cancel{144} \times \cancel{10^4}}}{\cancel{4} \times \cancel{10^4}} - 16$$

$$= 36 - 16 = 20 \text{ N/mm}^2 \quad \textbf{Ans.}$$

$$\sigma_r = \frac{144 \times 10^4}{(300)^2} - 16 \qquad \text{at outer surface}$$

$$= \frac{\overset{16}{\cancel{144} \times \cancel{10^4}}}{\cancel{9} \times \cancel{10^4}} - 16$$

$$= 16 - 16 = 0$$

Change in diameter at any radius r of the cylinder is given by formula.

$$\Delta D = \frac{2r}{E} [\sigma_c - v \, \sigma_r - v \sigma_l]$$

At inside cylinder $\sigma_c = 52 \, \text{N/mm}^2$

At outside cylinder $\sigma_c = 32 \, \text{N/mm}^2$

At inside cylinder $\sigma_r = 20 \, \text{N/mm}^2$

At outside cylinder $\sigma_r = 0$

Now, by formula, longitudinal stress $(\sigma_l) = \dfrac{p_i r_i^2 - p_o r_o^2}{r_o^2 - r_i^2}$

Since, at outer surface $p_o = 0$. So,

$$\sigma_l = \frac{p_i r_i^2}{r_o^2 - r_i^2}$$

$$= \frac{20 \times (200)^2}{(300)^2 - (200)^2}$$

$$= \frac{20 \times 4 \times 10^4}{500 \times 100}$$

$$= \frac{80 \times 10^4}{5 \times 10^4}$$

$$= 16 \, \text{N/mm}^2$$

Now, $\Delta D_i = \dfrac{2 r_i}{E} \left[\sigma_{c_i} + (-) v \, \sigma_{r_i} - v \cdot \sigma_l \right]$ $[\sigma_r = -20 \, \text{N/mm}^2]$

$$= \frac{2 \times 200}{2 \times 10^5} [52 + 0.3 \times 20 - 0.3 \times 16]$$

$$= \frac{4 \times 100}{2 \times 10^5} [52 + 6 - 4.8]$$

$$= 2 \times 10^{-3} \times 53.2 \, \text{mm}$$

$$= 0.0164 \, \text{mm}$$

$$\Delta D_o = \frac{2 r_o}{E} [\sigma_{c_0} - v \cdot \sigma_{r_0} - v \cdot \sigma_l]$$

$$= \frac{2 \times 300}{2 \times 10^5} [32 - 0.3 \times 0 - 0.3 \times 16]$$

$$= \frac{6 \times 100}{2 \times 10^5} [52 - 4.8]$$

$$= 3 \times 10^{-3} \times 27.2 \text{ mm}$$

$$= 0.0816 \text{ mm} \qquad \text{Ans.}$$

Now, rough graph can be plotted to show the finite value of stresses in the cylinder.
N.B.: To plot the exact graph, we will have to take more points like example-2 solved earlier.

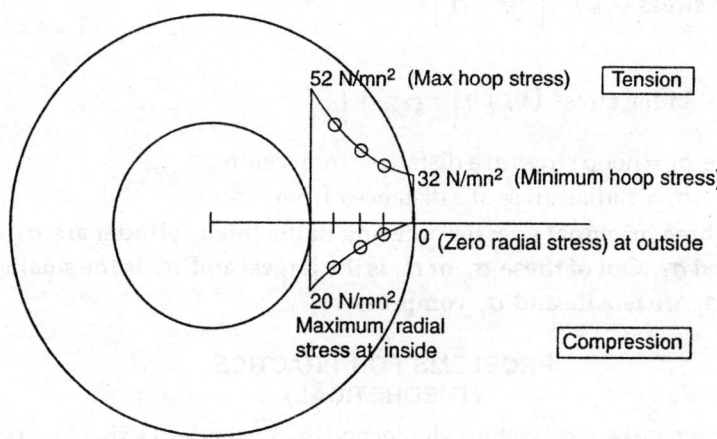

Fig. 17.27

HIGHLIGHTS

1. If $\dfrac{t}{D_i} > \dfrac{1}{20}$ then it is called thick cylinder.

2. The hoop stress is maximum at the inner circumference and the minimum at the outer circumference of a thick cylinder.

3. If a thick cylinder is subjected to internal fluid pressure, then

Hoop stress $(\sigma_x) = \dfrac{B}{x^2} + A$

at a distance 'x' from the centre $\qquad$ known as Lame's equation

and Radial stress $(p_x) = \dfrac{B}{x^2} - A$

at a distance 'x' from the centre

where, A and B are constants whose value can be obtained from the boundry conditions.

Lame's equation can be used to determine the stresses in compound thick cylinders.

The hoop stresses in a compound thick cylinder is the algebraic sum of the hoop stresses caused due to shrinkage and due to internal fluid pressure.

4. (a) The hoop stress in case of thin cylinders are reduced by wire winding on the cylinders.

(b) The hoop stress in case of thick cylinders are reduced by shrinking one cylinder over another cylinder.

5. **Hole on shaft:**

In shaft, hoop stress = radial stress = external pressure.

6. **For a thick spherical shell:**

Hoop stress $(\sigma_h) = \left(\dfrac{B}{r^3} + A \right)$

and, Radial stress $(\sigma_r) = \left(\dfrac{2B}{r^3} - A \right)$

where, σ_h = hoop stress at a distance r from centre.

and, σ_r = radial stress at a distance r from centre.

7. **The three principal stresses occuring in the thick cylinder are σ_h or σ_c; σ_r and σ_l. Out of these σ_h or σ_c is the largest and σ_r is the smallest. σ_c and σ_l are tensile and σ_r compressive.**

PROBLEMS FOR PRACTICE
(THEORETICAL)

1. Differentiate between a thin cylinder and thick cylinder. Derive an expression for the hoop stress; radial pressure at any point in case of thick cylinder.
2. Define compound thick cylinder. Why compounding is necessary?
3. What are the different methods of reducing hoop stress?
4. State and prove Lame's equation.

(NUMERICAL)

1. Find the thickness of metal necessary for a cylindrical shell of internal diameter 150 mm to withstand an internal pressure of $50 \, N/mm^2$, the maximum hoop stress in the section should not exceed $150 \, N/mm^2$.
2. A thick walled steel cylinder having an inside diameter of 150 mm is to be subjected to an internal pressure of $40 \, N/mm^2$. Find the nearest value, the outside diameter required, if the hoop stress in the cylinder wall is not to exceed $125 \, N/mm^2$.

   Calculate the actual hoop stresses at the inner and outer surfaces of the cylinder and plot a graph of the variation of hoop stress across the cylinder wall.
3. A compound tube of 10 cm internal diameter and 20 cm external diameter is made by shrinking one tube on to another.

   After cooling a radial stress of $20 \, N/mm^2$ is produced at the common surface, which is 15 cm in diameter. If the tube is now subjected to an internal pressure of $60 \, N/mm^2$, find the maximum hoop stress.
4. A compound cylinder is made by shrinking a cylinder of external diameter 300 mm and internal diameter of 250 mm over another cylinder of external diameter 250 mm and internal diameter 200 mm. The radial pressure at the junction after shrinking is $8 \, N/mm^2$.

Find the final stress set-up across the section, when the compound cylinder is subjected, to an internal fluid pressure of 84.5 N/mm².

5. A thin spherical vessel, 1.5 m in diameter and made up of 10 mm thick steel is first filled with water at atmospharic pressure (1.02×10^4 N/m²).
   What additional volume of water must be pumped into the vessel to raise the internal water pressure to 1.5 MPa?

ANSWERS

1. $t = 31$ mm
2. 210 mm; 124 N/mm²; 83.5 N/mm²
3. 127 N/mm²

OBJECTIVE QUESTIONS

1. If $\left(\dfrac{t}{D} \right) > \dfrac{1}{20}$ then the cylinder is:
   (a) thick cylinder (b) thin cylinder
   (c) either of the above (d) none of the above

2. In thick cylinder the radial stress in the wall is:
   (a) zero (b) negligibly small
   (c) not negligible (d) none of the above

3. In thick cylinders the circumferential stress:
   (a) is zero (b) varies along the thickness
   (c) does not vary along the thickness
   (d) none of the above

4. The error involved in the value of maximum stress by using thin cylinder formula instead of thick cylinder formula for cylinder with $\left(\dfrac{d}{t} \right) = 20$ is approximately.
   (a) 1 % (b) 5% (c) 10% (d) 20%

5. In thick cylinder, the radial stress at the inner surface is:
   (a) equal to the magnitude of the fluid pressure
   (b) less than the magnitude of the fluid pressure
   (c) more than the magnitude of the fluid pressure
   (d) independent of the magnitude of the fluid pressure

6. In a thick cylinder the radial stress at the outer surface is:
   (a) always more than zero (b) always less than zero
   (c) usually equal to zero (d) none of the above

7. For calculating change in radius of a thick cylinder due to internal pressure, the strain considered in the direction of:
   (a) hoop stress (b) radial stress
   (c) longitudinal stress (d) shear stress

8. The appropriate theory of failure for the design of thick cylinder is the:
   (a) maximum principal stress theory

(b) maximum shear stress theory   (c) maximum strain theory

(d) total strain energy theory

9. In case of a closed ends thick cylinder, the longitudinal stress (σ_l) is given by:

(a) $\sigma_l = \dfrac{p_i\, r_i^2}{r_o^2 - r_i^2}$

(b) $\sigma_l = \dfrac{p_i\, r_o^2}{r_o^2 - r_i^2}$

(c) $\sigma_l = \dfrac{2 p_i\, r_o^2}{r_o^2 - r_i^2}$

(d) $\sigma_l = \dfrac{r_o^2 - r_i^2}{p_i\, r_o^2}$

10. A thick cylinder is subjected to internal pressure (p) only. The radial stress is maximum at the inner surface of the cylinder, given by:

(a) zero   (b) p (c) $2 p$ (d) $3 p$

11. The variation of radial stress across the thickness of the cylinder is:

(a) linear   (b) cubic curve

(c) parabolic   (d) none of these

12. The volumetric strain ε_v is pressed as:

(a) $\varepsilon_v = 2\varepsilon_l + 2\varepsilon_h$

(b) $\varepsilon_v = 2\varepsilon_h + \varepsilon_l$

(c) $\varepsilon_h = 2\varepsilon_v + \varepsilon_l$

(d) $\varepsilon_v = 2\varepsilon_h + 2\varepsilon_i$

13. For a thick-walled pressure vessel, the (d/t) ratio is

(a) equal to 20   (b) greater than 20

(c) less than 20   (d) none of these

14. Which of the following statement (s) is/are true for a compound cylinder?

(a) it consists of two cylinder

(b) its purpose is to reduce hoop stress

(c) it has increased bearing capacity

(d) all of above

15. For a thick cylinder being subjected to external pressure only, the hoop stress is maximum:

(a) at the inner surface of the cylinder

(b) at the outer surface of the cylinder

(c) at the mid-point of thickness of the cylinder

(d) none of the above

16. For a thick cylinder being subjected to external pressure only, the hoop stress is minimum:

• (a) at the inner surface of the cylinder

(b) at the outer surface of the cylinder

(c) at the mid-point of the cylinder

(d) none of the above

ANSWERS

1. (a)	2. (c)	3. (b)	4. (b)	5. (a)	6. (c)
7. (a)	8. (b)	9. (a)	10. (b)	11. (c)	12. (b)
13. (c)	14. (d)	15. (a)	16. (b)		

— ❖❖ —

COLUMN AND STRUT

18.1 STRUT

A member of structure in any position other than vertical carrying an axial compressive load is called a strut.

Example of strut is connecting rod of I.C. engine.

18.2 COLUMN

A vertical strut is usually called column, carrying compressive load.

An ideal column is assumed to be a homogenous member of constant cross-section *i.e.* initially straight and subjected to axial compressive load.

Examples of columns are vertical pillar of a building and structural column in the form of I-beam or box column made-up of pipe etc.

Column in practice rarely experience concentric axial compresson alone, since columns are usually a part of a frame, these experience both bending moment and axial force.

Columns subjected to combined axial force and bending moment, are referred to as 'beam column'. A beam column may be subjected to single curvature bending over its length.

Nearly all members in a structure are not subjected to pure axial load or pure bending moment but to a combination of both.

The columns are usually classified according to their slenderness ratio.

18.3 SLENDERNESS RATIO (*l/k*)

$$\text{Slenderness ratio of a column} = \frac{\text{Length of column}}{\text{Least radius of gyration}}$$

$$= \left(\frac{l}{k}\right); \text{ where } k = \text{least radius of gyration.}$$

18.4 CLASSIFICATION OF COLUMNS

(i) When $(l/k) < 30$, it is called 'short column'. Such columns when subjected to axial compressive load, fails by yielding of the material due to direct compressive load, rather than buckling *i.e.* lateral deflection.

(ii) When $(l/k) > 120$, it is called 'long column'. Such column fails by buckling when loaded axially in compression.

(iii) When (l/k) lies between 30 and 120, it is termed intermediate column. In these column both buckling and direct compressive stress are significant.

18.5 BUCKLING LOAD 'OR' CRIPPLING LOAD 'OR' CRITICAL LOAD

The minimum axial load at which the column tends to have lateral displacement 'or' buckle is called the buckling 'or' crippling 'or' critical load.

Buckling always takes place about the axis having least moment of inertia (I_{XX} or I_{YY})

As an engineer, our attention should be to prevent the buckling by applying safe load.

$$\text{Safe load} = \frac{\text{Critical load}}{\text{Factor of safety}}$$

18.5.1 Euler's Theory of Buckling of Column

The following assumptions are considered for Euler's theory:
1. The column is initially perfectly straight and the load is applied axially.
2. The material of column is perfectly elastic, homogenous and isotropic. It obey's Hook's law.
3. The cross-section of the column is uniform.
4. Self weight of column is negligible.
5. The length of the column is very large as compared to its lateral dimensions.
6. The column will fail by buckling alone.

18.6 END CONDITION FOR COLUMN

End condition means ways in which the ends of columns are held.
There are four ways of holding column:
   (i)   Both ends are pinned.
   (ii) Both ends are fixed.
   (iii) One end fixed and other pinned.
   (iv) One end fixed and the other free.

18.7 SIGN CONVENTION FOR BENDING MOMENT (M)

The moment which bends the column with its convexity towards centre line of a column is considered positive moment.

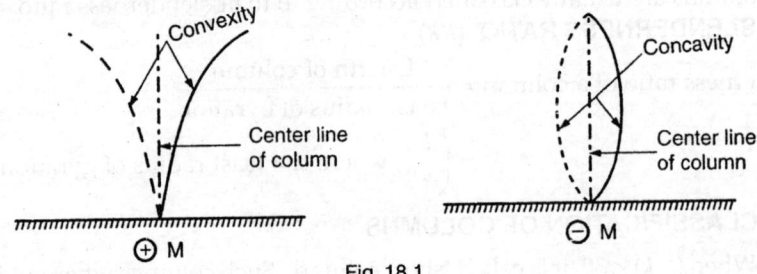

Fig. 18.1

Whereas, the moment that bends the column with its concavity towards the centre line of a column is considered negative.

18.8 COLUMNS WITH BOTH ENDS HINGED

Let us consider a column AB of the length l hinged at both ends A and B and carries an axial crippling load P at A.

The column bends due to crippling load in the manner are shown in the Fig. 18.2.

Let us take a section at a distance x from end B.

For x, let the corresponding deflection (lateral) by y.

Now, adopting the sign convention as per section 18.7.

$$B.M \ (M) = -P \cdot y$$

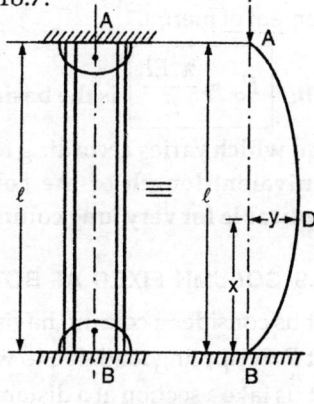

Fig. 18.2

But $M = EI \dfrac{d^2y}{dx^2}$

$\therefore$ $EI \cdot \dfrac{d^2y}{dx^2} = -P \cdot y$

or, $EI \cdot \dfrac{d^2y}{dx^2} + P \cdot y = 0$

or, $\dfrac{d^2y}{dx^2} + \left(\dfrac{P}{EI}\right) y = 0$

The solution of this differential equation is

$$y = C_1 \cos\left(x \cdot \sqrt{\dfrac{P}{EI}}\right) + C_2 \cdot \sin\left(x \sqrt{\dfrac{P}{EI}}\right) \qquad \qquad ...(1)$$

where, C_1 and C_2 are constant of integration.

The values of C_1 and C_2 can be evaluated by applying boundary condition.

B.C. are

At $x = 0$, $y = 0 \Rightarrow C_1 = 0$

At $x = l$; $y = 0$

$\therefore$ $0 = C_2 \sin\left(l \cdot \sqrt{\dfrac{P}{EI}}\right)$

$\therefore$ $\sin\left(l \sqrt{\dfrac{P}{EI}}\right) = 0 \sin 0$ or $\sin \pi$ or $\sin 2\pi$ or $\sin 3\pi$

or, $l \sqrt{\dfrac{P}{EI}} = 0$ or π or 2π or 3π

Taking the least value $i.e.$ π

$$l \sqrt{\dfrac{P}{EI}} = \pi$$

or, $l^2 \cdot \dfrac{P}{EI} = \pi^2$

$$\therefore P_{cr} = \frac{\pi^2 EI}{l_e^2}$$

P_{cr} is known as crippling load, l_e is known as equivalent length and I = least moment of Inertia.

N.B: $\boxed{P_{cr} = \frac{\pi^2 EI}{l_e^2}}$ is the basic formula known as Euler's Formula for crippling

load which varies according to the 'end condition' for which the value of l_e (*i.e.* equivalent length of the column) changes in every case. This formula is applicable for very long column which fails mainly due to buckling.

18.9 COLUMN FIXED AT BOTH ENDS   (UPTU 2014-15)

Let us consider a column having its both ends fixed at A and B.

Let P = crippling load due to which the column has buckled.

Let us take a section at a distance x from B and corresponding to this x, deflection is y.

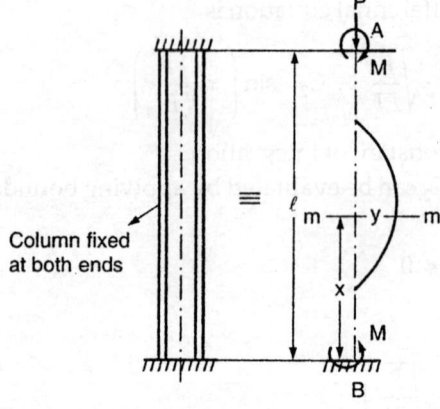

Fig. 18.3

Let M = fixed moment at A and B.

$\therefore$ B.M. at section $m - m = M - P.y$

Now, the differential equation of the elastic curve is

$$EI \cdot \frac{d^2 y}{dx^2} = M - P.y$$

$$\frac{d^2 y}{dx^2} + \frac{P}{EI} y = \frac{M}{EI}$$

$$\frac{d^2 y}{dx^2} + \left(\frac{P}{EI} \right) y = \frac{P}{EI} \times \frac{M}{P}$$

The general solution of the above differential equation is

$$y = C_1 \cos\left(x \cdot \sqrt{\frac{P}{EI}} \right) + C_2 \cdot \sin\left(x \cdot \sqrt{\frac{P}{EI}} \right) + \frac{M}{P} \qquad ...(1)$$

where, C_1 and C_2 are constants of integration and their values are obtained from boundary condition.

B.C are

At $\quad x = 0, y = 0$ also $\dfrac{dy}{dx} = 0$

$\therefore \qquad C_1 = -\dfrac{M}{P}$

Differentiating (1) w.r.t. x, we get

$$\left(\frac{dy}{dx} \right) = -C_1 \sin\left(x \cdot \sqrt{\frac{P}{EI}} \right) \cdot \sqrt{\frac{P}{EI}} + C_2 \cos\left(x \cdot \sqrt{\frac{P}{EI}} \right) \cdot \sqrt{\frac{P}{EI}} \qquad ...(2)$$

Substituting $x = 0$ and $\dfrac{dy}{dx} = 0$ in Equation (2), we get

$\qquad C_2 = 0$

Substituting the values of $C_1 = -\dfrac{M}{P}$ and $C_2 = 0$ in equation (1), we get

$$y = -\frac{M}{P} \cdot \cos\left(x\sqrt{\frac{P}{EI}} \right) + 0 + \frac{M}{P}$$

$$= -\frac{M}{P} \cos\left(x \sqrt{\frac{P}{EI}} \right) + \frac{M}{P}$$

At $x = l; y = 0$

$\therefore \qquad 0 = -\dfrac{M}{P} \cos\left(l \cdot \sqrt{\dfrac{P}{EI}} \right) + \dfrac{M}{P}$

or, $\qquad \dfrac{M}{P} \cos\left(l \sqrt{\dfrac{P}{EI}} \right) = \dfrac{M}{P}$

or, $\qquad \cos\left(l \sqrt{\dfrac{P}{EI}} \right) = \dfrac{\cancel{M}}{\cancel{P}} \times \dfrac{\cancel{P}}{\cancel{M}}$

or, $\qquad \cos\left(l \sqrt{\dfrac{P}{EI}} \right) = 1 = \cos 0, \cos 2\pi, \cos 4\pi, \cos 6\pi$

$$\therefore \qquad l\sqrt{\frac{P}{EI}} = 0, 2\pi, 4\pi, 6\pi$$

Considering least value *i.e.* 2π

$$l\sqrt{\frac{P}{EI}} = 2\pi$$

$$P = \left(\frac{4\pi^2 EI}{l^2}\right)$$

P is known as critical load denoted by P_{cr}

$$\boxed{\therefore P_{cr} = \frac{4\pi^2 EI}{l_e^2}}$$

where, $\quad l$ = effective length of the column;
here, $\quad l_e$ = equivalent length of the column = $(l/2)$ **(UPTU 3rd Sem. 2013-14)**

Expression for P_{cr} when one end is fixed and the other end is Hinged or Pinned
Let us consider column of length l fixed at B and hinged at end A.
Let P be the crippling load at which the column has buckled.
Let us consider a section mm at a distance of x from B.
Let y be the corresponding lateral deflection of the column.
$\qquad M_o$ = fixed moment at end B
$\qquad H$ = horizontal reaction at A
Hence, moment at the section

$$M_x = -P \cdot y + H(l-x)$$

We know that the differential equation of the moment is

$$M = \frac{d^2y}{dx^2} \cdot EI$$

$$\therefore \qquad EI \cdot \frac{d^2y}{dx^2} = -P \cdot y + H(l-x)$$

or, $\qquad \dfrac{d^2y}{dx^2} + \dfrac{P}{EI} \cdot y = \dfrac{H}{EI}(l-x)$

or, $\qquad \dfrac{d^2y}{dx^2} + \dfrac{P}{EI} \cdot y = \dfrac{P}{EI}(l-x) \cdot \dfrac{H}{P}$

The solution of the above differential equation is

$$y = C_1 \cos\left(x\sqrt{\frac{P}{EI}}\right) + C_2 \sin\left(x \cdot \sqrt{\frac{P}{EI}}\right) + \frac{M}{P}(l-x)$$

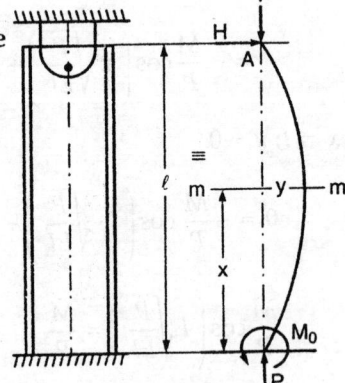

Fig. 18.4

where, C_1 and C_2 are constants and their values are obtained from boundary condition.

B.C. are

At $\quad x = 0, y = 0$ also $\dfrac{dy}{dx} = 0$

At $\quad x = l; y = 0$

Substituting the value $x = 0$ and $y = 0$ in eqn. (1)

$$0 = C_1 \times 1 + C_2 \times 0 + \frac{H}{P}(l - 0)$$

$$= C_1 + \frac{H \cdot l}{P}$$

$$C_1 = -\frac{H \cdot l}{P} \qquad \qquad ...(2)$$

Differentiating equation (1) w.r.t x

$$\frac{dy}{dx} = C_1(-1) \cdot \sin\left(x \cdot \sqrt{\frac{P}{EI}} \right) \cdot \sqrt{\frac{P}{EI}} + C_2 \cos\left(x \cdot \sqrt{\frac{P}{EI}} \right) \cdot \sqrt{\frac{P}{EI}} - \frac{H}{P}$$

$$= -C_1 \sin\left(x \cdot \sqrt{\frac{P}{EI}} \right) \cdot \sqrt{\frac{P}{EI}} + C_2 \cos\left(x \cdot \sqrt{\frac{P}{EI}} \right) \cdot \sqrt{\frac{P}{EI}} - \frac{H}{P}$$

At $x = 0, \dfrac{dy}{dx} = 0$

$\therefore \quad 0 = -C_1 \times 0 + C_2 \cdot 1 \cdot \sqrt{\dfrac{P}{EI}} - \dfrac{H}{P}$

$$= C_2 \cdot \sqrt{\frac{P}{EI}} - \frac{H}{P}$$

$\therefore \quad C_2 = \dfrac{H}{P} \cdot \sqrt{\dfrac{EI}{P}}$

Substituting the values of $C_1 = (-)\dfrac{H \cdot l}{P}$

and $\quad C_2 = \dfrac{H}{P} \cdot \sqrt{\dfrac{EI}{P}}$ in equation (1), we get

$$y = -\frac{H}{P} l \cos\left(x \cdot \sqrt{\frac{P}{EI}} \right) + \frac{H}{P} \cdot \sqrt{\frac{EI}{P}} \sin\left(x \cdot \sqrt{\frac{P}{EI}} \right) + \frac{H}{P}(l - x)$$

At $x = l; y = 0$

Therefore, the above equation reduces to

$$0 = -\frac{H}{P} l \cos\left(l \cdot \sqrt{\frac{P}{EI}}\right) + \frac{H}{P} \cdot \sqrt{\frac{EI}{P}} \sin\left(l \cdot \sqrt{\frac{P}{EI}}\right) + \frac{H}{P}(l - l)$$

$$0 = -\frac{H}{P} l \cos\left(l \cdot \sqrt{\frac{P}{EI}}\right) + \frac{H}{P} \cdot \sqrt{\frac{EI}{P}} \cdot \sin\left(l \cdot \sqrt{\frac{P}{Ei}}\right) + 0$$

$$\frac{H}{P} \cdot \sqrt{\frac{EI}{P}} \sin\left(l \cdot \sqrt{\frac{P}{EI}}\right) = \frac{H}{P} \cdot l \cos\left(l \cdot \sqrt{\frac{P}{EI}}\right)$$

$$\sin\left(l \cdot \sqrt{\frac{P}{EI}}\right) = \frac{H}{P} \cdot l \cdot \frac{P}{H} \times \sqrt{\frac{P}{EI}} \cdot \cos\left(l \cdot \sqrt{\frac{P}{Ei}}\right)$$

$$= l \cdot \sqrt{\frac{P}{EI}} \cdot \cos\left(l \cdot \sqrt{\frac{P}{EI}}\right)$$

$$\therefore \qquad \tan\left(l \cdot \sqrt{\frac{P}{EI}}\right) = l \cdot \sqrt{\frac{P}{EI}}$$

The solution to the above equation is

$$l \cdot \sqrt{\frac{P}{EI}} = 4.5 \text{ radian}$$

Squaring both sides, we get

$$l^2 \cdot \frac{P}{EI} = (4.5)^2 = 20.25$$

$$P = 20.25 \times \frac{EI}{l^2}$$

$$\therefore \qquad P = \frac{2\pi^2 EI}{l}$$

Therefore, critical load (P_{cr}) when one end of column is fixed and other is hinged is

$$P_{cr} = \frac{2\pi^2 EI}{l}$$

Crippling load (P_{cr}) when one end of the column is fixed and the other end is free

Let us consider a column AB of length 'l' and uniform cross-sectional area and fixed at end A and free at B.

Let P = crippling load at which the column buckles.

Due to crippling load P, the column will deflect as given in Fig. 18.5.

AB' is the deflected position of the column AB.

Let us take any section at a distance x from the fixed end A.

$\qquad y$ = deflection at a distance x

$\qquad a$ = deflection at free end B

Moment at section mm due to crippling load

$$M_X = P\,(a - y)$$

$$EI \cdot \frac{d^2 y}{dx^2} = P\,(a - y)$$

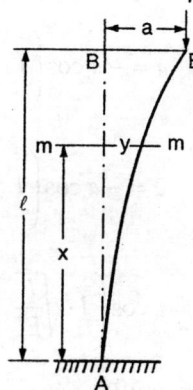

Fig. 18.5

or, $\qquad EI \cdot \dfrac{d^2 y}{dx^2} + Py = P \cdot a$

or, $\qquad \dfrac{d^2 y}{dx^2} + \left(\dfrac{P}{EI}\right) y = \dfrac{P}{EI} \cdot a$

The solution of this differential equation is

$$y = C_1 \cdot \cos\left(x\sqrt{\frac{P}{EI}}\right) + C_2 \sin\left(x\sqrt{\frac{P}{EI}}\right) + a \qquad \ldots(1)$$

where, C_1 and C_2 are constant of integration.

The value of C_1 and C_2 can be found by applying boundary condition. The boundary conditions are:

At $\qquad x = 0, y = 0 \Rightarrow C_1 = -a$

At $\qquad x = 0; \left(\dfrac{dy}{dx}\right) = 0$

Now, differentiating equation (1) w.r.t. x, we get

$$\left(\frac{dy}{dx}\right) = C_1 \cdot (-1) \cdot \sin\left(x\sqrt{\frac{P}{EI}}\right) \cdot \sqrt{\frac{P}{EI}} + C_2 \cos\left(x\sqrt{\frac{P}{EI}}\right) \cdot \sqrt{\frac{P}{EI}} + 0 \qquad \ldots(2)$$

$$0 = C_2 \cdot \sqrt{\frac{P}{EI}}$$

$\therefore \qquad C_2 = 0 \quad \text{As} \quad \sqrt{\dfrac{P}{EI}} \neq 0$

Substituting the values of C_1 and C_2 in eqn. (1)

$$\cdot\; y = -a \cdot \cos\left(x \cdot \sqrt{\frac{P}{EI}}\right) + a \qquad \ldots(3)$$

At $x = l, y = a$

Substituting these value in (3), we get

$$a = -a\cos\left(l \cdot \sqrt{\frac{P}{EI}}\right) + a$$

or, $$0 = -a\cos\left(l \cdot \sqrt{\frac{P}{EI}}\right)$$

or, $$a\cos\left(l \cdot \sqrt{\frac{P}{EI}}\right) = 0$$

$$a \neq 0$$

$\therefore$ $$\cos\left(l \cdot \sqrt{\frac{P}{EI}}\right) = 0 = \cos\frac{\pi}{2} \text{ or } \cos\frac{3\pi}{2} \text{ or } \cos\frac{5\pi}{2}$$

$\therefore$ $$l \cdot \sqrt{\frac{P}{EI}} = \frac{\pi}{2} \text{ or } \frac{3\pi}{2} \text{ or } \frac{5\pi}{2}$$

Taking the first practical value

$$l \cdot \sqrt{\frac{P}{EI}} = \frac{\pi}{2}$$

$$\sqrt{\frac{P}{EI}} = \left(\frac{\pi}{2l}\right)$$

$$\boxed{\therefore P = \frac{\pi^2 EI}{4l^2}} \text{ So, } P_{cr} = \frac{\pi^2 EI}{4l^2}$$

18.10 EQUIVALENT LENGTH 'OR' EFFECTIVE LENGTH

For a long column, the length actually involved in bending is called its equivalent length or effective length.

If l = actual length of a column.

Then equivalent length or effective length = l_e

$l_e = l \times C$, where, C is a constant factor

Crippling load 'or' buckling load = $P_{cr} = \dfrac{\pi^2 EI}{le^2}$

S. No	End condition	Value of factor (C)	Equivalent length (l_e)
1.	Both ends hinged	1	$l_e = 1$
2.	Both ends fixed	$\dfrac{1}{2}$	$l_e = \dfrac{l}{2}$
3.	One end fixed and other end hinged	$\dfrac{1}{\sqrt{2}}$	$l_e = \dfrac{l}{\sqrt{2}}$
4.	One end fixed and other end free	2	$l_e = 2l$

18.11 LIMITATIONS OF EULER'S FORMULA

Euler formula $(P_e) = \dfrac{\pi^2 EI}{l_e^2}$

where, l_e = effective length, here, in the above formula.

Euler's formula also shows that the critical load that causes buckling depends not on the strength of the material but only on its dimensions and modulus of elasticity.

The value of I in the column formula is always the least moment of inertia of the cross-section.

In order for Euler formula to be applicable, the stress accompanying the bending that occurs during buckling must not exceed the proportional limit. This stress may be found by replacing in Euler's formula, the moment of inertia $I = Ar^2$.

where, A = cross-sectional area

and r = least radius of gyration

This is substituted in the above Euler formula.

Hence, crippling load $(P) = \dfrac{\pi^2 E \cdot (Ar^2)}{l^2}$ $\qquad \left[\begin{array}{l} \because \text{Here, equivalent length } l_e = l \\[4pt] \therefore \left(\dfrac{P}{A} \right) = \dfrac{E\pi^2}{(l/r)^2} \text{ or, } \sigma = \dfrac{\pi^2 E}{(l/r)^2} \end{array} \right]$

Here, (P/A) is the average stress in the column when carrying its critical load. This stress is often called the 'critical stress'. It's limiting value is the stress at the proportional limit.

The ratio (l/r) is called the slenderness ratio of the column.

Since, an axially loaded column tend to buckle about the axis of least moment of inertia, the least radius of gyration should be used to determine the slenderness ratio.

We define long columns as those for which Euler's formula applies. The limiting (l/r) ratio that fixes the lower limit for Euler's formula is easily found out by substituting in above equation, the known values of the proportional limit and modulus of elasticity of the specified material.

This limiting ratio varies with different material and even with different grade of the same material.

If steel has a proportional limit of 200 MPa and for which $E = 200$ GPa, the limiting slenderness ratio is

$$\left(\frac{l}{r}\right)^2 = \frac{(200 \times 10^9)\,\pi^2}{200 \times 10^6}$$

$$\approx 10,000$$

or, $\quad \left(\dfrac{l}{r}\right) = 100$

Below this value, as shown in figure by the dashed portion of Euler's curve, the Euler unit load exceeds the proportional limit.

Hence, for $\left(\dfrac{L}{r}\right) < 100$, Euler's formula is not valid and the proportional limit is taken as the critical stress.

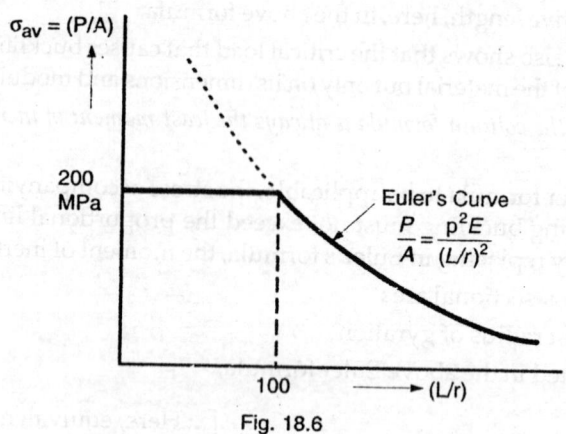

Fig. 18.6

(Critical 'or' allowable stress is given by the solid line,
Dashed portion of Euler's curve is not valid).

Euler's formula gives the critical load and not the working loads.

$$\text{Working load or allowable load} = \frac{\text{Critical load}}{\text{Factor of safety}}.$$

18.12 RANKINE FORMULA

Rankine devised an emperical formula for determining critical load which is applicable to all columns irrespective of whether they are short or long.

Let $\quad P_{cr} = $ The crippling load

$\quad P_c = $ Compressive load

$\quad = \sigma_c \times A$

$\quad \sigma_c = $ Ultimate compressive stress for the column material

$\quad A = $ Area of cross-section of the column

$\quad P_e = $ Euler's load $= \dfrac{\pi^2 EI}{l_e^2}$

$$\therefore \qquad P = \frac{P_e \times P_c}{P_e + P_c}$$

$$= \frac{P_c}{1 + \dfrac{P_c}{P_e}}$$

$$= \frac{\sigma_c \times A}{1 + \dfrac{\sigma_c \times A \times l_e^2}{\pi^2 EI}}$$

$$= \frac{\sigma_c \times A}{1 + \dfrac{\sigma_c \times A}{\pi^2 E} \times \left(\dfrac{l_e^2}{Ak^2}\right)} \qquad [\because I = Ak^2]$$

$$= \frac{\sigma_c \times A}{1 + \dfrac{\sigma_c \times \cancel{A}}{\pi^2 E} \times \dfrac{l_e^2}{\cancel{A}k^2}}$$

$$= \frac{\sigma_c \cdot A}{1 + a \cdot \left(\dfrac{l_e}{k}\right)^2}$$

where, $a = \left(\dfrac{\sigma_c}{\pi^2 E}\right)$ known as Rankine constant.

and $\left(\dfrac{l_e}{k}\right)$ = Buckling factor

The value of σ_c and 'a' are given below for some of the material:

Material	Compressive stress (σ_c) MPa	Young's modulus (E) G Pa	a (Rankine constant)
Cast Iron	562.5	91.189	1/1600
Wrought Iron	233.6	213	1/9000
Mild steel	276.3	210	1/7500
Medium carbon steel	414.5	210	1/5000
Aluminium	119.1	70	1/5000
Timber	474	96	1/2000

EXAMPLE 1 *A 1.5 m long column has a circular cross-section of 5 cm diameter. One of the ends of the column is fixed and the other end is free. Considering F.O.S as 3, calculate safe load using:*

(a) *Rankine's formula when* $\sigma_c = 560 \; N/mm^2$ *and* $a = \dfrac{1}{1600}$ *for pinned ends.*

(b) *Eular's formula, E for C.I* $= 1.2 \times 10^5 \; N/mm^2$

SOLUTION

Area $(A) = \dfrac{\pi}{4} \times 5^2$

$\qquad\qquad = 19.635 \; cm^2$

$\qquad\qquad = 19.635 \times 10^2 \; mm^2$

M.O.I $(I) = \dfrac{\pi}{64} \times 5^2$

$\qquad\qquad = 30.7 \; cm^4$

$\qquad\qquad = 30.7 \times 10^4 \; mm^4$

Least radius of gyration $(k) = \sqrt{\dfrac{I}{A}}$

$$= \sqrt{\dfrac{30.7 \times 10^4}{19.635 \times 10^2}}$$

$$= 12.5 \; mm$$

Since, as per given condition, one end is fixed and the other end is free.

Hence, effective length $(l_e) = 2l$

$$= 2 \times 1500$$

$$= 3000 \; mm$$

(a) Safe load by Rankine formula

Crippling load $(P_{cr}) = \dfrac{\sigma_c \cdot A}{1 + a \, (L/k)}$

$$= \dfrac{560 \times 1963.5}{1 + \dfrac{1}{1600} \times \left(\dfrac{3000}{12.5}\right)^2}$$

$$= 29708.1 \; Newton$$

$\therefore \qquad$ Safe load $= \left[\dfrac{P_{cr}}{F.O.S} \right]$

$$= \dfrac{29708.1}{3}$$

$$= 9902.7 \; Newton \qquad \textbf{Ans.}$$

(b) Safe load by Euler's formula

$$E = 1.2 \times 10^5 \text{ N/mm}^2$$

P_{cr} = Crippling load by Euler's formula

$$\therefore \quad P_{cr} = \frac{\pi^2 EI}{l_e^2} = \frac{\pi^2 \times (1.2 \times 10^5) \times (30.7 \times 10^4)}{3000^2}$$

$$= 40200 \text{ Newton}$$

$$\therefore \quad \text{Safe load} = \frac{\text{Crippling load}}{\text{Factor of safety}} = \left(\frac{40200}{3} \right)$$

$$= 1340 \text{ Newton} \quad \textbf{Ans.}$$

EXAMPLE 2 *A hollow C.I column whose outside diameter is 200 mm has thickness of 20 mm. It is 4.5 metre long and is fixed at both ends. Calculate the safe load by Rankine Gordon formula using factor of safety of 4.*

Assume: $\sigma_c = 550 \text{ MN/m}^2$

$$a = \frac{1}{1600} \qquad \textbf{(UPTU 2003-2004), (MTU 2011-12 3rd Sem.)}$$

SOLUTION Crippling load (P_{cr}) by Rankine Gordon formula

$$= \frac{\sigma_c \cdot A}{1 + a \left(\dfrac{l_e}{k} \right)^2}$$

As both ends of column are fixed

$$\therefore \quad l_e = \left(\frac{l}{2} \right)$$

$$= \frac{4.5 \times 1000}{2}$$

$$= \frac{4500}{2} = 2250 \text{ mm}$$

$$A = \frac{\pi}{4} (200^2 - 160^2)$$

$$= 11304 \text{ mm}^2$$

$$k^2 = \frac{D^2 + d^2}{16} = \frac{200^2 + 160^2}{16}$$

$$= 4100$$

$$\therefore \qquad P_{cr} = \frac{550 \times 11304}{1 + \dfrac{1}{1600} \times \dfrac{(2250)^2}{4100}}$$

$$= 3510559 \text{ N}$$

$$= 3510.56 \text{ kN}$$

Hence, safe load $= \dfrac{P_{cr}}{\text{Factor of safety}}$

$$= \left(\frac{3510.56}{4} \right)$$

$$= 877.64 \text{ kN}$$

EXAMPLE 3 *Calculate the critical load of a strut, which is made up of a bar circular in section and 5 cm long, which is pin-jointed at both ends. The same bar when freely supported gives mid span deflection of 10 mm with a 80 N load at the centre.* **(UPTU 2002-2003)**

SOLUTION Applied load $= W = 80$ N

Central deflection when freely supported $(y_{max}) = 10$ mm

For the given condition $y_{max} = \left[\dfrac{WL^3}{48 \, EI} \right]$

$$10 = \frac{80 \times (5000)^3}{48 \times EI}$$

$$\therefore \qquad EI = \frac{80 \times (5000)^3}{48 \times 10}$$

$$= 2.083 \times 10^{10} \text{ Nmm}^2$$

As the strut is pinned at the both ends,

$$\therefore \qquad l_e = l = 5 \text{ m} = 5000 \text{ mm}$$

Hence, $P_{cr} = \dfrac{\pi^2 EI}{l_e^2}$

$$= \frac{\pi^2 \, (EI)}{l^2}$$

$$= \frac{\pi^2 \times 2.083 \times 10^{10}}{(5000)^2}$$

$$= 8219.19 \text{ Newton}$$

EXAMPLE 4 *A rolled steel beam *ISMB 300 is to be used as a column of 3 metre length with both ends fixed. Find the safe axial load on the column. Assume F.O.S (factor of safety) = 3.*

$$\sigma_c = 320 \ N/mm^2 \ and \ a = \frac{1}{7500}$$

Properties of column are:

$$A = 5625 \ mm^2$$

$$I_{XX} = 8.603 \times 10^7 \ mm^4$$

$$I_{YY} = 4.539 \times 10^7 \ mm^4$$

SOLUTION Length of column (l) = 3 m = 3000 mm

Since, the column is fixed at both the ends.

∴   Effective length $(l_e) = \dfrac{l}{2}$

$$= \frac{3000}{2} = 1500 \ mm$$

As $I_{YY} < I_{XX}$, therefore, the column will tend to buckle about YY axis.

∴   Least moment of inertia of the column section

$$I = I_{min}$$

$$= I_{YY}$$

$$= 4.539 \times 10^7 \ mm^4$$

∴   Least radius of gyration of the column section

$$k = \sqrt{\frac{I}{A}}$$

$$= \sqrt{\frac{4.539 \times 10^7}{5625}}$$

$$= 89.82 \ mm.$$

By Rankine formula,

Crippling load $(P_{cr}) = \dfrac{\sigma_c \times A}{1 + a\left(\dfrac{l_e}{k}\right)^2}$

*ISMB stands for Indian Standard Medium Beam.

$$= \frac{320 \times 5626}{1 + \frac{1}{7500}\left(\frac{1500}{89.82}\right)^2}$$

$$= 1343522.38 \text{ Newton}$$

$\therefore$ Safe load $= \dfrac{P_{cr}}{F.O.S}$

$$= \frac{1343522.38}{3}$$

$$= 447840.79 \text{ Newton}$$

$$= 447.840 \text{ kN}$$

EXAMPLE 5 *A built-up section is made by 4 angles ISA 70 mm × 70 mm and four plates 250 mm × 10 mm as shown in figure 18.7.*

Find the safe load that the section can carry. Given $\sigma_c = 320 \text{ N/mm}^2$ $a = \dfrac{1}{7500}$.

Properties of angle : Area = 1302 mm^2 ; $I_x = I_y = 57.2 \times 10^4 \text{ mm}^4$. C.G. from the outer side = 21 mm.

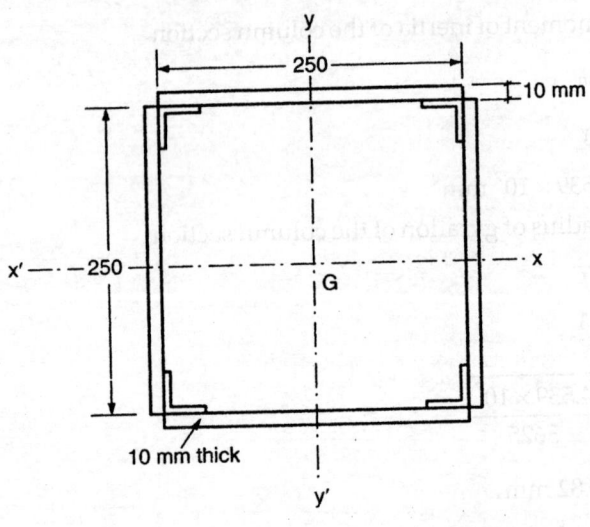

Fig. 18.7

SOLUTION Given, length of column $(l) = 4$ m $= 4000$ mm

Total area of built-up section

$$A = 4 \times 1302 + 4 \times (250 \times 10)$$

$$= 15208 \text{ mm}^2$$

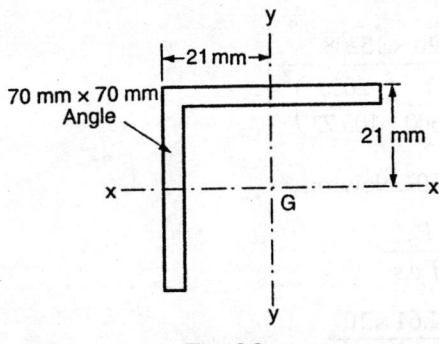

Fig. 18.8

The built-up section is symmetrical about both xx and yy axes.
Their intersection point is shown by G (centroid).

$$I_{xx} = 4\left[57.2 \times 10^4 + 1302\left(\frac{250}{2} - 21 \right)^2 \right.$$

$$\left. + 2\left[\frac{250 \times 10^3}{12} + (250 \times 10)\left(\frac{250}{2} + \frac{10}{2} \right)^2 \right] + 2 \times \frac{10 \times 250^3}{12} \right]$$

$$= 1.7 \times 10^8 \text{ mm}^4$$

Due to symmetry $I_{yy} = 1.7 \times 10^8 \text{ mm}^4 = I_{xx}$

As the column is fixed at both the ends.

$\therefore$ Effective length $(l_e) = \dfrac{l}{2}$

$$= \frac{4000}{2} = 2000 \text{ mm}$$

Least radius of gyration of the built up section

$$k = \sqrt{\frac{I}{A}}$$

$$= \sqrt{\frac{1.7 \times 10^8}{15208}}$$

$$= 105.73 \text{ mm}$$

By Rankine's formula
Crippling load or critical load or buckling load

$$P_{cr} = \left\{ \frac{\sigma_c \times A}{1 + a \cdot \left(\dfrac{l_e}{K} \right)^2} \right\}$$

$$= \left\{ \frac{320 \times 15208}{1 + \dfrac{1}{7500}\left(\dfrac{2000}{105.73}\right)^2} \right\}$$

$$= 4.64 \times 10^6 \text{ Newton}$$

$$\therefore \qquad \text{Safe load} = \frac{P_{cr}}{f.o.s}$$

$$= \frac{4.64 \times 10^6}{3}$$

$$= 1.54 \times 10^6 \text{ Newton}$$

EXAMPLE 6 *A mild steel hollow column, having 100 mm external diameter and 60 mm internal diameter and 4 m length is used as a column. Determine the crippling load by Rankine's formula when both ends are hinged.*

Take $\sigma_c = 320 \ N/mm^2$; $\alpha = \dfrac{1}{7500}$ **(UPTU 2006-07)**

SOLUTION Given end condition: Both ends are hinged.

Hence, equivalent length $l_e = l = 4\,\text{m} = 4000\ \text{mm}$

$$\sigma_c = 320\,\text{N/mm}^2$$

$$\alpha = \frac{1}{7500}$$

Now,

$$I = \frac{\pi}{64}\left[(d_o)^4 - (d_i)^4\right]$$

$$= \frac{\pi}{64}\left[(100)^4 - (60)^4\right]$$

$$= \frac{\pi}{64} \times 10^4\ [10000 - 36 \times 36]$$

$$= 427.428 \times 10^4 \text{ mm}^4$$

$$A = \frac{\pi}{4}\left[(d_o)^2 - (d_i)^2\right]$$

$$= \frac{\pi}{4}\left[(100)^2 - (60)^2\right]$$

$$= 5028.57 \text{ mm}^2$$

$$\therefore \qquad k = \sqrt{\frac{I}{A}}$$

$$= \sqrt{\frac{427.428 \times 10^4}{5028.57}} = 29.15 \text{ mm}$$

According to Rankine formula

$$P_c = \frac{\sigma_c \cdot A}{1 \times \alpha \cdot \left(\dfrac{le}{k}\right)^2}$$

$$= \frac{320 \times 5028.57}{1 + \dfrac{1}{7500} \times \left(\dfrac{4000}{29.15}\right)^2}$$

$$= 458363.69 \text{ Newton}$$

$$= 458.363 \text{ kN}$$

EXAMPLE 7 *Compare the strength of solid circular column of diameter 200 mm and hollow circular column of **same cross-sectional area** and thickness 30 mm. The other parameters are same for both the sections.*

SOLUTION Sectional area of solid circular section $= \dfrac{\pi}{4} \times 200^2 \text{ mm}^2$.

Thickness of the hollow circular column $(t) = 30 \text{ mm}$

Let external diameter of hollow circular column $= D$ mm

∴   Internal diameter of hollow circular column $= D - 2t$

$$= D - 2 \times 30$$

$$= (D - 60) \text{ mm}$$

Young's modulus of the material of both the column $= E$

∴   Sectional area of hollow circular section $= \dfrac{\pi}{4}[D^2 - (D - 60)^2]$

By question, sectional area of both the section is same.

∴ $\dfrac{\pi}{4}[D^2 - (D - 60)^2] = \dfrac{\pi}{4} \times 200^2$

or, $D^2 - (D - 60)^2 = 200^2$

or, $(D + D - 60)(\cancel{D} - \cancel{D} + 60) = 200^2$

or, $(2D - 60) \cdot 60 = 200^2$

∴ $D = 363.33 \text{ mm}$

∴   External diameter of hollow column $= 363.33 \text{ mm}$

        Internal diameter of hollow column $= (363.33 - 60) \text{ mm} = 303.33 \text{ mm}$

Least moment of inertia of hollow column = I_h

$$= \frac{\pi}{64}[D_o^4 - D_i^4]$$

$$= 4.34 \times 10^8 \text{ mm}^4$$

M.I. of Solid section $(I_s) = \dfrac{\pi}{64} \times 200^4 = 78.5 \times 10^6 \text{ mm}^4$

Assuming column hinged at both ends

$$\left(\frac{P_{\text{Cr Hollow}}}{P_{\text{Cr Solid}}}\right) = \left[\frac{\dfrac{\pi^2 E I_h}{l^2}}{\dfrac{\pi^2 E I_s}{l^2}}\right] = \left(\frac{I_h}{I_s}\right) = \frac{4 \times 9 \times 10^8}{78.5 \times 10^6} = 5.58 \qquad \textbf{Ans.}$$

18.13 ECCENTRIC LOADING IN COLUMN

While driving Euler's formula, we assumed that:

   (i) Load is acting centrally;

   (ii) Material is homogenous

But due to imperfection like eccentricity of loading, initial curvature etc., transverse deflection starts occurring right from the beginning of load application.

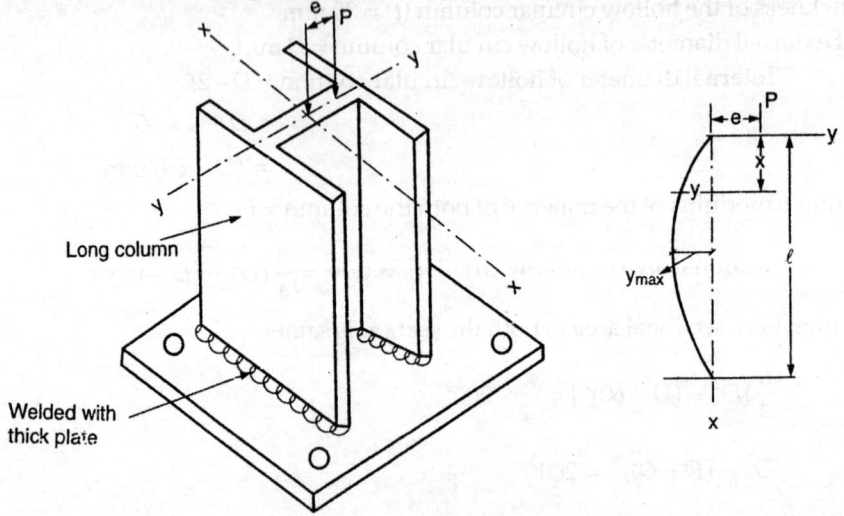

Fig. 18.9

So, when the load is eccentric then resultant stress (σ_r)

$$\sigma_r = \left\{\frac{P}{A} + \frac{(P \cdot y_{\max})}{Z}\right\} = \left\{\frac{P}{A} + \frac{(P \cdot y_{\max})}{I/y_c}\right\} \qquad \qquad ...(1)$$

where, $y_{\max}$ = lateral maximum deflection

z = section modulus

I = moment of inertia

y_c = distance of the outermost fibre in compression from the neutral axis of the column.

Now, we have to find out y_{max}.

Let the load P is applied to the column at eccentricity 'e'.

Then, at any arbitrary point x, Bending Moment

$$M = -P \cdot y$$

or, $$EI \cdot \frac{d^2y}{dx^2} = -P \cdot y$$

or, $$EI \cdot \frac{d^2y}{dx^2} + P \cdot y = 0$$

or, $$\frac{d^2y}{dx^2} + \left(\frac{P}{EI}\right) \cdot y = 0$$

or, $$\frac{d^2y}{dx^2} + m^2 y = 0 \quad \text{where } m = \left(\frac{P}{EI}\right)$$

The solution of this equation is

$$y = A \cos mx + B \sin mx \qquad \ldots(2)$$

where, A and B are constants.

Now, At $x = 0, y = e \Rightarrow A = e$

Differentiating equation (1), we get

$$\left(\frac{dy}{dx}\right) = -mA \sin mx + mB \cos mx$$

Further, at $x = \frac{l}{2}; \left(\frac{dy}{dx}\right) = 0$

∴ $$0 = -e \sin m \cdot \left(\frac{l}{2}\right) + B \cos m \cdot \left(\frac{l}{2}\right)$$

or, $$B = e \tan\left(\frac{ml}{2}\right)$$

∴ Equation (2) reduces to $y = e \cos mx + e \tan\left(\frac{ml}{2}\right) \cdot \sin mx$

$$= e\left[\cos mx + \tan\left(\frac{ml}{2}\right) \cdot \sin mx\right]$$

Now, from figure due to symmetry, we can say that maximum deflection occurs at centre i.e. $x = \frac{l}{2}$.

Now, substituting $x = \dfrac{l}{2}$ in the above equation,

$$y_{max} = e\left[\cos\frac{ml}{2} + \tan\left(\frac{ml}{2}\right)\cdot\sin\frac{ml}{2}\right]$$

$$= e\sec\frac{ml}{2}\left[\cos^2\frac{ml}{2} + \sin^2\frac{ml}{2}\right]$$

$$= e\sec\frac{ml}{2}$$

$\therefore \qquad \sigma_{max} = \dfrac{P}{A} + \dfrac{P\cdot y_{max}}{Z}$

$$= \frac{P}{A} + \frac{P\cdot e\sec\dfrac{ml}{2}}{Z}$$

$$= \frac{P}{A}\times\left[1 + \frac{A\cdot e}{Z}\cdot\sec\frac{ml}{2}\right]$$

$Z = \left(\dfrac{I}{y_c}\right)$ and $I = Ak^2$ where, k = radius of gyration.

Now, $\dfrac{A}{Z} = \dfrac{A}{I/y_c}$

$$= \frac{A\cdot y_c}{A\cdot k^2}$$

$$= \frac{y_c}{k^2}$$

$$\sigma_{max} = \frac{P}{A}\left[1 + \frac{e\cdot y_c}{k^2}\cdot\sec\sqrt{\frac{P}{EI}}\cdot\frac{l}{2}\right]$$

$$= \frac{P}{A}\left[1 + \frac{e\,y_c}{k^2}\cdot\sec\sqrt{\frac{P}{EI}}\,\frac{l}{2}\right]$$

For other end condition, we can write

$$\sigma_{max} = \frac{P}{A}\left[1 + \frac{e\cdot y_c}{k^2}\cdot\sec\sqrt{\frac{P}{EI}}\cdot\frac{l_e}{2}\right]$$

where, l_e is the equivalent length.

This is known as secant formula and is applicable for long columns.

EXAMPLE 1 *A tubular steel strut has 6.5 cm external and 5 cm internal diameter. It is 2.5 m long and has hinged ends. The load is parallel to the axis but eccentric.*

Find the maximum eccentricity for a buckling load of 0.75 of the Euler value.
Yield stress = 320 MPa and E = 210 GPa.

SOLUTION

$$A = \frac{\pi}{4}(6.5^2 - 5^2) = 13.55 \text{ cm}^2$$

$$I = \frac{\pi}{64}(6.5^4 - 5^4) = \frac{\pi}{64} \times 1160.06$$

$$= 56.94 \text{ cm}^4$$

Euler crippling or buckling load $(P_{cr}) = \dfrac{\pi^2 EI}{l^2}$

$$= \frac{\pi^2 \times 210 \times 10^9 \times 56.94 \times 10^{-8}}{(2.5)^2}$$

$$= 188.82 \text{ kN}$$

Eccentric load = $0.75 \, P_e$ = 141.615 kN

Now, $\quad \sigma_{max} = \dfrac{P}{A}\left[1 + \dfrac{ey_c}{k^2} \cdot \sec\sqrt{\dfrac{P}{EI}} \cdot \dfrac{l}{2}\right]$

$$320 \times 10^6 = \frac{141.615 \times 10^3}{13.55 \times 10^{-4}}\left[1 + \frac{e \times 3.25 \times 13.55 \times 10^{-2}}{56.94 \times 10^{-4}}\right.$$

$$\left. \times \sec\sqrt{\frac{141.615 \times 10^3}{210 \times 10^9 \times 56.94 \times 10^{-8}}} \times 1.25 \right]$$

$$320 \times 10^6 = 10.4513 \times 10^7 [1 + 77.34 \times e \times \sec 1.360]$$

Eccentricity $(e) = 5.57 \times 10^{-3}$ m **Ans.**

HIGHLIGHTS

1. A vertical member of a structure which is subjected to axial compressive load is known as column.
2. Strut is a member of a structure which is not vertical or whose one or both of its ends are hinged or pin-joined.
3. All short columns fails due to crushing whereas, long column fail due to buckling and crushing.
4. The load at which column just buckles is known as buckling load or critical load or crippling load.
5. The crippling load for a column by Euler's formula for different end conditions is given by

$P_{cr} = \dfrac{\pi^2 EI}{l^2}$ when both ends are hinged.

$\hspace{1.2cm} = \dfrac{\pi^2 EI}{4l^2}$ when one end is fixed and other is free.

$\hspace{1.2cm} = \dfrac{4\pi^2 EI}{l^2}$ when both end are fixed.

$\hspace{1.2cm} = \dfrac{2\pi^2 EI}{l^2}$ when one end is fixed and the other is hinged.

where, l = actual length of column.

$\hspace{1.2cm} E$ = Young's modulus of the material of column.

$\hspace{1.2cm} I$ = least moment of inertia of the column.

The crippling load for any type of end condition is given by

$$P_{cr} = \frac{\pi^2 EI}{l_e^{2}}$$

where, l_e = effective length.

$\hspace{1.2cm} = l$ when both ends are hinged.

$\hspace{1.2cm} = 2l$ when one end is fixed and other free.

$\hspace{1.2cm} = \dfrac{l}{2}$ when both ends are fixed.

$\hspace{1.2cm} = \dfrac{l}{\sqrt{2}}$ when one end fixed and other is hinged.

6. Crippling loads $(P_{cr}) = \dfrac{\pi^2 EA}{\left(\dfrac{l_e}{k}\right)^2}$

and, Crippling stress $(\sigma_{cr}) = \dfrac{\pi^2 E}{\left(\dfrac{l_e}{k}\right)^2}$

where, l_e = effective length.

$\hspace{1.2cm} k$ = least radius of gyration.

$$= \sqrt{\frac{I}{A}}$$

where, I = least M.I.

7. Slenderness ratio $= \left(\dfrac{l_e}{k}\right)$

8. Crippling load by **Rankine Formula** is

$$P_{cr} = \frac{\sigma_c \times A}{1 + a\left(\dfrac{l_e}{k}\right)^2}$$

where, σ_c = Ultimate crushing stress

A = Area of cross-section of column

a = Rankine constant

l_e = Effective length

k = Least radius of gyration.

9. **Gordon's Formula:** According to Gordon

$$P_{cr} = \frac{\sigma_c \cdot A}{1 + b \cdot \left(\dfrac{l_e}{d}\right)^2}$$

where, b = a constant

d = least diameter 'or' breadth of bar

$$b = \frac{\sigma_c \cdot A \cdot d^2}{\pi^2 \cdot E.I}$$

10. Straight line formula:

$$P = \sigma_c \times A\left(1 - c \cdot \frac{l_e}{k}\right)$$

where, c = a constant depending on the material

$$= \frac{\sigma_c}{4\pi^2 E}$$

PROBLEMS FOR PRACTICE
(THEORETICAL)

1. Differentiate between column and strut ? How do we classify column?
2. Define crippling load.
3. Derive an expression for the Euler's crippling load for a long column with following end condition.
   (a) Both ends are hinged.
   (b) Both ends are fixed.
4. Explain how the Rankine Gordon formula is used for calculating the intensity of stress in short, intermediate and long column?
5. Define slenderness ratio. What are the limitations of Euler's formula?

(NUMERICAL)

1. Compare the safe loads for two circular columns of same length, same material and equal area of cross-sections. One of them being hollow with diameters ratio 2 : 1 and the other a solid one.

   In each case one end of column is fixed and the other is hinged. Factor of safety is also same.

2. Compare the crippling loads given by Euler's and Rankine's formula for a tubular strut 2.3 m long having outer and inner diameters 38 mm and 33 mm respectively, loaded through pin-joints at each end. Take the yield stress as 335 N/mm², Rankine constant $a = \dfrac{1}{7500}$ and $E = 2 \times 10^5$ N/mm².

   For what length of this strut does the Euler's formula cease to apply?

3. A rolled steel joist ISMB 300 is to be used as a column of 3 metres length and both ends fixed. Find the safe axial load on the column. Take f.o.s 3;

   $\sigma_c = 320$ N/mm² and $a = \dfrac{1}{7500}$

   Properties of the column section:

   Area $= 5625$ mm²

   $I_{XX} = 8.603 \times 10^4$ min⁴

   $I_{YY} = 4.539 \times 10^7$ mm⁴

4. A column of diameter 10 cm and length 4 m is subjected to a load of 10 kN at an eccentricity of 5 mm from its geometric axis. If both the ends of the column are hinged, find the maximum stress induced in the column. Take $E = 1.8 \times 10^5$ N/mm². Also find the maximum deflection.

5. Using Euler's formula, calculate the critical stresses for a series of strut having slenderness ratio of 40, 80, 120, 160 and 200 under the following conditions and also state inference.

   (i) both ends hinged, and

   (ii) both ends fixed.

   Take $E = 2.05 \times 10^5$ N/mm²

ANSWERS

1. $\dfrac{P_{\text{hollow}}}{P_{\text{solid}}} = 1.67$ 2. $P_{\text{Euler}} = 16.88$ KN; $P_{\text{Rankine}} = 14.29; l = 978$ mm

5. (i) 316.135 N/mm²; 140.5 N/mm²; 79.03 N/mm²; 50.58 N/mm²

   Inference: (i) So, when both ends are hinged and the ratio of (l/k) increases, the value of crippling stress decreases.

   (ii) 5058.16 N/mm²; 1264.54 N/mm²; 562.02 N/mm²; 316.135 N/mm²; 202.32 N/mm².

   Inference: When both ends are fixed and the ratio of (l/k) increases, the value of critical stress decreases accordingly.

OBJECTIVE QUESTIONS

1. Euler's formula is valid for:
   (a) short column   (b) long columns
   (c) short and long columns both   (d) intermediate columns

2. Rankine formula is valid for:
   (a) long columns   (b) short columns
   (c) intermediate column   (d) none of the above

3. Euler's formula works for:
   (a) elastic limits only
   (b) plastic limit only
   (c) elastic and plastic limit-both
   (d) none of these

4. The critical load is the load at which:
   (a) the column breaks
   (b) the column loses its strength
   (c) the column buckls
   (d) none of these

5. Johnson formula is used for:
   (a) short column
   (b) long column
   (c) short and intermediate column
   (d) none of these

6. Slenderness ratio of a column is the ratio of its:
   (a) length and radius
   (b) length and diameter
   (c) length and least radius of gyration
   (d) length and least moment of inertia

7. For a long column, the slenderness ratio is more than:
   (a) 30
   (b) 60
   (c) 120
   (d) none of the above

8. Failure of column occurs due to:
   (a) Compressive stress
   (b) Bending stress
   (c) Stiffness
   (d) Instability

9. The failure of struts may occur:
   (a) by pure compression
   (b) by buckling
   (c) by combination of pure compression and buckling depending upon slenderness ratio
   (d) any of the above

10. For a short column the slenderness ratio is less than:
    (a) 30
    (b) 60
    (c) 120
    (d) none of the above

11. For a intermediate column the slenderness ratio is between:
    (a) 40 and 100
    (b) 30 and 120
    (c) 50 and 100
    (d) none of the above

12. When a member is acted upon simultaneously by an axial load and transverse load (causing bending) then, such members are referred to as:
    (a) Strut
    (b) Beam-column
    (c) Column
    (d) None of the above

13. The buckling in the case of a column, takes place about the axis having:
    (a) minimum radius of gyration
    (b) maximum radius of gyration
    (c) either of the above
    (d) none of the above

14. The radius of gyration of a circular column of diameter 'd' is:

    (a) $\dfrac{d}{4}$
    (b) $\dfrac{d}{2}$
    (c) $\dfrac{d^2}{4}$
    (d) $\dfrac{d^2}{16}$

15. Euler's critical load for a column of equivalent length l_e, moment of inertia I and modulus of elasticity E is given by:

(a) $\dfrac{\pi^2 EI}{l_e}$ (b) $\dfrac{\pi EI}{l_e^2}$ (c) $\dfrac{\pi^2 EI}{l_e^2}$ (d) $\dfrac{\pi EI}{l_e}$

16. Euler's buckling formula is applicable for columns:
    (a) subjected to eccentric loads   (b) having initial curvature
    (c) initially straight and subjected to only axial load
    (d) none of the above

17. The secant formula is used for:
    (a) long columns under eccentric loading
    (b) long columns under axial loading
    (c) short-columns under axial loading
    (d) short columns under eccentric loading

18. The effective length for Euler's formula in case of a strut of length L fixed at both ends is:
    (a) L (b) $L/2$
    (c) $2L$ (d) none of the above

19. The ratio of equivalent length of a column having one end fixed and the other end free to its length is:
    (a) 2   (b) $\sqrt{2}$ (c) $\dfrac{1}{2}$ (d) $\dfrac{1}{\sqrt{2}}$

20. The ratio of equivalent length of a column having both end fixed to its length is:
    (a) 2   (b) $\sqrt{2}$ (c) $\dfrac{1}{2}$ (d) $\dfrac{1}{\sqrt{2}}$

21. In the Rankine formula, the material constant for the mild steel is:
    (a) $\dfrac{1}{1200}$ (b) $\dfrac{1}{1600}$ (c) $\dfrac{1}{7500}$ (d) $\dfrac{1}{5000}$

22. Which of the following is the example of the strut?
    (a) piston rods   (b) connecting rods
    (c) side link in forging machines   (d) all of the above

23. A member of structure or bar which carries an axial compressive load is called:
    (a) strut   (b) tie
    (c) shaft   (d) none of the above

ANSWERS

1. (b)	2. (c)	3. (a)	4. (c)	5. (c)	6. (c)
7. (c)	8. (d)	9. (d)	10. (a)	11. (b)	12. (b)
13. (a)	14. (b)	15. (c)	16. (c)	17. (a)	18. (b)
19. (a)	20. (b)	21. (c)	22. (d)	23. (a)	

— ❖❖ —

CURVED BEAM

19.1 INTRODUCTION

Structural members such as arches, crane hooks, chain link and frame of some machines that have considerable initial curvature in the plane of loading are called **curved beam.** The flexural formula $\sigma = \dfrac{M}{I} \cdot y$ cannot be applied to them unless the depth of the beam is small compared with radius of curvature. A simple flexure formula may be used for curved beam for which radius of curvature $> 5h$ where h is the depth of beam.

For more deep curved beam, the Centroidal axis and Neutral axis do not meet together as is met in the case of straight beam. **Winkler,** therefore, devised a formula which is capable to calculate the stress in a curved beam subjected to load.

19.2 WINKLER-BATCH THEORY

Assumptions for this theory are —
  (i) Plane Transverse Section before bending remains plane after bending.
  (ii) Limit of proportionality is not exceeded.
  (iii) Radial strain is negligible.
  (iv) The material is considered elastic; isotropic; homogenous and obeys Hook's law.

[N.B.: Although the stress and strain variation along the cross-section of the curved beam are hyperbolic, Hook's law is still valid because material is linearly elastic.]

Let us consider a Curved Beam *ABCD* Subjected to moment M as shown in Fig. 19.1.

Let r_0 = outer radius of the curved beam;
      r_i = inner radius of the curved beam;
      $\bar{r}$ = centroidal radius of the curved beam;
      R_N = radius of neutral axis;
      r = radius of element having elemental area dA.

We know that when any elastic body is subjected to load, deformation takes place *i.e.* strain occurs as such B shifts to B', C shifts to C' and m on the element shift to m'. The new shape of the beam becomes AB'C'D. Here load (M) causes to decrease the curvature.

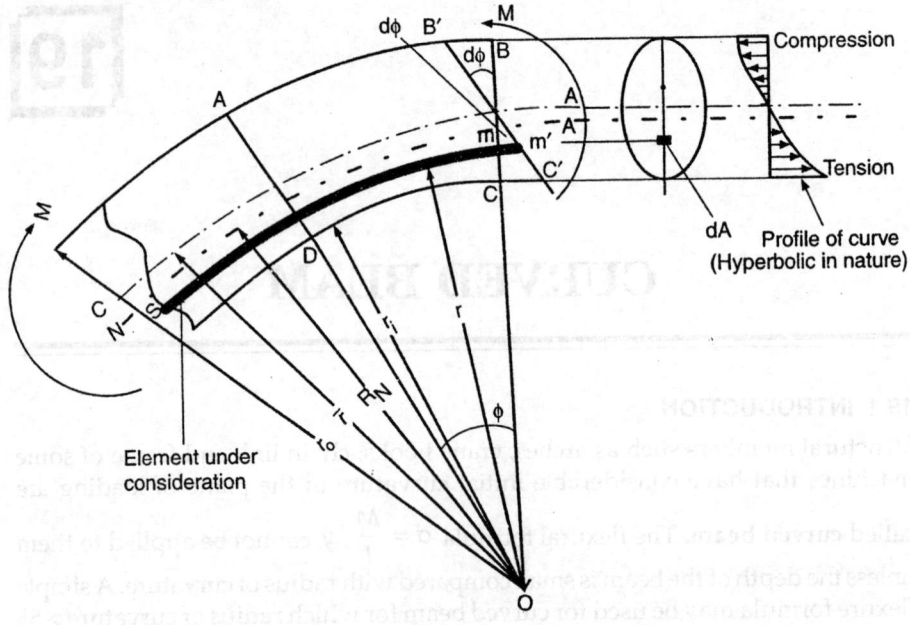

Fig. 19.1 Curved Beam subjected to moment M

The non-linear stress distribution over the cross-section causes shift in the neutral axis towards the centre of curvature (O)*.

$$\epsilon \text{ for the element} = \left(\frac{\text{change in arc}}{\text{original arc}} \right) = \frac{mm'}{S\,m}$$

$$= \frac{(R_N - r)\,d\phi}{r\phi} \qquad \qquad ...(1) \qquad \left[\because \theta = \frac{l}{r} \quad \therefore l = r\theta \atop \text{So, } mm' = (R_N - r)\,d\phi \right]$$

where, $d\phi$ is the angle subtended by the differential element (shown by black colour) of the beam.

$$\because \qquad \sigma = \epsilon E$$

$$\therefore \qquad E = \left(\frac{\sigma}{\epsilon} \right)$$

$$\therefore \qquad E = \frac{\sigma r \phi}{(R_N - r)\,d\phi} \qquad \qquad ...(2)$$

---

*It has been found from the result of photoelastic experiment that is the case of curved beam, the neutral surface does not coincide with the centroidal axis but is shifted towards the centre of curvature.

At the Neutral Axis $\Sigma F_n = 0$

or, $\int \sigma \cdot dA = 0$

or, $\int E \cdot \in \cdot dA = 0$

or, $\int \dfrac{E(R_N - r)d\phi}{r\phi} dA = 0$

or, $\dfrac{Ed\phi}{\phi} \int \left(\dfrac{R_N - r}{r} \right) dA = 0$

$\left(\dfrac{Ed\phi}{\phi} \right) \neq 0$

So $\int \left(\dfrac{R_N - r}{r} \right) dA = 0$

or, $R_N \int \dfrac{dA}{r} - \int dA = 0$ ...(3)

or, $R_N \int \dfrac{dA}{r} - A = 0$

Hence, location of *neutral Axis $\boxed{R_N = \dfrac{A}{\int \dfrac{dA}{r}}}$

Further, in equilibrium condition, for the element taken for study.
Applied moment = Restoring Moment

i.e, $M = \int (\sigma \cdot dA)(R_N - r)$

$= \int E \in dA (R_N - r)$

$= \int \dfrac{E(R_N - r) \cdot d\phi \cdot dA (R_N - r)}{r\phi}$

[Substituting the value of $\in$ from equation (1)]

$= \int \dfrac{E(R_N - r)^2 d\phi}{r\phi} \cdot dA$

E, R, ϕ and $d\phi$ are constant at a section.

$\therefore$ $M = \left\{ \dfrac{E \, d\phi}{\phi} \int \dfrac{(R_N - r)^2 \, dA}{r} \right\}$

$= \dfrac{E \, d\phi}{\phi} \int \dfrac{(R_N^2 - R_N r - R_N r + r^2) \, dA}{r}$

---

*This is the general formula for R_N, however, it will be different for different type of section as discussed in the section 19.3.

Now, substituting the value of E from eqn. (2)

$$M = \frac{\sigma \cdot r \cdot \phi}{(R_N - r) \, d\phi} \times \frac{d\phi}{\phi} \int \frac{(R_N^2 - R_N \, r - R_N \, r + r^2) \, dA}{r}$$

$$= \frac{\sigma \cdot r}{(R_N - r)} \left[R_N^2 \int \frac{dA}{r} - R_N \int dA - R_N \int dA + \int r \cdot dA \right] \qquad \text{...(4)}$$

From equation (3) $R_N \int \dfrac{dA}{r} - \int dA = 0$

Multiplying by R_N both sides,

$$R_N^2 \int \frac{dA}{r} - R_N \int dA = 0$$

Therefore, equation (4) reduces to

$$= \frac{\sigma \cdot r}{(R - r)} \left[\int r dA - R_N \int dA \right]$$

$$= \frac{\sigma r}{(R_N - r)} [\bar{r} \cdot A - R_N \cdot A] \qquad \left[\begin{array}{l} \text{By formula } \bar{r} = \dfrac{\int r \cdot dA}{\int dA} = \dfrac{\int r \cdot dA}{A} \\[2mm] \qquad \therefore \qquad \int r dA = \bar{r} \cdot A \end{array} \right]$$

$$\therefore \qquad M = \frac{\sigma \cdot r \cdot A \, (\bar{r} - R_N)}{(R_N - r)}$$

$$\therefore \qquad \boxed{\sigma = \frac{M \, (R_N - r)}{r \, A \, (\bar{r} - R_N)}} \qquad \text{...(5)}$$

This is the general formula for stress in a curve beam irrespective of any type of section (rectangular, square, circular, elliptical, T-section, I-section etc.).
Stress at innermost fibre of the specimen of curved beam.

$$\sigma_i = \left\{ \frac{M \, (R_N - r_i)}{r_i \cdot A \cdot (\bar{r} - R_N)} \right\}$$

Similarly, at outmost fibre of the specimen of curved beam

$$\sigma_o = \left\{ \frac{M \, (R_N - r_o)}{r_o \cdot A \cdot (\bar{r} - R_N)} \right\}$$

Total stress at inner surface $= \left(\dfrac{P}{A} + \sigma_i \right)$

Total stress at outer surface $= \left(\dfrac{P}{A} + \sigma_o \right)$

N.B.: We will see that the value of Bending stress (Tensile in nature) is (+) ve and the Bending Stress (Compressive in nature) is (–)ve

$$(\bar{r} - R_N) = \text{Shift of N.A. from centroidal axis}$$

$$\therefore \qquad (\bar{r} - R_N) = e \text{ (eccentricity)}$$

e must always be positive. This indicates that shift of N.A. with respect to the centroidal axis is always towards the centre of curvature. Further, 'e' must be computed carefully otherwise correct value of stress will not be obtained.

Further, M will be (+)ve for tensile loading and $\left(\dfrac{P}{A}\right)$ will also be (+)ve for tensile loading.

Similarly, M will be (–)ve for compressive loading and $\left(\dfrac{P}{A}\right)$ will also be (–)ve for compressive loading.

19.3 FORMULA TO SOLVE THE PROBLEM OF CURVED BEAM

We will use suffix 'i' for the stress developed inside the section under study, and suffix 'o' for the stress developed outside the section under study.

Normally, we will come across following types of sections in curved beam:

  (i) Rectangular section/square section

  (ii) Trapezoidal section   (iii) Circular section

  (iv) Triangular section   (v) T-section

  (vi) I-section

Steps for Solving Problems of Rectangular Section

(i) **Find the radius of the N.A.**

$$R_N = \text{radius of N.A.} = \frac{A}{\int \left(\dfrac{dA}{r}\right)}$$

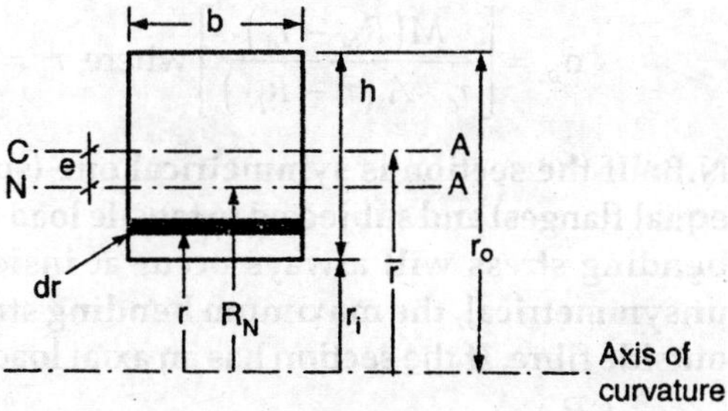

Let h = depth and b = width

$\therefore \qquad A = \text{area} = b \cdot h$

Let us take an element at a distance r from the axis of curvature having thickness dr.

Hence, Elemental Area; $dA = b.dr$

Fig. 19.2

$$\therefore \qquad R_N = \frac{b \cdot h}{\displaystyle\int_{r_i}^{r_o} \left(\frac{b \cdot dr}{r}\right)}$$

$$= \frac{b \cdot h}{b \cdot \log_e \left(\dfrac{r_o}{r_i}\right)}$$

$$R_N = \frac{h}{\log_e \left(\dfrac{r_o}{r_i} \right)}$$

Once, the radius of the neutral axis is evaluated, the following formula will be used to find the stress developed (owing to application of load) at the inner or outer surface of the beam.

$$\sigma = \frac{M.(R_N - r)}{r.A.(\bar{r} - R_N)}$$

Where

M = applied moment = $P \times$ distance between *C.A.* and Axis of loading

R_N = Radius of neutral axis.

r = Radius of the element (having elemental area dA) under consideration

A = Area of cross-section

$\bar{r}$ = Centroidal radius of the Curved beam.

(The difference between $\bar{r}$ and R_N i.e. $(\bar{r} - R_N)$ is denoted by *'e'* also, known as eccentricity).

Now, bending stress at innermost fibre of the section.

$$\sigma_i = \left[\frac{M(R_N - r_i)}{r_i \cdot A.(\bar{r} - R_N)} \right] \text{where, } r_i = \text{radius of innerside}$$

Bending Stress at outermost fibre of the section.

$$\sigma_o = \left[\frac{M(R_N - r_o)}{r_o \cdot A.(\bar{r} - R_N)} \right] \text{where, } r_o = \text{radius of outerside}.$$

N.B: If the section is symmetrical one (such as circle; rectangle, I-beam with equal flanges) and subjected to tensile load OR compressive load then maximum bending stress will always occur at inside fibre. However, if the section is unsymmetrical, the maximum bending stress may occur at either the inside or outside fibre. If the section has an axial load in addition to the bending, the axial stress $\left(\dfrac{P}{A} \right)$ must be added to the bending stress.

These two formule for σ_i and σ_o will be used for all types of sections whether it is

(a) Rectangular/square
(b) Trapezoidal
(c) Circular
(d) Triangular
(e) T-section
(f) I-section

However, the derivation/expression for 'R_N' will be different for different types of sections. Let us see one by one.

Square Section

Let 'b' is the side of square section.

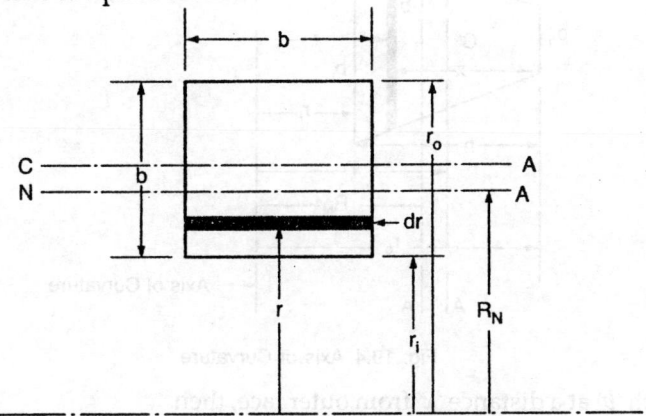

Fig. 19.3 Axis of Curvature

By formula (R_N) = radius of neutral axis

$$= \frac{A}{\int \frac{dA}{r}}$$

$$\left[\begin{array}{l} A = b \cdot b, \ \ dA = b \cdot dr \\ dA = \text{Area of Element} \\ \text{taken for analysis of } R_N \end{array} \right]$$

$$= \frac{b \cdot b}{\int_{r_i}^{r_o} \frac{b \cdot dr}{r}}$$

$$= \frac{b}{\int_{r_i}^{r_o} \frac{dr}{r}}$$

$$\therefore R_N = \frac{b}{\ln\left(\dfrac{r_o}{r_i}\right)}$$

Trapezoidal Cross-Section

A trapezoidal section of curved beam of width b_i at the inner surface, b_o at the outer surface and depth 'h' is shown in Fig. 19.4.

Consider a strip of width 'b' and depth 'dr' at a distance r from the axis of curvature.

Let r_i = distance of the inner radius of the section from the axis of curvature.

and r_o = distance of the outer radius of the section from the axis of curvature.

Let $\bar{r}$ = distance of centroidal axis from the axis of curvature.

and R_N = distance of neutral axis from the axis of curvature.

Our aim is to derive R_N.

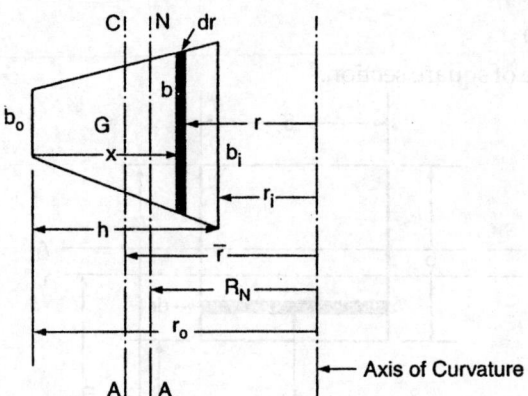

Fig. 19.4 Axis of Curvature

Now, width 'b' at a distance 'x' from outer face, then

$$b = b_o + \left(\frac{b_i - b_o}{h}\right) \times x$$

$$\because \qquad x = (r_o - r)$$

Hence, $b = b_o + \left(\dfrac{b_i - b_o}{h}\right)(r_o - r)$

Now, $\displaystyle\int \frac{dA}{r}$

$$= \int \frac{b \times dr}{r}$$

$$= \int_{r_i}^{r_o} \left[\frac{b_o + \left(\dfrac{b_i - b_o}{h}\right)(r_o - r)}{r}\right] dr$$

$$= b_o \int_{r_i}^{r_o} \frac{dr}{r} + \int_{r_i}^{r_o} \left[\frac{(b_i - b_o)\, r_o}{h \cdot r}\right] dr - \int_{r_i}^{r_o} \left[\frac{(b_i - b_o)\, \cancel{r}}{h \cdot \cancel{r}}\right] dr$$

$$= b_o \cdot \ln\left(\frac{r_o}{r_i}\right) + \frac{(b_i - b_o)\, r_o}{h} \cdot \ln\left(\frac{r_o}{r_i}\right) - \frac{(b_i - b_o)}{\cancel{h}} \times (r_o \cancel{- r_i}) \quad [\because h = (r_o - r_i)]$$

$$= \ln\left(\frac{r_o}{r_i}\right) \left[b_o + \frac{r_o (b_i - b_o)}{h}\right] - (b_i - b_o)$$

$$= \ln\left(\frac{r_o}{r_i}\right) \left[\frac{b_o h + r_o (b_i - b_o)}{h}\right] - (b_i - b_o)$$

$$= \ln\left(\frac{r_o}{r_i}\right)\left[\frac{b_o\,(r_o - r_i) + r_o\,(b_i - b_o)}{h}\right] + b_o - b_i$$

$$= \ln\left(\frac{r_o}{r_i}\right)\left[\frac{b_o\,\cancel{r_o} - b_o r_i + b_i r_o - b_o\,\cancel{r_o}}{h}\right] + (b_o - b_i)$$

$$= \ln\left(\frac{r_o}{r_i}\right)\left[\frac{b_i r_o - b_o r_i}{h}\right] + (b_o - b_i)$$

$$\therefore \qquad R_N = \frac{A}{\displaystyle\int \frac{dA}{r}}$$

$$\therefore\ R_N = \frac{A}{(b_o - b_i) + \left(\dfrac{b_i r_o - b_o r_i}{h}\right)\cdot \ln\left(\dfrac{r_o}{r_i}\right)}$$

N.B.: If $b_o = 0$ then R_N turns into triangular section.

So, R_N for triangular section $= \dfrac{A}{-b_i + \dfrac{b_i r_o}{h}\cdot \ln\left(\dfrac{r_o}{r_i}\right)}$

Triangular Section

Let us consider an elementary strip at a distance r from the axis of curvature.

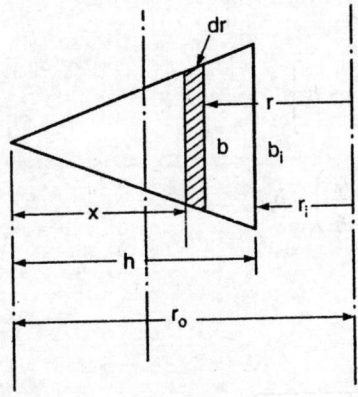

Fig. 19.5

Let the width of the strip $= b$
and depth of strip $= dr$
Hence, elemental area $(dA) = b \times dr$
Now, from similar triangle, we have

$$\frac{b}{x} = \frac{b_i}{h}$$

$$\therefore \qquad b = \left(\frac{b_i x}{h}\right)$$

Hence, $dA = b \times dr$

$$= \left(\frac{b_i x}{h}\right) dr$$

But $\qquad x = (r_o - r)$

Therefore, $dA = \dfrac{b_i (r_o - r)}{h} dr$

Now, $\displaystyle\int \frac{dA}{r}$

$$= \int_{r_i}^{r_o} \left[\frac{b_i (r_o - r)}{h}\right] \times \frac{1}{r} \times dr$$

$$= \frac{b_i}{h} \int_{r_i}^{r_o} \frac{(r_o - r)}{r} dr$$

$$= \frac{b_i}{h} \left[r_o \int_{r_i}^{r_o} \frac{dr}{r} - \int_{r_i}^{r_o} dr \right]$$

$$= \frac{b_i}{h} \left[r_o \cdot \ln\left(\frac{r_o}{r_i}\right) - (r_o - r_i) \right]$$

$$= \frac{b_i}{h} \left[r_o \cdot \ln\left(\frac{r_o}{r_i}\right) - h \right]$$

$$\therefore \qquad \int \frac{dA}{r} = \frac{b_i r_o}{h} \cdot \ln\left(\frac{r_o}{r_i}\right) - b_i$$

$$\therefore \qquad R_N = \frac{A}{\displaystyle\int \frac{dA}{r}}$$

$$\boxed{R_N = \frac{A}{\dfrac{b_i r_o}{h} \cdot \ln\left(\dfrac{r_o}{r_i}\right) - b_i}} \qquad \textbf{(Form I)}$$

$$\therefore \qquad R_N = \frac{\dfrac{1}{2} \times b_i \times h}{\dfrac{b_i r_o}{h} \cdot \ln\left(\dfrac{r_o}{r_i}\right) - b_i}$$

$$R_N = \frac{\dfrac{h}{2}}{\dfrac{r_o}{h}\ln\left(\dfrac{r_o}{r_i}\right) - 1}$$ **(Form II)**

Form I or II may be used to compute R_N for triangular section.

Now stresses at inside and outside surface of triangular section can be computed by applying formula derived on Page 19.4 *i.e.,* by equation (5).

Circular Section

Let us consider a circular section of diameter 'd'.

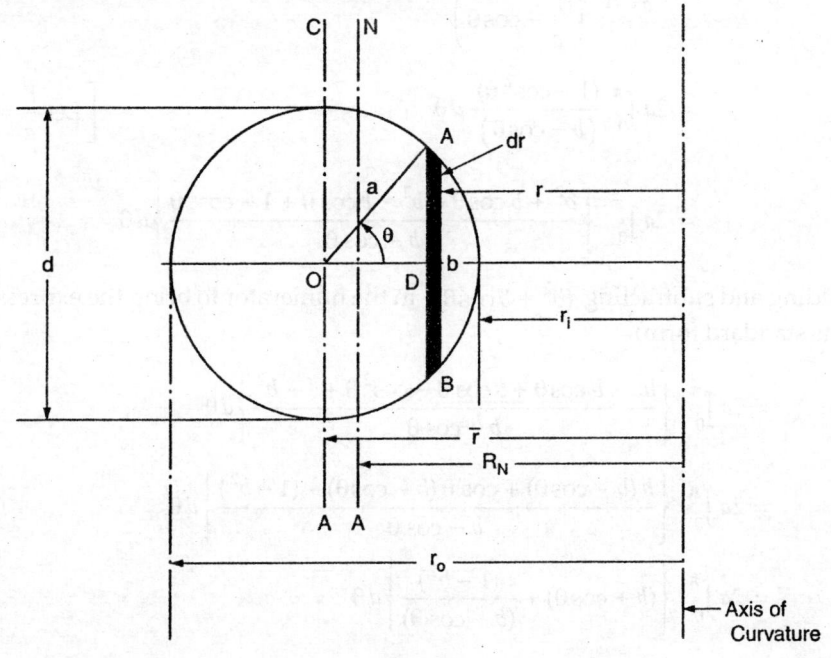

Fig. 19.6

Let us consider a small elementary strip of width 'b' and depth 'dr' at a distance 'r' from the axis of curvature.

Let r_i = inner radius of curvature of the circular section

       r_o = outer radius of curvature of the circular section

       $\bar{r}$ = radius of centroidal axis

     R_N = radius of neutral axis

       b = width of the strip = $2AD = 2a \sin\theta$

                 (Considering $OA = a$ for simplifying the derivation)

Elemental area (dA) of the strip = $b \times dr$

                         = $2a \sin\theta \times dr$

Now, $r = (\bar{r} - a\cos\theta)$

$\therefore \qquad dr = a\sin\theta\, d\theta$

$\therefore \qquad dA = 2a^2 \sin^2\theta \cdot d\theta$

Now, $\qquad \displaystyle\int \frac{dA}{r} = \int_0^\pi \frac{2a^2 \sin^2\theta\, d\theta}{(\bar{r} - a\cos\theta)}$

$\qquad\qquad = 2a^2 \int_0^\pi \frac{(1 - \cos^2\theta)\, d\theta}{(\bar{r} - a\cos\theta)}$

$\qquad\qquad = \dfrac{2a^2}{a} \displaystyle\int_0^\pi \frac{(1 - \cos^2\theta)}{\left(\dfrac{\bar{r}}{a} - \cos\theta\right)}\, d\theta$

$\qquad\qquad = 2a \displaystyle\int_0^\pi \frac{(1 - \cos^2\theta)}{(b - \cos\theta)}\, d\theta \qquad\qquad \left[\text{Let } \dfrac{\bar{r}}{a} = b\right]$

$\qquad\qquad = 2a \displaystyle\int_0^\pi \left\{\frac{b^2 + b\cos\theta - b^2 - b\cos\theta + 1 - \cos^2\theta}{b - \cos\theta}\right\}\, d\theta$

(Adding and subtracting $(b^2 + b\cos\theta)$ in the numerator to bring the expression in its standard form)

$\qquad\qquad = 2a \displaystyle\int_0^\pi \left\{\frac{b^2 - b\cos\theta + b\cos\theta - \cos^2\theta + 1 - b^2}{b - \cos\theta}\right\}\, d\theta$

$\qquad\qquad = 2a \displaystyle\int_0^\pi \left\{\frac{b(b - \cos\theta) + \cos\theta(b - \cos\theta) + (1 - b^2)}{b - \cos\theta}\right\}\, d\theta$

$\qquad\qquad = 2a \displaystyle\int_0^\pi \left\{(b + \cos\theta) + \frac{(1 - b^2)}{(b - \cos\theta)}\right\}\, d\theta$

$\qquad\qquad = 2ab \displaystyle\int_0^\pi d\theta + 2a \int_0^\pi \cos\theta\, d\theta + 2a \cdot (1 - b^2) \int_0^\pi \frac{d\theta}{(b - \cos\theta)}$

$\qquad\qquad = 2ab\pi + 2a \times 0 + 2a(1 - b^2) \displaystyle\int_0^\pi \frac{d\theta}{(b - \cos\theta)}$

$\qquad\qquad = 2ab\pi + 2a(1 - b^2) \displaystyle\int_0^\pi \frac{\left(\cos^2\dfrac{\theta}{2} + \sin^2\dfrac{\theta}{2}\right)}{b\left(\cos^2\dfrac{\theta}{2} + \sin^2\dfrac{\theta}{2}\right) - \left(\cos^2\dfrac{\theta}{2} - \sin^2\dfrac{\theta}{2}\right)}\, d\theta$

$\qquad\qquad = 2ab\pi + 2a(1 - b^2) \displaystyle\int_0^\pi \frac{\left(1 + \tan^2\dfrac{\theta}{2}\right) d\theta}{b\left(1 + \tan^2\dfrac{\theta}{2}\right) - \left(1 - \tan^2\dfrac{\theta}{2}\right)}\, d\theta$

$$= 2ab\pi + 2a\,(1-b^2)\int_0^\pi \frac{\sec^2\dfrac{\theta}{2}\,d\theta}{b + b\tan^2\dfrac{\theta}{2} - 1 + \tan^2\dfrac{\theta}{2}}$$

$$= 2ab\pi + 2a\,(1-b^2)\int_0^\pi \frac{\sec^2\dfrac{\theta}{2}\,d\theta}{(b-1) + \tan^2\dfrac{\theta}{2}(b+1)}$$

$$= 2ab\pi + \frac{2a\,(1-b^2)}{(b+1)}\int_0^\pi \frac{\sec^2\dfrac{\theta}{2}\,d\theta}{\tan^2\dfrac{\theta}{2} + \left(\dfrac{b-1}{b+1}\right)}$$

$$= 2ab\pi + 2a\,(1-b)\int_0^\pi \frac{\sec^2\dfrac{\theta}{2}\,d\theta}{\tan^2\dfrac{\theta}{2} + \left(\sqrt{\dfrac{b-1}{b+1}}\right)^2}$$

Let $\tan\left(\dfrac{\theta}{2}\right) = t$

$\therefore \qquad \sec^2\dfrac{\theta}{2}\cdot\dfrac{1}{2}\cdot d\theta = dt$

$\Rightarrow \qquad \sec^2\dfrac{\theta}{2}\,d\theta = 2dt$

When, $\theta = 0, t = 0$

When, $\theta = \pi; t = \infty$

Hence, the above expression reduces to

$$2ab\pi + 2a\,(1-b)\int_0^\infty \frac{2dt}{t^2 + \left(\sqrt{\dfrac{b+1}{b-1}}\right)^2}$$

$$= 2ab\pi + 4a\,(1-b)\left[\sqrt{\frac{b+1}{b-1}}\,\tan^{-1}\left(t + \sqrt{\frac{b+1}{b-1}}\right)\right]_0^\infty$$

$$= 2ab\pi + 4a\,(1-b)\sqrt{\frac{b+1}{b-1}}\,[\tan^{-1}(\infty) - \tan^{-1}(0)]$$

$$= 2ab\pi - 4a\,\sqrt{b^2 - 1}\times\frac{\pi}{2}$$

$$= 2ab\pi - 2a\left(\sqrt{b^2 - 1}\right)\pi$$

$$= 2\bar{r} + \frac{\bar{r}}{\bar{r}}\pi - 2a\left(\sqrt{b^2 - 1}\right)\pi$$

$$= 2\bar{r}\pi - \left\{2a\sqrt{\frac{\bar{r}^2}{a^2} - 1}\right\}\pi$$

$$= 2\bar{r}\pi - \left\{2\sqrt{\bar{r}^2 - a^2}\right\}\pi$$

$$= 2\bar{r}\pi - \left\{2\sqrt{\bar{r}^2 - \frac{d^2}{4}}\right\}\pi$$

$$= 2\bar{r}\pi - \sqrt{4\bar{r}^2 - d^2}\ \pi$$

$$= \pi(2\bar{r} - \sqrt{4\bar{r}^2 - d^2})$$

$$\therefore \quad \int\frac{dA}{r} = \pi\,(2\bar{r} - \sqrt{4\bar{r}^2 - d^2})$$

Hence, R_N for circular section $= \dfrac{A}{\displaystyle\int\frac{dA}{r}}$

$$= \frac{\dfrac{\pi}{4}d^2}{\pi\,(2\bar{r} - \sqrt{4\bar{r}^2 - d^2})}$$

$$\boxed{\therefore \ R_N = \frac{d^2}{4\,(2\bar{r} - \sqrt{4\bar{r}^2 - d^2})}} \qquad \text{Form I}$$

Once the R_N is derived/evaluated, we can compute bending stress at inner most fibre and outermost fibre by applying the following formula

$$\sigma_{b_i} = \frac{M\,(R_N - r_i)}{A\cdot r_i\,(\bar{r} - R_N)}$$

$$= \frac{M\cdot(R_N - r_i)}{A\cdot r_i\cdot e}$$

Similarly, $\sigma_{b_o} = \dfrac{M\cdot(R_N - r_o)}{A\cdot r_o\,(\bar{r} - R_N)}$

$$= \frac{M\cdot(R_N - r_o)}{A\cdot r_o\cdot e}$$

We can derive R_N for circular section in terms of r_i and r_o as below:

$$R_N \text{ for circular section} = \frac{d^2}{4\left(2\bar{r} - \sqrt{4\bar{r}^2 - d^2}\right)}$$

From figure we have, $d = (r_o - r_i)$

and $\quad \bar{r} = \left(r_i + \frac{d}{2}\right)$

$$= \left\{r_i + \frac{(r_o - r_i)}{2}\right\}$$

$$= \left\{\frac{(r_i + r_o)}{2}\right\}$$

Now, substituting the value of $\bar{r}$ and d, we get

$$R_N = \frac{(r_o - r_i)^2}{4\left\{\frac{2(r_i + r_o)}{2} - \sqrt{4\left(\frac{r_i + r_o}{2}\right)^2 - (r_o - r_i)^2}\right\}}$$

$$= \frac{(r_o - r_i)^2}{4\left\{(r_o + r_i) - \sqrt{(r_o + r_i)^2 - (r_o - r_i)^2}\right\}}$$

$$= \frac{(r_o - r_i)^2}{4\left\{r_i + r_o - 2\sqrt{r_i r_o}\right\}}$$

$$= \frac{\left\{\left(\sqrt{r_o}\right)^2 - \left(\sqrt{r_i}\right)^2\right\}^2}{4\left(\sqrt{r_o} - \sqrt{r_i}\right)^2}$$

$$= \frac{(\sqrt{r_o} + \sqrt{r_i})^2 \, (\sqrt{r_o} - \sqrt{r_i})^2}{4\left(\sqrt{r_o} - \sqrt{r_i}\right)^2}$$

$$\boxed{\therefore \ R_N = \frac{(\sqrt{r_i} + \sqrt{r_o})^2}{4}} \qquad \text{Form II}$$

R_N can be computed from Form I or from Form II.

N.B.: Readers may prefer formula Form-II for R_N for circular section, being easy to remember for solving problem.

T-section

The given figure 19.7, shows a T-section of curved beam. Consider a strip of width '*b*' and depth *dr* at a distance *r* from axis of curvature, then

$$R_N = \frac{A}{\int \frac{dA}{r}}$$

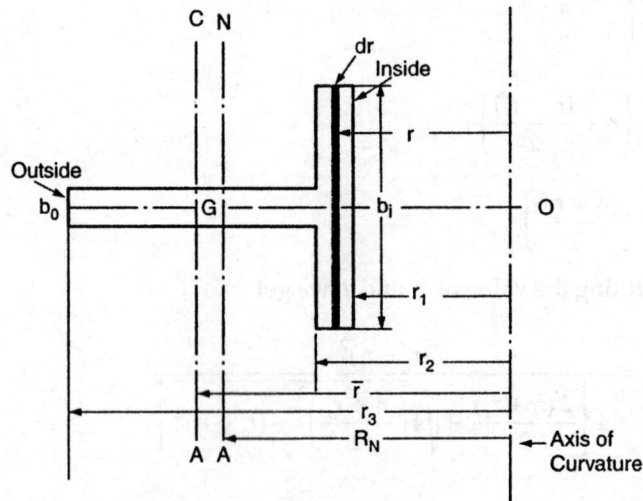

Fig. 19.7

Total area of T-section $(A) = b_i \, (r_2 - r_1) + b_o \, (r_3 - r_2)$

$$\int \frac{dA}{r} = \int_{r_1}^{r_2} \frac{b_i \cdot dr}{r} + \int_{r_2}^{r_3} \frac{b_o \cdot dr}{r}$$

$$= b_i \cdot \ln\left(\frac{r_2}{r_1}\right) + b_o \cdot \ln\left(\frac{r_3}{r_2}\right)$$

∴ R_N for T- section $= \dfrac{b_i \, (r_2 - r_1) + b_c \, (r_3 - r_2)}{b_i' \cdot \ln\left(\dfrac{r_2}{r_1}\right) + b_o \cdot \ln\left(\dfrac{r_3}{r_2}\right)}$

Now, stresses at inside and outside surfaces of the T-section can be computed by applying the formula derived on Page 19.4 by equation (5).

I-section

The given figure 19.8 shows the I-section of a curved beam. Consider a strip of width '*b*' and depth *dr* at a distance *r* from axis of curvature.

$$R_N = \frac{A}{\int \frac{dA}{r}}$$

$$\int \frac{dA}{r} = \int_{r_1}^{r_2} \frac{b_1 \cdot dr}{r} + \int_{r_2}^{r_3} \frac{b_2 \cdot dr}{r} + +\int_{r_3}^{r_4} \frac{b_3 \cdot dr}{r}$$

$$= b_1 \cdot \ln\left(\frac{r_2}{r_1}\right) + b_2 \cdot \ln\left(\frac{r_3}{r_2}\right) + b_3 \cdot \ln\left(\frac{r_4}{r_3}\right)$$

A = Total area of the I-section

$$= b_1 (r_2 - r_1) + b_2 (r_3 - r_2) + b_3 (r_4 - r_3)$$

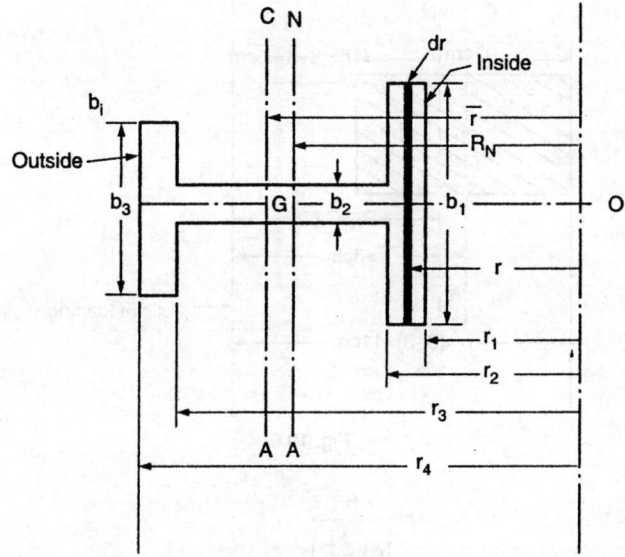

Fig. 19.8

$$\therefore \quad R_N = \frac{A}{\int \frac{dA}{r}}$$

$$= \frac{b_1 (r_2 - r_1) + b_2 (r_3 - r_2) + b_3 (r_4 - r_3)}{b_1 \cdot \ln\left(\frac{r_2}{r_1}\right) + b_2 \cdot \ln\left(\frac{r_3}{r_2}\right) + b_3 \cdot \ln\left(\frac{r_4}{r_3}\right)}$$

Now, stresses at inside and outside surfaces can be computed as discussed earlier by equation (5) on Page 19.4.

SOLVED EXAMPLES

EXAMPLE 1 *Determine the ratio of maximum and minimum values of the stresses for a curved bar of rectangular section in pure bending. Radius of Curvature is 8 cm and depth of the beam is 6 cm. Locate neutral axis.* [UPTU 2001-2002]

SOLUTION Here, $h = 6$ cm

$$\therefore \quad r_i = \bar{r} - \frac{h}{2}$$

$$= (8-3) = 5 \text{ cm}$$

$$r_o = r_i + h = 5 + 6 = 11 \text{ cm} \quad \text{or} \quad \bar{r} + \frac{h}{2} = 8 + 3 = 11 \text{ cm}$$

Location of N.A $(R_N) = \dfrac{h}{\ln\left(\dfrac{r_o}{r_i}\right)}$

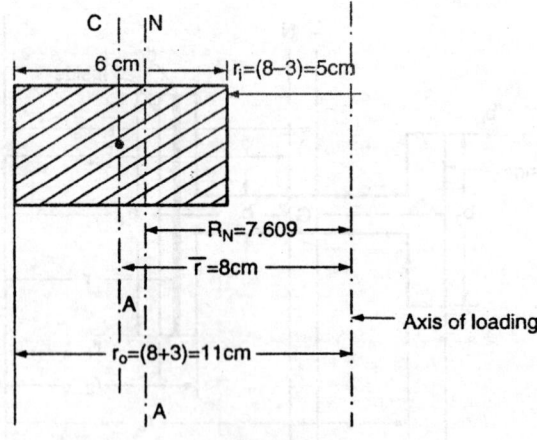

Fig. 19.9

$$= \frac{6}{\ln\left(\dfrac{11}{5}\right)}$$

$$= 7.609$$

$\therefore$ $\quad R_N = 7.609$

$\therefore$ $\quad$ Eccentricity $(e) = (\bar{r} - R_N)$

$$= (8 - 7.6) = 0.4 \text{ cm}$$

$$e = 4 \text{ mm}$$

From the Figure 19.9, it is obvious that maximum stress will develop at inner surface and minimum stress will develop at the outer surface.

Stress developed at innerside surface $(\sigma_i) = \dfrac{M(R_N - r_i)}{A \cdot r_i (\bar{r} - R_N)}$

$$= \frac{M(7.6 - 5)}{A \times 5 \times 0.4}$$

Similarly, stress at outerside surface $(\sigma_o) = \dfrac{M(R_N - r_o)}{A \cdot r_o (\bar{r} - R_N)} = \dfrac{M(7.6 - 11)}{A \times 11 \times 0.4}$

$$\therefore \quad \frac{\sigma_i}{\sigma_o} = \frac{M(7.6-5)}{A \times 5 \times 0.4} \times \frac{A \times 11 \times 0.4}{M(7.6-11)} = -\left(\frac{2.6 \times 11}{5 \times 3.4}\right)$$

= 1.682. Neglecting $\ominus$ minus sign as ratio is always positive. **Ans.**

EXAMPLE 2 *Compare stress and state your comment for the following:*

(i) *A straight beam 50 mm × 50 mm subjected to 2085 NM.*

(ii) *beam curved to radius 250 mm.*

(iii) *beam curved to radius $\bar{r} = 75$ mm.*

SOLUTION

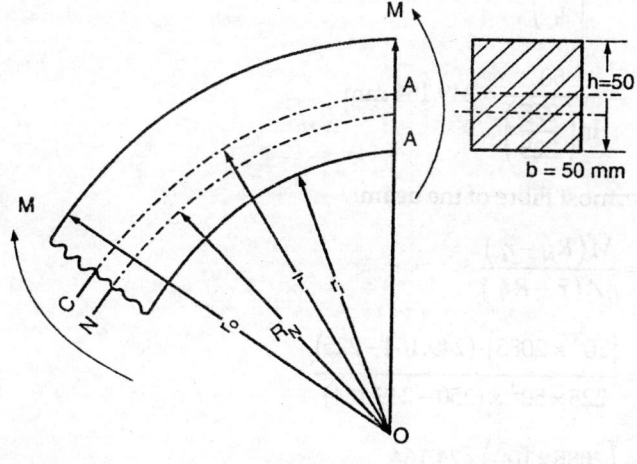

Fig. 19.10

(i) Section Modulus $(z) = \dfrac{bh^2}{6}$

$$= \left[\frac{50 \times (50)^2}{6}\right]$$

$$= 20.83 \times 10^3 \text{ mm}^3$$

$$\sigma_{max} = \left[\frac{M}{Z}\right]$$

$$= \frac{2085 \times 10^3}{20.83 \times 103}\left[\frac{N \text{ mm}}{\text{mm}^3}\right] = 100.09 \text{ N/mm}^2$$

$$= 100 \text{ N/mm}^2$$

$$= 100 \text{ MPa} \qquad\qquad \left[1 \text{ MPa} = 1 \text{ N/mm}^2\right]$$

(ii) Given, $h = 50$ mm

$\bar{r} = 250$ mm

$r_i = 225$ mm

$r_o = 275$ mm

Location of neutral axis

$$R_N = \frac{h}{\ln\left(\dfrac{r_o}{r_i}\right)}$$

$$= \frac{50}{\ln\left(\dfrac{275}{225}\right)} = 249.164 \text{ mm}$$

Stress at innermost Fibre of the beam

$$\sigma_i = \frac{M(R_N - r_i)}{r_i A(\bar{r} - R_N)}$$

$$= \frac{\left(10^3 \times 2085\right) \cdot (249.164 - 225)}{225 \times 50^2 \times (250 - 249.164)}$$

$$= \frac{\left(2085 \times 10^3\right) \times 24.164}{225 \times 0.836 \times 2500} \text{ N/mm}^2$$

$$= 107.13 \text{ N/mm}^2$$

$$= 107 \text{ MPa} \quad \textbf{Ans.}$$

Stress at outermost Fibre of the beam,

$$\sigma_o = \frac{M(R_N - r_o)}{r_o A(\bar{r} - R_N)}$$

$$= \frac{\left(10^3 \times 2085\right) \times (249.164 - 275)}{275 \times 50^2 \times 0.836}$$

$$= -\frac{2085 \times 25.836 \times 10^3}{275 \times 2500 \times 0.836}$$

$$= -93.72 \text{ N/mm}^2$$

$$\simeq -94 \text{ MPa}$$

Thus, tensile stress of magnitude 107 MPa is developed at the inner surface and compressive stress of magnitude 94 MPa is developed at the outer surface.

(iii) In this case $h = 50$ mm

$$\overline{r} = 75 \text{ mm}$$
$$r_i = 50 \text{ mm}$$
$$r_o = 100 \text{ mm}$$

Location of N.A $(R_N) = \dfrac{h}{\ln\left(\dfrac{r_o}{r_i}\right)}$

$$= \dfrac{50}{\ln\left(\dfrac{100}{50}\right)}$$

$$= \dfrac{50}{\ln(2)}$$

$$= 72.134 \text{ mm}$$

Eccentricity $(e) = (\overline{r} - R_N)$

$$= (75 - 72.13) \text{ mm}$$

$$= 2.87 \text{ mm}$$

Stress at inner surface $(\sigma_i) = \dfrac{M \cdot (R_N - r_i)}{r_i \cdot A \cdot (\overline{r} - R_N)}$

$$= \dfrac{\left(2085 \times 10^3\right) \times (72.13 - 50)}{50 \times 50^2 \times 2.87} \text{ N/mm}^2$$

$$= \dfrac{2085 \times 10^3 \times 22.13}{50 \times 2500 \times 2.87} \text{ N/mm}^2$$

$$= 128.6 \text{ MPa}$$

$$\simeq 129 \text{ MPa}$$

Stress at outer surface $(\sigma_o) = \dfrac{M(R_N - r_o)}{r_o \cdot A \cdot (\overline{r} - R_N)}$

$$= \dfrac{\left(2085 \times 10^3\right) \times (72.13 - 100)}{100 \times 50^2 \times 2.87}$$

$$= \dfrac{(-)\, 2085 \times 10^3 \times 27.87}{2500 \times 287} \text{ N/mm}^2$$

$$= -80.98 \text{ N/mm}^2$$

$$= -81 \text{ MPa}$$

Inference

(i) Flexural formula is good for beam of large radius $(r = \infty)$

(ii) In part (ii) $\sigma = 107$ MPa.

Hence, $\left(\dfrac{107-100}{100}\right) \times 100 = 7\%$ error was found in the maximum stress.

(iii) In part (ii) $\sigma = 129$ MPa

Hence, 29% error occurs.

Summary of the solution: As the Curvature of beam increases the stress on the concave side rapidly increases.

EXAMPLE 3 *A Cranehook has a trapezoidal cross-section as shown below.*
Determine the maximum load to be carried by the hook if the working stress is 150 MN/M^2.

SOLUTION

$\qquad$ $CA \Rightarrow$ Controidal Axis

$\qquad$ $NA \Rightarrow$ Neutral Axis

Let b_i and b_0 are width of inside and outside section.

We have, $\qquad h = (r_0 - r_i)$

$\qquad\qquad\qquad = (90 - 50)$

$\qquad\qquad\qquad = 40$ mm

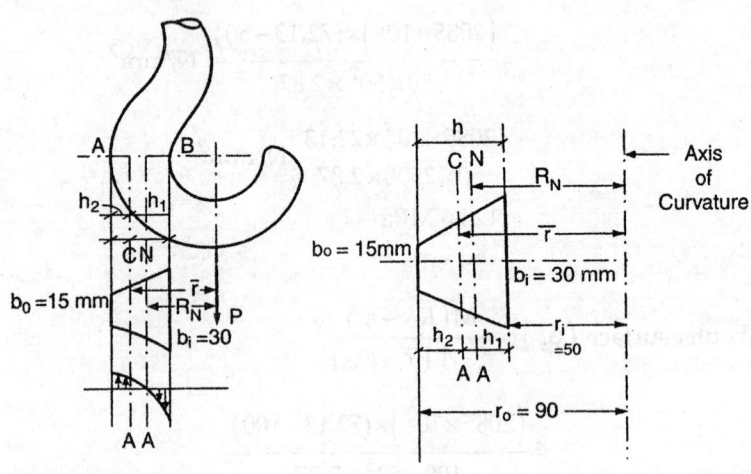

Fig. 19.11

$$h_1 = \frac{h}{3} \cdot \left(\frac{b_i + 2b_0}{b_i + b_0} \right)$$

$$= \frac{40}{3} \cdot \left(\frac{30 + 2 \times 15}{30 + 15} \right)$$

$$= \left(\frac{160}{9} \right) mm$$

$$\bar{r} = (r_i + h_i)$$

$$= \left(50 + \frac{160}{9} \right)$$

$$= \left(\frac{610}{9} \right)$$

$$= 67.77 \text{ mm}$$

R_N = Radius of Neutral Axis of trapezoidal section.

$$= \frac{A}{(b_o - b_i) + \left(\dfrac{b_i r_o - b_o r_i}{h} \right) \cdot \ln\left(\dfrac{r_o}{r_i} \right)}$$

$$= \frac{\dfrac{1}{2} \times h (b_o + b_i)}{(b_o - b_i) + \left(\dfrac{b_i r_o - b_o r_i}{h} \right) \cdot \ln\left(\dfrac{r_o}{r_i} \right)}$$

$$= \frac{\dfrac{1}{2} \times 40 \times (30 + 15)}{(15 - 30) + \left(\dfrac{30 \times 90 - 15 \times 50}{40} \right) \cdot \ln\left(\dfrac{90}{50} \right)}$$

$$= \frac{20 \times 45}{-15 + \dfrac{1950}{40} \times \ln\left(\dfrac{9}{5} \right)}$$

$$= \frac{900}{-15 + 48.75 \times \ln\left(\dfrac{9}{5} \right)}$$

$R_N = 65.91 \text{ mm}$.

Shifting of N.A *i.e.* eccentricity $(e) = (\bar{r} - R_N)$

$$= (67.77 - 65.91) \text{ mm}$$

$$= 1.86 \text{ mm}$$

Now, bending stress at inner surface

$$\sigma_{b_i} = \left\{ \frac{M \cdot (R_N - r_i)}{A \cdot r_i \cdot e} \right\}$$

$$= \frac{(P \cdot \bar{r}) \cdot (R_N - r_i)}{A \cdot r_i \cdot e}$$

$$= \frac{(P \times 67.77) \times (65.91 - 50)}{900 \times 50 \times 1.86}$$

$$= \frac{P \times 67.77 \times 15.91}{900 \times 50 \times 1.86}$$

$$= 0.01288 \ P \ \text{N/mm}^2$$

Direct stress at the inner surface

$$\sigma_{d_i} = \frac{P}{A}$$

$$= \frac{P}{900} \ \text{N/mm}^2$$

∴   Total stress (Tensile) at the inner surface

$$= \sigma_{bi} + \sigma_{di}$$

$$= \left[0.01288 \ P + \frac{P}{900} \right] \ \text{N/mm}^2 \qquad \qquad \text{...(i)}$$

Given, working stress $= 150 \ \text{MN/m}^2$

$$= 150 \times 10^6 \ \text{N/m}^2$$

$$= 150 \ \text{N/mm}^2 \qquad \qquad \text{...(ii)}$$

Equating these two

$$0.01288 \ P + \frac{P}{900} = 150$$

$$P = 10791.36 \ \text{N}$$

$$= 10.791 \ \text{kN}.$$

$$\boxed{\therefore \ P_{max} = 10.8 \ \text{kN}} \quad \textbf{Ans.}$$

EXAMPLE 4 *A Crane hook whose horizontal cross-section is trapezoidal, 50 mm wide at the inside and 25 mm wide at the outside, thickness 50 mm carries a vertical load of 1000 Kg whose line of action is 38 mm from the inside edge of this section.*

The centre of Curvature is 50 mm from the inside edge. Calculate the maximum tensile and compressive stresses set-up.

SOLUTION

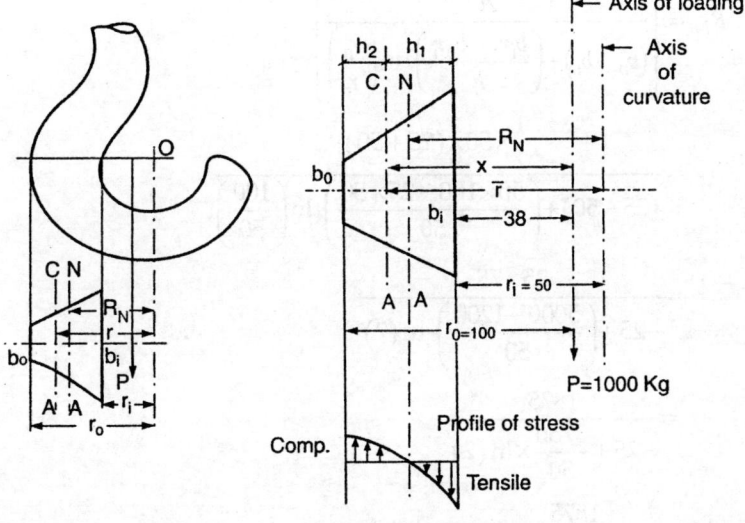

Fig. 19.12

Given, $r_i = 50$ mm

$\quad\quad r_o = 100$ mm

$\quad\quad b_i = 50$ mm

$\quad\quad b_o = 25$ mm

$\quad\quad \bar{r} = (50 + h_1)$ mm

$\quad\quad h = (100 - 50) = 50$ mm

$\quad\quad P = 1000$ Kg

$\quad\quad\quad = (1000 \times 9.81)$ Newton

$\quad\quad\quad = 9810$ Newton.

Now,

By formula, $h_1 = \dfrac{h}{3}\left(\dfrac{b_i + 2b_o}{b_i + b_o}\right)$

$\quad\quad\quad = \dfrac{50}{3}\left(\dfrac{50 + 2 \times 25}{50 + 25}\right)$

$\quad\quad\quad = 22.2$ mm.

Location of Centroidal axis $(\bar{r}) = (r_i + h_1)$

$\quad\quad\quad\quad\quad\quad = (50 + 22.2)$

$\quad\quad\quad\quad\quad\quad = 72.2$ mm

Location of Neutral axis

$$RN = \left\{ \frac{A}{(b_o - b_i) + \left(\frac{b_i r_o - b_o r_i}{h} \right) \cdot \ln\left(\frac{r_o}{r_i} \right)} \right\}$$

$$= \frac{\frac{1}{2} \times 50 \times (25 + 50)}{(25 - 50) + \left(\frac{50 \times 100 - 25 \times 50}{50} \right) \cdot \ln\left(\frac{100}{50} \right)}$$

$$= \frac{25 \times 75}{-25 + \left(\frac{5000 - 1200}{50} \right) \cdot \ln(2)}$$

$$= \frac{1875}{-25 + \frac{3750}{50} \times \ln(2)}$$

$$= \frac{1875}{-25 + 75 . \ln(2)}$$

$$= 69.48 \text{ mm} .$$

$\therefore$ Shift of the neutral axis $(e) = (\bar{r} - R_N)$

$$= (72.22 - 69.48)$$

$$= 2.74 \text{ mm}$$

Moment $= P \cdot x$ Nmm

$$= (1000 \times 9.81) x \text{ Nmm}$$

$$= 9810 (38 + h_1)$$

$$= 9810 (38 + 22.2)$$

$$= 590562 \text{ N.mm}$$

At the inside edge

$$\sigma_b = \frac{M(R_N - r_i)}{A \cdot r_i \cdot e}$$

$$= \left\{ \frac{(9810 \times 60.2)(69.5 - 50)}{1875 \times 50 \times 2.75} \right\}$$

$$= 44.66 \text{ N/mm}^2$$

$$\sigma_d = \frac{P}{A}$$

$$= \left(\frac{1000 \times 9.81}{1875} \right) = 5.23 \text{ N/mm}^2$$

$\therefore \qquad \sigma_{max} = \sigma_b + \sigma_d$

$$= \left(44.66 + 5.23 \right) \ \text{N/mm}^2$$

$$= 49.89 \ \text{N/mm}^2 \ \text{(Tensile)} \ \textbf{Ans.}$$

At the outside edge

$$\sigma_o = \frac{M \cdot (R_N - r_o)}{A \cdot r_o \cdot e}$$

$$= \frac{(9810 \times 62.2) \times (69.45 - 100)}{1875 \times 100 \times 2.75}$$

$$= -36.15 \ \text{N/mm}^2$$

$\therefore \qquad \sigma_{min} = \sigma_o + \dfrac{P}{A}$

$$= -36.15 + 5.23$$

$$= -30.92 \ \text{N/mm}^2 \ \ \text{(Compressive)} \ \ \textbf{Ans.}$$

EXAMPLE 5 *Calculate the extreme intensities of stress when the hook carries a load of 30 kN, the load line passing 40 mm from the inside edge of the section and the centre of curvature being in the load line.* **[UPTU 2002-2003]**

SOLUTION

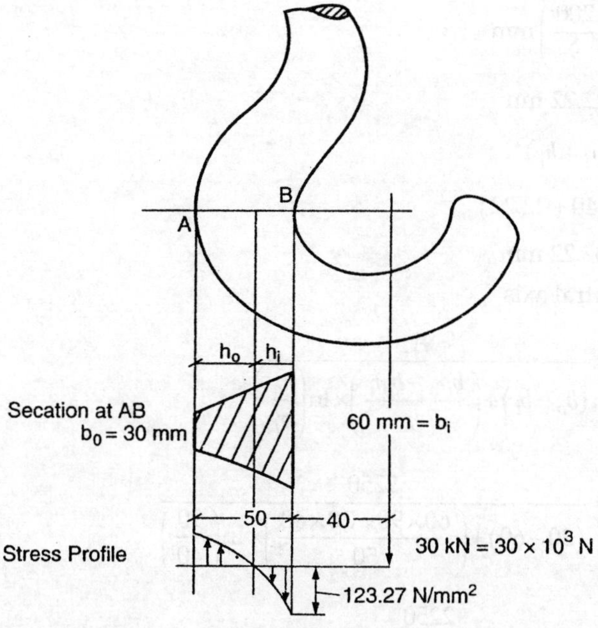

Fig. 19.13

The section of hook at *AB* is shown in Fig. 19.13. It is trapezium in shape.

So, the area of the section,

$$A = \frac{1}{2} \times h \left(b_i + b_o \right)$$

$$= \frac{1}{2} \times 50 \left(60 + 30 \right)$$

$$= 25 \times 90 \ \text{mm}^2$$

$$= 2250 \ \text{mm}^2$$

Further, it is given $r_i = 40$ mm

$$r_o = 90 \ \text{mm}$$

$$\bar{r} = \left(40 + h_i \right) \text{mm}$$

Now, $h_i = \dfrac{h}{3} \left(\dfrac{b_i + 2b_o}{b_o + b_i} \right)$

$$= \frac{50}{3} \left(\frac{60 + 2 \times 30}{30 + 60} \right)$$

$$= \frac{50}{3} \times \frac{120}{90}$$

$$= \left(\frac{200}{9} \right) \text{mm}$$

$$= 22.22 \ \text{mm}$$

$$\therefore \qquad \bar{r} = \left(r_i + h_i \right)$$

$$= \left(40 + 22.22 \right)$$

$$= 62.22 \ \text{mm}$$

Radius of neutral axis

$$R_N = \frac{A}{\left(b_o - b_i \right) + \left(\dfrac{b_i r_o - b_o r_i}{h} \right) \times \ln \left(\dfrac{r_o}{r_i} \right)}$$

$$= \frac{2250}{\left(30 - 60 \right) + \left(\dfrac{60 \times 90 - 30 \times 40}{50} \right) \times \ln \left(\dfrac{90}{40} \right)}$$

$$= \frac{2250}{-30 + \left(\dfrac{5400 - 1200}{3} \right) \times \ln \left(\dfrac{9}{4} \right)}$$

$$= \frac{2250}{-30 + 68.12}$$

$$= 59.024 \text{ mm}.$$

Eccentricity $(e) = (\bar{r} - R_N)$

$$= (62.22 - 59.02)$$

$$= 3.19$$

$$\simeq 3.2 \text{ mm}$$

Bending stress at inside of hook

$$\sigma_{bi} = \frac{M(R_N - r_i)}{A \cdot r_i \cdot e}$$

$$= \frac{(P \cdot \bar{r}) \cdot (R_N - r_i)}{A \cdot r_i \cdot e}$$

$$= \frac{(30 \times 10^3 \times 62.22)(59.024 - 40)}{2250 \times 40 \times 3.2} \qquad \left[\begin{array}{l} \bar{r} = 40 + h_i = 40 + 22.22 \\ = 62.22 \end{array} \right]$$

$$= 123.27 \text{ N/mm}^2$$

$$\sigma \text{ direct} = \left(\frac{P}{A} \right)$$

$$= \left(\frac{30 \times 10^3}{2250} \right)$$

$$= 13.33 \text{ N/mm}^2$$

$\therefore \qquad \sigma \text{ total} = (123.27 + 13.33)$

$$= 136.60 \text{ N/mm}^2$$

$$= 136.6 \text{ MPa}. \textbf{ Ans.}$$

This is the maximum stress developed (tensile in nature) inside fibre of hook.

[**N.B**: Minimum stress will be induced at outside surface (compressive in nature) and its magnitude will be

$$\sigma_{min} = \left[\sigma_{b_o} + \frac{P}{A} \right]$$

$\therefore \qquad \sigma_{b_o} = \frac{M(R_N - r_o)}{A \cdot r_o \cdot e}$

$$= \frac{(30 \times 10^3 \times 62.22) \times (59.02 - 90)}{2250 \times 100 \times 3.2}$$

$$= -80.315 \text{ N/mm}^2$$

$\therefore$ $\sigma_{min} = \sigma_{b_o} + \dfrac{P}{A}$

$$= -80.315 + 13.33 = -66.98 \text{ N/mm}^2]$$

EXAMPLE 6 *A Curved beam with circular Centre line has inverted T-Section as shown in Fig. 19.11 and subjected to pure bending in the two planes of symmetry.*
Find the dimension (b_i) in order to have equal tensile and compressive stress in the extreme fibre.

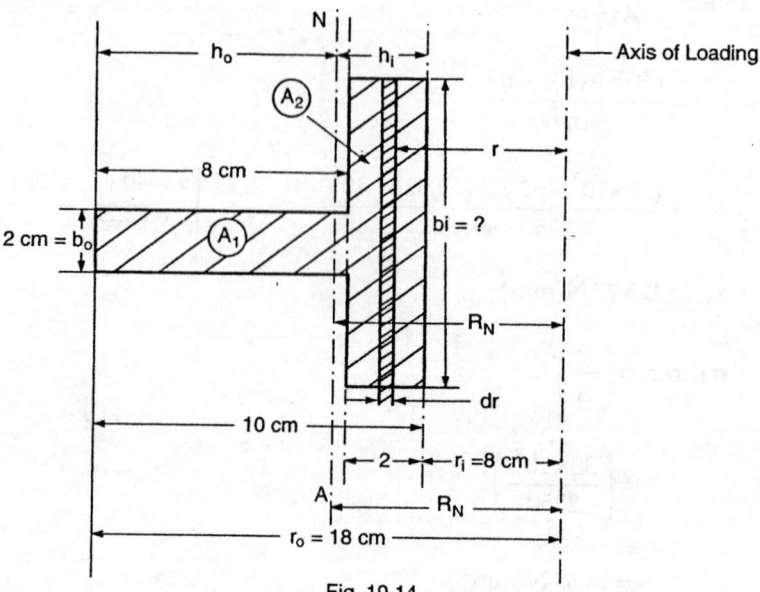

Fig. 19.14

SOLUTION Given $|\sigma_{max}| = |\sigma_{min}|$

$\Rightarrow$ $\dfrac{M(R_N - r_i)}{A \cdot r_i \cdot e} = \dfrac{M(R_N - r_o)}{A \cdot r_o \cdot e}$

$\Rightarrow$ $\dfrac{R_N - r_i}{R_N - r_o} = \dfrac{r_i}{r_o}$

$\Rightarrow$ $\dfrac{h_i}{h_o} = \dfrac{r_i}{r_o} = \dfrac{8}{18} = \dfrac{4}{9}$

Also, $(h_i + h_o) = 10$ cm (given)

As, $\dfrac{h_i}{h_o} = \dfrac{4}{9}$

$\therefore \qquad \dfrac{h_i + h_o}{h_o} = \dfrac{4+9}{9}$

$\dfrac{10}{h_o} = \dfrac{13}{9}$

$h_o = \left(\dfrac{90}{13}\right)$

$\therefore \qquad h_i = (10 - h_o)$

$\qquad\quad = \left(10 - \dfrac{90}{13}\right)$

$\qquad\quad = \left(\dfrac{40}{13}\right)$

$\qquad\quad = 3.07$ cm. $\simeq 3$ cm (let)

Now, $\qquad \displaystyle\int \dfrac{dA}{r} = \int_8^{10} \dfrac{b_i dr}{r} + \int_{10}^{18} \dfrac{b_o dr}{r}$

$\qquad\qquad\quad = b_i \left[\log r\right]_8^{10} + b_o \left[\log r\right]_{10}^{18}$

$\qquad\qquad\quad = \left[b_i \log\left(\dfrac{10}{8}\right) + b_o \log\left(\dfrac{18}{10}\right)\right]$

$\qquad\qquad\quad = (0.223\, b_i + 0.588 \times 2)$

In this problem,

$R_N = \dfrac{(A_1 + A_2)}{\displaystyle\int \dfrac{dA}{r}}$

For Rectangular Section here $R_N = \dfrac{2 \times 8 + 2\, b_i}{0.223\, b_i + 0.588 \times 2}$ ...(1)

From Fig. 19.14 $R_N = (r_i + h_i)$

$\qquad\qquad = 8 + 3$

$\qquad\qquad = 11$ cm ...(2)

From (i) and (ii)

$\qquad \dfrac{16 + 2\, b_i}{0.223\, b_i + 0.588 \times 2} = 11$

$\Rightarrow \qquad b_i = 6.76$ cm

$\qquad\qquad = 67.6$ mm   **Ans.**

EXAMPLE 7 *A hook of circular section 25 mm diameter and radius of curvature of its central axis is 25 mm carries a load of 5 kN. Calculate the maximum stress in the hook.*

SOLUTION   Given: $d = 25$ mm

$$\bar{r} = 25 \text{ mm}$$

$$P = 5 \text{ kN}$$

$$r_A = \left(\bar{r} - \frac{d}{2} \right) = (25 - 12.5)$$

$$= 12.5 \text{ mm}$$

$$r_B = \left(\bar{r} + \frac{d}{2} \right) = 37.5 \text{ mm}$$

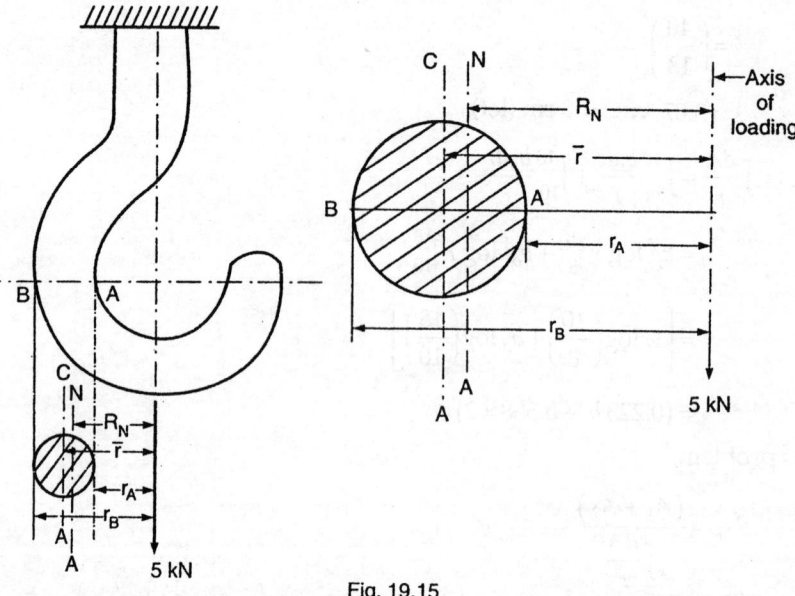

Fig. 19.15

First, radius of neutral axis will be computed. We know that for circular cross-section,

$$R_N = \frac{d^2}{4 \left(2 \times \bar{r} - \sqrt{4 \times \bar{r}^2 - d^2} \right)}$$

[**N.B.:** To compute R_N, we can also use form-II *i.e.*, $R_N = \dfrac{(\sqrt{r_i} + \sqrt{r_o})^2}{4}$ which will give the same result as above.]

$$\therefore \qquad R_N = \frac{(25)^2}{4 \left(2 \times 25 - \sqrt{4 \times (25)^2 - (25)^2} \right)}$$

$$= \frac{625}{4\left(50 - \sqrt{4 \times 625 - 625}\right)}$$

$$= \frac{625}{4\left(50 - 25\sqrt{3}\right)}$$

$$= \frac{625}{4 \times (50 - 25 \times 1.732)}$$

$$= \frac{625}{4 \times 6.7}$$

$$= 23.32 \text{ mm}$$

Eccentricity $(e) = (\bar{r} - R_N) = (25 - 23.32) = 1.68$ mm

$$\therefore \qquad \sigma_A = \frac{M(R_N - r_A)}{A \cdot r_A \cdot e} + \frac{P}{A}$$

$$= \frac{(P \cdot \bar{r})(R_N - r_A)}{A \cdot r_A \cdot e} + \frac{P}{A} \qquad\qquad [\because \ M = P\bar{r}]$$

$$= \frac{\left(5 \times 10^3 \times 25\right)(23.32 - 12.5)}{\frac{\pi}{4} \times (25)^2 \times 12.5 \times 1.68} + \frac{5 \times 10^3}{\frac{\pi}{4} \times (25)^2}$$

$$= \frac{125 \times 10^3 \times 10.82 \times 4}{3.14 \times 625 \times 12.5 \times 1.68} + \frac{5 \times 4 \times 10^3}{3.14 \times 625}$$

$$= \frac{125 \times 10820 \times 4}{3.14 \times 625 \times 12.5 \times 1.68} + \frac{20 \times 10^3}{3.14 \times 625}$$

$$= 131.27 + 10.19 \text{ N/mm}^2$$

$$= 141.46 \text{ N/mm}^2$$

$$\boxed{\sigma_A = 141.46 \text{ MPa (Tensile)}.} \quad \textbf{Ans.}$$

$$\sigma_B = \frac{M(R_N - r_B)}{A \cdot r_B \cdot e} + \frac{P}{A}$$

$$= \frac{\left(5 \times 10^3 \times 25\right)(23.32 - 37.5)}{\frac{\pi}{4} \times (25)^2 \times 37.5 \times 1.68} + \frac{5 \times 10^3}{\frac{\pi}{4} \times (25)^2}$$

$$= -\frac{125 \times 10^3 \times 14.18 \times 4}{3.14 \times 625 \times 37.5 \times 1.68} + \frac{5000 \times 4}{3.14 \times 625}$$

$$= -57.34 + 10.19$$

$$= -47.15 \text{ N/mm}^2$$

$$\boxed{\sigma_B = -47.15 \text{ MPa Compressive}} \qquad \textbf{Ans.}$$

EXAMPLE 8 *Calculate the stress at A and B in the given ring when the internal diameter is 100 mm.*

SOLUTION Given: *ID* of ring = 100 mm

$\therefore$ $r_i = r_A = 50$ mm

$$\bar{r} = r_A + \frac{d}{2}$$

$$= 50 + \frac{80}{2}$$

$$= 90 \text{ mm}$$

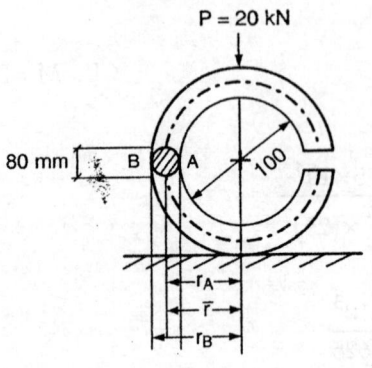 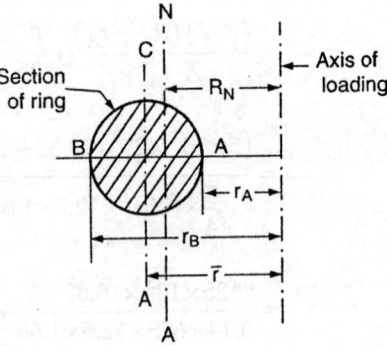

Fig. 19.16

$r_B = r_A + d$

     $= 50 + 80$

     $= 130$ mm

We will find out R_N (*i.e.* radius of neutral axis of ring)

$$R_N = \frac{d^2}{4\left(2 \times \bar{r} - \sqrt{4\bar{r}^2 - d^2}\right)}$$

$$= \frac{(80)^2}{4\left(2 \times 90 - \sqrt{4 \times (90)^2 - (80)^2}\right)}$$

$$= \frac{6400}{4\left(180 - \sqrt{4 \times 8100 - 6400}\right)}$$

$$= \frac{6400}{4\left(180 - \sqrt{32400 - 6400}\right)}$$

$$= 85.31 \text{ mm}$$

$$e = \left(\bar{r} - R_N\right)$$

$$= (90 - 85.31) \text{ mm}$$

$$= 4.69 \text{ mm}$$

Total compressive stress at A

$$\sigma_A = \left[\frac{-M(R_N - r_A)}{A \cdot r_A \cdot e} - \frac{P}{A}\right]$$

$$= \frac{(-P \times \bar{r})(R_N - r_A)}{A \cdot r_A \cdot e} - \frac{P}{A}$$

$$= \frac{\left(-20 \times 10^3 \times 90\right)(85.31 - 50)}{\frac{\pi}{4}(80)^2 \times 50 \times 4.69} - \frac{20 \times 10^3}{\frac{\pi}{4}(80)^2}$$

$$= -53.95 - 3.98$$

$$= -57.93 \text{ N/mm}^2$$

$$\approx -58 \text{ N/mm}^2$$

$$= -58 \text{ MPa} \quad \textbf{Ans.}$$

By the compressive load $(P) = 20$ kN, tensile stress will be develop at B.

Since, the nature of loading is compressive, so, M will be $(-)$ ve, and direct stress $\left(\dfrac{P}{A}\right)$ will also be $(-)$ ve.

Total tensile at B

$$\sigma_B = \frac{-M(R_N - r_B)}{A \cdot r_B \cdot e} - \frac{P}{A}$$

$$= \frac{\left(-20 \times 10^3 \times 90\right)(85.31 - 130)}{\frac{\pi}{4}(80)^2 \times 130 \times 4.69} - \frac{1000}{\frac{\pi}{4}(80)^2}$$

$$= 26.26 - 3.98$$

$$= 22.27 \text{ N/mm}^2$$

$$= 22.27 \text{ MPa} \quad \textbf{Ans.}$$

EXAMPLE 9 *The Curved member shown in figure has a Solid Circular Cross-section 100 mm in diameter. If the maximum tensile and compressive stress in the members are not to exceed 150 N/mm² and 200 N/mm² respectively, determine the value of load P that can safely be carried by the member.*

SOLUTION

Given: $d = 100$ mm

$$r_i = r_A = 50 \text{ mm} \qquad\qquad \bar{r} = r_i + \frac{d}{2}$$

$$r_o = r_B = (r_i + d) \qquad\qquad\quad = 50 + \frac{100}{2}$$

$$= (50 + 100) \qquad\qquad\qquad\quad = 100 \text{ mm}$$

$$= 150 \text{ mm}$$

$$l = 150 \text{ mm}$$

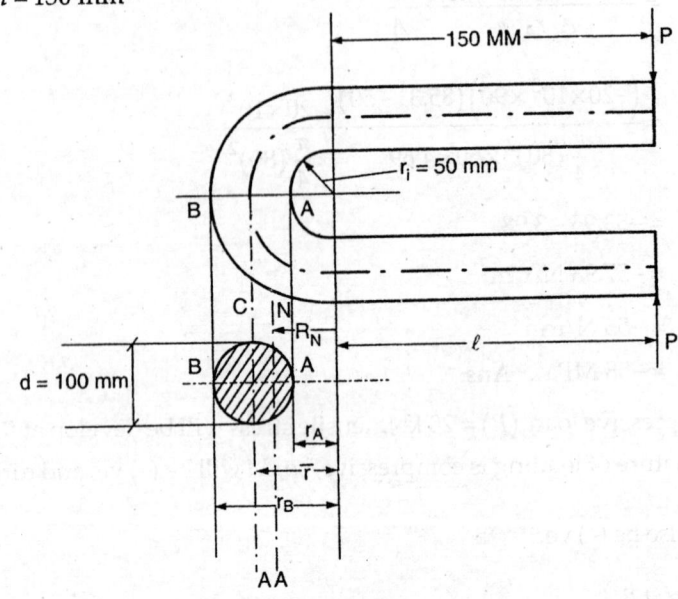

Fig. 19.17

Since load is compressive, hence, $M = -P(\bar{r} + l)$

$$R_N = \frac{d^2}{4\left(2\bar{r} - \sqrt{4\bar{r}^2 - d^2}\right)}$$

$$= \frac{(100)^2}{4\left(2 \times 100 - \sqrt{4 \times (100)^2 - (100)^2}\right)}$$

$$= \frac{10000}{4\left(200 - 100 \times \sqrt{3}\right)}$$

$$= \frac{10000}{4(200 - 173.2)}$$

$$= 93.28 \text{ mm}$$

Shifting of neutral axis $(e) = (\bar{r} - R_N)$

$$= (100 - 93.28)$$

$$= 6.72 \text{ mm}$$

[N.B: Since Compressive load P is acting on the Curve beam so at 'A', Compressive stress will develop and at 'B' tensile stress will develop. Further, M will be $(-)$ ve and direct stress $\left(\dfrac{P}{A}\right)$ will also be $(-)$ ve]

Now, total stress at A will be compressive in nature,

$$\therefore \qquad 200 = \frac{-M(R_N - r_A)}{A \cdot r_A \cdot e} - \frac{P}{A}$$

$$\text{or,} \qquad 200 = \frac{-P(\bar{r} + l)(R_N - r_A)}{\dfrac{\pi}{4}d^2 \cdot r_A \cdot e} - \frac{P}{A}$$

$$\text{or,} \qquad 200 = \frac{-P(100 + 150)(93.28 - 50) \times 4}{3.14 \times (100)^2 \times 50 \times 6.72} - \frac{4P}{3.14 \times (100)^2}$$

$$\text{or,} \qquad 200 = -P\left[\frac{250 \times 43.28 \times 4}{3.14 \times 50 \times 672} + \frac{4}{31400}\right]$$

$$\text{or,} \qquad 200 = -P\left[4.10221 \times 10^{-3} + 1.27388 \times 10^{-4}\right]$$

$$\text{or,} \qquad 200 = -P\left[\frac{4.10221}{10^3} + \frac{1.27388}{10^4}\right]$$

$$\text{or,} \qquad 200 = -P\left[\frac{4.10221 \times 10 + 1.27388}{10^4}\right]$$

$$\therefore \qquad P = -\left[\frac{200 \times 10^4}{41.02210 + 1.27388}\right]$$

$$= 47285.817 \text{ N}$$

$$= 47.285 \text{ kN}$$

Stress at B will be tensile in nature

So, $150 = \left\{ \dfrac{-M(R_N - r_B)}{A \cdot r_B \cdot e} - \dfrac{P}{A} \right\}$

$150 = \dfrac{-P(150+100)\cdot(93.28-150)\times 4}{\pi \times (100)^2 \times 150 \times 6.72} - \dfrac{P\times 4}{\pi \times (100)^2}$

or, $150 = P\left[\dfrac{250\times 56.72\times 4}{3.14\times 10000 \times 150 \times 6.72} - \dfrac{4}{31400} \right]$

or, $150 = P\left[1.792\times 10^{-3} - 1.273\times 10^{-4} \right]$

or, $150 = P\left[\dfrac{1.792}{10^3} - \dfrac{1.273}{10^4} \right]$

or, $150 = P\left[\dfrac{17.920 - 1.273}{10^4} \right]$

$\therefore$ $P = \left(\dfrac{150\times 10^4}{16.647} \right)$

        $= 90106.325 \text{ N}$

        $= 90.106 \text{ kN}$

P will be less of the two *i.e.* 47.285 kN for safe work.

EXAMPLE 10 *A curved beam, rectangular in cross-section is subjected to pure bending with couple of + 40 kN-cm. The beam has width of 2 cm and depth of 4 cm and is curved in plane parallel to width. The mean radius of curvature is 5 cm. Find the position of the neutral axis, and the ratio of the maximum to the minimum stress.* **(UPTU 2006-07)**

SOLUTION

        Given: $M = 40$ kN-cm $= 40 \times 10^4$ Nmm

                $\bar{r} = 2$ cm $= 50$ mm

                $h = 40$ mm

Hence, $r_i = \bar{r} - \dfrac{40}{2}$

        $= 50 - 20 = 30$ mm

and $r_o = \bar{r} + \dfrac{40}{2}$

        $= 50 + 20 = 70$ mm

Position of neutral axis $(R_N) = \dfrac{h}{\ln\left(\dfrac{r_o}{r_i}\right)}$

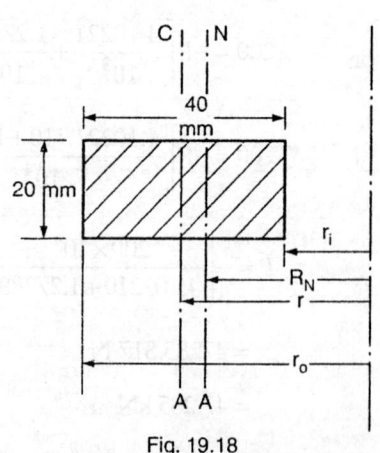

Fig. 19.18

$$= \frac{40}{\ln\left(\frac{70}{30}\right)}$$

$$= \frac{40}{0.847} = 47.20 \text{ mm}$$

Eccentricity $(e) = \bar{r} - R_N$

$$= (50 - 47.2) = 2.8 \text{ mm}$$

$$\sigma_i = \text{Stress at inner surface} = \frac{M(R_N - r_i)}{A \cdot r_i \cdot e}$$

$$\sigma_o = \text{Stress at outer surface} = \frac{M(R_N - r_o)}{A \cdot r_o \cdot e}$$

Hence, $\dfrac{\text{Max Stress}}{\text{Min Stress}} = \dfrac{\sigma_i}{\sigma_o}$

$$= \frac{M(R_N - r_i)}{A \cdot r_i \cdot e} \times \frac{A \cdot r_o \cdot e}{M(R_N - r_o)}$$

$$= \frac{R_N - r_i}{R_N - r_o} \times \frac{r_o}{r_i}$$

$$= \frac{47.2 - 30}{47.2 - 70} \times \frac{70}{30}$$

$$= -\frac{17.2}{22.8} \times \frac{70}{30}$$

$$= -\frac{1204}{684}$$

$$= -1.76$$

Ratio of $\left(\dfrac{\sigma_i}{\sigma_o}\right) = 1.76$ (neglecting negative sign).   **Ans.**

EXAMPLE 11 *A curved bar of rectangular cross-section has a width 40 mm and depth 60 mm and radius of curvature 80 mm about the centroidal axis parallel to width. Find the bending stress at the inner and outer faces caused by a moment of 500 Nm tending to increase the curvature.*   **(UPTU 3rd Sem 2009-10)**

SOLUTION

Given: $M = 500 \text{ Nm}$

$$\bar{r} = 80 \text{ mm}$$

$$h = 60 \text{ mm}$$

$$r_i = \bar{r} - \frac{h}{2}$$

$$= 80 - 30 = 50 \text{ mm}$$

and $\quad r_o = \bar{r} - \frac{h}{2}$

$$= 80 + 30 = 110 \text{ mm}$$

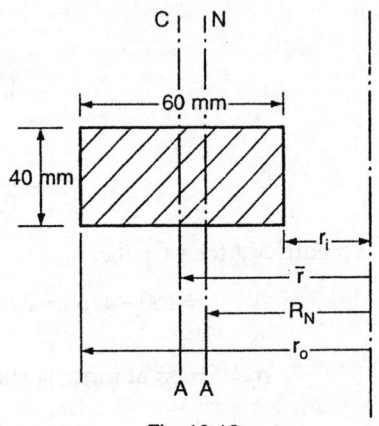

Fig. 19.19

$$(R_N) = \frac{h}{\ln\left(\dfrac{r_o}{r_i}\right)}$$

$$= \frac{60}{\ln\left(\dfrac{110}{50}\right)}$$

$$= \frac{60}{0.788} = 76.14 \text{ mm}$$

$$(e) = (\bar{r} - R_N) = (80 - 76.14) = 3.86 \text{ mm}$$

Given $M = 500 \text{ Nm} = 500 \times 10^3 \text{ N mm}$

Bending stress at inner face $= \dfrac{M\,(R_N - r_i)}{A \cdot r_i \cdot e}$

$$= \frac{500 \times 10^3 \,(76.14 - 50)}{(60 \times 40) \times 50 \times 3.86}$$

$$= 28.216 \text{ N/mm}^2 \text{ (Tensile in nature)}$$

Bending stress at outer face $= \dfrac{M\,(R_N - r_o)}{A \cdot r_o \cdot e}$

$$= \frac{500 \times 10^3 \,(76.14 - 110)}{(60 \times 40) \times 110 \times 3.86}$$

$$= -16.613 \text{ N/mm}^2 \text{ (Compressive in nature) } \textbf{Ans.}$$

EXAMPLE 12 *For the curved beam of triangular section, determine:*
   (a) Centroidal radius of curvature
   (b) Neutral axis location
   (c) The maximum stress when the beam is subjected to moment 80 Nm as shown in Fig. 19.20.

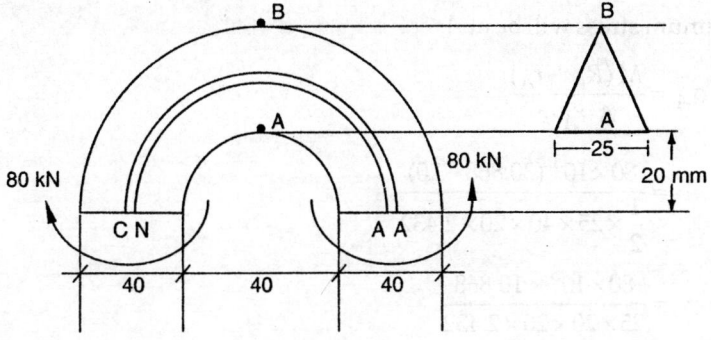

Fig. 19.20

SOLUTION

Given $r_A = 20$ mm

$r_B = 60$ mm

$h = 40$ mm

$M = +80$ Nm

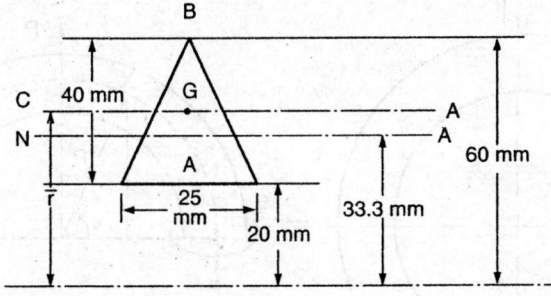

Fig. 19.21

(a) Radius of curvature $(\bar{r}) = AG + 20$

$$= \frac{40}{3} \div 20 = 33.3 \text{ mm}$$

(b) Location of neutral axis $(R_N) = \dfrac{h/2}{\dfrac{r_B}{h} \cdot \ln\left(\dfrac{r_B}{r_A}\right) - 1}$

$$= \frac{40/2}{\dfrac{60}{40} \cdot \ln\left(\dfrac{60}{20}\right) - 1} = 30.868 \text{ mm}$$

$e = (\bar{r} - R_N)$

$= (33.3 - 30.868) = 2.432$ mm

(c) Maximum stress will be at A,

i.e., $\sigma_A = \dfrac{M\,(R_N - r_A)}{A \cdot r_A \cdot e}$

$= \dfrac{80 \times 10^3\,(30.868 - 20)}{\dfrac{1}{2} \times 25 \times 40 \times 20 \times 2.432}$

$= \dfrac{80 \times 10^3 \times 10.868}{25 \times 20 \times 20 \times 2.432}$

$= 35.74\ \text{N/mm}^2$

$= 35.74\ \text{MPa (Tensile in nature)}$ **Ans.**

19.4 DETERMINATION OF BENDING MOMENT IN A RING

Let M_o = B.M. on cross-section perpendicular to P.

There will be a normal pull of $\dfrac{P}{2}$ on these sections shown in Fig. 19.22 (b).

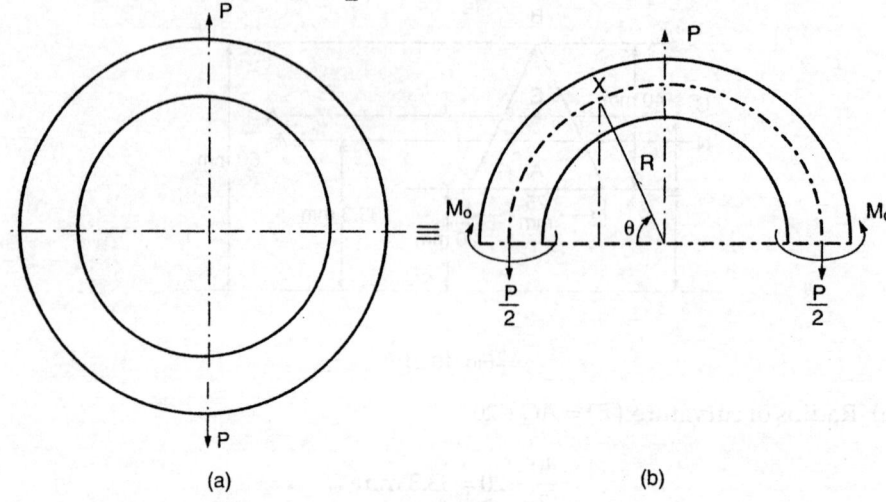

(a)   (b)

Fig. 19.22

At any point 'X' which is at an angle θ.

$$M\,(\theta) = -\frac{P}{2}\,(R - R\cos\theta) + M_o \qquad \left[\begin{array}{l}\text{As moment reducing} \\ \text{curvature is positive}\end{array}\right]$$

$$= -\frac{PR}{2}\,(1 - \cos\theta) + M_o \qquad \qquad \dots(1)$$

Now, strain energy stored in the ring

$$U = \int \frac{M^2\,ds}{2EI}$$

$$= 4 \times \int_0^{\pi/2} \frac{\left[-\dfrac{PR}{2}(1-\cos\theta) + M_o \right]^2 (R\, d\theta)}{2\, EI}$$

$$= \frac{2R}{EI} \int_0^{\pi/2} \frac{\left[-PR(1-\cos\theta) + 2M_o \right]^2}{4} d\theta \qquad\qquad [\because ds = R\, d\theta]$$

$$= \frac{R}{2EI} \int_0^{\pi/2} \left[-PR(1-\cos\theta) + 2M_o \right]^2 d\theta \qquad\qquad \ldots(2)$$

$$\therefore \qquad \left(\frac{\partial U}{\partial M_o} \right) = \frac{R}{2EI} \int_0^{\pi/2} 2\left[-PR(1-\cos\theta) + 2M_o \right](2)\, d\theta$$

$$= \frac{2R}{EI} \int_0^{\pi/2} \left[-PR(1-\cos\theta) + 2M_o \right] d\theta$$

$$= 0 \quad \text{(Since the ring does not rotate in the direction of } M_o)$$

$$\therefore \qquad \int_0^{\pi/2} \left[-PR(1-\cos\theta) + 2M_o \right] d\theta = 0$$

or, $\qquad \displaystyle\int_0^{\pi/2} PR\, d\theta - \int_0^{\pi/2} PR \cos\theta\, d\theta - 2M_o \int_0^{\pi/2} d\theta = 0$

or, $\qquad PR\left(\dfrac{\pi}{2} \right) - PR - 2M_o\left(\dfrac{\pi}{2} \right) = 0$

or, $\qquad M_o = \dfrac{PR}{2} - \dfrac{PR}{\pi}$

$$= \frac{PR}{2}\left[1 - \frac{2}{\pi} \right]$$

B.M. at any point X

$$M(\theta) = (-)\frac{PR}{2}(1-\cos\theta) + M_o$$

$$= -\frac{PR}{2}(1-\cos\theta) + \frac{PR}{2}\left(1 - \frac{2}{\pi} \right)$$

$$\therefore \qquad M(\theta) = (-)\frac{PR}{2}\left[\frac{2}{\pi} - \cos\theta \right]. \text{ This is the general formula of } M(\theta).$$

M will be maximum when $\theta = \dfrac{\pi}{2}$

$$\therefore \qquad M_{max} = -\frac{PR}{2}\left[\frac{2}{\pi} - 0 \right]$$

$$= -\frac{PR}{\pi}$$

$$\boxed{i.e.\ M_{max} = (-)\,\frac{PR}{\pi}}\ .\ \text{This is used as a formula for ring}$$

When $\theta = \dfrac{\pi}{2}$, M will be maximum along the load line and minimum at $\theta = 0°$

EXAMPLE 1 *A ring made up of 20 mm diameter steel bar carries a pull of 10 kN. Calculate the maximum tensile and compressive stresses in the material of the ring if the mean diameter of the ring is 200 mm.*

SOLUTION $\quad r_A = \left(\bar{r} - \dfrac{d}{2}\right)$

$$= 100 - \frac{20}{2}$$

$$= 90\ mm$$

$$r_B = \left(\bar{r} + \frac{d}{2}\right)$$

$$= 100 + 10 = 110\ mm$$

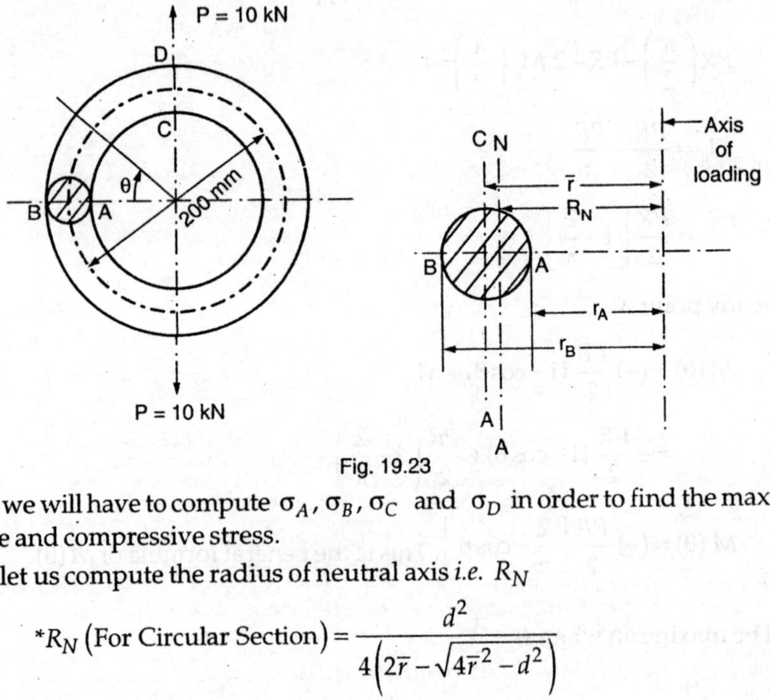

Fig. 19.23

Here, we will have to compute σ_A, σ_B, σ_C and σ_D in order to find the maximum tensile and compressive stress.

First, let us compute the radius of neutral axis *i.e.* R_N

$$*R_N\ (\text{For Circular Section}) = \frac{d^2}{4\left(2\bar{r} - \sqrt{4\bar{r}^2 - d^2}\right)}$$

----

*We may also use $R_N = \dfrac{(\sqrt{r_i} + \sqrt{r_o})^2}{4}$ for any circular section problem.

Here $r_i = r_A = 90$ mm and $r_o = r_B = 110$ mm.

where, d = dia. of the steel bar

$$\bar{r} = \left(\frac{200}{2}\right) = 100 \text{ mm}$$

$\therefore$
$$R_N = \frac{(20)^2}{4\left(2 \times 100 - \sqrt{4 \times (100)^2 - (20)^2}\right)}$$

$$= \frac{400}{4\left(200 - \sqrt{40000 - 400}\right)}$$

$$= \frac{100}{200 - \sqrt{39600}}$$

$$= \frac{100}{200 - 198.99748}$$

$$= 99.748$$

$$\simeq 99.75 \text{ mm}$$

$\therefore$
$$e = (\bar{r} - R_N)$$

$$= (100 - 99.75)$$

$$= 0.25 \text{ mm}$$

Here, M is min. at $\theta = 0$ and M is max. at $\theta = 90$.

$$M_{\min} = \frac{P\bar{r}}{2}\left(1 - \frac{2}{\pi}\right)$$

$$= 0.181 \, P\bar{r}$$

$$= 0.181 \times 10 \times 10^3 \times 100$$

$$= 181000 \text{ Nmm}$$

(will be used to compute σ_A and σ_B i.e. $\perp$ to the load line)

$$M_{\max} = (-)\frac{P\bar{r}}{\pi}$$

$$= (-)\frac{10 \times 10^3 \times 100 \times 7}{22}$$

$$= (-) \, 318181.81 \text{ Nmm}$$

(will be used to compute σ_C and σ_D i.e. along the load line)

$$\sigma_A = \frac{M_{\min} \, (R_N - r_A)}{A \cdot r \cdot e} + \frac{P}{2A}$$

$$= \frac{181000\,(99.75-90)}{\dfrac{\pi}{4}\,(20)^2 \times 90 \times 0.25} + \frac{10}{2\times\dfrac{\pi}{4}\,(20)^2}$$

$\therefore \qquad \sigma_A = 265.46 \text{ N/mm}^2$

$$\sigma_B = \frac{M_{\min}\,(R_N - r_B)}{A \cdot r_B \cdot e} + \frac{P}{2A}$$

$$= \frac{181000\,(99.75-110)}{\dfrac{\pi}{4}\times(20)^2 \times 110 \times 0.25} + \frac{10}{2\times\dfrac{\pi}{4}\times(20)^2}$$

$= (-)\,214.65 + 15.92$

$= (-)\,198.73 \text{ N/mm}^2 \text{ (Compressive in nature)}$

$$\sigma_C = \frac{M_{\max}\,(R_N - r_C)}{A \cdot r_C \cdot e}$$

$$= \frac{(-)318181.81\,(99.75-90)}{\cdot\dfrac{\pi}{4}\times(20)^2 \times 90 \times 0.25}$$

$= (-)\,438.70 \text{ N/mm}^2$

$= (-)\,438.70 \text{ MPa \ (Compressive in nature)}$

$$\sigma_D = \frac{M_{\max}\,(R_N - r_D)}{A \cdot r_D \cdot e}$$

$$= \frac{(-)318181.81\,(99.75-110)}{\dfrac{\pi}{4}\times(20)^2 \times 110 \times 0.25}$$

$$= \frac{318181.81 \times 10.25 \times 4 \times 7}{22 \times 400^2 \times 110 \times 0.25}$$

$= (+)\,377.34 \text{ N/mm}^2$

$= (+)\,377.34 \text{ MPa \quad (Tensile in nature)}$

$\sigma_A = 265.46 \text{ N/mm}^2 \text{ or MPa}; \ \sigma_B = (-)\,198.73 \text{ N/mm}^2 \text{ or MPa};$

$\sigma_C = (-)\,438.70 \text{ N/mm}^2 \text{ or MPa}; \ \sigma_D = (+)\,377.34 \text{ N/mm}^2 \text{ or MPa};$

From the calculated value we find that max. tensile stress is developed at '*D*' and maximum compressive stress is developed at *C*.

EXAMPLE 2 *A ring, made up of 25 mm diameter steel bar carries a pull of 10 kN. Calculate the maximum tensile and compressive stresses in the material of the ring. The mean radius of the ring is 150 mm.*

SOLUTION Since, here, we have shown AB to the right side of the ring, so, after applying load the neutral axis will shift to the left side (towards the centre of curvature of the ring).

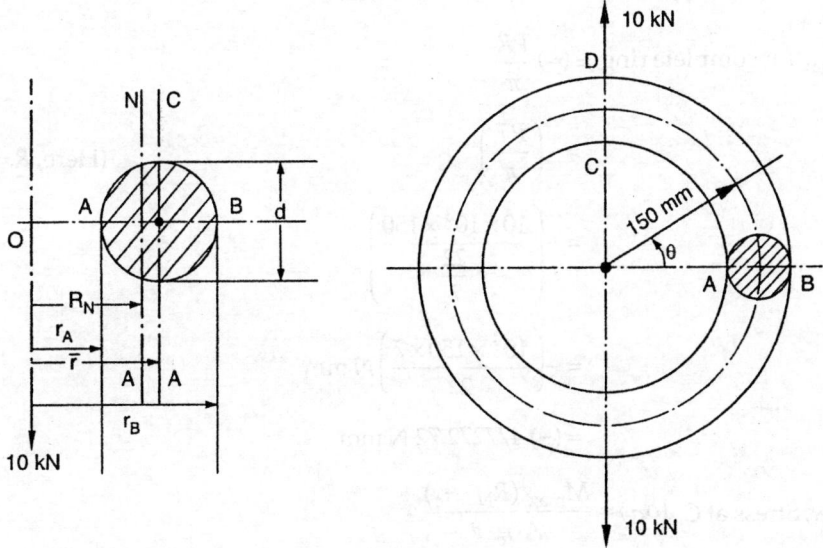

Fig. 19.24

We know that in the case of complete ring or chain, M will be maximum along load line *i.e.*, along CD and M will be minimum perpendicular to CD *i.e.*, along AB.

Given: $\bar{r} = 150$ mm

$$r_A = r_C = \bar{r} - \frac{d}{2}$$

$$= 150 - \left(\frac{25}{2}\right)$$

$$= 137.5 \text{ mm} = r_i$$

$$r_B = r_D = \bar{r} + \frac{d}{2}$$

$$= 150 + \frac{25}{2}$$

$$= 162.5 \text{ mm} = r_o$$

Now, $R_N = \dfrac{(\sqrt{r_i} + \sqrt{r_o})^2}{4}$

$$= \frac{(\sqrt{137.5} + \sqrt{162.5})^2}{4}$$

$$= 149.739$$

$$= 149.74 \text{ mm}$$

$$(\bar{r} - R_N) = e = (150 - 149.74) = 0.26 \text{ mm}$$

M_{max} for complete ring $= (-) \dfrac{PR}{\pi}$

$$= -\left(\frac{P\bar{r}}{\pi}\right) \hspace{3cm} \text{(Here, } R = \bar{r}\text{)}$$

$$= -\left(\frac{10 \times 10^3 \times 150}{\frac{22}{7}}\right)$$

$$= -\left(\frac{10^4 \times 150 \times 7}{22}\right) \text{N mm}$$

$$= (-) \, 477272.72 \text{ N mm}$$

Now, Stress at C, $(\sigma_C) = \dfrac{M_{max} (R_N - r_c)}{A \cdot r_c \cdot e}$

$$= (-) \frac{477272.72 \times (149.74 - 137.5)}{\frac{22}{7 \times 4} \times (25)^2 \times 137.5 \times 0.26}$$

$$= (-) \frac{477272.72 \times 28 \times 12.24}{22 \times 625 \times 137.5 \times 0.26}$$

$$= (-)332.75 \text{ MPa} \quad \text{(Compressive)}$$

Stress at D, $(\sigma_D) = \dfrac{M_{max} (R_N - r_D)}{A \cdot r_D \cdot e}$

$$= (-) \frac{477272.72 \times (149.74 - 162.5)}{\frac{22}{7 \times 4} \times (25)^2 \times 162.5 \times 0.26}$$

$$= \frac{477272.72 \times 12.76 \times 7 \times 4}{22 \times 625 \times 162.5 \times 0.26}$$

$$= 293.52 \text{ N/mm}^2$$

$$= 293.52 \text{ MPa} \quad \text{(Tensile) Maximum}$$

N.B. Maximum stress will develop along the load line in a ring.

19.5 DETERMINATION OF BENDING MOMENT IN A CHAIN LINK WITH STRAIGHT SIDES

At any point X (Angle θ)

B.M; $M(\theta) = -\dfrac{P}{2}(R - R\cos\theta) + M_o$

$\qquad\qquad = -\dfrac{P}{2}(1 - \cos\theta) + M_o$

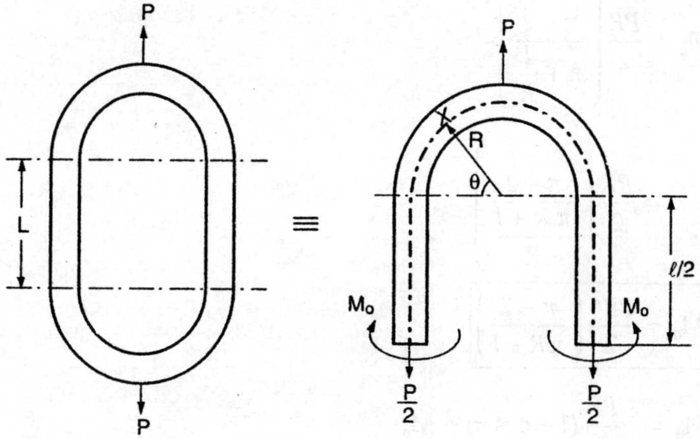

Fig. 19.25

Strain Energy $(U) = \displaystyle\int \frac{M^2 ds}{2EI}$

$$= 4\left[\int_0^{\pi/2} \frac{\left[-\dfrac{PR}{2}(1-\cos\theta) + M_o\right]^2 [R\,d\theta]}{2EI} + \int_0^{L/2} \frac{M_o^{\,2} dx}{2EI}\right]$$

$\therefore \qquad \dfrac{\partial U}{\partial M_o} = 4\dfrac{\left[\displaystyle\int_0^{\pi/2}(-)\dfrac{PR}{2}(1-\cos\theta) + M_o\right]}{2EI} R\,d\theta + \displaystyle\int_0^{L/2}\dfrac{2\,M_o\,dx}{2EI}$

$$= -\frac{4R}{EI}\int_0^{l/2}\left[\frac{PR}{2}(1-\cos\theta) - M_o\right]d\theta + 4\int_0^{l/2}\frac{M_o\,dx}{EI}$$

$$= 0 \qquad\qquad\qquad\qquad\text{(By Castigliano's Theorem)}$$

$\therefore \qquad -R\displaystyle\int_0^{\pi/2}\left[\frac{PR}{2}(1-\cos\theta) - M_o\right]d\theta + M_o\cdot\frac{l}{2} = 0$

or, $\qquad -R\left[\displaystyle\int_0^{\pi/2}\frac{PR}{2}d\theta - \frac{PR}{2}\int_0^{\pi/2}\cos\theta\,d\theta - M_o\int_0^{\pi/2}d\theta\right] + \frac{M_o\,l}{2} = 0$

or, $\quad \dfrac{PR}{2} \cdot \left(\dfrac{\pi}{2}\right) - \dfrac{PR}{2} - M_o\left(\dfrac{\pi}{2}\right) = \dfrac{M_o\,l}{2R}$

or, $\quad M_o\left(\pi + \dfrac{l}{R}\right) = PR\left(\dfrac{\pi}{2} - 1\right)$

$\therefore \qquad M_o = \dfrac{PR}{2}\left(\dfrac{\pi - 2}{\pi + \dfrac{l}{R}}\right)$

$$= \dfrac{PR}{2}\left(\dfrac{\pi - 2}{\dfrac{\pi R + l}{R}}\right)$$

$$\boxed{\therefore M_o = \dfrac{PR^2}{2}\left(\dfrac{\pi - 2}{\pi R + l}\right)} \qquad\qquad \text{...(I)}$$

$\therefore \qquad M_\theta = -\dfrac{PR}{2}(1 - \cos\theta) + M_o$

$$= -\dfrac{PR}{2}(1 - \cos\theta) + \dfrac{PR^2}{2}\left(\dfrac{\pi - 2}{\pi R + l}\right) \qquad\qquad \text{...(II)}$$

This is maximum when $\theta = \dfrac{\pi}{2}$

$\therefore \qquad M_{\max} = -\dfrac{PR}{2} + \dfrac{PR^2}{2}\left(\dfrac{\pi - 2}{\pi R + l}\right)$

$$= -\dfrac{PR}{2}\left[1 - \dfrac{R(\pi - 2)}{\pi R + l}\right]$$

$$= -\dfrac{PR}{2}\left[\dfrac{\pi R + l - \pi R + 2R}{\pi R + l}\right]$$

$$\boxed{\therefore M_{\max} = -\dfrac{PR}{2}\left[\dfrac{l + 2R}{l + \pi R}\right]}$$

N.B: This is the general formula for $M_{\max}$ for a chain having radius R and straight length 'l'

To compute stress perpendicular to the load line (when $\theta = 0$) of **chain, equation (II)** will be used to get M_o which will be substituted in the bending stress equation.

Further, $\left(\dfrac{P}{2A}\right)$ will also be added. So, total stress will be = $(\sigma_b + \sigma_d)$.

Readers must remember this formula to find M_{max} in a chain 'or' ring.

To find M_{max} for complete ring put $l = 0$

Then $$M_{max} = -\frac{PR}{\cancel{2}}\left[\frac{2\cancel{R}}{\pi \cancel{R}}\right]$$

$$\boxed{M_{max} = -\frac{PR}{\pi} \text{ for complete ring.}}$$

EXAMPLE 1 *Determine the maximum compressive stress and tensile stress at the same junction of the given chain link.*

(UPTU 2005-06)

SOLUTION

$$r_B = \bar{r} - \frac{d}{2}$$

$$= 45 - 7.5 = 37.5 \text{ mm}$$

$$r_A = \bar{r} + \frac{d}{2}$$

$$= 45 + 7.5 = 52.5 \text{ mm}$$

Maximum tensile stress will be produced at A and Maximum compressive stress will be produced at B

$$M_{max} = -\frac{PR}{2}\left[\frac{l + 2R}{l + \pi R}\right]$$

$$= (-)\frac{P\bar{r}}{2}\left[\frac{l + 2\bar{r}}{l + \pi\bar{r}}\right] \qquad [\text{As } R = \bar{r}]$$

$$= (-)\frac{1.5 \times 10^3 \times 4.5}{2}\left[\frac{75 + 2 \times 45}{75 + \frac{22}{7} \times 45}\right]$$

$$= (-)1.5 \times 22.5 \times 10^3\left[\frac{75 + 90}{75 + 141.42}\right]$$

$$= (-)25731.21 \text{ N mm}$$

$$^*R_N = \frac{d^2}{4\left(2\bar{r} - \sqrt{4\bar{r}^2 - d^2}\right)}$$

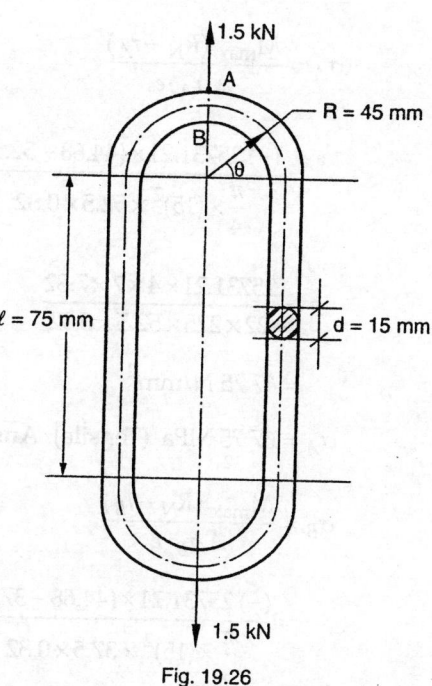

1.5 kN

A

R = 45 mm

B

θ

ℓ = 75 mm

d = 15 mm

1.5 kN

Fig. 19.26

---

*Formula $R_N = \dfrac{(\sqrt{r_i} + \sqrt{r_o})^2}{4}$ can also be used for circular cross-section object.

$$= \frac{(15)^2}{4\left(2 \times 45 - \sqrt{4 \times (45)^2 - (15)^2}\right)}$$

$$= \frac{225}{4\left(90 - \sqrt{8100 - 225}\right)} = \frac{225}{4 \times \left(90 - \sqrt{7825}\right)}$$

$$= \frac{225}{4\left(90 - 88.74\right)}$$

$$= +44.68 \text{ mm}$$

$$e = (\bar{r} - R_N)$$

$$= (45 - 44.68) = 0.32 \text{ mm}$$

$$\sigma_A = \frac{M_{max}\,(R_N - r_A)}{A \cdot r_A \cdot e}$$

$$= \frac{(-)\,25731.21 \times (44.68 - 52.5)}{\dfrac{\pi}{4} \times (15)^2 \times 52.5 \times 0.32}$$

$$= \frac{25731.21 \times 4 \times 7 \times 7.82}{22 \times 225 \times 52.5 \times 0.32}$$

$$= 67.75 \text{ N/mm}^2$$

$$\therefore \qquad \sigma_A = 67.75 \text{ MPa (Tensile) } \textbf{Ans.}$$

$$\sigma_B = \frac{M_{max}\,(R_N - r_B)}{A \cdot r_B \cdot e}$$

$$= \frac{(-)\,25731.21 \times (44.68 - 37.5)}{\dfrac{\pi}{4} \times (15)^2 \times 37.5 \times 0.32}$$

$$= (-)\,\frac{25731.21 \times 4 \times 7 \times 7.18}{22 \times 225 \times 37.5 \times 0.32}$$

$$= (-)\,87.08 \text{ N/mm}^2$$

$$= (-)\,87.08 \text{ MPa (Compressive) } \textbf{Ans.}$$

EXAMPLE 2 *An open ring has T-section. It is subjected to a tensile load of 80-kN as shown in Fig. 19.27. Find the stresses at A and B.*

[Similar Problem UPTU-2010-11 3rd Sem]

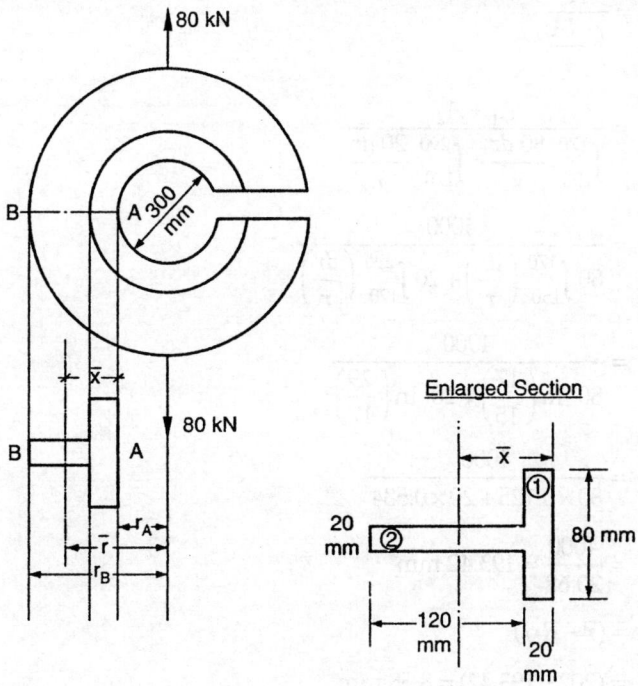

Fig. 19.27

SOLUTION

Given: $r_A = 150$ mm

$r_B = 290$ mm

$\bar{r} = (r_A + \bar{x})$

$\bar{x}$ = C.G. of T-section

A = Area of T-section

$= 80 \times 20 + 120 \times 20$

$= 4000$ mm^2

$\bar{x} = \left(\dfrac{A_1 x_1 + A_2 x_2}{A_1 + A_2} \right)$

$= \dfrac{20 \times 80 \times 10 + 120 \times 20 \times 80}{20 \times 80 + 120 \times 20}$

$= \dfrac{16000 + 192000}{4000} = 52$ mm

$\therefore \qquad \bar{r} = (r_A + \bar{x}) = (150 + 52) = 202$ mm

$$R_N = \frac{A}{\int \frac{dA}{r}}$$

$$= \frac{A_1 + A_2}{\int_{150}^{170} \frac{80\, dr}{r} + \int_{170}^{290} \frac{20\, dr}{r}}$$

$$= \frac{4000}{80 \int_{150}^{170} \left(\frac{dr}{r}\right) + 20 \int_{170}^{290} \left(\frac{dr}{r}\right)}$$

$$= \frac{4000}{80 \cdot \ln\left(\frac{17}{15}\right) + 20 \cdot \ln\left(\frac{29}{17}\right)}$$

$$= \frac{4000}{80 \times 0.125 + 20 \times 0.534}$$

$$= \frac{4000}{20.68} = 193.42 \text{ mm}$$

$$e = (\bar{r} - R_N)$$

$$= (202 - 193.42) = 8.58 \text{ mm}$$

$$\sigma_A = \frac{M(R_N - r_A)}{A \cdot r_A \cdot e} + \frac{P}{A}$$

$$= \frac{(P \times \bar{r})(R_N - r_A)}{A \cdot r_A \cdot e} + \frac{P}{A}$$

$$= \frac{P}{A}\left[\frac{\bar{r}(R_N - r_A)}{r_A \cdot e} + 1\right]$$

$$= \frac{80 \times 10^3}{4000}\left[\frac{202(193.42 - 150)}{150 \times 8.58} + 1\right]$$

$$= 20\left[\frac{202 \times 43.42}{150 \times 8.58} + 1\right]$$

$$= 156.29 \text{ N/mm}^2$$

$\therefore \qquad \sigma_A = 156.3 \text{ MPa}$ (Tensile in nature) **Ans.**

$$\sigma_B = \frac{M(R_N - r_B)}{A \cdot r_B \cdot e} + \frac{P}{A}$$

$$= \frac{(P \times \bar{r})(R_N - r_B)}{A \cdot r_B \cdot e} + \frac{P}{A}$$

$$= \frac{P}{A}\left[\frac{\bar{r}(R_N - r_B)}{r_B \cdot e} + 1\right]$$

$$= \frac{\overset{20}{\cancel{80}} \times \cancel{1000}}{\underset{A}{\cancel{4000}}}\left[\frac{202(193.42 - 290)}{290 \times 8.58} + 1\right]$$

$$= 20\left[(-)\frac{202 \times 96.58}{290 \times 8.58} + 1\right]$$

$$= (-)\,136.81 \text{ N/mm}^2$$

$\therefore \qquad \sigma_B = 136.81 \text{ MPa (Compressive in nature) } \textbf{Ans.}$

EXAMPLE 3 *An open ring has I-section, as shown in Fig. 19.28. Find the stresses at A and B.*
SOLUTION

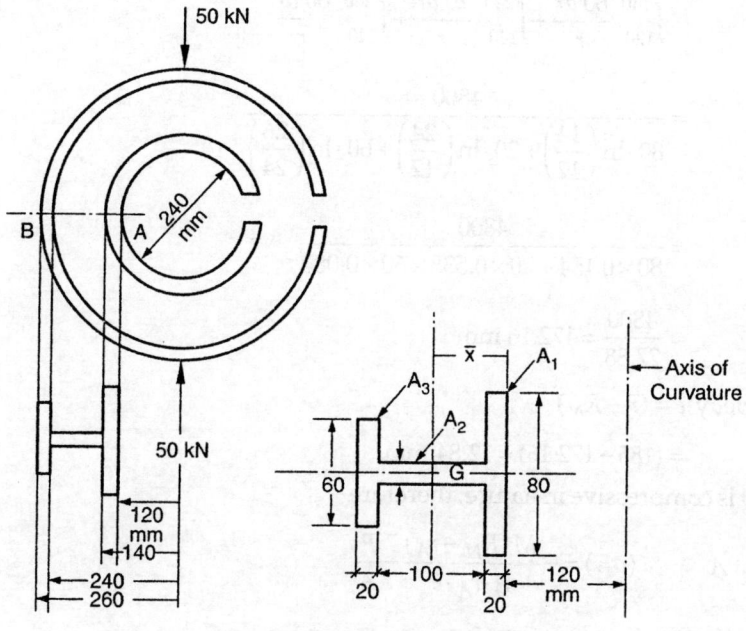

Fig. 19.28 Section at *AB* with Dimension

$$\bar{r} = (r_A + \bar{x})$$

$$\bar{x} = \left(\frac{A_1 x_1 + A_2 x_2 + A_3 x_3}{A_1 + A_2 + A_3} \right)$$

$$= \frac{(20 \times 80) \times \dfrac{20}{2} + (120 \times 20) \times \left(\dfrac{100}{2} + 20 \right) + (20 \times 60)(120 + 10)}{80 \times 20 + 100 \times 20 + 20 \times 60}$$

$$= \frac{16000 + 140000 + 156000}{1600 + 2000 + 1200}$$

$$= \frac{312000}{4800} = 65 \text{ mm}$$

$$\therefore \qquad \bar{r} = (r_A + \bar{x}) = 120 + 65 = 185 \text{ mm}$$

$$R_N = \frac{A}{\displaystyle\int \frac{dA}{r}}$$

Here, R_N for I-section

$$= \frac{A_1 + A_2 + A_3}{\displaystyle\int_{120}^{140} \frac{80 \, dr}{r} + \int_{140}^{240} \frac{20 \, dr}{r} + \int_{240}^{260} \frac{60 \, dr}{r}}$$

$$= \frac{4800}{80 \cdot \ln\left(\dfrac{14}{12} \right) + 20 \cdot \ln\left(\dfrac{24}{12} \right) + 60 \cdot \ln\left(\dfrac{26}{24} \right)}$$

$$= \frac{4800}{80 \times 0.154 + 20 \times 0.538 \times 60 \times 0.080}$$

$$= \frac{4800}{27.88} = 172.16 \text{ mm}$$

Eccentricity $e = (\bar{r} - R_N)$

$$= (185 - 172.16) = 12.84 \text{ mm}$$

As load is compressive in nature, therefore

Stress at A $\qquad (\sigma_A) = -\dfrac{M (R_N - r_A)}{A \cdot r_A \cdot e} - \dfrac{P}{A}$

$$= -\frac{P}{A} \left[\frac{\bar{r} (R_N - r_A)}{r_A \cdot e} + 1 \right] \qquad\qquad (\because M = P \cdot \bar{r})$$

$$= (-)\frac{50 \times 10\,00}{48\,00} \left[\frac{185 (172.16 - 120)}{120 \times 12.84} + 1 \right]$$

$$= (-)\frac{500}{48}\left[\frac{185 \times 52.16}{120 \times 12.84}+1\right]$$

$$= (-)\,75.65 \text{ N/mm}^2$$

$$= (-)\,75.65 \text{ MPa} \quad \text{(Compressive)}$$

Stress at $B \qquad (\sigma_B) = \dfrac{-M(R_N - r_B)}{A \cdot r_B \cdot e} - \dfrac{P}{A}$

$$= (-)\frac{P}{A}\left[\frac{\bar{r}\,(R_N - r_B)}{r_B \cdot e}+1\right]$$

$$= (-)\frac{50 \times 10^3}{4800}\left[\frac{185\,(172.16 - 260)}{260 \times 12.84}+1\right]$$

$$= (-)\frac{500}{48}\left[\frac{185 \times (-87.84)}{260 \times 12.84}+1\right]$$

$$= (-)\frac{500}{48}\,[-4.867+1]$$

$$= 40.28 \text{ N/mm}^2$$

$$= 40.28 \text{ MPa} \quad \text{(Tensile)}$$

PROBLEMS FOR PRACTICE

1. What do you mean by Curved beam?

2. Derive Winkler-Bach theory with the assumptions.

or

Prove that $\sigma = \dfrac{M \cdot y}{A \cdot e(r - y)}$

where r = radius of N.A.

y = distance of the element (under consideration) from N.A.

e = distance from centroidal axis to the neutral axis.

A = area of cross-section of the beam.

3. Compare stresses in a 50×50 mm rectangular bar subjected to end moment 2083 Nm in three special cases.

   (a) straight beam

   (b) beam Curved to radius of 250 mm along the centroidal axis

$(i.e.\ \bar{r} = 250\ \text{mm}\ ).$

(c) beam Curved to $\bar{r} = 75$ mm .

What inference do you get from these?

4. Determine the numerical value of ratio $\sigma_{max} / \sigma_{min}$ for the case of curved beam of rectangular cross-section in pure bending of $R = 15$ cm and $h = 10$ cm.

5. An open ring having T-section is subjected to a compressive load of 100 kN. Determine stress at A and B.

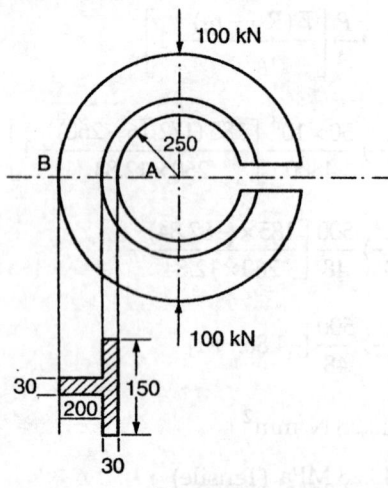

Fig. 19.29

6. Given $r_i = b = h = 2$ cm. and $P = 500$ Kg. Find σ_A and σ_B (Fig. 19.30).

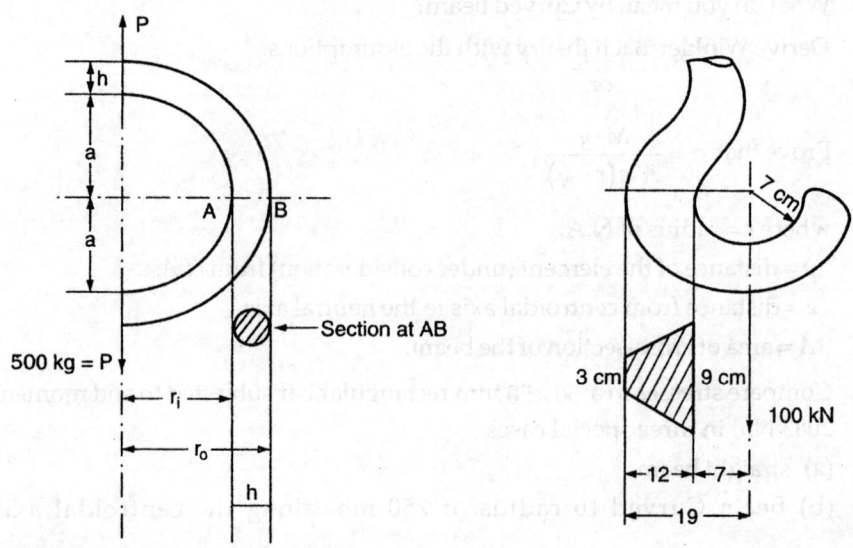

Fig. 19.30   Fig. 19.31

7. The dimensions of 100 kN crane hook is shown in the Fig. 19.31. Determine stress at the inside and outside fibre of the hook.

8. A Crane hook has trapezoidal cross-section. Determine the maximum load to be carried by the hook, if the working stress is 150 MN/M^2

Given, $r_i = 50$ mm

$\qquad r_0 = 90$ mm

$b_i = 30$ mm

$b_0 = 15$ mm

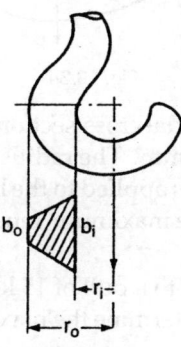

Fig. 19.32

9. An open ring is made of 5 cm diameter round bar as shown in Fig. 19.33. Calculate stresses at point A and B.

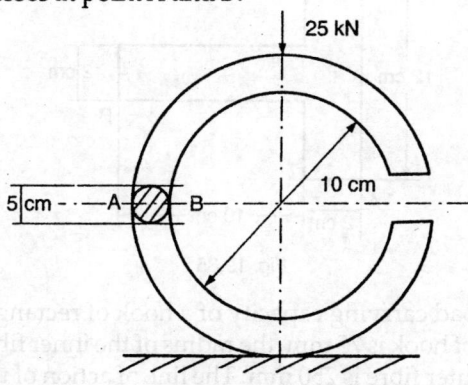

Fig. 19.33

10. For the hook of circular section:
   (a) Determine the maximum load P that may be supported without exceeding a stress of 120 MPa.
   (b) Find σ_B.

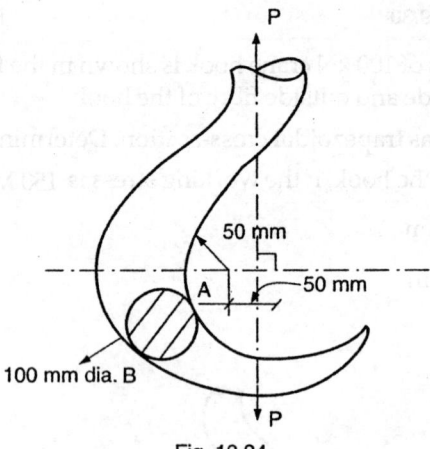

Fig. 19.34

11. A Crane hook is of trapezoidal cross-section having inner side 80 mm; outer side 30 mm and depth 120 mm. The radius of curvature of the inner side is 80 mm. If a load of 100 kN is applied to the hook passing through the centre of curvature, determine the maximum Tensile and Compressive stresses at the critical cross-section

12. A circular ring is subjected to a pull of 15 kN. The ring is T-section and the internal radius is 10 cm. Determine the maximum and minimum stresses in the ring.

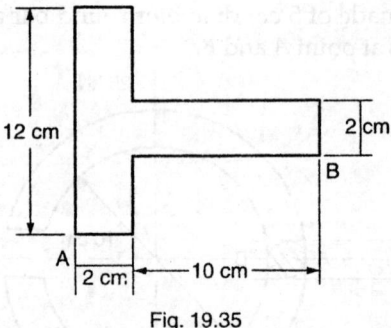

Fig. 19.35

13. Evaluate the load carrying capacity of a hook of rectangular cross-section. The thickness of hook is 75 mm, the radius of the inner fibre is 150 mm while the radius of outer fibre is 250 mm. The line of action of the force passes at a distance of 75 mm from the inner fibres. The allowable stress is 70 MN/m².

ANSWERS

4. 1.58

5. $\bar{x}$ = c.g. of T-section = 80.71 mm; R_N = 317.31 mm; $e = (\bar{r} - R_N)$

= 13.4 mm; σ_A = (–) 72.8 MPa (Comp); σ_B = (+) 70.14 MPa (Tensile)

6. $\sigma_A = \dfrac{P}{A} + \dfrac{M(R_N - r_A)}{A \cdot r_A \cdot e} = 241.24 \, \text{MPa}$;

$\sigma_B = \dfrac{P}{A} + \dfrac{M(R_N - r_B)}{A \cdot r_B \cdot e} = (-)120.61 \, \text{MPa}$

9. $R_N = 72.8 \, \text{mm}; e = 2.15 \, \text{mm}; \sigma_A = 107.81 \, \text{MPa}; \sigma_B = (-) \, 215.62 \, \text{MPa}$

10. $P = 46.1 \, \text{KN};$ 11. $141.9 \, \text{MN/M}^2; \, -74.8 \, \text{MN/M}^2$

12. $\bar{x} = 37.27 \, \text{mm}; \, \bar{r} = r_A + \bar{x} = (100 + 37.27) \, \text{mm}; \, R_N = 129.71 \, \text{mm};$

$e = 7.56 \, \text{mm}; \, \sigma_A = \left[\dfrac{P}{A} + \dfrac{M(R_N - r_A)}{A \cdot r_A e} \right] = 21.78 \, \text{MPa}; \, \sigma_B = -22 \, \text{MPa}.$

13. 52.51 kN

OBJECTIVE QUESTIONS

1. The theory of curved beam was given by:
   (a) Rankine   (b) Mohr
   (c) Castigliano   (d) Winkler-Bach
2. The bending equation in case of initially straight beams is similar to the bending equation in case of curved bar with:
   (a) small initial curvature   (b) large initial curvature
   (c) infinite initial curvature   (d) none of the above
3. The distribution of bending stress across the section of a curved bar with large initial curvature is:
   (a) linear   (b) parabolic
   (c) expotential   (d) hyperbolic
4. For a crane hook, the most appropriate section is:
   (a) triangular   (b) trapezoidal
   (c) circular   (d) rectangular
5. The maximum stress in a ring under tension occurs:
   (a) along the line of action of load
   (b) perpendicular to the line of action of load
   (c) at 45° with the line of action of the load
   (d) none of the above
6. In the case of curved bar with large initial curvature subjected to bending moment, the neutral axis:
   (a) coincides with the centroidal axis
   (b) is pulled towards the centre of curvature of the bar
   (c) is pushed away from the centre of curvature of the bar
   (d) none of the above

ANSWERS

1. (d)   2. (a)   3. (d)   4. (b)   5. (a)   6. (b)

UNSYMMETRICAL BENDING AND SHEAR CENTRE

20.1 INTRODUCTION

We have studied beam, symmetrical with respect to the neutral axis. In such type of beam, **Flexural Stresses** (σ_b) vary directly with distance from the neutral axis—which is the centroidal axis. Such types of beam sections are desirable for materials that are equally strong in tension and compression.

Materials which are weak in tension and strong in compression, such as Cast Iron, it is desirable to use beam that is unsymmetrical with respect to the neutral axis.

With such type of cross-section, the stronger fibres can be located at a greater distance from the neutral axis than the weaker fibres. In such type of material, the centroidal or neutral axis is selected in such a way that the ratio of the distances from it to the fibres in tension and compression is exactly the same as the ratio of the allowable stresses in tension and in compression.

20.2 UNSYMMETRICAL BENDING (For Symmetrical Body)

Unsymmetrical bending is defined as bending caused by loads that are inclined to the principal planes of bending.

Example of Unsymmetrical Bending is roof purlin.

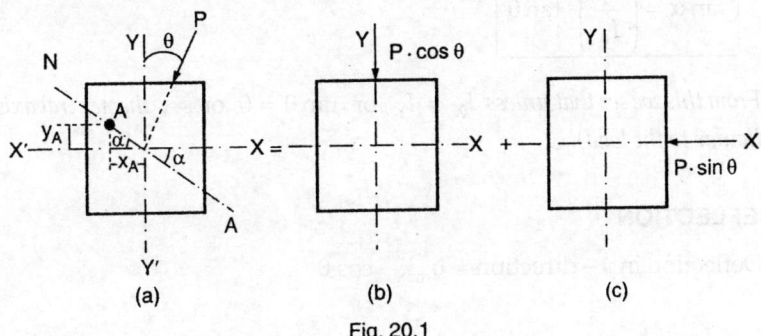

Fig. 20.1

In the above figure, Unsymmetrical bending has been resolved into symmetrical bending about x and y axes.

Let us consider a situation in which a *'Symmetrical Section'* is subjected to load (P) inclined (θ) to the axis of symmetry.

Now, resolving the inclined loading into horizontal and vertical component *i.e.* $P \sin \theta$ and $P \cos \theta$ respectively.

In Fig. 20.1 (b) x-axis is the neutral axis.

In Fig. 20.1 (c) y-axis is the neutral axis.

Each loading *i.e.* $P \cos \theta$ and $P \sin \theta$ produces flexural stresses that are normal to the cross-section.

Therefore, the resultant stress $(\sigma_R) = \dfrac{M_X}{I_X} \cdot y + \dfrac{M_Y}{I_Y} \cdot x$

$$\therefore \quad \boxed{\sigma_{Resultant} = \frac{M \cos \theta}{I_X} \cdot y + \frac{M \sin \theta}{I_Y} \cdot x}$$

20.3 LOCATION OF NEUTRAL AXIS

Neutral axis is the axis passing through the centroid in the plane of cross-section along which the bending stress and strains are zero.

Let $\alpha =$ Inclination of Neutral Axis (N.A.) with the x-axis then for point A,
$x_A = \ominus$ ve and $y_A = \oplus$ ve

Hence,

As we know that at N.A, $\sigma = 0$

$$\therefore \quad 0 = \frac{M \cos \theta \cdot y_A}{I_X} - \frac{M \sin \theta \cdot x_A}{I_Y}$$

$$\therefore \quad \left(\frac{y_A}{x_A}\right) = \left(\frac{I_X}{I_Y}\right) \cdot \tan \theta$$

$$\boxed{\tan \alpha = \left(\frac{I_x}{I_y}\right) \cdot \tan \theta}$$

N.B: *(From this we see that unless $I_X = I_Y$ or $\tan \theta = 0$ or ∞, the neutral axis is not perpendicular to the load).*

20.4 DEFLECTION

$(\delta_y) =$ Deflection in y – direction $= \delta_{max} \cdot \cos \theta$

$(\delta_x) = $ Deflection in x direction $= \delta_{max} \cdot \sin \theta$

Now, δ_{max} depends upon the type of loading *i.e.* whether

(i) Beam is simply supported
(ii) Simply supported with U.D.L.
(iii) Cantilever etc.

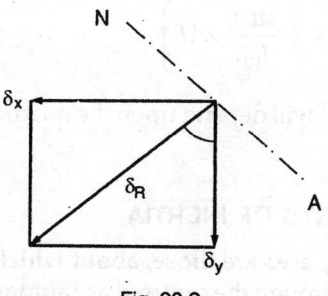

Fig. 20.2

Once the deflections, δ_x and δ_y are known, the resultant deflection can be known

by, $\delta_{resultant} = \sqrt{\delta_x^2 + \delta_y^2}$.

20.5 STRESSES IN BEAMS DUE TO UNSYMMETRICAL BENDING (For Unsymmetrical Body)

In the given Fig. 20.3, there is a uniform cross-section beam under the action of a bending moment M acting in plane YY which is inclined with the principal axis VV at the angle θ .

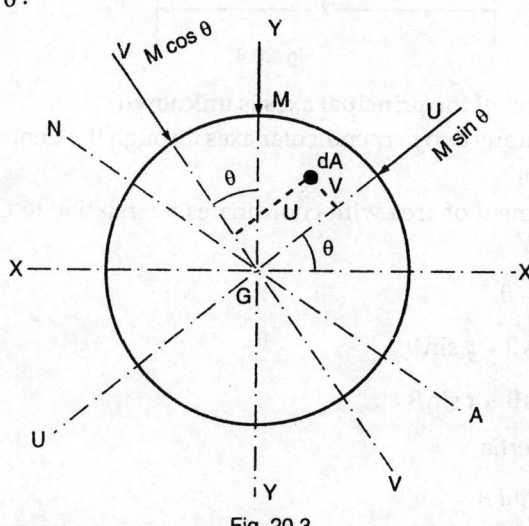

Fig. 20.3

Our aim is to find the stress distribution over the section.

Moment along the plane $VV = M_x = M \cos \theta$

Moment along the plane $UU = M_y = M \sin \theta$

The resultant bending stress at the arbitrary point P having (U, V) as its coordinates with respect to GU and GV axes is given by σ_b.

$$\sigma_b = \frac{(M \cos\theta)}{I_{uu}} \times V + \frac{(M \sin\theta)}{I_{vv}} \times U$$

$$= M\left[\frac{\cos\theta}{I_{uu}} \times V + \frac{\sin\theta}{I_{vv}} \times U\right]$$

The nature of σ_b at a point will depend upon the quadrant with respect to GU and GV axes in which it lies.

20.6 PRINCIPAL MOMENTS OF INERTIA

The principal axes of any area are those, about which the product of Inertia is zero. Axes of symmetry through the centroid are automatically principal axes, the product moments for opposite quadrants cancel each other out.

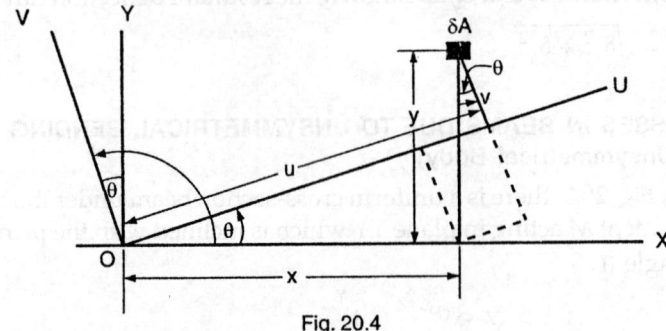

Fig. 20.4

When the direction of the principal axes is unknown

Let, OX and OY be any two perpendicular axes through the Centroid and OU, OV the principal axes.

Let, δA be an element of area with coordinates u,v relative to OU, OV and x, y relative to OX ; OY

$$\angle UOX = \theta$$

Then $u = x \cos\theta + y \sin\theta$

and, $v = y \cos\theta - x \sin\theta$

The product of inertia

$$I_{uv} = \int uv\, dA$$

$$= \int (x \cos\theta + y \sin\theta)(y \cos\theta - x \sin\theta)\, dA$$

$$= \sin\theta \cdot \cos\theta \left[\int y^2 dA - \int x^2 dA\right] + \left(\cos^2\theta - \sin^2\theta\right)\int xy\, dA$$

$$= \left(\frac{1}{2} \sin 2\theta \right) \cdot \left(I_X - I_Y \right) + \cos 2\theta \cdot I_{XY} \qquad \ldots(1)$$

Condition for principal axes is $I_{UV} = 0$

i.e. $\qquad \tan 2\theta = \dfrac{2I_{XY}}{I_Y - I_X}$ $\qquad \ldots(2)$

Now, $\quad I_U = \int v^2 \cdot dA = \int (y \cos\theta - x \sin\theta)^2 \, dA$

$$= \cos^2\theta \cdot I_X + \sin^2\theta \cdot I_Y - \sin 2\theta \cdot I_{XY}$$

and, subsitituting for I_{XY} from (2)

$$= \frac{1}{2}(I_X + I_Y) + \frac{1}{2}\cos 2\theta \, (I_X - I_Y) + \frac{1}{2}\left(\frac{\sin^2 2\theta}{\cos 2\theta} \right)(I_X - I_Y)$$

$$= \frac{1}{2}(I_X + I_Y) + \frac{1}{2}(I_X - I_Y)\sec 2\theta \qquad \ldots(3)$$

$$I_V = \int u^2 \cdot dA = \int (x \cos\theta + y \sin\theta)^2 \, dA$$

$$= \cos^2\theta \cdot I_Y + \sin^2\theta \cdot I_X + \sin 2\theta \cdot I_{XY}$$

$$= \frac{1}{2}(I_X + I_Y) - \frac{1}{2}(I_X - I_Y)\sec 2\theta \qquad \ldots(4)$$

Adding (3) and (4)

$$I_U + I_V = I_X + I_Y \qquad \ldots(5)$$

If I_X, I_Y and I_{XY} are calculated 'or' determined graphically, θ can be found from equation (2), I_U from (3) and I_V from (5).

For a rectangle of dimensions b and d with sides parallel to the axes OX and OY

$$I_{XY} = \iint xy \, dy \, dx$$

$$= \left[\frac{x^2}{2} \right]_{h-b/2}^{h+b/2} \times \left[\frac{y^2}{2} \right]_{k-d/2}^{k+d/2}$$

Where, h and k are the centroid

$\therefore \qquad I_{XY} = hd \times kd$

$\qquad\qquad = bd \times hk$

$\qquad\qquad = Ahk$

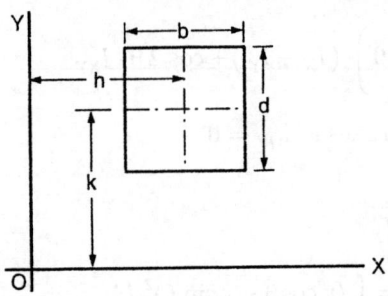

Fig. 20.5

20.7 PROCEDURE FOR SOLVING PROBLEMS ON UNSYMMETRICAL BENDING FOR SYMMETRICAL BODY OR SECTION

— If the given section is symmetrical about both axes X and Y as shown in figure 20.6, then apply formula for stress as given below.
— Find M. Resolve M
— Apply formula to get the stress at the point desired.

$$\sigma = \frac{M \cos \theta}{I_X} \cdot y + \frac{M \sin \theta}{I_Y} \cdot x$$

to get the value of σ_A, σ_B, σ_C and σ_D
— Evalute the inclination (α) of neutral axis by applying formula,

$$\tan \alpha = \left(\frac{I_X}{I_Y} \right) \tan \theta$$

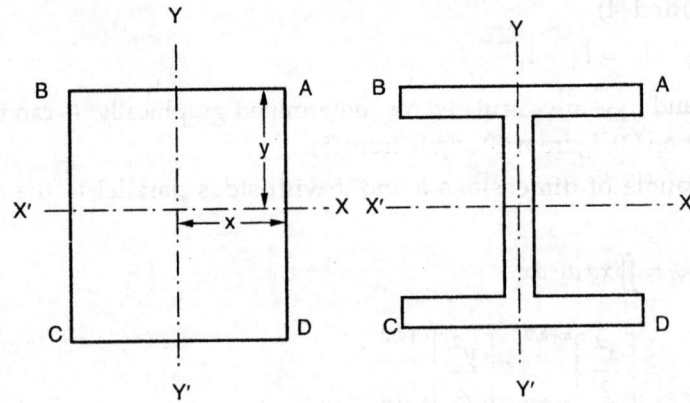

Fig. 20.6

20.8 PROCEDURE FOR SOLVING PROBLEM ON 'UNSYMMETRICAL BENDING' FOR UNSYMMETRICAL BODY (*i.e.* L, T AND Z SECTION)

— Choose X and Y axes
— Calculate I_X; I_Y; I_{XY}

— Locate U-axis by using equation $\tan 2\theta = \dfrac{2\,I_{XY}}{I_X - I_Y}$

From this equation we will get the value of θ.

If θ comes to be positive, then, U-axis is in the anticlockwise direction with x-axis.

If θ comes to be negative, then, U-axis is in the clockwise direction with x-axis.

— Find $I_u = \int V^2 \, dA$

$$= \frac{1}{2}\left[(I_X + I_Y) + \sec 2\theta\,(I_X - I_Y)\right]$$

— Find M and its components M_U and M_V.

— Use relation $\sigma = \dfrac{M_U}{I_U} \times V + \dfrac{M_V}{I_V} \times U$ to find the stress at any point in the quadrant.

— To find the inclination of the neutral axis (N.A) apply $\tan\alpha = \left(\dfrac{v}{u}\right)$.

A negative value of α indicates that the axes passes through quadrants in which u and v is negative.

— It is observed that one side of N.A. the stress will be tensile and compressive on the other side.

EXAMPLE 1 *A rectangular section 80 mm × 50 mm is arranged as a cantilever 1.3 metre long and loaded at the free end with a load of 5 kN inclined at an angle of 30° to the vertical. Determine the position and magnitude of the greatest tensile stress in the section.*

What will be the vertical deflection at the end? $E = 200 \, GN/m^2$

SOLUTION $I_{XX'} = \dfrac{bd^3}{12}$

$$= \frac{50 \times (80)^3}{12} \, mm^4$$

$$= \frac{50 \times (80)^3}{12 \times 10^{-12}} \, mm^4$$

$I_{YY'} = \dfrac{bd^3}{12}$

$$= \frac{80 \times (50)^3}{12} \, mm^4$$

$$= \frac{80 \times (50)^3}{12 \times 10^{-12}} \, m^4$$

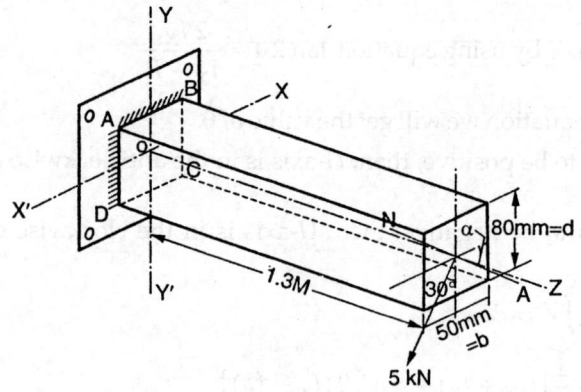

Fig. 20.7

$$M_{XX'} = 5 \times 10^3 \times \cos 30° \times 1.3 \text{ Nm}$$

$$= 5629 \text{ Nm in the plane } YY'$$

$$M_{YY'} = 5 \times 10^3 \times \sin 30° \times 1.3 \text{ Nm}$$

$$= 3250 \text{ Nm in the plane } XX'$$

Maximum stress will occur at B.

$$\therefore \qquad \sigma_B = \left[\frac{M_{XX'}}{I_{XX'}} \times y_B + \frac{M_{YY'}}{I_{YY'}} \times x_B \right]$$

$$= \frac{5629 \times \left(40 \times 10^{-3} \right)}{\dfrac{50 \times 80^3 \times 10^{-12}}{12}} + \frac{3250 \times \left(25 \times 10^{-3} \right)}{\dfrac{80 \times 50^3 \times 10^{-12}}{12}}$$

$$= 105.5 + 97.5$$

$$= 203 \text{ MN/m}^2 \quad \text{(Tensile in nature).}$$

Vertical deflection is given by

$$\delta_V = \frac{WL^3}{3EI_{XX'}}$$

where, W = vertical load

L = span length

and, I_{XX} = M.I about $I_{XX'}$

$$\therefore \qquad \delta_V = \frac{(W \cos 30°) \cdot L^3}{3EI_{XX}}$$

$$= \frac{5000 \times 0.866 \times (1.3)^3}{3 \times 210 \times 10^9 \times \left(\dfrac{50 \times 80^3}{12}\right) \times 10^{-12}}$$

$= 7.1$ mm   **Ans.**

EXAMPLE 2 *A rectangular section beam 80 mm × 50 mm is used as a cantilever 1.5 m long and loaded at its free end with a load of 5 kN inclined at an angle of 30° to the vertical in the third quadrant.*

Determine the greatest tensile stress in the section.

Evaluate the vertical deflection at the free end. Given $E = 200$ GN / m^2.

SOLUTION

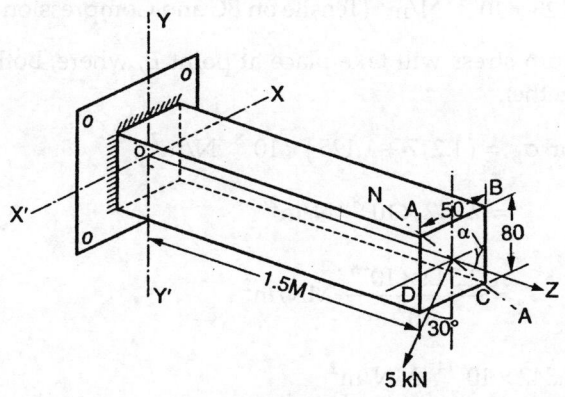

Fig. 20.8

$M_{XX} = 5000 \cos 30° \times 1.5 = 6495$ Nm

$M_{YY} = 5000 \sin 30° \times 1.5 = 3750$ Nm

Stresses on edges *AB* and *CD* due to M_{XX}

$$\sigma = \frac{M_{XX}}{I_{XX}} \times y$$

$$= \frac{6495 \times 12}{\dfrac{50}{1000} \times \left(\dfrac{80}{1000}\right)^3} \times \left(40 \times 10^{-3}\right) \text{N/m}^2$$

$$= \frac{6495 \times 12}{0.05 \times (80)^3} \times 40 \times 10^6 \ \text{N/m}^2$$

$= 10^6 \times 121.78 \ \text{N/m}^2$ (Tensile on *AB* and compression on *DC*).

$= 1.217 \times 10^{-8} \ \text{N/m}^2$

Stresses on edges AD and BC due to M_{YY}

$$\sigma = \frac{M_{YY}}{I_{YY}} \cdot x$$

$$= \frac{3750 \times 12}{\left(\dfrac{80}{1000}\right) \times \left(\dfrac{50}{1000}\right)^3} \times \left(\frac{25}{1000}\right)$$

$$= \frac{3750 \times 12}{0.08 \times (0.05)^3} \times 0.025 \ \text{N/m}^2$$

$$= 1.125 \times 10^{-8} \ \text{N/m}^2 \ (\text{Tensile on } BC \text{ and Compression stress on } AD).$$

$\therefore$ Maximum stress will take place at point B, where, both tensile stress add together.

$\therefore$ σ_{max} 'or' $\sigma_B = (1.217 + 1.125) \times 10^{-8} \ \text{N/m}^2$

$$= 2.342 \times 10^{-8} \ \text{N/m}^2$$

$$= \frac{2.342 \times 10^{-8}}{10^6} \ \text{MN/m}^2$$

$\sigma_B = 2.342 \times 10^{-14} \ \text{MN/m}^2$

Vertical deflection $(\delta_V) = \dfrac{Wl^3 \cos\theta}{3EI_{XX'}}$

$$= \frac{5000 \times (1.5)^3 \times \cos 30° \times 12}{3 \times 200 \times 10^9 \times \left(\dfrac{50}{1000}\right) \times \left(\dfrac{80}{1000}\right)^3}$$

$$= \frac{5000 \times (1.5)^3 \times 0.866 \times 12}{3 \times 2 \times 0.05 \times (80)^3 \times 100}$$

$$= \frac{600 \times (1.5)^3 \times 0.866}{6 \times 0.05 \times (80)^3}$$

$$= 0.0114 \ \text{metre}$$

$$= 11.41 \ \text{mm}$$

EXAMPLE 3 *The figure 20.9 shows a simply supported beam having span of 4 metre and loaded at an angle 30° to the vertical. The magnitude of load is 2 kN. Modulus of elasticity (E) of beam is 210 GPa.*

Evaluate the maximum deflection and stress at point A and B.

SOLUTION

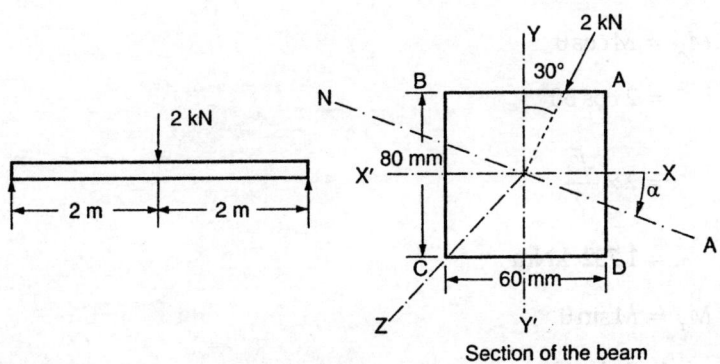

Section of the beam

Fig. 20.9 (i)

Let, N.A. makes angle α with the x-axis

Now, Stress at A, $\sigma_A = \left(\dfrac{M_X}{I_X}\right) \cdot y_A + \left(\dfrac{M_Y}{I_Y}\right) \cdot x_A$ ...(1)

and, that at B; $\sigma_B = \left(\dfrac{M_X}{I_X}\right) \cdot y_B + \left(\dfrac{M_Y}{I_Y}\right) \cdot x_B$ ...(2)

Now, $I_{XX'} = \left(\dfrac{bd^3}{12}\right)$

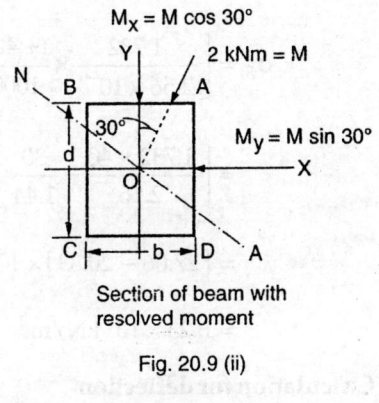

$M_X = M \cos 30°$

$M_Y = M \sin 30°$

Section of beam with resolved moment

Fig. 20.9 (ii)

$= \dfrac{0.06 \times (0.08)^3}{12}$

$\cdot = 2.56 \times 10^{-6} \ \text{m}^4 = I_X$

$I_{YY'} = \left(\dfrac{db^3}{12}\right)$

$= \dfrac{0.08 \times (0.06)^3}{12}$

$= 1.44 \times 10^{-6} \ \text{m}^4 = I_Y$

Maximum B.M for the given simply supported beam $= \dfrac{2 \times 4}{4}$ kNm

$$\left[\because M_{max} = \dfrac{W \cdot l}{4} \right]$$

$\therefore \qquad M_{max} = 2 \ \text{kNm}$

Now, $\qquad M_X = M \cos \theta$

$\qquad\qquad = 2 \cos 30°$

$\qquad\qquad = 2 \times \dfrac{\sqrt{3}}{2}$

$\qquad\qquad = 1.732 \ \text{kNm}$

$\qquad M_Y = M \sin \theta$

$\qquad\qquad = 2 \sin 30°$

$\qquad\qquad = 2 \times 0.5$

$\qquad\qquad = 1 \ \text{kNm}$

Therefore, from equation (1)

$$\sigma_A = \left[\dfrac{1.732}{2.56 \times 10^{-6}} \times \dfrac{40}{1000} + \dfrac{1}{1.44 \times 10^{-6}} \times \dfrac{30}{1000} \right]$$

$$= [27.06 + 20.83]$$

$$= 47.89 \ \text{kN/m}^2 \qquad\qquad\qquad\qquad \text{(Tensile in nature)}$$

$$\sigma_B = \left[\dfrac{1.732}{2.56 \times 10^{-6}} \times \dfrac{(+40)}{1000} + \dfrac{(+)1}{1.44 \times 10^{-6}} \times \dfrac{(-)30}{1000} \right]$$

$$= \left[\dfrac{1.732 \times 40}{2.56} - \dfrac{30}{1.44} \right] \times \dfrac{10^6}{1000}$$

$$= [27.06 - 20.83] \times 10^3 \ \text{kN/m}^2$$

$$= 6.23 \times 10^3 \ \text{kN/m}^2 \qquad \text{(Tensile)}$$

Calculation for deflection

Deflection in y direction $= \delta y$

$$= \delta_{max} \cdot \cos \theta$$

$$= \frac{Wl^3}{48\,EI_{XX'}} \times \cos\theta$$

$$= \frac{2 \times 10^3 \times (4)^3}{48 \times 210 \times 10^9 \times 2.56 \times 10^{-6}} \times \cos 30°$$

$$= \left[\frac{2 \times 64}{48 \times 2.56 \times 210} \right] m \times \frac{\sqrt{3}}{2}$$

$$= 4.295 \times 10^{-3} \text{ meter}$$

$$= 4.295 \text{ mm}$$

Deflection in x-direction $= \delta x$

$$= \delta_{max} \cdot \sin\theta$$

$$= \left[\frac{Wl^3}{48\,EI_{YY'}} \times \sin\theta \right]$$

$$= \frac{2 \times 10^3 \times (4)^3 \times \sin 30°}{48 \times 210 \times 10^9 \times 1.44 \times 10^{-6}} \text{ meter}$$

$$= \frac{2 \times 64 \times 0.5}{48 \times 210 \times 1.44} \text{ meter}$$

$$= 4.409 \times 10^{-3} \text{ meter}$$

$$= 4.409 \text{ mm}$$

Location of Neutral Axis

$$\tan\alpha = \frac{I_X}{I_Y} \cdot \tan\theta$$

$$= \frac{256}{144} \times \tan 30°$$

$$= 1.0264$$

$$= \tan 45.748°$$

$$\boxed{\therefore \ \alpha = 45.7°}$$

EXAMPLE 4 *A Cantilever beam of rectangular section is subjected to a load of 1000 Newton which is inclined 30° to the vertical. Find the stress at C.*

SOLUTION

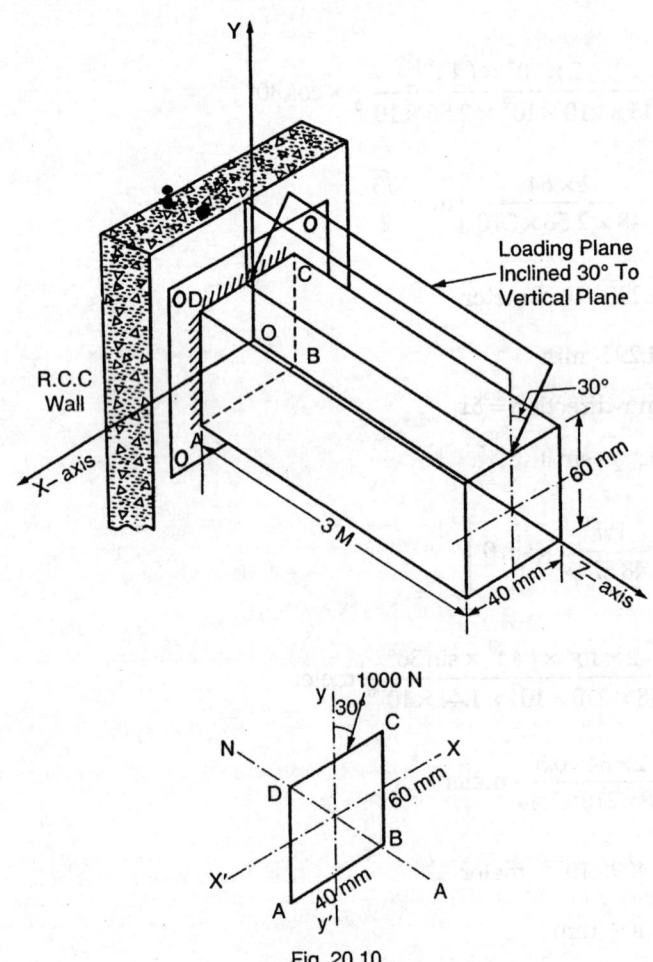

Fig. 20.10.

Resolving the oblique load into their x and y component

$$M_X = \left(1000 \cos 30°\right) \times 3 = +3000 \times \frac{\sqrt{3}}{2} \text{ Nm}$$

$$= 1500\sqrt{3} \text{ Nm}$$

$$M_Y = \left(1000 \sin 30° \times 3\right) = 1500 \text{ Nm}$$

$$I_{XX}' = \frac{bd^3}{12}$$

$$= \frac{40 \times 10^{-3} \times \left(60 \times 10^{-3}\right)^3}{12} \text{ meter}^4$$

$$= \frac{0.040 \times (0.060)^3}{12} \text{ meter}^4$$

$$= 7.2 \times 10^{-7} \text{ m}^4 = I_X$$

$$I_{YY'} = \frac{db^3}{12}$$

$$= \frac{10^{-3} \times 60 \times (40 \times 10^{-3})^3}{12}$$

$$= \frac{0.060 \times (0.040)^3}{12} \text{ meter}^4$$

$$= 3.2 \times 10^{-7} \text{ meter}^4 = I_Y$$

Stress at C, $\sigma_C = \left\{ \dfrac{M_X}{I_X} \times y_C + \dfrac{M_Y}{I_Y} \times x_C \right\} \text{ N/m}^2$

$$= \left\{ \frac{+1500\sqrt{3}}{7.2 \times 10^{-7}} \times \left(+\frac{30}{1000} \right) + \frac{(+)1500}{3.2 \times 10^{-7}} \times \left(\frac{20}{1000} \right) \right\} \begin{bmatrix} x_C = + \text{ ve} \\ y_C = + \text{ ve} \end{bmatrix}$$

$$= \left(+\frac{15 \times 1.732 \times 30}{7.2 \times 10^{-4}} + \frac{30,000}{3.2 \times 10^{-4}} \right)$$

$$= +\frac{450 \times 17320}{7.2} + \frac{30000 \times 10^4}{3.2}$$

$$= +\frac{45 \times 173200}{7.2} + \frac{3 \times 10^8}{3.2}$$

$\therefore \quad \sigma_C = 1082500 + 93750000 = 94832500 \text{ N/m}^2$

$$= 94.832 \text{ MN/m}^2 \qquad \textbf{Ans.}$$

EXAMPLE 5 *A steel bar of rectangular section 60 mm × 40 mm is arranged as Cantilever having length one meter. The face having 60 mm side of the cantilever is making 30° with the horizontal.*

A concentrated load of 200 N is acting from the free end. Find the N.A and the maximum stress produced. Modulus of elasticity (E) of the cantilever = 200 GPa.

SOLUTION

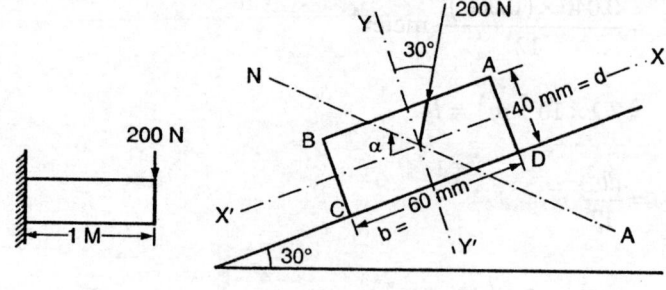

Fig. 20.11

$$I_{XX} = \frac{bd^3}{12}$$

$$= \frac{60 \times 10^{-3} \times \left(40 \times 10^{-3}\right)^3}{12} \, m^4$$

$$= \frac{60 \times 64 \times 10^3 \times 10^{-3} \times 10^{-9}}{12} \, m^4$$

$$= 320 \times 10^{-9} \, m^4$$

$$I_{YY} = \frac{db^3}{12}$$

$$= \frac{40 \times 10^{-3} \times \left(60 \times 10^{-3}\right)^3}{12}$$

$$= \frac{40 \times 216 \times 10^{-3} \times 10^3 \times 10^{-9}}{12}$$

$$= 720 \times 10^{-9} \, m^4$$

$$M_X = M_{max} \cdot \cos\theta$$

$$= (200 \times 1) \times \cos 30° \, Nm$$

$$= 200 \times \frac{\sqrt{3}}{2} \, Nm$$

$$= 100\sqrt{3} \, Nm$$

$$= 173.2 \, Nm$$

$$M_y = M_{max.} \cdot \sin\theta$$

$$= (200 \times 1) \times \sin 30° \, Nm$$

$$= 200 \times 1 \times \frac{1}{2} \text{ Nm}$$

$$= 100 \text{ N-m}$$

Now, stress at a point, $\sigma = \left\{ \dfrac{M_{XX}}{I_{XX}} \cdot y + \dfrac{M_{YY}}{I_{YY}} \cdot x \right\}$

at N.A, $\sigma = 0 \Rightarrow \dfrac{y}{x} = -\left(\dfrac{I_{XX}}{I_{YY}} \right) \tan 30°$

$$\tan \alpha = -\left(\frac{320 \times 10^{-9}}{720 \times 10^{-9}} \right) \times \tan 30°$$

$$= -0.2566$$

$$\alpha = -14.39° \text{ clockwise} \qquad \text{(Anticlockwise angle is positive)}$$

Maximum stress will be at A.

Now, from stress formula

$$\sigma_A = \left\{ \frac{M_X}{I_X} \times y_A + \frac{M_Y}{I_Y} \times x_A \right\}$$

$$= \left\{ \frac{173.2}{320 \times 10^{-9}} \times \frac{40}{2 \times 1000} + \frac{100}{720 \times 10^{-9}} \times \frac{30}{2 \times 1000} \right\}$$

$$= \left\{ \frac{173.2 \times 40}{32 \times 10^{-10}} + \frac{100 \times 30}{72 \times 10^{-10}} \right\}$$

$$= 10^5 \left\{ \frac{173.2 \times 40}{32 \times 2} + \frac{3000}{72 \times 2} \right\} \text{ N/m}^2$$

$$= 10^5 \{ 108.25 + 20.83 \}$$

$$= 10^5 \times 129.08 \text{ N/m}^2$$

$$\sigma_A = 12.90 \text{ MN/m}^2$$

$\therefore$ Maximum stress $= 12.90 \text{ MN/m}^2$ **Ans.**

EXAMPLE 6 *A I-Section beam of 2.4 meter is used as cantilever beam to support the load of 200 N at the free end which makes 30° with the vertical. Determine the resulting bending stresses at corner A and B.*

SOLUTION

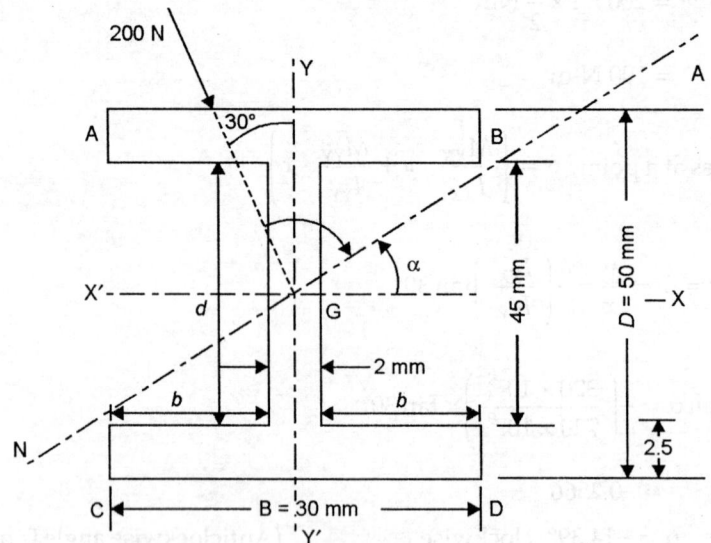

Fig. 20.12

$$I_{XX} = \Sigma \frac{BD^3}{12}$$

$$= \left\{ \frac{BD^3}{12} - \frac{bd^3}{12} \times 2 \right\}$$

$$= \left\{ \frac{30 \times 50^3}{12} - 2 \times \frac{14 \times 45^3}{12} \right\}$$

Here $B = 30$ mm
   $D = 50$ mm
   $b = 14$ mm
   $d = 45$ mm

$$= 99875 \text{ mm}^4$$

$$= 9.99 \times 10^{-8} \text{ m}^4$$

$$= 1 \times 10^{-8} \text{ m}^4$$

$$I_{YY} = \frac{2 \times 2.5 \times 30^3}{12} + \frac{45 \times (2)^3}{12}$$

$$= 1.128 \times 18^{-8} \text{ m}^4$$

Now, $M_{max} = W \times l$

$$= 200 \times 2.4 \text{ N·m}$$

$$= 480 \text{ Nm}$$

$$M_X = M_{max} \cdot \cos \theta$$

$$= 480 \cos 30° \text{ N·m}$$

$$= 240 \times \sqrt{3} \text{ N·m}$$

$$M_Y = M_{max} \cdot \sin\theta$$

$$= 480 \sin 30°$$

$$= 240 \times \frac{1}{2} \text{ Nm}$$

$$= 120 \text{ Nm}$$

Stress at A, $(\sigma_A) = \left\{ \dfrac{M_{XX}}{I_{XX}} \cdot y_A + \dfrac{M_{YY}}{I_{YY}} \cdot x_A \right\}$

$$= \left\{ \frac{M\cos\theta}{I_{XX}} \times y_A + \frac{M\sin\theta}{I_{YY}} \times x_A \right\}$$

$$\sigma_A = \left\{ \frac{240\sqrt{3}}{1 \times 10^{-8}} \times \left(\frac{25}{1000}\right) + \frac{120}{1.13 \times 10^{-8}} \times \left(+\frac{15}{1000}\right) \right\}$$

$$= \left\{ +\frac{25 \times 240 \times 1.732}{10^{-5}} + \frac{120 \times 15}{1.13 \times 10^{-5}} \right\}$$

$$= 10^5 \left\{ \frac{120 \times 15}{1.13} + \frac{25 \times 240 \times 1.732}{1} \right\}$$

$$= 10^5 \left\{ 1593 + 10392 \right\}$$

$$= 11985 \times 10^5 \text{ N/m}^2 \quad \text{(Tensile in nature)} \quad \textbf{Ans.}$$

Stress at B, $(\sigma_B) = \left\{ \dfrac{M_{XX}}{I_{XX}} \times y_B + \dfrac{M_{YY}}{I_{YY}} \times x_B \right\}$

$$= \left\{ +\frac{25 \times 240 \times 1.732}{10^{-5}} - \frac{120 \times 15}{1.13 \times 10^{-5}} \right\}$$

$$= 10^5 \left\{ +25 \times 240 \times 1.732 - \frac{120 \times 15}{1.13} \right\}$$

$$= 10^5 \left\{ +10392 - 1593 \right\} = 8799 \times 10^5 \text{ N/m}^2 \text{ (Tensile in nature)} \quad \textbf{Ans.}$$

Position of neutral axis (NA) is given by

$$\tan\alpha = \left(\frac{I_X}{I_Y}\right) \cdot \tan\theta$$

$$= \frac{1 \times 10^{-8}}{1.128 \times 10^{-8}} \times \tan 30°$$

$$= 0.515$$

$\therefore \alpha = 27.27°$ Anticlockwise with XX'

Since, point A is at a longer distance from neutral axis (NA) so, $\sigma_A > \sigma_B$.

N.B: Readers should check the point at which stress has been computed. Remember the point farthest from neutral axis will have greater stress. Further, one should check that one side of neutral axis will induce tensile stress and otherside will induce compressive stress.

EXAMPLE 7 *A (50 mm × 30 mm × 5 mm) angle is used as a cantilever of length 500 mm with the 30 mm leg (horizontal). A load of 1000 N is applied at the free end. Determine the position of the neutral axis and the maximum stress set up.*
SOLUTION

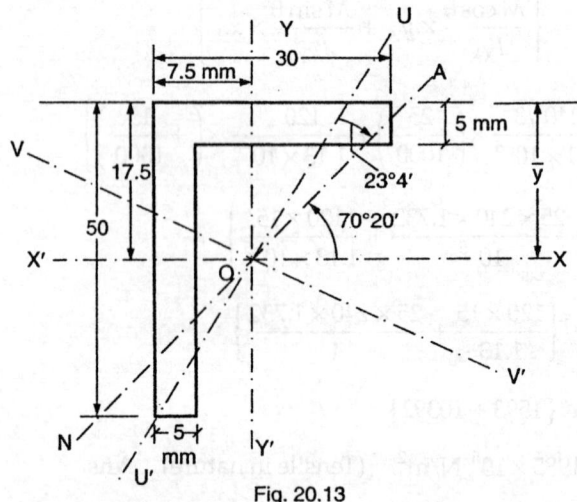

Fig. 20.13

The position of the centroid O and the inclination of the principal axes UU' and VV' can be determined as below.

Let us first calculate centroid 'O'

$$\bar{x} = \frac{(45 \times 5) \times 2.5 + (30 \times 5) \times 15}{(45 + 30) \times 5}$$

$$= 7.5 \text{ mm}$$

$$\bar{y} = \frac{(45 \times 5) \times 2.75 + (30 \times 5) \times 0.25}{(45 + 30) \times 5}$$

$$= 17.5 \text{ mm} \qquad \left[\because \bar{x} = \frac{A_1 x_1 + A_2 x_2}{A_1 + A_2} \text{ and } \bar{y} = \frac{A_1 y_1 + A_2 y_2}{A_1 + A_2} \right]$$

$$I_X = \frac{0.5 \times 4.5^3 \times 10^4}{12} + (45 \times 5) \times 10^2 + \frac{30 \times 5^3}{12} + (30 \times 15) \times 15^2$$

$$= 94400 \text{ mm}^4$$

$$I_Y = \Sigma \left(\frac{bd^3}{12} + Ad^2 \right)$$

$$= \frac{45 \times 5^3}{12} + (45 \times 5) \times 5^2 + \left(\frac{5 \times 30^3}{12} \right) + (5 \times 30) \times 7.5^2$$

$$= 25800 \ \text{mm}^4$$

$$I_{XY} = (45 \times 5) \times (-5)(-1) + (30 \times 5)(2.5) \times (15) \text{mm}^4$$

$$= 28130 \ \text{mm}^4$$

Now, $\tan 2\theta = \left(\dfrac{2 \tan \theta}{I_y - I_x} \right)$

$$= -0.820$$

Given, $2\theta = 140° 40'$

$$\theta = 70°20'$$

By formula $I_U = \dfrac{1}{2}(94.4 + 25.8) + \dfrac{1}{2}(94.4 - 25.8) \times \sec 140°40'$

$$= 15900 \ \text{mm}^4$$

and, $I_V = I_X + I_Y - I_U$

$$= 104300 \ \text{mm}^4$$

The maximum bending moment about XX' is

$$1000 \times 500 \ \text{Nmm} = 5 \times 10^5 \ \text{N mm}$$

Resolving about VV' and UU' respectively

$$M_V = 500000 \sin 70° 20'$$

$$= 470080 \ \text{N mm}$$

and, $M_U = 500000 \cos 70° 20'$

$$= 160830 \ \text{N mm}$$

The combined bending stress at any point defined by coordinates U, V mm is

$$\sigma = \frac{M_v}{I_v} \times u + \frac{M_u}{I_u} \times v \qquad \left[\begin{array}{l} \text{where, } U \text{ and } V \text{ are both positive} \\ \text{in the quadrant } UOV) \end{array} \right]$$

$$= \left(\frac{470,080}{104300} \right) u + \left(\frac{160,830}{15900} \right) v$$

$$= 4.51 \, u + 10.6 \, v$$

The equation of the neutral axis is $\sigma = 0$

i.e. $4.51\, u + 10.6\, v = 0$

or, $\left(\dfrac{4.51}{10.6}\right) u + v = 0$

or, $0.426\, u + v = 0$

This is a line through O inclined at $\tan^{-1}(-0.426)$.

or, $-23°4'$ to UU'

The Stress will be tensile above the N.A and the compressive below N.A.

The maximum tensile stress is at the outside of the corner of the angle, where, U and V are both positive and is given by

$$4.51\,(17.5 \sin 70°\,20' - 7.5 \cos 70°\,20')$$

$$+ 10.6\,(17.5 \cos 70°\,20' + 7.5 \sin 70°\,20')$$

$$= 4.51 \times 13.9 + 10.6 \times 13$$

$\therefore$ $\sigma_t = 203\ \text{N/mm}^2$ **Ans.**

The maximum compressive stress occurs at the inside bottom edge of the vertical leg, where, U and V are negative.

$$\sigma_c = -4.51\,(32.5 \sin 70°20' + 2.5 \cos 70°20')$$

$$-10.6\,(32.5 \cos 70°20' + 2.5 \sin 70°20')$$

$$= -4.51 \times 31.4 - 10.6 \times 8.62$$

$$= -233\ \text{N/mm}^2 \qquad \textbf{Ans.}$$

20.9 SHEAR CENTRE

Shear centre is the point in or outside a section through which the shear force applied, produces no torsion or twist of the member.

In the case of a beam having two axes of symmetry, the shear centre coincides with the centroid.

It the case of section having one axis of symmetry, the shear centre does not coincide with the centroid but lies on the axis of symmetry.

When the load passes through the shear centre there will be only bending in the cross-section and no twisting.   **Similar Problem**

Shear centre for channel section   **(UPTU 3rd Sem. 2013-14)**

For the channel section as shown in Fig. 20.14, let, F_1, F_2 and F_3 be the shear forces in the three legs of the channel.

$$F_1 = \int \tau\, dA$$

$$= \int \frac{F\, A\, \bar{y}}{I t}\, dA$$

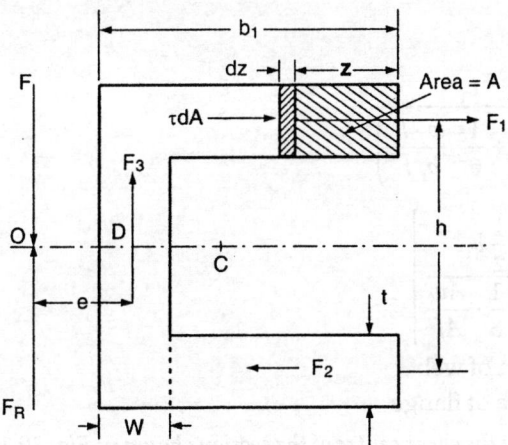

Fig. 20.14

$$A = t \cdot z$$

$$dA = t \, dz$$

$$\bar{y} = \left(\frac{h}{2}\right)$$

$$F_1 = \frac{F}{It} \int_0^{b_1} tz \cdot \frac{h}{2} \cdot t \, dz$$

$$= \frac{Fth}{4I} b_1^2$$

$$I = 2 b_1 t \left(\frac{h}{2}\right)^2 + \frac{1}{12} wh^3$$

$$= \frac{1}{2} b_1 t h^2 \left[1 + \frac{1}{6} \cdot \frac{wh}{b_1 t} \right]$$

$$\therefore \qquad F_1 = \frac{F \cdot b_1}{2h \left[1 + \dfrac{1}{6} \dfrac{wh}{b_1 t} \right]} = F_2$$

Taking moment about D, we get,

$$F_R \times e = F_1 \times \frac{h}{2} + F_2 \times \frac{h}{2}$$

$$= F_1 \cdot h$$

$$= \frac{F b_1}{2 \left(1 + \dfrac{1}{6} \cdot \dfrac{wh}{b_1 t} \right)}$$

Since, $F_R = F$

$\therefore$ $e = \dfrac{b_1}{2\left(1 + \dfrac{1}{6} \cdot \dfrac{w \cdot h}{b_1 t}\right)}$

$= \left\{\dfrac{\dfrac{1}{2} b_1}{1 + \dfrac{1}{6} \cdot \dfrac{Aw}{Af}}\right\}$

where, A_w = Area of web

A_f = Area of flange

EXAMPLE 1 *Locate the shear centre of the section shown in Fig. 20.15.*

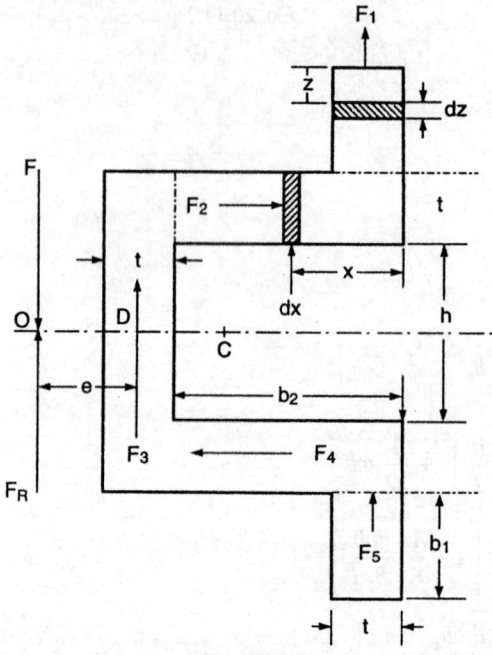

Fig. 20.15

SOLUTION Due to symmetry of the cross-section,

$F_1 = F_5$ and $F_2 = F_4$

$F_1 = \int \tau \cdot dA$

$= \int \dfrac{F A \overline{y}}{It} dA$

$= \dfrac{F}{It} \int_0^{b_1} tz \cdot \left(\dfrac{h}{2} + t + b_1 - \dfrac{z}{2}\right) t\, dZ$

$$= \frac{F \cdot t}{I} \int_0^{b_1} \left(z \cdot \frac{h}{2} + z \cdot t + z \cdot b_1 - \frac{z^2}{2} \right) dZ$$

$$= \frac{F \cdot t}{I} \left[\frac{h}{2} \cdot \frac{b_1^2}{2} + \frac{t b_1^2}{2} + b_1 \cdot \frac{b_1^2}{2} - \frac{1}{6} \cdot b_1^3 \right]$$

$$= \frac{F \cdot t \cdot b_1^2}{I} \left[\frac{h}{4} + \frac{t}{2} + \frac{b_1}{3} \right]$$

$$F_2 = \frac{F}{It} \int_0^{b_2} \left\{ tx \left(\frac{h}{2} + \frac{t}{2} \right) + b_1 t \times \left(\frac{h}{2} + t + \frac{b_1}{2} \right) \right\} t \, dx$$

$$= \frac{Ft}{I} \int_0^{b_2} \left\{ x \left(\frac{h}{2} + \frac{t}{2} \right) + b_1 \times \left(\frac{h}{2} + t + \frac{b_1}{2} \right) \right\} dx$$

$$= \frac{Ft}{It} \left[\left(\frac{h+t}{2} \right) \times \frac{b_2^2}{2} + b_1 \left(\frac{h}{2} + t + \frac{b_1}{2} \right) b_2 \right]$$

$$= \frac{Ft}{I} \left[\frac{h b_2^2}{4} + \frac{t b_2^2}{4} + \frac{b_1 b_2 h}{2} + b_1 b_2 \cdot t + \frac{b_1^2 b_2}{2} \right]$$

$$I = 2 \left[\frac{t b_1^3}{2} + t b_1 \left(\frac{h}{2} + t + \frac{b_1}{2} \right)^2 \right] + \frac{b_2 t^3}{12} + b_2 t \left(\frac{h}{2} + \frac{t}{2} \right)^2 + \frac{t(h+2t)^3}{12}$$

Taking moment about F_3, we get

$$F_R \times e = 2 F_1 \times b_2 - 2 F_2 \times \frac{h}{2}$$

$$F \times e = 2 F_1 b_2 - 2 F_2 \times \frac{h}{2}$$

$$= 2 F_1 b_2 - F_2 h$$

$$= \frac{2 Ft b_1^2 b_2}{I} \left[\frac{h}{4} + \frac{t}{2} + \frac{b_1}{3} \right]$$

$$- \frac{Fth}{I} \left[\frac{h b_2^2}{4} + \frac{t b_2^2}{4} + \frac{b_1 b_2 h}{2} + b_1 b_2 t + \frac{b_1^2 b_2}{2} \right]$$

$$\therefore \quad e = \frac{2 t b_1^2 b_2}{I} \left[\frac{h}{4} + \frac{t}{2} + \frac{b_1}{3} \right] - \frac{th}{I} \left[\frac{h b_2^2}{4} + \frac{t b_2^2}{4} + \frac{b_1 b_2 h}{2} + b_1 b_2 t + \frac{b_1^2 b_2}{2} \right]$$

PROBLEMS FOR PRACTICE

1. If the maximum bending stress allowed in the cross-section of the beam is 15 MPa, determine the value of P.

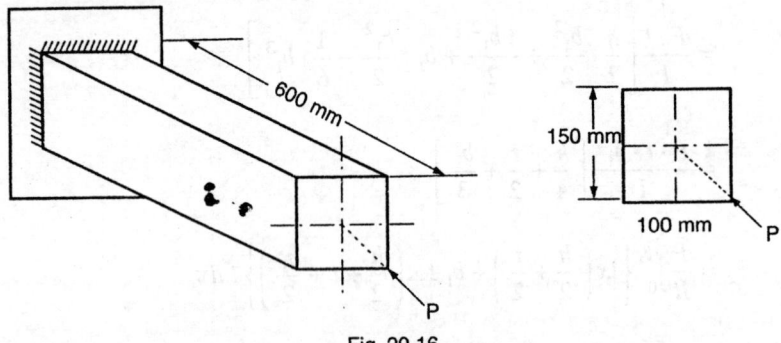

Fig. 20.16

2. A beam simply supported at the ends has the cross-section and is loaded with a concentrated load P as shown in figure. If the maximum flexural stress is not to exceed 20 MPa, determine the safe value of P.

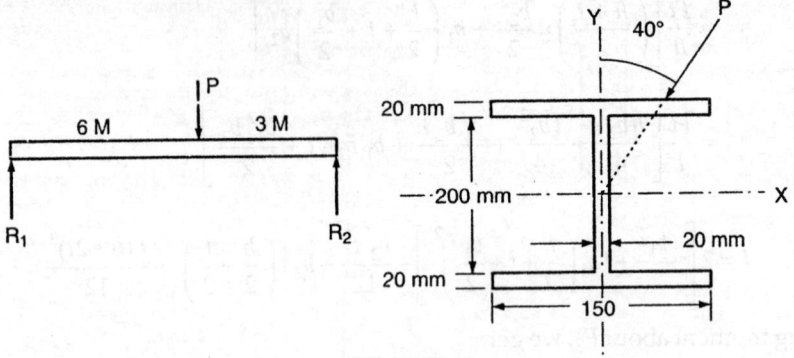

Fig. 20.17

3. A horizontal cantilever of an angle section (100 mm × 80 mm × 20 mm) carries a load $P = 2$ kN at the free end. The length of cantilever is 2 meter from the fixed end. The line of action of the load passes through the centroid of the section and is inclined at 30° to the vertical. Determine the maximum normal stress set up in the beam.

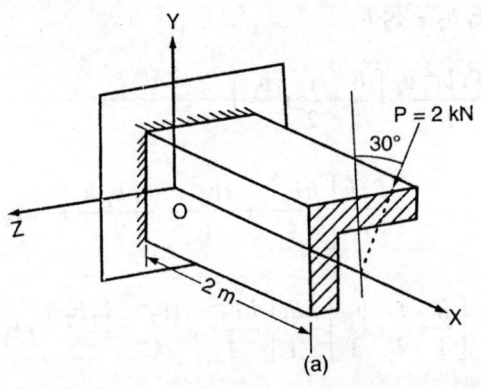

(a)

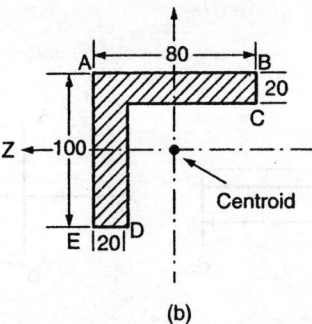

(b)

Fig. 20.18

4. A cantilever beam consists of 10 cm × 10 cm × 1.5 cm angle with the top face *AB* horizontal. It carries a load of 5 kN at 2 meter from the fixed end. The line of action of the load passes through the centroid and inclined at 30° to the vertical. Determine σ_A, σ_B and σ_C and the position of the neutral axis.

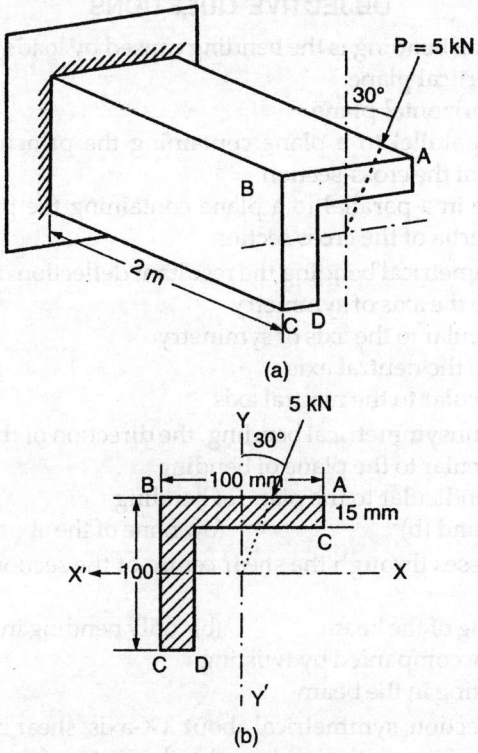

(a)

(b)

Fig. 20.19

5. A horizontal beam, 5 m long is simply supported at ends carries a load of 8 kN at the mid span. The load is inclined 30° to the vertical plane. The line of action of load passes through the centroid of the rectangular section of the beam (100 mm × 120 mm). Find the stresses at all the corners of the section and final max stress also. Locate the neutral axis.

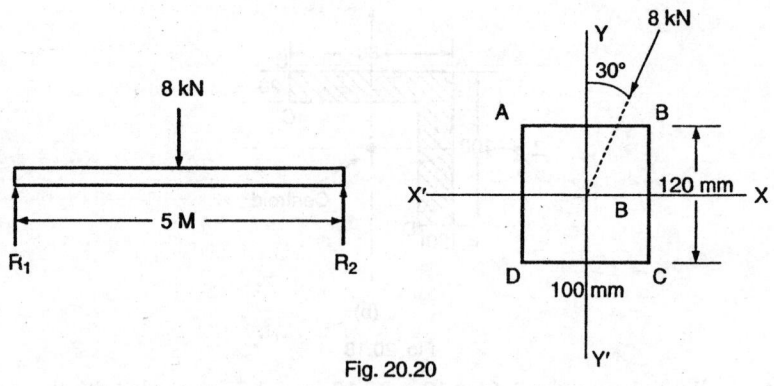

Fig. 20.20

ANSWERS

1. $P = 5.63$ KN   **3.** $\sigma_E\,(max) = -76.54$ MN/m^2 (compressive)

OBJECTIVE QUESTIONS

1. Unsymmetrical bending is the bending caused by loads that
    (a) lie in a vertical plane
    (b) lie in a horizontal plane
    (c) lie in or parallel to a plane containing the principal centroidal axis of inertia of the cross-section
    (d) do not lie in a parallel to a plane containing the principal centroidal axis of inertia of the cross section

2. Under unsymmetrical bending the resultant deflection of a beam is
    (a) parallel to the axis of symmetry
    (b) perpendicular to the axis of symmetry
    (c) parallel to the neutral axis
    (d) perpendicular to the neutral axis

3. In the case of unsymmetrical bending, the direction of the neutral axis is
    (a) perpendicular to the plane of bending
    (b) not perpendicular to the plane of bending
    (c) either (a) and (b)   (d) none of the above

4. If the load passes through the shear centre of the section of the beam then there will be
    (a) no bending of the beam   (b) only bending in the beam
    (c) bending accompanied by twisting
    (d) only twisting in the beam

5. In a channel section, symmetrical about XX-axis, shear centre lies at
    (a) the centre of the vertical web   (b) the centre of the top flange
    (c) the centroid of the section   (d) none of the above

ANSWERS

1. (d)   **2.** (d)   **3.** (b)   **4.** (b)   **5.** (d)

— ❖❖ —

21

ROTATIONAL STRESSES

21.1 INTRODUCTION

In engineering we come across many machine members which are of rotating type. Due to rotation centrifugal stresses are set up in these members.

Derivation for the stress set up in the rotating rim 'OR' ring:

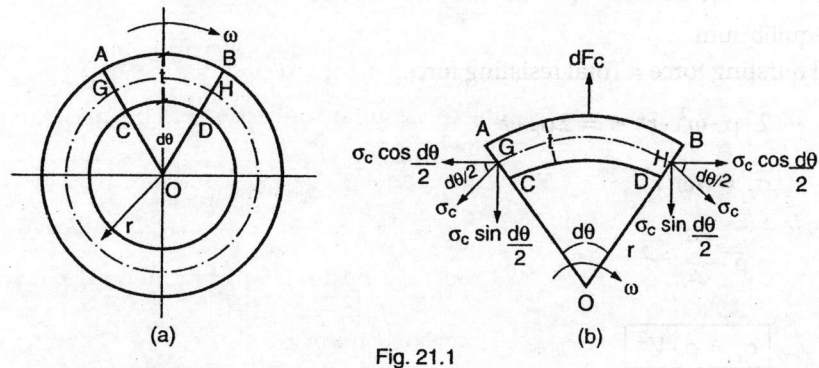

Fig. 21.1

Let us consider a thin ring rotating about its C.G. 'O'.

Let ρ = density of the ring. (Kg/m³)

$OG = OH = r$ = mean radius of the ring in meter

ω = Angular speed (m/sec)

t = thickness of ring, (meter).

Consider an element $ABCD$ of the ring between θ and $\theta + d\theta$

Then $GH = r \cdot d\theta$

Volume of the element per unit length = $r \cdot d\theta \cdot t$.

As a result of rotation each and every element of the ring $ABCD$ will experience centrifugal force F_c which will tend to expand the ring radially outward. This will induce centrifugal stress (or hoop stress) σ_c in the ring which will be tensile in nature.

Centrifugal force on the element

$$dF_c = \rho \cdot (r \cdot d\theta) \cdot t \cdot w^2 r \qquad\qquad (\because F_c = m\omega^2 r)$$

Vertical component of $dF_c = dF_c \sin\theta$

$$= \rho \cdot r \, d\theta \cdot t \cdot \omega^2 r \sin\theta$$

Total vertical or bursting force along xx'

$$= \int_0^\pi dF_c \sin\theta$$

$$= \int_0^\pi \rho \, r \, d\theta \, t \cdot \omega^2 r \sin\theta$$

$$= \rho \omega^2 \, r^2 t \int_0^\pi \sin\theta \, d\theta$$

$$= \rho \omega^2 \, r^2 \, t \left[-\cos\theta\right]_0^\pi$$

$$= 2\,\rho\omega^2 r^2 t \qquad\qquad\qquad\qquad ...(1)$$

Total Resisting force $= 2\sigma_c \cdot t \cdot 1 \qquad\qquad ...(2)$

For equilibrium,

Total bursting force = Total resisting force

$$2 \cdot \rho \cdot \omega^2 \cdot r^2 \cdot t = 2\sigma_c \cdot t$$

$$\sigma_c = \rho \omega^2 \, r^2$$

$$= \rho \cdot \frac{V^2}{r^2} \cdot r^2$$

$$\boxed{\sigma_c = \rho \cdot V^2}$$

where V = peripheral velocity $= \omega \cdot r$

21.2 ROTATING DISC

Let us consider a disc having inner radius $= r_i$

Outer radius $= r_o$

Density of element of disc $= \rho$

Thickness $= t$

Further, let stress at radius $r = \sigma_r$

Stress at radius $(r + dr) = \sigma_r + d\sigma_r$

Circumferential stress or hoop stress $= \sigma_c$

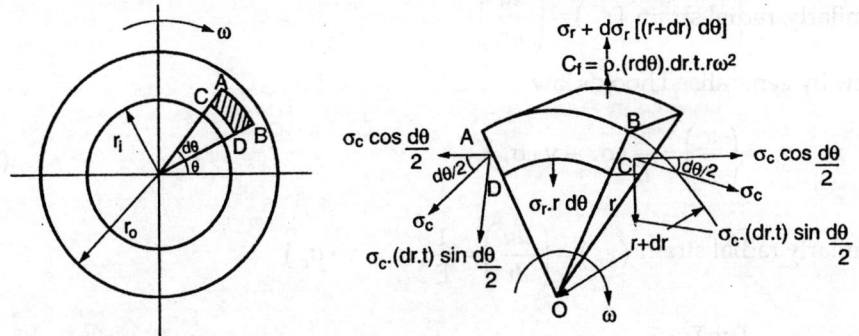

Fig. 21.2

Radial Stress = σ_r

The spinning disc rotating at speed ω produces centrifugal stress which in turn produces strain.

Let unit shift at $r = u$

and radial shift at $(r + dr) = (u + du)$

For equilibrium of the element $ABCD$

Inward force = outward force.

$$2\sigma_c \cdot dr \cdot t \cdot \sin\left(\frac{d\theta}{2}\right) = C_f + (\sigma_r + d_r)\left[(r + dr)d\theta\right] \cdot t - \sigma_r (r d\theta) \cdot t$$

or, $$\sigma_c \cdot dr \cdot t \cdot d\theta = \left[(r d\theta) \cdot dr \cdot t \cdot \rho\right] r \omega^2$$

$$+ (\sigma_r + d_r)(r + dr) d\theta \cdot t - \sigma_r \cdot r \cdot d\theta \cdot t$$

Dividing by $d\theta \cdot t$ both sides

$$\sigma_c \cdot dr = r^2 dr \cdot \rho \cdot \omega^2 + \sigma_r \cdot r + \sigma_r \cdot dr + r \cdot dr - \sigma_r \cdot r$$

(Neglecting small terms)

or, $$(\sigma_c - \sigma_r) dr = \rho w^2 r^2 dr + r \cdot d\sigma_r$$

$$(\sigma_c - \sigma_r) = \rho \omega^2 r^2 + r \cdot \left(\frac{d\sigma_r}{dr}\right) \qquad \qquad \ldots(1)$$

Let us now derive strain. Circumferential 'or' hoop strain

$$(\varepsilon_c) = \frac{2\pi(r + u) - 2\pi r}{2\pi r}$$

$$= \left(\frac{u}{r}\right)$$

Similarly, radial strain $(\varepsilon_r) = \left(\dfrac{du}{dr}\right)$

Now by generalised hook's law

$$\varepsilon_c = \left(\frac{u}{r}\right) = \frac{1}{E}\left(\sigma_c - v \cdot \sigma_r\right) \qquad \ldots(2)$$

Similarly radial strain $(\varepsilon_r) = \left(\dfrac{du}{dr}\right) = \dfrac{1}{E}\left(\sigma_r - v \cdot \sigma_c\right)$

$$\text{As } \left(\frac{u}{r}\right) = \frac{1}{E}\left(\sigma_c - v \cdot \sigma_r\right) \qquad \ldots(3)$$

$$\therefore \quad u = \frac{1}{E}\left(r \cdot \sigma_c - r \cdot v \cdot \sigma_r\right)$$

$$\therefore \quad \left(\frac{du}{dr}\right) = \frac{1}{E}\left(1 \cdot \sigma_c + r \cdot \frac{d\sigma_c}{dr} - 1 \cdot v \cdot \sigma_r - v \cdot r \cdot \frac{d\sigma_r}{dr}\right) \qquad \ldots(4)$$

From (3), $\left(\dfrac{du}{dr}\right) = \dfrac{1}{E}\left(\sigma_r - v \cdot \sigma_c\right)$

Hence, from (3) and (4)

$$\sigma_c + r \cdot \frac{d\sigma_c}{dr} - v \cdot \sigma_r - v \cdot r \cdot \frac{d\sigma_r}{dr} = \sigma_r - v \cdot \sigma_c$$

or, $\quad (\sigma_c - \sigma_r) + v(\sigma_c - \sigma_r) + r \cdot \dfrac{d\sigma_c}{dr} - v \cdot r \cdot \dfrac{d\sigma_r}{dr} = 0$

or, $\quad (\sigma_c - \sigma_r)(1 + v) + r \cdot \dfrac{d\sigma_c}{dr} - v \cdot r \cdot \dfrac{d\sigma_r}{dr} = 0 \qquad \ldots(5)$

Substituting the value of $(\sigma_c - \sigma_r)$ in equation (5) from equation (1)

$$\left\{\rho\omega^2 r^2 + r \cdot \left(\frac{d\sigma_r}{dr}\right)\right\}(1 + v) + r \cdot \left(\frac{d\sigma_c}{dr}\right) - v \cdot r \cdot \left(\frac{d\sigma_r}{dr}\right) = 0$$

or, $\quad \rho\omega^2 r^2 (1+v) + r\left(\dfrac{d\sigma_r}{dr}\right) + r\left(\dfrac{d\sigma_r}{dr}\right) \cdot v + r\left(\dfrac{d\sigma_c}{dr}\right) - v \cdot r \cdot \left(\dfrac{d\sigma_r}{dr}\right) = 0$

or, $\quad \rho\omega^2 r^2 (1+v) + r\left(\dfrac{d\sigma_r}{dr}\right) + r\left(\dfrac{d\sigma_c}{dr}\right) = 0$

or, $\quad \rho\omega^2 r (1+v) + \left(\dfrac{d\sigma_r}{dr}\right) + \left(\dfrac{d\sigma_c}{dr}\right) = 0$

or, $\quad \rho \omega^2 r (1+v) + \dfrac{d}{dr} \times (\sigma_r + \sigma_c) = 0$

or, $\quad \dfrac{d}{dr} (\sigma_r + \sigma_c) = -\rho \omega^2 r (1+v)$

Integrating we get

$$(\sigma_r + \sigma_c) = -\dfrac{\rho \omega^2 r}{2} (1+v) + 2A \qquad \qquad \text{...(6)}$$

where $2A$ is constant of integration

Subtracting (1) from (6)

$$2\sigma_r = -(1+v) \cdot \dfrac{\rho \omega^2 r^2}{2} + 2A - \rho \omega^2 r^2 - r \cdot \left(\dfrac{d\sigma_r}{dr} \right)$$

or, $\quad 2\sigma_r + r \cdot \left(\dfrac{d\sigma_r}{dr} \right) = -\dfrac{(3+v)}{2} \rho \omega^2 r^2 + 2A$

or, $\quad 2r \cdot \sigma_r + r^2 \cdot \left(\dfrac{d\sigma_r}{dr} \right) = -\dfrac{(3+v)}{2} \rho \omega^2 r^3 + 2Ar \qquad \left[\begin{array}{l} \text{Multiplying by} \\ r \text{ both sides} \end{array} \right]$

$$\dfrac{d}{dr} \left(r^2 \cdot \sigma_r \right) = -\dfrac{(3+v)}{2} \rho \omega^2 r^3 + 2Ar$$

Integrating both sides

$$\sigma_r \cdot r^2 = -\left(\dfrac{3+v}{8} \right) \rho \omega^2 r^4 + Ar^2 - B$$

where 'B' is constant of Integration

$$\sigma_r = -\left(\dfrac{3+v}{8} \right) \rho \omega^2 r^2 + A - \dfrac{B}{r^2}$$

$$\therefore \boxed{ \sigma_r = \left(A - \dfrac{B}{r^2} \right) - \left(\dfrac{3+v}{8} \right) \rho \omega^2 r^2 } \qquad \qquad \text{...(7)}$$

Similarly we can derive

$$\boxed{ \sigma_c = \left(A + \dfrac{B}{r^2} \right) - \left(\dfrac{1+3v}{8} \right) \rho \omega^2 r^2 } \qquad \qquad \text{...(8)}$$

The constants A and B can be evaluated from boundary condition

21.3 SOLID DISC

For solid disc constant B in the above equation is zero otherwise stress would become infinite at $r = 0$

For the constant 'A', we have

$$\sigma_r = 0 \text{ at } r = r_o \text{ (outside diameter)}$$

$$\therefore \qquad 0 = A - \left(\frac{3+v}{8}\right)\rho \cdot \omega^2 \cdot r_o^2$$

$$A = \left(\frac{3+v}{8}\right)\cdot \rho \cdot \omega^2 \cdot r_o^2$$

Therefore, $$\boxed{\sigma_r = \left(\frac{3+v}{8}\right)\rho\omega^2\left[r_o^2 - r^2\right]}$$

and $$\sigma_c = A - (1+3v)\cdot\frac{\rho\omega^2 r_o^2}{8}$$

$$= \left(\frac{3+v}{8}\right)\rho\omega^2 r_o^2 - (1+3v)\cdot\frac{\rho\omega^2 r_o^2}{8}$$

$$= \frac{\rho\omega^2 r_o^2}{8}(3 + v - 1 - 3v)$$

$$\boxed{\sigma_c = \frac{\rho\omega^2 r_o^2 (1-v)}{4}}$$

Maximum stress occurs at the centre and are

$$\sigma_{r(\max)} = \sigma_{c(\max)} \text{ at } r = 0$$

$$= \left(\frac{3+v}{8}\right)\rho\omega^2 r_o^2$$

21.4 DISC WITH CENTRAL HOLE

Here the boundary conditions are

$$\text{At } r = r_i, \ \sigma_r = 0$$

and $$\text{At } r = r_o; \ \sigma_r = 0$$

Hence from equation (8)

$$0 = A - \frac{B}{r^2} - \left(\frac{3+v}{8}\right)\cdot \rho \cdot r_i^2 \cdot \omega^2$$

and $$0 = A - \frac{B}{r^2} - \left(\frac{3+v}{8}\right)\cdot \rho \cdot r_o^2 \omega^2$$

Solving, $$B = \left(\frac{3+v}{8}\right)\cdot \rho\omega^2 \cdot r_i^2 \cdot r_o^2$$

and $\quad A = \left(\dfrac{3+v}{8}\right) \cdot \rho\omega^2 \left(r_i^2 + r_o^2\right)$

Now, putting values of 'A' and 'B' in equation (7) and (8) we can get the values of σ_r and σ_c respectively.

$$\therefore \qquad \sigma_r = \left(\dfrac{3+v}{8}\right)\rho\omega^2 \left[r_i^2 + r_o^2 - \dfrac{r_i^2 r_o^2}{r^2} - r^2 \right] \qquad \qquad \dots(9)$$

and $\quad \sigma_c = \left(\dfrac{3+v}{8}\right) \cdot \rho\omega^2 \left[r_i^2 + r_o^2 + \dfrac{r_i^2 r_o^2}{r^2} - \dfrac{1+3v}{3+v} r^2 \right] \qquad \dots(10)$

For σ_r to be maximum, $\left(\dfrac{d\sigma_r}{dr}\right) = 0$

Let the value of r at which σ_r in maximum is R_1.

Now, differentiating equation (9) and equating the same to zero

We have, $\dfrac{d\sigma_r}{dr} = \left(\dfrac{3+v}{8}\right)\rho\omega^2 \left[\dfrac{2r_i^2 \, r_o^2}{R_1^3} - 2R_1 \right] = 0$

i.e. $\qquad R_1^4 = r_i^2 \, r_o^2$

$\therefore \qquad R_1 = \sqrt{r_i \, r_o}$

σ_r is maximum at the value of radius which is the geometric mean of the inner and outer radii of the disc.

Substituting $r = \sqrt{r_i \, r_o}$ in equation (9)

$$\sigma_{r \, max} = \dfrac{3+v}{8}\rho\omega^2 \left[r_i^2 + r_o^2 - \dfrac{r_i^2 \, r_o^2}{r_i \, r_o} - r_i \, r_o \right]$$

$$= \dfrac{3+v}{8}\rho\omega^2 \left(r_o - r_i \right)^2 \qquad \qquad \dots(11)$$

It can be seen from equation (10) that σ_c is maximum when r is minimum i.e. when $r = r_i$

$$\therefore \qquad \sigma_{c \, max} = \dfrac{3+v}{8}\rho\omega^2 \left[r_i^2 + r_o^2 + \dfrac{r_i^2 \, r_o^2}{r_i^2} - \dfrac{1+3v}{3+v} r_i^2 \right]$$

$$= \dfrac{3+v}{8}\rho\omega^2 \left[r_o^2 + \dfrac{1-v}{3+v} \cdot r_i^2 \right]$$

The stress distribution *i.e.* σ_r and σ_c as given by equation (9) and (10) is shown in the fig. below.

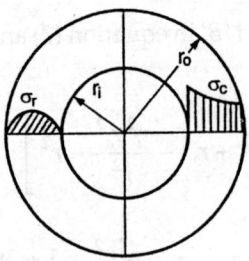

Fig. 21.3

Comparison of maximum stresses in solid and hollow discs

We have seen earlier that maximum stress occurs at the centre in solid disc

and $\sigma_{r(max)} = \left(\dfrac{3+v}{8} \right) \rho \omega^2 r_o^2$ for solid disc

Similarly for hollow disc whose inner radius $= r_i$ and outer radius $= r_o$,

$$\sigma_{r\ max} = \left(\frac{3+v}{8} \right) \rho \omega^2 \left(r_o - r_i \right)^2 \text{ for hollow disc}$$

∴ $\dfrac{(\sigma_r) \text{max, hollow}}{(\sigma_r) \text{max, solid}} = \dfrac{\dfrac{3+v}{8} \rho \omega^2 \left(r_o - r_i \right)^2}{\dfrac{3+v}{8} \rho \omega^2 r_o^2}$

$$= \frac{\left(r_o - r_i \right)^2}{r_o^2}$$

$$= \left[1 - \frac{r_i}{r_o} \right]^2$$

$$\equiv 1 \text{ if } r_i \ll r_o$$

Hence a small hole at the centre of a solid disc does not affect the radial stress in the disc.

For comparing the hoop stresses,

$$\frac{\left(\sigma_{c\ max} \right) \text{hollow}}{\left(\sigma_{c\ max} \right) \text{solid}} = \frac{\dfrac{3+v}{4} \rho \omega^2 \left[r_o^2 + \dfrac{1-v}{3+v} r_i^2 \right]}{\dfrac{3+v}{8} \rho \omega^2 r_o^2}$$

$$= 2\left[1 + \frac{1-v}{3+v} \cdot \frac{r_i^2}{r_o^2}\right]$$

$$\equiv 2 \text{ if } r_i \ll r_o$$

This shows that a small hole at the centre of a solid disc doubles the maximum hoop stress in the disc.

EXAMPLE 1 *A thin steel disc of uniform thickness and of 250 mm diameter with a central hole of 50 mm diameter rotates at 10,000 rpm. Calculate the maximum principal stress and the maximum shear stress in the disc.*

$$\text{Given } \rho = 7000 \ Kg/m^3$$

$$v = 0.3$$

SOLUTION

We know that Radial stress $(\sigma_r) = A - \dfrac{B}{r^2} - \left(\dfrac{3+v}{8}\right)\rho\omega^2 r^2$

and Hoop stress $(\sigma_c) = A + \dfrac{B}{r^2} - \left(\dfrac{1+3v}{8}\right)\rho\omega^2 r^2$

$$\omega = \frac{2\pi \times 10,000}{60}$$

$$= 1046.66 \text{ rad/sec}$$

$$\left(\frac{3+v}{8}\right)\rho\omega^2 = \left(\frac{3+0.3}{8}\right) \times 7000 \times (1046.66)^2$$

$$= \frac{3.3}{8} \times 7000 \times (1046.66)^2$$

$$= 3.163 \times 10^9$$

$$\left(\frac{1+3v}{8}\right)\rho\omega^2 = \left(\frac{1+3\times0.3}{8}\right) \times 7000 \times (1046.66)^2$$

$$= \left(\frac{1+0.9}{8}\right) \times 7000 \times (1046.66)^2$$

$$= \frac{1.9}{8} \times 7000 \times (1046.66)^2$$

$$= 1.821 \times 10^9$$

$$\therefore \qquad \sigma_r = A - \frac{B}{r^2} - 3.163 \times 10^9 \, r^2 \ \text{N/m}^2$$

$$\text{and} \qquad \sigma_c = A + \frac{B}{r^2} - 1.821 \times 10^9 r^2 \ \text{N/m}^2$$

Now, $\sigma_r = 0$ when $r = 25$ mm and $r = 125$ mm

$\therefore$ $0 = A - \dfrac{B}{(0.025)^2} - 3.163 \times 10^9 \times (0.025)^2$

and $0 = A - \dfrac{B}{(0.125)^2} - 3.163 \times 10^9 \times (0.125)^2$

On solving we get

$\quad\quad B = 30918$

and $A = 51.447 \times 10^6$

Maximum principal stress is the 'Hoop Stress' at the inner surface.

$$\sigma_{max} = \sigma_c = \left\{ 51.447 \times 10^6 + \dfrac{(30918)^2}{(0.025)^2} - 1.821 \times 10^9 \times (0.025)^2 \right\}$$

at $r = 25$ mm

$$= 99.77 \times 10^6 \ \ N/m^2$$

$$= 99.77 \ \ MPa \quad \textbf{Ans.}$$

Maximum shear stress

$$\tau_{max} = \dfrac{\sigma_{max}}{2}$$

$$= \dfrac{99.77}{2}$$

$$= 49.88 \ MPa \quad\quad \textbf{Ans.}$$

EXAMPLE 2 *Compute the largest value of 'radial' and 'hoop stress' for a rotating disc of internal diameter 150 mm and external diameter 300 mm.*
The disc is rotating at 1500 rpm.
For the disc material, density $\rho = 7000 \ Kg/m^3$ and $v = 0.3$.
SOLUTION   We have,

$$\sigma_r = A - \dfrac{B}{r^2} - \left(\dfrac{3+v}{8} \right) \rho \omega^2 r^2$$

and $$\sigma_c = A + \dfrac{B}{r^2} - \left(\dfrac{1+3v}{8} \right) \rho \omega^2 r^2$$

$$\omega = \dfrac{2\pi \times 1500}{60}$$

$$= 157.08 \ rad/sec$$

Now, $\sigma_r = 0$ when $r = 0.075$ m

and   when $r = 0.150$ m

$$\therefore \qquad 0 = A - \frac{B}{(0.075)^2} - \left(\frac{3.3}{8}\right)\left(7 \times 10^3\right)(157.08)^2 (0.075)^2$$

and $\qquad 0 = A - \dfrac{B}{(0.15)^2} - \left(\dfrac{3.3}{8}\right)\left(7 \times 10^3\right)(157.08)^2 (0.150)^2$

Solving these two equations we get

$$B = 9014.6$$

and $\qquad A = 2003298$

$$\therefore \qquad \sigma_r = 2003298 - \frac{9014.6}{r^2} - \frac{3.3}{8}\left(7 \times 10^3\right)(157.08)^2 r^2$$

and $\qquad \sigma_c = 2003298 + \dfrac{9014.6}{r^2} - \dfrac{1.9}{8}\left(7 \times 10^3\right)(157.08)^2 r^2$

i.e. $\qquad \sigma_r = 2003298 - \dfrac{9014.6}{r^2} - 71246539\, r^2$

and $\qquad \sigma_c = 2003298 + \dfrac{9014.6}{r^2} - 41020734\, r^2$

Further σ_r is maximum when,

$$r^2 = r_i\, r_o$$

$$= 0.075 \times 0.150$$

$$= 0.01125 \text{ m}^2$$

$$\therefore \qquad \sigma_{r(max)} = 20032928 - \frac{9014.6}{0.01125} - 71246539 \times 0.1125$$

$$= 400476 \text{ N/m}^2$$

$$= 0.4 \text{ MPa} \qquad \textbf{Ans.}$$

σ_c is maximum when

$$r = 75 \text{ mm} = 0.075 \text{ m}$$

$$\therefore \qquad \sigma_{c\,max} = 2003298 + \frac{9014.6}{5.625 \times 10^{-3}} - 41020734 \times (0.075)^2$$

$$= 3375.52 \text{ N/m}^2$$

$$= 3.37 \text{ MPa} \qquad \textbf{Ans.}$$

21.5 DISC OF UNIFORM STRENGTH

It is observed that the hoop stress in the disc due to rotation is maximum at the centre and decreases towards the periphery.

Even the radial stress is zero at the periphery. Therefore, it is uneconomical if the thickness of the disc is kept constant.

The most economical section of the disc is the one which results in the same value of the stresses radial or hoop, throughout the disc.

Such a disc a called the disc of uniform strength, and in this disc $\sigma_r = \sigma_c = \sigma$ constant.

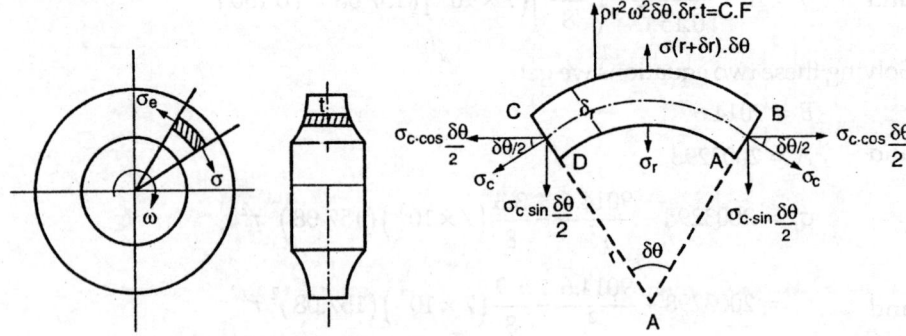

Fig. 21.4

Let t = thickness of the disc at radius r

and $(t + \delta t)$ = thickness at radius $(r + \delta r)$

           ρ = density of material.

Outward radial force on face BC

$$= \sigma(t + \delta t)(r + \delta r)\,\delta\theta$$

$$= \sigma(t \cdot r + t \cdot \delta r + r\,\delta t) \cdot \delta\theta$$

Centrifugal force acting on the element $ABCD$ is

$$\rho \cdot (r \cdot \delta\theta \cdot \delta r \cdot t) \cdot \omega^2 r$$

Inward radial force on the face AD

$$= \sigma \cdot t \cdot r \cdot \delta\theta$$

Inward radial force due to component of force

on faces AB and $CD = (\sigma \cdot t \cdot \delta r \cdot \delta\theta)$

For equilibrium of the element

Total inward radial force = Total outward radial force

$$\sigma \cdot t \cdot r \cdot \delta\theta + \sigma \cdot t \cdot \delta r \cdot \delta\theta = \sigma(t \cdot r + r \cdot \delta t + t \cdot \delta r)\delta\theta$$
$$+ \rho(r \cdot \delta\theta \cdot \delta r \cdot t)\omega^2 r$$

$\therefore$ $\sigma \cdot r \cdot \delta t \cdot \delta\theta + \rho \cdot \delta\theta \cdot \delta r \cdot t \cdot \omega^2 r^2 = 0$

$$\frac{\delta t}{t} = -\rho \cdot \frac{\omega^2}{\sigma} \cdot r \cdot \delta r$$

Taking limit both sides.

$$\left(\frac{dt}{t}\right) = -\rho \cdot \frac{\omega^2}{\sigma} \cdot r \cdot dr$$

Integrating both sides

$$\ln(t) = -\rho \cdot \frac{\omega^2}{\sigma} \cdot \frac{r^2}{2} + \ln A$$

$$\ln\left(\frac{t}{A}\right) = -\rho \cdot \left(\frac{\omega^2 r^2}{2\sigma}\right)$$

$$\frac{t}{A} = e^{-\frac{\rho \cdot \omega^2 r^2}{2\sigma}}$$

$$\therefore \quad t = A \cdot e^{-\frac{\rho \cdot \omega^2 r^2}{2\sigma}}$$

Let $t = t_0$ at $r = r_i$ then we have

$$t_0 = A \cdot e^{-\frac{\rho \cdot \omega^2 r_i^2}{2\sigma}}$$

$$\boxed{\therefore \quad t = t_0 \cdot e^{-\rho \cdot \frac{\omega^2}{2\sigma}\left(r^2 - r_i^2\right)}}$$

For solid uniform disc $r_i \to 0$

$$\boxed{\therefore \quad t = t_0 \cdot e^{-\frac{\rho \omega^2 r^2}{2\sigma}}}$$

EXAMPLE 3 *A solid circular disc of radius 3 m is of uniform strength. It rotates at 1000 rpm and the permissible stress is restricted to 100 MPa.*
Find out the equation for the thickness of the disc and hence evaluate the values of minimum thickness.
Assume density of steel $(\rho) = 7850 \ Kg/m^3$ *and* $t_0 = 100 \ mm$.
SOLUTION

$$\omega = \frac{2\pi N}{60}$$

$$= \frac{2\pi \times 1000}{60}$$

$$= 104.7 \ \text{rad/sec}$$

$$\sigma_{permissible} = 100 \ \text{MPa}$$

$$= 100 \times 10^6 \ \text{N/mm}^2$$

Density $(\rho) = 7850 \ \text{Kg/m}^3$

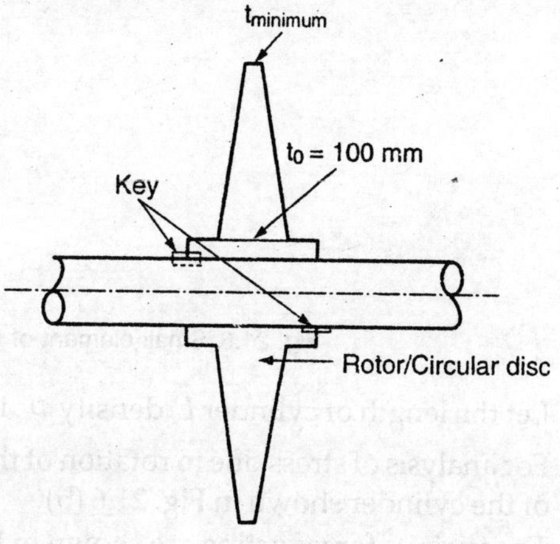

Equation for thickness $t = t_0 \cdot e^{\left(\frac{\rho \omega^2 r^2}{2\sigma}\right)}$

Fig. 21.5

$\therefore$ $\qquad$ $\dfrac{\rho\omega^2}{2\sigma} = \dfrac{7850 \times (104.7)^2}{2 \times (100 \times 10^6)} = 0.43$

$\therefore$ $\qquad$ Required thickness at any distance, $r(t) = t_0 \cdot e^{-0.43\, r^2}$

$\therefore$ $\qquad$ Minimum thickness which occurs at circumference where $r = 3$ m

$\therefore$ $\qquad$ $t_{min} = \left(100 \times e^{-0.43 \times 3^2}\right)$

$\qquad\qquad$ $= 2.09$ mm.   **Ans.**

21.6 ROTATING CYLINDER

Consider a circular cylinder of inside radius r_i outside radius r_o, rotating at speed w.

Assume that plane section of the cylinder remain plane during rotation, therefore, the axial strain (ε_z) along z-axis will be independent of radius r of the cylinder and will be constant.

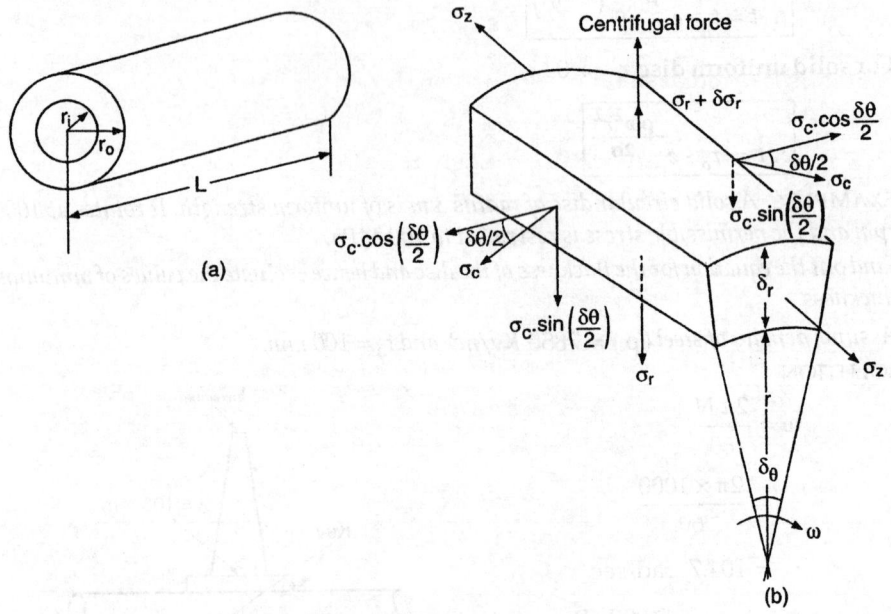

Fig. 21.6 Small element of the cylinder and forces acting

Let the length of cylinder L, density ρ, inner radius r_i, outer radius r_o.

For analysis of stress due to rotation of the cylinder let us consider a small element of the cylinder shown in Fig. 21.6 (b).

The various forces acting are shown in Fig. 21.6 (b).

Let $\qquad$ σ_r = Radial stress at radius r

$$\sigma_r + \delta\sigma_r = \text{Radial stress at radius } (r + \delta r)$$

$$\sigma_c = \text{Circumferential stress at radius } r$$

$$\sigma_z = \text{Axial stress (constant) over cylinder cross section.}$$

$$u = \text{Radial displacement at radius } r$$

$$(u + \delta u) = \text{Radial displacement at radius } (r + \delta r)$$

Circumferential strain $(\varepsilon_c) = \dfrac{2\pi(r + u) - 2\pi r}{2\pi r} = \left(\dfrac{u}{r}\right)$

Also applying generalized Hook's law

$$\varepsilon_c = \frac{1}{E}[\sigma_c - \nu(\sigma_r + \sigma_z)]$$

$$\therefore \qquad \frac{1}{E}[\sigma_c - \nu(\sigma_r + \sigma_z)] = \frac{u}{r}$$

$$\Rightarrow \qquad E_u = r[\sigma_c - \nu(\sigma_r + \sigma_z)] \qquad\qquad \text{...(i)}$$

Radial strain $= \dfrac{\delta u}{\delta r}$

By Hook's law, radial strain $= \dfrac{1}{E}[\sigma_r - \nu(\sigma_c + \sigma_z)]$

$$\therefore \qquad E \cdot \frac{\delta u}{\delta r} = \sigma_r - \nu(\sigma_c + \sigma_z)$$

In the limit, $\delta r \to 0$

$$E \cdot \frac{du}{dr} = \sigma_r - \nu(\sigma_c + \sigma_z) \qquad\qquad \text{...(ii)}$$

Now, diffrerentiating equation (i), we get

$$E \cdot \frac{du}{dr} = r \cdot \frac{d\sigma_c}{dr} + \sigma_c - \nu(\sigma_r + \sigma_z) - \nu r\left(\frac{d\sigma_r}{dr} + \frac{d\sigma_z}{dr}\right)$$

$$= \sigma_r - \nu(\sigma_c + \sigma_z) \qquad\qquad\qquad \text{[From equation (i)]}$$

$$\therefore \qquad (\sigma_c - \sigma_r)(1 + \nu) + r\left[\frac{d\sigma_c}{dr} - \nu\left(\frac{d\sigma_r}{dr} + \frac{d\sigma_z}{dr}\right)\right] = 0 \qquad \text{...(iii)}$$

Contrifugal force on the element $= \rho(r\delta\theta \cdot \delta rL)\omega^2 r$

$$= \rho\omega^2 r^2 L\delta\theta \cdot \delta r$$

Now equating forces on the element in the direction of centrifugal force we have,

$$\rho\omega^2 r^2\,\delta\theta \cdot \delta r \cdot L + (\sigma_r + \delta\sigma_r)[(r + \delta r)\,\delta\theta \cdot L]$$

$$= \sigma_r \cdot r \cdot \delta\theta \cdot L + 2\sigma_c \cdot \delta_r \cdot \frac{\delta\theta}{2} \cdot L \qquad \left[\text{As } \sin\frac{\delta\theta}{2} = \frac{\delta\theta}{2}\right]$$

On simplification, we get

$$(\sigma_c - \sigma_r) = \rho\omega^2 r^2 + r \cdot \frac{d\sigma_r}{dr} \qquad\qquad \text{...(iv)}$$

Substituting values of $(\sigma_c - \sigma_r)$ into equation (iii), we get

$$\left(\rho\omega^2 r^2 + r \cdot \frac{d\sigma_r}{dr}\right)(1+v) + r\left\{\frac{d\sigma_c}{dr} - v\left(\frac{d\sigma_r}{dr} + \frac{d\sigma_z}{dr}\right)\right\} = 0$$

or, $$\rho\omega^2 r^2 (1+v) + r \cdot \frac{d\sigma_r}{dr} + vr\frac{d\sigma_r}{dr} + r \cdot \frac{d\sigma_c}{dr} - rv\frac{d\sigma_r}{dr} - rv \cdot \frac{d\sigma_z}{dr} = 0$$

or, $$\frac{d\sigma_c}{dr} + \frac{d\sigma_r}{dr} = (-)\rho\omega^2 r^2(1+v) + v \cdot \frac{d\sigma_z}{dr} \qquad\qquad \text{...(v)}$$

Now, $$\varepsilon_z = \frac{1}{E}[\sigma_z - v(\sigma_c + \sigma_r)]$$

∴ $$E \cdot \varepsilon_z = \sigma_z - v(\sigma_c + \sigma_r) = \text{constant} = c \text{ (let)}$$

∴ $$\sigma_z = c + v(\sigma_c + \sigma_r)$$

or, $$\left(\frac{d\sigma_z}{dr}\right) = v\left[\frac{d\sigma_c}{dr} + \frac{d\sigma_r}{dr}\right] \qquad\qquad \text{...(vi)}$$

Substituting this in eqn. (v), we get

$$\frac{d\sigma_c}{dr} + \frac{d\sigma_r}{dr} = -\rho\omega^2 r(1+v) + v^2\left[\frac{d\sigma_c}{dr} + \frac{d\sigma_r}{dr}\right]$$

∴ $$\frac{d\sigma_c}{dr} + \frac{d\sigma_r}{dr} = (-)\frac{\rho\omega^2 r(1+v)}{(1-v^2)}$$

or $$\frac{d\sigma_c}{dr} + \frac{d\sigma_r}{dr} = (-)\frac{\rho\omega^2 r}{(1-v)}$$

Integrating, we get

$$\sigma_c + \sigma_r = \frac{\rho\omega^2 r^2}{2(1-v)} + 2A \qquad\qquad \text{...(vii)}$$

where $2A$ is constant of Integration.

From equation (iv) and (vii), we get

$$2\sigma_r = \frac{\rho\omega^2 r^2}{2(1-v)} + 2A - \rho\omega^2 r^2 - r \cdot \frac{d\sigma_r}{dr}$$

or, $$\left(2\sigma_r + r \cdot \frac{d\sigma_r}{dr}\right) = -\rho\omega^2 r^2\left[\frac{3-2v}{2(1-v)}\right] + 2A$$

or, $\dfrac{1}{r} \cdot \dfrac{d}{dr}(\sigma_r \cdot r^2) = -\rho \cdot \omega^2 r^2 \left[\dfrac{3 - 2v}{2(1 - v)} \right] + 2A$

or, $\dfrac{d}{dr}(\sigma_r \cdot r^2) = -\rho \cdot \omega^2 r^3 \left[\dfrac{3 - 2v}{2(1 - v)} \right] + 2Ar$

Integerating

$$\sigma_r \cdot r^2 = -\dfrac{\rho \cdot \omega^2 r^3}{8} \left[\dfrac{3 - 2v}{2(1 - v)} \right] + A r^2 - B$$

where (–) B is constant of integration.

$$\therefore \; \sigma_r = A - \dfrac{B}{r^2} - \left[\dfrac{3 - 2v}{2(1 - v)} \right] \rho \omega^2 r^2$$ ...(viii)

Substituting this value of σ_r in equation (vii), we get

$$\sigma_c = -\dfrac{\rho \omega^2 r^2}{2(1 - v)} + 2A - A + \dfrac{B}{r^2} + \dfrac{3 - 2v}{8(1 - v)} - \rho \omega^2 r^2$$

or, $\sigma_c = A + \dfrac{B}{r^2} - \dfrac{\rho \omega^2 r^2}{2(1 - v)} \left[1 - \dfrac{3 - 2v}{4} \right]$

$$\therefore \; \sigma_c = A + \dfrac{B}{r^2} - \left[\dfrac{1 + 2v}{8(1 - v)} \right] \rho \omega^2 r^2$$ ...(ix)

For the evaluation of σ_z, we substitute σ_c and σ_r in equation (vi) and differentiate w.r.t. r.

$$\dfrac{d\sigma_z}{dr} = v \left[\dfrac{d\sigma_c}{dr} + \dfrac{d\sigma_r}{dr} \right]$$

$$= v \left[\left\{ -\dfrac{2B}{r^3} - \dfrac{1 + 2v}{4(1 - v)} \times \rho \omega^2 r \right\} + \left\{ -\dfrac{2B}{r^3} - \dfrac{3 + 2v}{4(1 - v)} \times \rho \omega^2 r \right\} \right]$$

$$= (-) \left(\dfrac{v}{1 - v} \right) \rho \omega^2 r$$

$$\therefore \qquad \sigma_z = (-) \dfrac{v}{1 - v} , \dfrac{\rho \omega^2 r^2}{2} + C$$

where C is constant of integration.

To evaluate C, consider the equilibrium of cylinder in the axial direction

$$\int_{r_i}^{r_o} \sigma_z \, (2\pi r \, dr) = 0$$

$$\int_{r_i}^{r_o} \sigma_z \cdot r\, dr = 0$$

or, $$\int_{r_i}^{r_o} \left\{ -\frac{\nu}{1-\nu} \cdot \frac{\rho\omega^2 r^3}{2} + Cr \right\} dr = 0$$

or, $$-\frac{\nu}{1-\nu} \cdot \frac{\rho\omega^2}{8} (r_o^4 - r_i^4) + \frac{C}{2}(r_o^2 - r_i^2) = 0$$

or, $$C = \left(\frac{\nu}{1-\nu}\right) \cdot \frac{\rho\omega^2}{4}(r_o^2 + r_i^2)$$

$$\therefore \quad \sigma_z = \left(\frac{\nu}{1-\nu}\right) \cdot \frac{\rho\omega^2 r^2}{2} + \left(\frac{\nu}{1-\nu}\right) \cdot \frac{\rho\omega^2}{4}(r_o^2 + r_i^2)$$

$$\boxed{\therefore \quad \sigma_z = \frac{\nu}{4(1-\nu)} \cdot \rho\omega^2 \cdot [r_i^2 + r_o^2 - 2r^2]} \qquad \ldots(x)$$

21.7 SOLID CYLINDER

For the solid cylinder constant B in eqn (viii) and (ix) is zero because stresses become infinite at $r = 0$.

Now, for solid cylinder boundary condition is

at $r = r_0$; $\sigma_r = 0$

Hence from equation (viii)

$$0 = A - \frac{3-2\nu}{8(1-\nu)} \rho\omega^2 r_o^2$$

$$\therefore \quad A = \frac{3-2\nu}{8(1-\nu)} \rho\omega^2 r_o^2$$

Now, substituting the value of A in eqn (viii) and (ix) and putting $B = 0$, we get

$$\sigma_r = \frac{3-2\nu}{8(1-\nu)} \rho\omega^2 (r_o^2 - r^2)$$

and $$\sigma_c = \frac{\rho\omega^2}{8(1-\nu)} [(3-2\nu) r_o^2 - (1+2\nu) r^2]$$

Putting $r_i = 0$ in equation (x)

$$\sigma_z = \frac{\nu}{1-\nu} \cdot \frac{\rho\omega^2}{4} [r_o^2 - 2r^2]$$

Maximum values of σ_r, σ_c and σ_z occur when $r = 0$ i.e., at the centre of solid cylinder.

$$\therefore \qquad \sigma_{r_{max}} = \frac{3-2\nu}{8(1-\nu)} \rho\omega^2 r_o^2$$

$$\sigma_{c_{max}} = \frac{3-2\nu}{8(1-\nu)} \rho\omega^2 r_o^2$$

Hence, $\sigma_{r_{max}} = \sigma_{c_{max}}$

and $\sigma_{z_{max}} = -\dfrac{\nu}{4(1-\nu)} \rho\omega^2 r_o^2$ (Tensile in nature)

Also, at $r = r_o$; σ_z is maximum

$$\therefore \qquad \sigma_{z_{max}} = -\frac{\nu}{4(1-\nu)} \rho\omega^2 r_o^2 \text{ (compressive in nature)}$$

The nature of graph $\sigma_r, \sigma_c, \sigma_z$ is shown in Fig. 21.7.

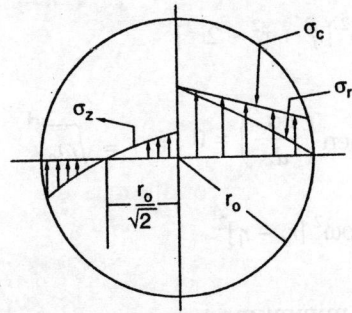

Fig. 21.7 Stress distribution in rotating solid cylinder

Further when $\sigma_z = 0$ then $2r^2 = r_o^2$

$$\therefore \qquad r = \left(\frac{r_o}{\sqrt{2}}\right)$$

21.8 HOLLOW CYLINDER

Here constants A and B can be determined from the boundary condition $\sigma_r = 0$ when $r = r_i$ and $r = r_o$.

$\therefore$ From eqn. (viii)

$$0 = A - \frac{B}{r_i^2} - \frac{3-2\nu}{8(1-\nu)} \rho\omega^2 r_i^2$$

and $0 = A - \dfrac{B}{r_o^2} - \dfrac{3-2v}{8(1-v)}\rho\omega^2 r_o^2$

Then, from these two, we get

$$B = \frac{3-2v}{8(1-v)}\rho\omega^2 r_i^2 r_o^2$$

and $A = \dfrac{3-2v}{8(1-v)}\rho\omega^2(r_i^2 + r_o^2)$

$\therefore$ $\sigma_r = \dfrac{3-2v}{8(1-v)}\rho\omega^2\left[r_i^2 + r_o^2 - \dfrac{r_i^2 r_o^2}{r^2} - r^2\right]$

and $\sigma_c = \dfrac{3-2v}{8(1-v)}\rho\omega^2\left[r_i^2 + r_o^2 - \dfrac{r_i^2 r_o^2}{r^2} - \dfrac{1+2v}{3-2v}r^2\right]$

We have derived that

$$\sigma_z = \frac{v}{4(1-v)}\rho\omega^2\,[r_i^2 + r_o^2 - 2r^2]$$

Now, σ_r is maximum when $\left(\dfrac{d\sigma_r}{dz}\right) = 0$ i.e. $r = \sqrt{r_i r_o}$

$\therefore$ $\sigma_{r_{max}} = \dfrac{3-2v}{8(1-v)}\rho\omega^2\,[r_o - r_i]^2$

σ_c is maximum when r is minimum i.e. $r = r_i$

$\therefore$ $\sigma_{c_{max}} = \dfrac{3-2v}{4(1-v)}\rho\omega^2 r_o^2\left[1 + \dfrac{1-2v}{3-2v}\cdot\dfrac{r_i^2}{r_o^2}\right]$

and σ_z is maximum at $r = r_i$ and $r = r_o$

$\therefore$ $\sigma_{z_{max}} = \dfrac{v}{4(1-v)}\rho\omega^2\,(r_o^2 - r_i^2)$ Tensile in nature at $r = r_i$

and $\sigma_{z_{max}} = (-)\dfrac{v}{4(1-v)}\rho\omega^2\,(r_o^2 - r_i^2)$ Compressive in nature at $r = r_o$

Also when $\sigma_z = 0$ then $2r^2 = r_i^2 + r_o^2$

$\therefore$ $r = \sqrt{\dfrac{r_i^2 + r_o^2}{2}}$

Stress distribution in rotating hollow cylinder

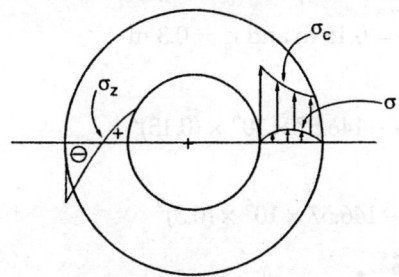

Fig. 21.8

EXAMPLE *A steel cylinder of 300 mm internal and 600 mm external diameters is rotating at 2000 rpm. Compute the maximum value of radial, circumferential and longitudinal stresses. Also determine the maximum shear stress in the cylinder. Take $\rho = 7800 \ kg/m^3$ and $v = 0.3$.*

SOLUTION The formulae for the stresses (to be computed) are :

$$\text{Radial stress } (\sigma_r) = A - \frac{B}{r^2} - \frac{3 - 2v}{8(1 - v)} \rho\omega^2 r^2$$

$$\text{Circumferential stress } (\sigma_c) = A + \frac{B}{r^2} - \frac{1 + 2v}{8(1 - v)} \rho\omega^2 r^2$$

$$\text{Longitudinal stress } (\sigma_z) = \frac{v}{4(1 - v)} \rho\omega^2 \left(r_i^2 + r_o^2 - 2r^2 \right)$$

$$\omega = \frac{2\pi N}{60} = \frac{2\pi \times 2000}{60}$$

$$= 209.43 \simeq 209.4 \ \text{rad/sec}$$

Now, $\sigma_r = A - \dfrac{B}{r^2} - \dfrac{3 - 2 \times 0.3}{8(1 - 0.3)} \times 7800 \times 209.4 \times r^2$

$$= A - \frac{B}{r^2} - 146.57 \times 10^6 \cdot r^2 \qquad \qquad \text{...(i)}$$

Similarly,

$$\sigma_c = A + \frac{B}{r^2} - 97.72 \times 10^6 \, r^2 \qquad \qquad \text{...(ii)}$$

and $\sigma_z = 36.64 \times 10^6 \, (0.1125 - 2r^2)$

$$= 4.122 \times 10^6 - 73.28 \times 10^6 r^2 \qquad \qquad \text{...(iii)}$$

Now, substituting the value of r_i and r_o in (i), we have

$$\sigma_r = 0 \text{ when } r_i = 0.15 \text{ m and } r_o = 0.3 \text{ m}$$

From (i)

$$0 = A - \frac{B}{(0.15)^2} - 146.57 \times 10^6 \times (0.15)^2$$

and

$$0 = A - \frac{B}{(0.3)^2} - 146.57 \times 10^6 \times (0.3)^2$$

which gives $A = 16.489 \times 10^6$

$$B = 296804$$

∴ Putting value of A and B in (i) and (ii), we have

$$\sigma_r = 16.489 \times 10^6 - \frac{296804}{r^2} - 146.57 \times 10^6 r^2 \qquad \text{...(iv)}$$

and

$$\sigma_c = 16.489 \times 10^6 + \frac{296804}{r^2} - 97.72 \times 10^6 r^2 \qquad \text{...(v)}$$

(a) Now σ_r is maximum when $r^2 = r_i r_o$

$$= (0.15)(0.3)$$
$$= 0.045 \text{ m}^2$$

From (iv)

$$\sigma_{r_{max}} = 16.489 \times 10^6 - \frac{296804}{r^2} - 146.57 \times 10^6 \times 0.045$$

$$= 3.3 \times 10^6 \text{ N/m}^2$$

$$\boxed{\therefore \sigma_{r_{max}} = 3.3 \text{ MPa}}$$

Ans.

(b) σ_c is maximum at $r = r_i = 0.15$ m

Hence, from (v)

$$\sigma_c = 16.489 \times 10^6 + \frac{296804}{(0.15)^2} - 97.72 \times 10^6 \times (0.15)^2$$

$$\boxed{\therefore \sigma_{c_{max}} = 27.48 \text{ MPa}}$$

Ans.

(c) σ_z is maximum at $r = r_i = 0.15$ m (Tensile)

$$r = r_o = 0.3 \text{ m (Compressive)}$$

Hence, from eqn. (iii), we get

$$\sigma_{z_{max}} = \pm [4.122 \times 10^6 - 73.28 \times 10^6 (0.15)^2]$$

$$= \pm 2.47 \text{ MPa}$$

(d) Now, at the inner surface of the cylinder, we have

$$\sigma_c = 27.48 \text{ MPa}, \ \sigma_r = 0; \ \sigma_z = 2.47 \text{ MPa}$$

Hence, $\tau_{max} = \dfrac{\sigma_{max} - \sigma_{min}}{2}$

$$= \dfrac{27.48 - 0}{2}$$

$$\boxed{\therefore \ \tau_{max} = 13.74 \text{ MPa}}$$ **Ans.**

HIGHLIGHTS

1. For a ring of main radius r rotating at an angular speed ω, circum-ferential stress $\sigma_c = \rho v^2$

where ρ = density of material, kg/m^3

v = linear velocity of the ring m/s.

2. Rotating disc

(a) Solid disc: $\sigma_r = \left(\dfrac{3+v}{8}\right)\rho\omega^2 \ (r_o^2 - r^2)$

and $\sigma_c = \dfrac{\rho\omega^2 \, r_o^2 (1 - v)}{4}$

Maximum stress occurs at the centre and its magnitude.

$$\sigma_r = (\text{max}) = \sigma_c \ (\text{max}) \ \text{at} \ r = 0 = \left(\dfrac{3+v}{8}\right)\rho\omega^2 r_o^2$$

(b) Disc with central hole 'or' hollow disc:

$$\sigma_r = \left(\dfrac{3+v}{8}\right)\rho\omega^2 \cdot \left[r_i^2 + r_o^2 + \dfrac{r_i^2 \, r_o^2}{r^2} - r^2 \right]$$

$$\sigma_c = \left(\dfrac{3+v}{8}\right) \cdot \rho\omega^2 \cdot \left[r_i^2 + r_o^2 + \dfrac{r_i^2 \, r_o^2}{r^2} - \dfrac{1+3v}{3+v} r^2 \right]$$

$$R = \sqrt{r_i \, r_o}$$

$$\sigma_r \ (\text{max}) = \dfrac{3+v}{8}\rho\omega^2 \cdot (r_o - r_i)^2$$

$$\sigma_c \ (\text{max}) = \left(\dfrac{3+v}{8}\right)\rho\omega^2 \cdot \left[r_o^2 + \dfrac{1-v}{3+v} r_i^2 \right]$$

$$\dfrac{\sigma_c(\text{max}) \text{ hollow}}{\sigma_c(\text{max}) \text{ solid}} = 2 \text{ if } r_i \gg r_o$$

3. **Disc of uniform strength :**

   Thickness at any radius $t = t_o \cdot e^{-\frac{\rho \omega^2 r^2}{2\sigma}}$

   where t_o = thickness at the centre

   and σ = uniform stress in the radial and circumferential direction.

4. **For rotating cylinder:**

$$\sigma_r = A - \frac{B}{r^2} - \left[\frac{3-2v}{8(1-v)}\right]\rho\omega^2 r^2$$

$$\sigma_C = A + \frac{B}{r^2} - \left[\frac{1+2v}{8(1-v)}\right]\rho\omega^2 r^2$$

$$\sigma_z = (-)\frac{v}{1-v} \cdot \frac{\rho\omega^2 r^2}{2} + C$$

where A, B and C are constant of integration.

   (a) For Solid cylinder:

$$A = \frac{3-2v}{8(1-v)}\rho\omega^2 r_0^2$$

   and $B = 0$

   Therefore, $\sigma_r = \frac{3-2v}{8(1-v)}\rho\omega^2(r_0^2 - r^2)$

$$\sigma_C = \frac{\rho\omega^2}{8(1-v)}[(3-2v)\,r_0^2 - (1+2v)\,r^2]$$

   and $\sigma_z = \frac{v}{1-v} \cdot \frac{\rho\omega^2}{4}[r_0^2 - 2r^2]$

   (b) For Hollow Cylinder:

$$A = \frac{3-2v}{8(1-v)}\rho\omega^2\,(r_i^2 + r_o^2)$$

$$B = \frac{3-2v}{8(1-2v)}\rho\omega^2\,r_i^2 \cdot r_o^2$$

   Therefore, $\sigma_r = \frac{3-2v}{8(1-v)}\rho\omega^2\left[r_i^2 + r_o^2 - \frac{r_i^2 r_o^2}{r^2} - r^2\right]$

$$\sigma_C = \frac{3-2v}{8(1-v)}\rho\omega^2\left[r_i^2 + r_o^2 + \frac{r_i^2 r_o^2}{r^2} - \frac{1+2v}{3-2v}r^2\right]$$

   and $\sigma_z = \frac{v}{4(1-v)}\rho\omega^2\left[r_i^2 + r_o^2 - 2r^2\right]$

PROBLEMS FOR PRACTICE
(THEORETICAL)

1. Find the expression for the circumferential stress developed in a rotating ring.

2. Prove that the maximum radial and circumferential stress in a rotating solid disc is given by

$$\sigma_r \text{ (max)} = \left(\frac{3 + v}{8} \right) \rho \omega^2 r_o^2$$

and $\quad \sigma_c \text{ (max)} = \left(\frac{3 + v}{4} \right) \rho \omega^2 r_o^2$

3. Prove that the maximum circumferential stress in a disc with a pin hole at the centre is two times the maximum circumferential stress in a solid disc.

4. Prove that the thickness of a disc of uniform strength is given by $t = t_0 \cdot e^{\frac{-\rho \omega^2 r^2}{2\sigma}}$ where t_0 is the thickness at $r = 0$.

5. For a rotating disc with a central hole the radial stress is maximum at the radius $R = \sqrt{r_i \, r_o}$.

6. A hollow circular cylinder is rotating at a uniform velocity. Derive the expressions for the radial, hoop and axial stresses developed.

   Derive their maximum value.

   How will these expressions be affected in case of solid rotating shaft.

(NUMERICAL)

1. A thin uniform disc of 250 mm diameter with a central hole of 50 mm diameter runs at 10,000 r.pm. Calculate the maximum principal stresses and the maximum shearing stress in the disc. Poisson's ratio = 0.3 and density of material = 7470 Kg/m^3.

2. The maximum radial pressure in a circular disc of uniform thickness when rotating at a certain speed is 20 MPa. The external diameter of the disc is 800 mm, whereas internal diameter is 200 mm. Determine the corresponding maximum hoop stress. Density of the disc material = 7000 Kg/m^3 Poission's ratio = 0.3.

3. A solid disc of 500 mm diameter is made up with a material for which various properties are: ρ = 6000 Kg/m^3; v = 0.25; σ_0 = 250 MPa . Determine the maximum permissible the speed for the disc to rotate. Use all theories of failure.

4. A disc of 150 mm diameter and 40 mm thick at the centre is to be designed for uniform strength. The maximum speed at which the disc is to run is 3000 radian/sec.

   Calculate the thickness of the disc at a radius of 50 mm if the material density is 7000 Kg/m^3 and the maximum permissible stress in the disc material is 150 MPa.

5. A long hollow cylinder is made of steel having 250 mm internal and 300 mm external diameters.
    It is rotating at a speed of 3000 rpm.
    Compute the maximum values of various stresses produced in the cylinder due to rotation.
    Plot the variation of stressess across the cylinder cross-section.
    Compare the maximum stress value in the cylinder with the case when it is assumed to be a disc of uniform thickness.

$$\rho = 7800 \text{ kg/m}^3 ; v = 0.3$$

ANSWERS

1. 33.79; 106.49; 36.55 MPa

2. 72 MPa

3. 11053 r.p.m

4. 23.6 mm

5. For Hollow Cylinder

$$\sigma_{r\,max} = 5.3 \text{ MPa}, \ \sigma_{z\,max} = \pm\,4 \text{ MPa}, \sigma_{c\,max} = 44 \text{ MPa}$$

For disc, $\sigma_{r\,max} = 5 \text{ MPa} \ \ \sigma_{c\,max} = 43 \text{ MPa}$

OBJECTIVE QUESTIONS

1. A rotating thin disc of uniform thickness is a case of
    (a) plane strain   (b) plane stress
    (c) three dimensional stress   (d) none of these.
2. In case of a solid rotating circular disc the radial stress is maximum at
    (a) the mean radius   (b) the outer surface
    (c) square root of the radius   (d) the centre.
3. The circumferential stress in a solid rotating disc is maximum at
    (a) the mean radius   (b) the inner radius
    (c) the centre   (d) the geometric mean radius.
4. The radial stress in a hollow circular rotating disc is at
    (a) the inner radius   (b) the outer radius
    (c) the mean radius   (d) the geometric mean radius
5. The ratio of the maximum values of the hoop and the radial stresses in a thin solid rotating disc is
    (a) equal to 1   (b) less than 1
    (c) more than 1   (d) none of the above

ANSWERS

1. (b)   2. (d)   3. (c)   4. (d)   5. (a)

— ❖❖ —

SOLVED QUESTIONS
(IAS, IES and GATE)

Q. 1 *A steel bolt having nominal diameter of 20 mm and pitch of 2.4 mm is used to connect two plates of 10 mm thickness each. An aluminium tube of inner diameter 22 mm and outer diameter of 44 mm is separating the plate as shown in figure. The nut is pulled sung (just tight) and then given one third additional turn.*

Find the resulting stresses in bolt and the tube neglecting the deformation of the plates.

Young's modulus of steel and aluminium are 207 × 10³ MPa and 67.5 × 10³MPa respectively. **(GATE 2001)**

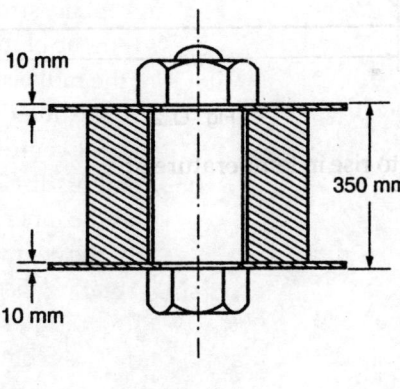

Fig. Q.1

SOLUTION

Movement of nut $= \left(\dfrac{2.4}{3} \right) = 0.8$ mm

Tensile force in steel bolt = Compressive force in aluminium tube

$$\frac{\pi}{4}(20)^2 \times \sigma_s = \frac{\pi}{4}(44^2 - 22^2) \times \sigma_a$$

$$\left(\frac{\sigma_s}{\sigma_a} \right) = 3.63 \qquad \qquad \dots (1)$$

Total movement of nut = Extension of bolt + Compression of tube

$$\therefore \quad 0.8 = \frac{\sigma_s \cdot l_s}{E_s} + \frac{\sigma_a \cdot l_a}{E_a}$$

$$= \frac{\sigma_s \times 350}{207 \times 10^3} + \frac{\sigma_a \times 330}{67.5 \times 10^3}$$

$$= 1.69 \times 10^{-3} \times \sigma_s + 4.89 \times 10^{-3} \, \sigma_a$$

$$0.8 = (6.1347 + 4.89) \times 10^{-3} \times \sigma_a$$

$$\sigma_a = 72.56 \, \text{N/mm}^2$$

$$\sigma_s = 263.4 \, \text{N/mm}^2 \qquad \textbf{Ans}$$

Q. 2 *Determine the temperature rise necessary to induce buckling in a 1 m long circular rod of diameter 40 mm.*

Assuming the rod to be pinned at its ends and the coefficient of thermal expansion as 20 × 10⁻⁶/°C (Assume uniform heating of the bar). **(GATE 1993)**

SOLUTION Let P = buckling load.

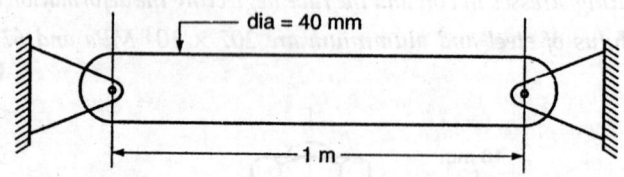

Fig. Q. 2

Change in length due to rise in temperature Δt

$$\delta l = \alpha \cdot \Delta t \cdot l$$

$$\Delta t = \frac{\delta l}{l \cdot \alpha} \qquad \qquad \dots (1)$$

Further, $\delta l = \dfrac{P \cdot l}{A \cdot E} \qquad \qquad \dots (2)$

and, $\quad P_{cr} = \dfrac{\pi^2 EI}{l^2}$

$$\therefore \quad \frac{\pi^2 EI}{l^2} = A \cdot E \cdot \frac{\delta l}{l}$$

$$\delta l = \left(\frac{\pi^2 I}{l \cdot A} \right)$$

$$= \frac{\pi^2}{l} \times k^2 \qquad \qquad \dots (3)$$

From (1) $\delta t = \dfrac{\pi^2 k^2}{\alpha \cdot l^2}$ [Substituting the value of dl from (iii)]

$$K^2 = \frac{d^2}{16}$$

$$= \frac{(40)^2}{16} = 100$$

$\therefore$ $\delta t = \dfrac{\pi^2}{\alpha l^2} \times k^2$

$$= \frac{\pi^2 \times 100}{20 \times 10^{-6} \times (1000)^2}$$

$$= 49.35\,°C \qquad \textbf{Ans.}$$

Q. 3 *At a point in an elastic material the stresses on three mutually perpendicular planes are as follows:*
First plane : 50 MPa tensile and 40 MPa shear
Second plane: 30 MPa compressive and 40 MPa shear
Third plane: No stress.
Find (i) the position of principal planes and the magnitude of principal stresses.
(ii) The position of planes on which maximum shear stress acts and calculate the normal and shear stresses on them.   **(IAS 1992)**
SOLUTION

$$\sigma_x = 50\,MPa; \ \sigma_y = -30\,MPa$$

$$\tau_{xy} = 40\,MPa$$

(i) $\sigma_{1,2} = \dfrac{1}{2}(\sigma_x + \sigma_y) \pm \dfrac{1}{2}\sqrt{(\sigma_x - \sigma_y)^2 + 4\,\tau_{xy}^2}$

$$= \frac{1}{2}(50 - 30) \pm \frac{1}{2}\sqrt{(50 + 30)^2 + 4 \times 40^2}$$

$$= 10 \pm 56.5685$$

$$= 66.5685\,MPa; \ (-)46.56\,MPa$$

$$\tan 2\theta = \left(\frac{2\,\tau_{xy}}{\sigma_x - \sigma_y}\right)$$

$$= \left(\frac{2 \times 40}{50 + 30}\right) = 1$$

$$\theta_1 = 225°; \ \theta_2 = 112.5°$$

(ii)   Planes on which maximum shear stress acts are:

$$\theta_3 = 45° + 22.5°$$

$$= 67.5°$$

$$\theta_4 = 112.5 + 45°$$

$$= 157.5°$$

$$\sigma_n = \frac{1}{2}(\sigma_x + \sigma_y) + \frac{1}{2}(\sigma_y - \sigma_x)\cos 2\theta - \tau_{xy}\sin 2\theta$$

At $\theta = \theta_3$: $\sigma_n = \frac{1}{2}(50 - 30) + \frac{1}{2}(-30 - 50)\cos 135° - 40\sin 135°$

$$= 10 \text{ MPa}$$

$$\tau = \frac{1}{2}(\sigma_y - \sigma_x)\sin 2\theta + \tau_{xy}\cos 2\theta$$

$$= \frac{1}{2}(-30 - 50)\sin 135° + 40\cos 135°$$

$$= -56.56 \text{ MPa} \qquad \textbf{Ans.}$$

At $\theta = \theta_4$: $\sigma_n = 10 - 28.28 + 28.28 = 10 \text{ MPa}$

$$\tau = 28.28 + 28.28 = 56.56 \text{ MPa} \quad \textbf{Ans.}$$

Q. 4 *A circular rod of diameter 'd' and length 3 d is subjected to a compressive force F acting on the top point as shown in figure.*

Calculate the stress at the bottom support A.   **(GATE 1994)**

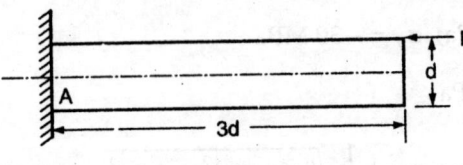

Fig. Q 3

SOLUTION

Direct stress $(\sigma_d) = -\dfrac{4F}{\pi d^2}$ (As the load is compressive)

Bending moment in the rod $(M) = F \times \left(\dfrac{d}{2}\right)$

Bending stress in the rod $(\sigma_b) = \dfrac{32M}{\pi d^3}$

$$= \frac{32}{\pi d^3} \times \frac{Fd}{2}$$

$$= \frac{16\,F}{\pi d^2}$$

Hence resultant stress at A,

$$\sigma = -\frac{4F}{\pi d^2} - \frac{16F}{\pi d^2}$$

$$= -\left(\frac{20F}{\pi d^2}\right) \qquad \textbf{Ans.}$$

Q. 5 *The stresses in the element of an elastic body are :*
  (i) 60 N/mm² tensile;
  (ii) 30 N/mm² tensile in a direction at right angles to (i) and; (ii)
  (iii) Complementary shear stress of 45 N/mm² in the direction of (i) and (ii).
Calculate the normal and tangential stress on two planes which are equally inclined to (i) and (ii).   **(IES 1999)**

SOLUTION

$$\sigma_x = 30\,\text{N/mm}^2$$

$$\sigma_y = 60\,\text{N/mm}^2$$

$$\tau_{xy} = 45\,\text{N/mm}^2$$

$$\sigma_{1,2} = \frac{1}{2}(\sigma_x + \sigma_y) \pm \frac{1}{2}\sqrt{(\sigma_x - \sigma_y)^2 + 4\tau_{xy}^2}$$

$$= \frac{1}{2}(30 + 60) \pm \frac{1}{2}\sqrt{(30 - 60)^2 + 4 \times 45^2}$$

$$= 45 \pm 47.43$$

$$= 92.43\,\text{N/mm}^2 ; -2.43\,\text{N/mm}^2$$

$$\sigma_n = \frac{1}{2}(\sigma_x + \sigma_y) + \frac{1}{2}(\sigma_y - \sigma_x)\cos 2\theta - \tau_{xy}\sin 2\theta$$

At $\theta = 45°$:

$$\sigma_n = \frac{1}{2}(30 + 60) + \frac{1}{2}(60 - 30)\cos 90° - 45\sin 90°$$

$$= 45 - 45 = 0$$

$$\tau = \frac{1}{2}(\sigma_y - \sigma_x)\sin 2\theta + \tau_{xy}\cos 2\theta$$

$$= \frac{1}{2}(60 - 30)\sin 90° + 45\cos 90°$$

$$= \frac{1}{2} \times \overset{15}{\cancel{30}} \times 1 + 45 \times 0$$

$$= 15\,\text{N/mm}^2$$

At $\theta = 135°$:

$$\sigma_n = \frac{1}{2}(30 + 60) + 45$$

$$= 90 \text{ N/mm}^2$$

$$\tau = \frac{(-)1}{2}(30 + 60)$$

$$= -45 \text{ N/mm}^2 \qquad \textbf{Ans.}$$

Q. 6 *The pulley A exerts a torque on the shaft 'B' as shown in figure. The total vertical tension in both sides of the belt on each pulley is 4 kN. The diameter of the shaft is 60 mm. If the tensile and shear stress intensities are not to exceed 320 N/mm² and 160 N/mm² respectively. What is the maximum power that can be transmitted by the shaft when running at 150 rpm? The shaft may be assumed simply supported at the bearings.*

(IAS-1989)

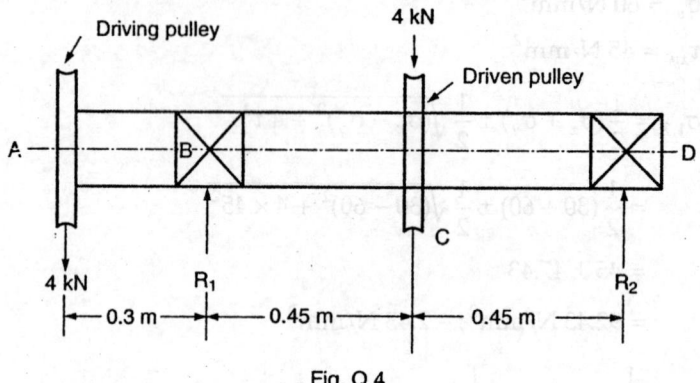

Fig. Q.4

SOLUTION

$$R_1 \times 0.9 = 4 \times 1.2 - 4 \times 0.45$$

$$\Sigma M_D = 0 \quad \text{gives}$$

$$R_1 = \left(\frac{10}{3}\right) \text{kN}$$

$$M_1 = -4 \times 0.3 = -1.2 \text{ kNm}$$

$$M_c = \left(\frac{10}{3}\right) \times 0.45 - 0.75 \times 4$$

$$= -1.5 \text{ kNm}$$

$$M_{max} = 1.5 \text{ kNm}$$

Let T Nm be the torque on the shaft.

$\therefore$ 　　　Equivalent torque $T_e = \sqrt{M^2 + T^2} = \dfrac{\pi}{16} d^3 \cdot \tau$

$$\sqrt{(1500)^2 + T^2} = \frac{\pi}{16} \times (60)^3 \times 10^{-9} \times 160 \times 10^6$$

or,　　　$\sqrt{(1500)^2 + T^2} = 6785.84$

or,　　　$225 \times 10^4 + T^2 = 6785.84$

$$\boxed{T = 6618 \text{ Nm}}$$

Equivalent bending moment,

$$M_e = \frac{1}{2}\left[M + \sqrt{M^2 + T^2} \right] = \frac{\pi}{32} d^3 \sigma$$

$$\frac{1}{2}\left[1500 + \sqrt{(1500)^2 + T^2} \right] = \frac{\pi}{32} d^3 \sigma$$

$$\frac{1}{2}\left[1500 + \sqrt{(1500)^2 + T^2} \right] = \frac{\pi}{32} \times (60)^3 \times 10^{-9} \times 320 \times 10^6$$

$$= 6785.84$$

On solving, 　　$\boxed{T = 11978 \text{ Nm}}$

$\therefore$ 　　　Permissible Torque $= 6618$ Nm

$\therefore$ 　　　Power transmitted $= \left(\dfrac{2\pi NT}{60 \times 10^3} \right)$

$$= \left(\frac{2\pi \times 150 \times 6618}{60 \times 10^3} \right)$$

$$P = 103.95 \text{ kW} \qquad \textbf{Ans.}$$

Q. 7 *A 500 × 180 mm rolled steel beam is simply supported over a span of 6 metre. A load of 20 kN is dropped on the middle of the beam from a height of 12.5 m.*

Find the maximum instantaneous deflection and maximum stress induced. The section modulus is equal to 45218×10^{-8} m^4 and the Young's modulus is 200 GPa.

(IAS - 1980)

SOLUTION

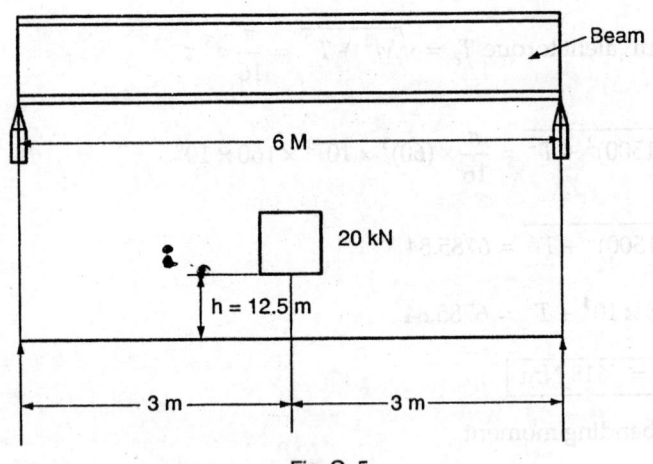

Fig. Q. 5

Here we have,

$$W(h + \delta) = \frac{1}{2} \times W \times \delta \qquad \qquad \ldots(1)$$

Here δ for simply supported beam is equal to $\dfrac{Wl^3}{48\,EI}$

$$\therefore \qquad \delta = \frac{W \times l^3}{48 \times (200 \times 10^9) \times (45218 \times 10^8)}$$

$$= 4.9 \times 10^{-8}\ W \text{ metre}$$

Now substituting the value of δ in eqn. (1)

$$20 \times 10^3 \, (12.5 \times 10^3 + 4.9 \times 10^{-8}\ W) = \frac{1}{2}\,W \times 4.9 \times 10^{-8}\ W$$

Rearranging we get

$$W^2 - 40 \times 10^3\ W - 102.04 \times 10^8 = 0$$

This is euadratic in We

$$W = \frac{40 \times 10^3 \pm \sqrt{1600 \times 10^6 + 4 \times 102.04 \times 10^8}}{2}$$

$$= 20 \pm 102.976$$

$$= 122.976 \text{ kN}$$

$$\therefore \qquad \text{Instantaneous deflection} = \frac{Wl^3}{48\,EI}$$

$$= 4.9 \times 10^{-8} \times 122.97 \times 10^3$$

$$= 6.026 \text{ mm}$$

By formula, $M_{max} = \left[\dfrac{W \cdot l}{4} \right]$

$$= \dfrac{6.026 \times 6}{4} = 184.469 \text{ kNm}$$

$$\sigma_{max} = \dfrac{M}{Z}$$

$$= \left(\dfrac{184.469 \times 10^3 \times 90 \times 10^{-3}}{45218 \times 10^{-8}} \right)$$

$$= 36.715 \text{ MPa} \qquad \textbf{Ans.}$$

Q. 8 *The figure shows a hollow shaft of 150 mm external diameter and 80 mm internal diameter. At its free end a pulley of 500 mm diameter is rigidly fixed. A force of 25 kN is applied tangential to the pulley as shown in figure. Determine the principal stresses and the absolute maximum shear stress at point A located 1 m from the free end and at the top shaft surface* **(IES 1986)**

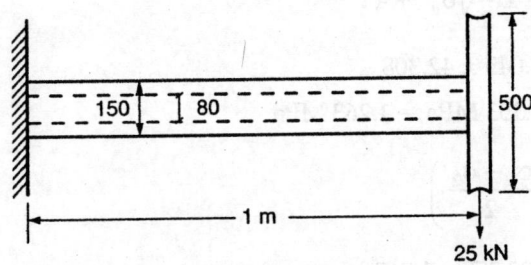

Fig. Q.6

Objective to find σ_1, σ_2 and τ_{max} at A.

SOLUTION Torque $(T) = 25 \times \dfrac{D_{pulley}}{2}$

$$= 25 \times \dfrac{500 \times 10^3}{2 \times 10^3} = 6250 \text{ Nm}$$

Moment $(M) = 25 \times 10^3 \times 1$

$$= 25000 \text{ Nm}$$

Now, bending stress for hollow shaft

$$\sigma_b = \dfrac{32M}{\pi d_0^3 \left[1 - \left(\dfrac{di}{do} \right)^4 \right]}$$

$$= \frac{32 \times 25000}{\pi \times 150^3 \left[1 - \left(\frac{80}{150}\right)^4\right] \times 10^{-9}}$$

$$= 82.09 \text{ MPa}$$

$$\tau = \frac{16T}{\pi \, d_0^{\,3} \left[1 - \left(\dfrac{di}{do}\right)^4\right]}$$

$$= \frac{16 \times 6250}{\pi \times 150^3 \left[1 - \left(\dfrac{80}{150}\right)^4\right] \times 10^{-9}}$$

$$= 10.26 \text{ MPa}$$

$$\sigma_{1,2} = \frac{\sigma_b}{2} \pm \frac{1}{2}\sqrt{\sigma_b^{\,2} + 4\tau^2}$$

$$= 41.045 \pm 42.308$$

$$= 83.353 \text{ MPa}; -1.263 \text{ MPa}$$

$$\tau_{max} = \left(\frac{\sigma_1 - \sigma_2}{2}\right)$$

$$= \left(\frac{83.353 + 1.263}{2}\right)$$

$$= 42.308 \text{ MPa} \qquad \textbf{Ans.}$$

Q. 9 *Find the maximum principal stress developed in a cylindrical shaft; 8 cm in diameter and subjected to a bending moment of 2.5 kNm and twisting moment of 4.2 kNm. If the yield stress of the material is 300 MPa, determine the factor of safety of the shaft according to the maximum stress theory of failure.* **(GATE 1994)**
SOLUTION

Equivalent torque $(T_e) = \sqrt{M^2 + T^2}$

$$= \sqrt{(2.5)^2 + (4.2)^2}$$

$$= 4.887 \text{ kNm}$$

Shear stress developed in the shaft $(\tau) = \left(\dfrac{16 T_e}{\pi \, d^3}\right)$

$$= \frac{16 \times 4.887 \times 10^3}{\pi \times 83 \times 10^{-6}}$$

$$= 48.61 \, MPa$$

Permissible shear stress $= \left(\dfrac{300}{2} \right)$

$$= 150 \, MPa$$

Factor of safety $(fos) = \left(\dfrac{150}{48.61} \right) = 3$ **Ans.**

Q. 10 *Determine the reaction at the supports of the beam.*   **(GATE 1995)**

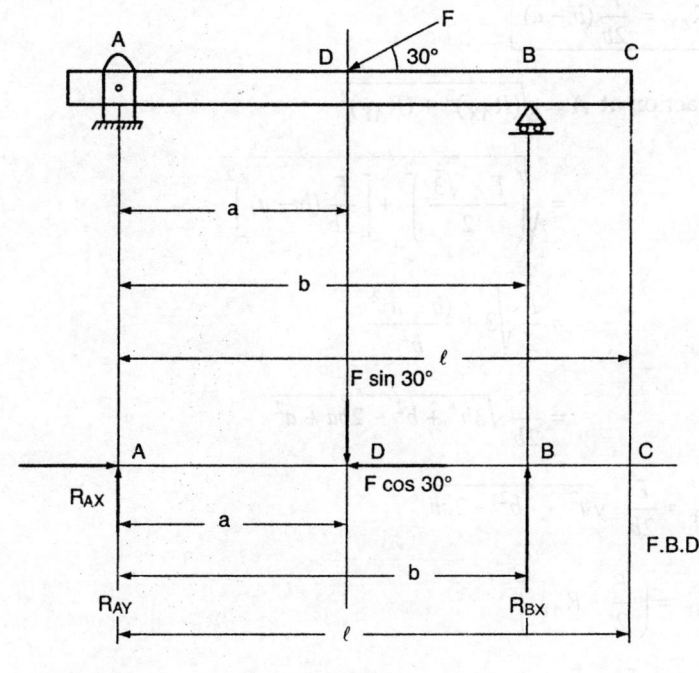

Fig. Q.7

SOLUTION *Draw FBD first*

Applying $\Sigma F_x = 0$

$$R_{AX} - F \cos 30° = 0$$

$$R_{AX} = F \cos 30°$$

$$R_{AX} = \frac{F \times \sqrt{3}}{2} \qquad \qquad \dots (1)$$

Applying $\Sigma F_y = 0$

$$R_{AY} - F \sin 30° + R_{BY} = 0$$

$$R_{Ay} + R_{BY} = F \sin 30°$$

$$R_{AY} + R_{BY} = \frac{F}{2} \qquad\qquad \dots (2)$$

Applying $\Sigma M_B = 0$

$$R_{AY} \cdot b - F \sin 30° \cdot (b - a) = 0$$

$$R_{AY} \cdot b = F \sin 30° (b - a) = \frac{F}{2} (b - a)$$

$$\boxed{R_{AY} = \frac{F}{2b} (b - a)}$$

$\therefore$ Reaction at $A = \sqrt{(R_{AX})^2 + (R_{AY})^2}$

$$= \sqrt{\left(\frac{F \times \sqrt{3}}{2} \right)^2 + \left[\frac{F}{2b} (b - a) \right]^2}$$

$$= \frac{F}{2} \sqrt{3 + \frac{(b - a)^2}{b^2}}$$

$$= \frac{F}{2b} \sqrt{3b^2 + b^2 - 2ba + a^2}$$

$$R_A = \frac{F}{2b} \cdot \sqrt{a^2 + 4b^2 - 2ab}$$

$$R_{BY} = \left(\frac{F}{2} - R_{AY} \right)$$

$$= \frac{F}{2} - \frac{F}{2b} (b - a)$$

$$= \frac{F}{2} - \left[1 - \frac{(b - a)}{b} \right]$$

$$= \frac{F}{2} - \left[\frac{b - b + a}{b} \right]$$

$$\boxed{R_{BY} = \frac{F \cdot a}{2b}} \quad \textbf{Ans.}$$

Q. 11 *A truck weighing 25 kN and moving at 2.5 m/s has to be brought to rest by a buffer. Find how many springs each of 25 coils will be required to store energy of motion during compression of 0.2 m. The spring is made of 25 mm diameter steel coiled to a mean diameter of 0.2 m. (G = 100 GPa).* **(IES - 1989)**

SOLUTION

$$\text{K.E of the truck} = \frac{1}{2} \cdot \left(\frac{W}{g} \right) \cdot v^2$$

$$= \frac{1}{2} \times \left(\frac{25 \times 10^3}{9.81} \right) \times (2.5)^2$$

$$= 7963.81 \text{ Nm}$$

$$\delta = \frac{8 W D^3 n}{G d^4}$$

Stiffness of spring $(K) = \left(\frac{W}{\delta} \right)$

$$= \left(\frac{G d^4}{8 D^3 n} \right)$$

$$= \frac{(100 \times 10^9) \times 25^4 \times 10^{-12}}{8 \times (0.2)^3 \times 25}$$

$$= 24414 \text{ N/m}$$

Energy stored by spring $= \frac{1}{2} K \delta^2$

$$= \frac{1}{2} \times 24414 \times (0.2)^2$$

$$= 488.28 \text{ Nm}$$

Number of springs required $= \left(\dfrac{7963.81}{488.28} \right) = 16.3 = 17$ **Ans.**

Q. 12 *Find the maximum shear stress and deflection induced in a helical spring of the following specification, if it has to absorb 1 kNm of energy.*

     Mean dia. of spring = 100 mm

     Dia. of spring steel wire = 20 mm

     No. of coils = 30

     Modulus of regidity of steel = 85 GPa. **(IES 1982)**

SOLUTION

Strain energy $(U) = \dfrac{\tau^2}{4G} \times \text{Volume}$

$$10^3 = \dfrac{\tau^2}{4 \times (85 \times 10^9)} \times \dfrac{\pi}{4} \times 20^2 \times 10^{-6} \times \pi \times 100 \times 10^{-3} \times 30$$

$\therefore$ $\tau = 338.66 \text{ MPa}$

$\because$ $\tau = \dfrac{8WD}{\pi d^3}$

$$338.66 = \dfrac{8W \times 100 \times 10^{-3}}{\pi \times 20^3 \times 10^{-9}}$$

$\therefore$ $W = 10.645 \text{ kN}$

$$\delta = \left(\dfrac{8WD^3\eta}{Gd^4} \right)$$

$$= \left(\dfrac{8 \times 10.645 \times 10^3 \times 100^3 \times 10^{-9} \times 30}{85 \times 10^9 \times 20^4 \times 10^{-12}} \right)$$

$$= 187.86 \text{ mm} \qquad \textbf{Ans}$$

Q. 13 *A steel tube is of 18 mm internal diameter and 3 mm thick. Its one end is closed and the other end is screwed into a pressure vessel. The projected length is 300 mm. Neglecting any constraints due to the ends, calculate the safe internal pressure for the tube if allowable stress is not to exceed 150 N/mm². Calculate the increase in its internal volume under this pressure.*

Assume Young's modulus for the tube material as 200 GPa. Poission's ratio 0.3.

(IAS - 1981)

SOLUTION

Hoop stress $(\sigma_h \text{ or } \sigma_c) = \dfrac{pd}{2t}$

$$150 = \dfrac{p \times 18}{2 \times 3}$$

$$= 50 \text{ N/mm}^2$$

Longitudinal stress $(\sigma_l) = \dfrac{\sigma_b}{2}$

$$= 75 \text{ N/mm}^2$$

$$\varepsilon_h = \frac{1}{E}\left[\sigma_h - v \cdot \sigma_l\right]$$

$$= \frac{1}{200 \times 10^9}\left[150 - 0.3 \times 75\right] \times 10^6$$

$$= 637.5 \times 10^{-6}$$

$$\varepsilon_l = \frac{1}{E}\left[\sigma_l - v\,\sigma_h\right]$$

$$= \frac{1}{200 \times 10^9}\left[75 - 0.3 \times 150\right] \times 10^6$$

$$= 150 \times 10^{-6}$$

Now, volumetric strain $(\varepsilon_v) = 2\,\varepsilon_h + \varepsilon_l$

$$= (2 \times 637.5 + 150) \times 10^{-6}$$

$$= 1425 \times 10^{-6}$$

$$V = \frac{\pi}{4}d^2\,l$$

$$= \frac{\pi}{4} \times (18)^2 \times 300 \times 10^{-9}$$

$$= 76.34 \times 10^{-6}\,\text{m}^3$$

$$\delta_V = \varepsilon_v \cdot V$$

$$= 1425 \times 10^{-6} \times 76.34 \times 10^{-6}$$

$$= 108.78 \times 10^{-9}\,\text{m}^3 \qquad \textbf{Ans.}$$

Q. 14 *What should be the ratio of a thin cylindrical shell to the thickness of its hemispherical end for a pressure vessel subjected to internal fluid pressure so that the junction section remains free from unequal deformation?*   **(IAS-1995)**

SOLUTION

For cylinder:

$$\sigma_h = \frac{pd}{2t_1}$$

and $\quad \sigma_l = \dfrac{pd}{4t_1} \qquad$ where t_1 = wall thickness

$$(\varepsilon_h) = \frac{1}{E}\left[\sigma_h - v \cdot \sigma_l\right]$$

$$= \frac{pd}{2t_1 E}\left[1 - 0.5v\right] \qquad\qquad\qquad \dots (1)$$

For sphere:

$$\sigma_h = \frac{pd}{4t_2} \qquad \text{where } t_2 = \text{thickness of wall of sphere}$$

$$\sigma_h = \frac{1}{E}\left[\sigma_h - v \cdot \sigma_h\right]$$

$$= \frac{pd}{4t_2 E}\left[1 - v\right] \qquad\qquad\qquad \text{...(2)}$$

For $\varepsilon_h = \sigma_h$

$$\left(\frac{t_1}{t_2}\right) = \left(\frac{2-v}{1-v}\right) \qquad \textbf{Ans.}$$

Q. 15 *Find the shortest length of a hinged-highed steel column having a rectangular cross-section 60 mm × 100 mm for which the Euler's formula applies. Take yield strength and modulus of elasticity (E) for steel as 250 MPa and 200 GPa respectively.*

(GATE 1995)

SOLUTION

$$\text{M.I. } (I) = \frac{bd^3}{12}$$

$$= \frac{100 \times 60^3}{12} \times 10^{-12}$$

$$\therefore \qquad I = 1.8 \times 10^{-6} \, m^4$$

$$P_{cr} = \frac{\pi^2 EI}{l^2}$$

$$\sigma_{cr} \times A = \frac{\pi^2 EI}{l^2}$$

$$\sigma_{cr} \times \cancel{A} = \frac{\pi^2 E \times \cancel{A} \, k^2}{l^2}$$

$$k^2 = \left(\frac{I}{A}\right)$$

$$= \frac{1.8 \times 10^{-6}}{6 \times 10^{-3}} = 0.3 \times 10^{-3} \, m^2$$

$$l^2 = \frac{\pi^2 E K^2}{\sigma_{cr}}$$

$$l = \sqrt{\frac{\pi^2 E K^2}{\sigma_{cr}}}$$

$$= \sqrt{\frac{\pi^2 \times 200 \times 10^9 \times 0.3 \times 10^{-3}}{250 \times 10^6}}$$

$l = 1.54 \text{ m}$ **Ans.**

Q. 16 *An overhanging pulley of 1 m diameter and weighing 1 kN transmits 45 HP at 140 rpm, the sides of the belt being vertical.*

The ratio of tension is 2 : 1 and the maximum tensile and shear stresses are limited to 120 and 60 MPa respectively. Find the diameter of the shaft. The centre of pulley is 0.35 m from the nearest bearing. **(IES - 1989)**

SOLUTION

$$HP = \frac{2\pi NT}{4500}$$

$$45 = \frac{2\pi \times 140 \times T}{4500}$$

(Torque) $T = 230.2 \text{ Kgm}$

$$= 2258.26 \text{ Nm}$$

Let F_1 and F_2 be the belt tension.

$$T = (F_1 - F_2) R$$

or, $$F_1 - F_2 = \frac{T}{R}$$

$$= \left(\frac{2258.26}{0.5}\right) = 4516.52 \text{ Newton}$$

$$\frac{F_1}{F_2} = 2$$

$\therefore$ $F_1 = 9033.04 \text{ Newton}$

and $F_2 = 4516.52 \text{ Newton}$

Resultant force on pulley $= F_1 + F_2 + W$

$$= 9033.04 + 4516.52 + 1000$$

$$= 14549.56 \text{ N}$$

Maximum bending moment $(M) = 14549.56 \times 0.35$

$$= 5092.346 \text{ Nm}$$

Equivalent twisting moment $(T_e) = \sqrt{M^2 + T^2}$

$$= \sqrt{(5092.346)^2 + (2258.26)^2}$$

$$= 5570.61 \text{ Nm}$$

By formula, $\dfrac{\pi}{16} d^3 \tau = T_e$

$\therefore \qquad \dfrac{\pi}{16} \times d^3 \times 10^{-9} \times (60 \times 10^6) = 5570.61$

$\qquad d = 77.9 \text{ mm} \qquad$ **Ans.**

UNIVERSITY QUESTIONS

UNIT - I

COMPOUND STRESS AND STRAIN

2001-2002

1. Fill in the blanks with suitable word(s): A member is subjected to a tensile force 'P' and its normal cross-section perpendicular to the line of force is 'A'. The resulting normal stress on an oblique plane inclined at an angle θ to the transverse section will be_____ (2 Marks)

$$\text{Ans. } \sigma = \frac{P}{A}\cos^2\theta$$

2. At a point in a stressed material, the principal stresses are 1000, – 600 and zero. If the maximum principal stress is increased to 1200 and the maximum shear stress is to remain the same, the minimum principal stress should be changed to_____ (2 Marks)

Ans. –1200 MPa

3. Write short note on: Mohr's stress circle. (3 Marks)

2003-2004

4. Write a short note on: Principal stresses. (2 Marks)

2005-2006

5. Draw Mohr's circle for:
   (i) Pure shear
   (ii) Pure biaxial tension
   (iii) Pure uniaxial compression
   (iv) Pure uniaxial tension
   In a two-dimensional stress field. (10 Marks)

2006-2007

6. A point in a strained material is subjected to a tensile stress of 65 N/mm² and a compressive stress of 45 N/mm², acting on two mutually perpendicular planes and a shear stress of 10 N/mm² are acting on these planes. Find the normal stress, tangential stress and resultant stress on a plane inclined to 30° with the plane of the compressive stress. (10 Marks)

2008-2009

7. At a point in a body the normal and shear stresses on two mutually perpendicular planes are given as $\sigma_x = -100 \text{ MN/m}^2$.

$\sigma_y = 40 \text{ MN/m}^2$, $\tau_{xy} = 50 \text{ MN/m}^2$

Using Mohr's circle determine principal stresses and their planes. (7½ Marks)

ELASTIC CONSTANT

2002-2003

1. Show that if E is assumed correct, an error of 1% in the determination of G will involve an error of about 5% in the calculation of Poisson's ratio when its correct value is 0.25.   (6 Marks)

2004-2005

2. While testing on a metallic rod, it is observed that the diameter of rod is reduced by 0.00025 mm under an axial pull of 20 KN. The original diameter of the rod is 15 mm. If rigidity modulus for the rod metal be 50 KN/mm². Find the Young's modulus and Bulk modulus.   (6 Marks)

Carry Over 2005-2006

3. The bulk modulus for a material is $0.5 \times 10^5 \, N/mm^2$. A 12 mm diameter rod of the material was subjected to an axial pull of 14 kN and the change in diameter was observed to be 3.6×10^{-3} mm. Calculate Poisson's ratio and modulus of elasticity.   (6 Marks)

2006-2007

4. Write short note on: Airy's stress function.   (5 Marks)
5. The stresses in the three principal direction are $+ 65$ MN/mm², $+ 20$ MN/m², -85 MN /m². Find the principal strain. Take $\mu = 0.3$ and $E = 200 \, GN/m^2$ (5 Marks)

2007-2008

6. State the generalized Hook's law and prove for an anisotropic elastic material the maximum number of elastic constants is 21only. Also, show that for isotropic materials it is 2.   (6 Marks)
7. Derive the equation of equilibrium in z-direction, by considering the equilibrium of an infinitestimal rectangular element of size $dx \, dy \, dz$ in the Cartesian co-ordinate system as

$$\frac{\partial \sigma_z}{\partial z} + \frac{\partial \tau_{xz}}{\partial x} + \frac{\partial \tau_{yz}}{\partial z} + \overline{z} = 0$$ (6 Marks)

8. At a point in a body, the displacement field is linear and is given by the following expressions. Find all the strains
   $u = 0.07x + 0.05y + 0.01z, v = 0.01y - 0.04x, w = 0.02x + 0.02z$ (6 Marks)

2008-2009

9. What is significance of strain compatibility equations? Write down these compatibility equations.   (5 Marks)

THEORY OF FAILURE

2001-2002

1. At a point in a steel member, the major principal stress is 200 N/mm², find the minor principal stress which is compressive. If the tensile yield stress is

250 N/mm², find the minor principal stress at which yielding will commence, using:

(i) maximum total strain energy theory,

(ii) maximum shear strain energy theory.

Take Poisson's ratio = 0.25 (6 Marks)

2. Write short note on: Necessity and significance of theories of failure. (3 Marks)

2002-2003

3. Briefly explain theories of failure.(6 Marks)

2003-2004

4. If the principal stresses at a point in an elastic material are $2f$ tensile, f tensile and $\frac{1}{2}f$ compressive, calculate the value of f at failure according to:

(i) Maximum principal stress theory

(ii) Maximum shear stress theory

(iii) Maximum strain energy theory

The elastic limit in simple tension is 200 N/mm² and Poisson's ratio = 0.3. (6 Marks)

2004-2005

5. What is the necessity of a theory of failure? Explain briefly theories of failure. (6 Marks)

Carry Over 2005-2006

6. The load on a bolt consists of an axial pull of 15 kN together with a transverse shear of 7.5 kN. Calculate the diameter of the bolt according to

(i) Maximum principal stress theory, and

(ii) Maximum principal strain theory, taking elastic limit in tension 285 MPa, μ = 0.3 amd factory of safety = 3.

(6 Marks)

2006-2007

7. A mild steel shaft, 100 mm diameter is subjected to a maximum torque of 15 kN-m and a maximum bending moment of 10 kN-m. at a particular section. Find the factor of safety according to maximum shear stress theory of failure if the elastic limit in simple tension is 240 MN/m². (5 Marks)

2008-2009

8. The three principal stresses at a point in a body subjected to a system of loading are 2.5σ (tensile), 1.2σ (tensile) and 0.8σ (compressive). If yield stress for the material is 280 MN/m², using factor of safely = 2, Poisson's ratio = 0.3, determine the maximum value of σ so that failure may not occur according to principal stress theory and shear stress theory. (7½ Marks)

IMPACT LOAD AND STRESSES

2003-2004

1. Write briefly on: Castigliano's theorem. (3½ Marks)

2005-2006

2. What do you understand by strain energy absorbed by a system, complimentary strain energy, and elastic strain energy? Explain these with the help of a diagram.   (2 Marks)

2006-2007

3. Write short note on: Castigliano's theorem.   (5 Marks)

2007-2008

4. State Castigliano's first and second theorems for strain energy. What are their uses?   (6 Marks)

5. Derive an expression for strain energy in cantilever due to bending and shear under a concentrated edge load?   (6 Marks)

2008-2009

6. State and explain Castigliano's theorem with an example.   (7½ Marks)

UNIT - II

STRESS IN BEAMS

2001-2002

1. The algebraic sum of moments taken about a section x-x of all the transverse forces acting on a beam is_____.   (2 Marks)

                                                                                            Ans. Bending moment.

2. _____ the measure of the strength of the beam in bending. (2 Marks)

                                                                                            Ans. Sectional modulus.

3. A cantilever, length L having square cross-section of side 'a', is subjected to transverse load of w per unit length. The maximum bending stress in the beam, caused for section as shown in Fig. 1(a) is f. Find the maximum bending stress in the beam if the section is placed as shown in Fig. 1(b).   (6 Marks)

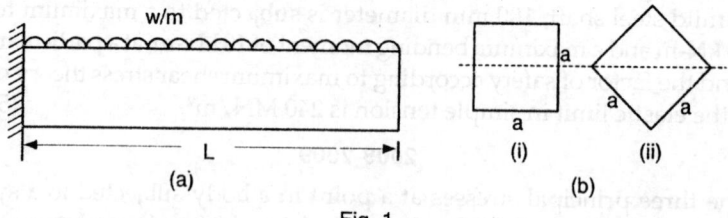

Fig. 1

2002-2003

4. Calculate the dimensions of the strongest section, that can be cut, of a circular log of wood 25 cm in diameter.   (6 Marks)

2003-2004

5. A cantilever 2.5 m long carries a U.D.L. of 20 kN/m run. The breath of the section remains constant and is equal to 100 mm. Determine the depth of the

section at the middle of the length of the cantilever and at fixed end if stress remains the same throughout and equal to 120 MN/m². (6 Marks)

2004-2005

6. Deduce a formula for the shear stress at the junction of flange and web in the I-Section of a beam. (6 Marks)

2005-2006

7. What assumptions are made in simple theory of bending? (5 Marks)
8. Determine the maximum compressive stress set up in a 200 mm × 60 mm I-section girder carrying load of 100 kN with an eccentricity of 6 mm from the critical axis of the section. The ends of the struct are pin-jointed and overall length is 4 m.
   Take $T_{yy} = 3 \times 10^{-6}$ m⁴
   $A = 6 \times 10^{-3}$ m²
   $E = 207$ GPa (10 Marks)

Carry Over 2005-2006

9. A cast iron water pipe of 500 mm inside diameter and 20 mm thick is supported over a span of 10 meter. Determine the maximum stress in the pipe material, when the pipe is running full. Take Density of C.I. as 70.6 kN/m³ and that of water as 9.8 kN/m³. (6 Marks)
10. A flitched beam consists of two 50 mm × 200 mm wooden beam and a 12 mm × 80 mm steel plate. The plate is placed centrally between the wooden beams and recused into each so that, when rigidly joined, the three units form a 100 mm × 200 mm section as shown in Fig. 2. Determine the moment of resistance of the flitched beam when the maximum bending stress in the timber is 12 MN / m². What will then be the maximum bending stress in the steel? For steel $E = 200$ GPa, for wood $E = 10$ GPa. (10 Marks)

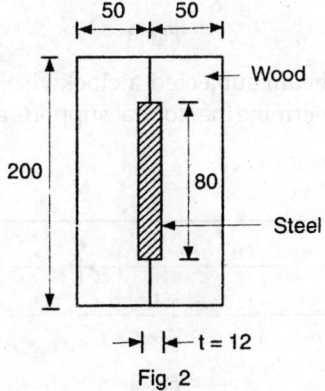

Fig. 2

2006-2007

11. A timber beam of 3 m span carries a uniformly distributed load of 5 kN/m and a point load 1 kN at the center of the span. If the permissible bending stress be 100 N/mm², determine the section taking depth as twice the breadth. (10 Marks)

2007-2008

12. What are the assumptions made in the simple theory of bending? (10 Marks)
13. In a thin circular tube show that the maximum shear stress is twice the average shear stress over the cross-section.   (7 Marks)

DEFLECTION OF BEAMS

2001-2002

1. The maximum deflection in a cantilever beam due to an end load P is δ. If the depth of the beam is doubled, the maximum deflection due to the same load will be _____.   (6 Marks)
2. Derive an expression for the slope and deflection of a simple supported beam, span L, carrying a uniformly distributed load w per unit length and a point load P at the mid span. Hence, find the slope and deflection at a point $L/4$ from the left support.   (6 Marks)

2002-2003

3. A simply supported prismatic beam AB carries a uniform distributed load of intensity w over its span 'l'. Develop the equation of the elastic line and find the maximum deflection at the middle of the span.   (6 Marks)

2003-2004

4. Cantilever beam of span L and subjected to udL 'w' over it's entire length. Determine slope and deflection at free end.   (6 Marks)

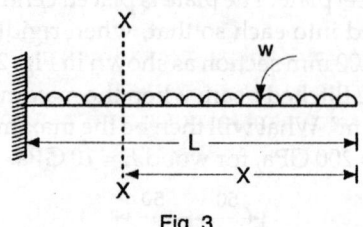

Fig. 3

5. Simply supported beam subjected a clockwise couple M at a distance 'a' from left support. Determine the slope at supports and deflection under couple.   (6 Marks)

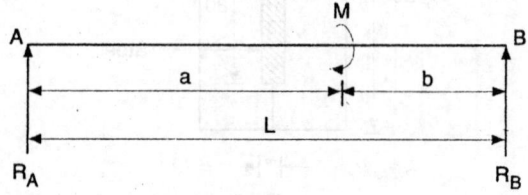

Fig. 4

2004-2005

6. A simply supported beam of 'L' carrying two equal point load W at $L/4$ from each support. Find slope at support and maximum deflection (at centre).   (6 Marks)

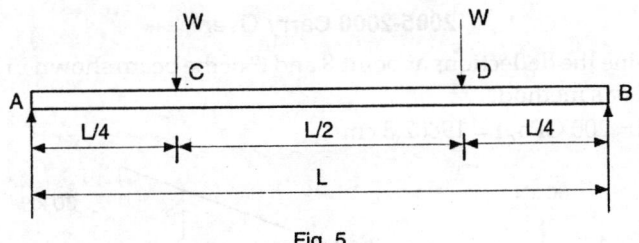

Fig. 5

(For detailed solution See page 10.9)

[Hints: For checking Answers

$$y_{max} = (-)\frac{P \cdot a}{24\, EI}(3L^2 - 4a^2)$$

Here $P = W$

$$a = \frac{L}{4}$$

$$\therefore \quad y_{max} = (-)\frac{W \cdot \dfrac{L}{4}}{24\, EI}\left(3L^2 - 4 \cdot \frac{L^2}{16}\right)$$

$$= (-)\frac{W \cdot L}{96\, EI}\left(3L^2 - \frac{L^2}{4}\right) = (-)\frac{W \cdot L}{96\, EI}\times\frac{11L^2}{4} = (-)\frac{11WL^3}{384\, EI}\ ]$$

7. Derive an expression for the slope and deflection of a simple supported beam, span L, carrying a uniformly distributed load w per unit length and a point load P at the mid span. Hence, find the slope and deflection at a point $L/4$ from the left support. (6 Marks)

2005-2006

8. A cantilever subject to uvL in such a way that zero at free end and maximum load intensity w kN/m at fixed end. Determine maximum slope and deflection. (10 Marks)

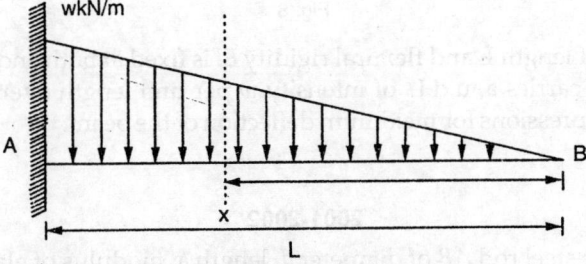

Fig. 6

2005-2006 Carry Over

9. Determine the deflections at point B and C of the beam shown in Fig. 7 using Macaulay's method.   (6 Marks)

Take; $E = 200$ GPa, $I = 19802.8$ cm^4

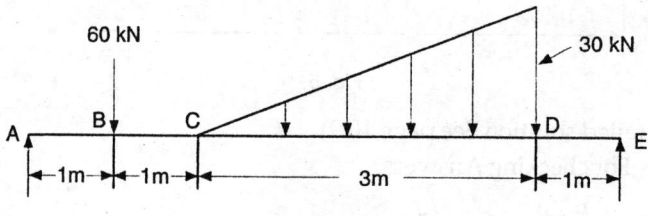

Fig. 7

2006-2007

10. A beam of uniform section, 10 m long is simply supported at the ends. It carries point loads of 150 kN and 65 kN at distances of 2.5 m and 5.5 m respectively from the left end. Calculate:

(i) Deflection under each load

(ii) Maximum deflection.

Take $E = 200$ GN/m^2 and $I = 118 \times 10^{-4}$ m^4 (10 Marks)

2007-2008

11. Derive the deflection equation for cantilever beam with uniformly distributed load.   (7 Marks)

2008-2009

12. A simple supported beam has a flexural rigidity of 24 MN/m^2 and is loaded as shown in Fig. 8. Determine the deflections at mid-span.   (10 Marks)

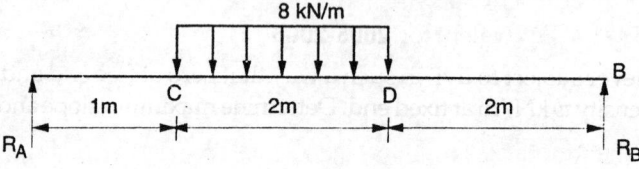

Fig. 8

13. A beam of length L and flexural rigidity EI is fixed at both ends at the same level and carries a. u.d.L. of intensity w per unit length over whole span. Obtain expressions for maximum deflection of the beam.   (10 Marks)

TORSION

2001-2002

1. A circular steel rod AB of diameter d, length a, modulus of elasticity E and modulus of rigidity G, is loaded as shown in Fig. 9 rigid bar BC of length b is rigidly fixed to AB at B such that BC is perpendicular to AB and lies in the horizontal plane. Find the deflection at point C due to:

(i) bending of AB (ii) torsion of AB (6 Marks)

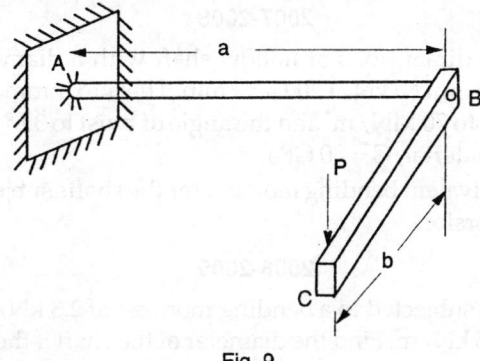

Fig. 9

(Solved in Chapter 13)
2. Fill in the blanks with suitable word(s):
   A shaft is subjected to a torque 'T' and bending moment 'T' (both equal) and another similar shaft is subjected to a single torque $T\sqrt{2}$. The ratio of maximum principal stresses in these two cases will be _____.(3 Marks)
3. Write brief note on: Equivalent torque.   (3 Marks)

2002-2003

4. Compare the weight of hollow and solid shaft of equal length to transmit a
• given torque of the same maximum shear stress, if the inside diameter is 2/3 of the outside.   (6 Marks)

2003-2004

5. A flywheel weighing 500 kg is mounted on a shaft 75 mm diameter and midway between bearings 0.6 m apart. If the shaft is transmitting 30 kW at 360 rpm, calculate the principal stresses and the maximum shear stress at the ends of a vertical diameter in a plane close to the flywheel.   (6 Marks)
6. Write briefly on: Equivalent torque.   (3 Marks)

2005-2006

7. A solid shaft of 80 mm diameter is to be replaced by a hollow shaft of external diameter 100 mm. Determine the internal diameter of hollow shaft if the same power is to be transmitted by both the shaft at same angular velocity and shear stress.   (6 Marks)
8. Derive the relation to obtain polar modulus for hollow circular section. Also, derive the equation for the power transmitted by shaft.   (6 Marks)

2006-2007

9. In a shaft of hollow circular section, has external diameter 100 mm and internal diameter is 60 mm. The allowable shear stress in the shaft material is 55 N/mm². Determine the angle of twist in a length of twenty times the external diameter of the shaft. Take: $G = 8.5 \times 10^4 \text{N/mm}^2$.   (10 Marks)

2007-2008

10. Determine the dimensions of hollow shaft with a diameter ratio of 3 : 4, which is to transmit 60 kN at 200 rev/min. The maximum shear stress in the shaft is limited to 70 MN/m² and the angle of twist to 3.8° in a length of 4 m. For the shaft material, G = 80 GPa. (7 Marks)

11. Determine equivalent bending moment for the shafts subjected to combined bending and torsion. (7 Marks)

2008-2009

12. A solid shaft is subjected to a bending moment of 2.3 kN/m and a twisting moment of 3.45 kN/m. Find the diameter of the shaft if the allowable tensile and shear stresses for shaft material are limited to 703 MN/m² and 421.8 MN/m² respectively. (10 Marks)

UNIT - III

HELICAL AND LEAF SPRING

2005-2006

1. Deduce an expression for the extension of an open-coiled helical spring carrying an axial load W. Take 'a' as the inclination of the coils, d as the diameter of the wire and R as the mean radius of the coils. Find by what percentage the axial extension is underestimated if the inclination of the coil is neglected for a spring in which $\alpha = 25°$, Assume n and R remain constant. (10 Marks)

2006-2007

2. A helical spring having 12 coils of mean coil diameter of 20 cm is made of 10 mm diameter steel rod. The helix angle is 25°.
   Find the angular twist and the axial deflection of one end of the spring relative to the other if it is subjected to an axial couple of 14 Nm. Calculate the maximum bending stress and maximum torsional stress in the wire.
   Take $E = 200$ GN/m² and $G = 80$ GN/m² (10 Marks)

2007-2008

3. An open coiled spring carries an axial load W, show that the deflection is related to W by $\delta = \dfrac{8\,Wn\,D^3}{Gd^u}\,K$ where K is a corrective factor which allows for the inclination of the coils, n = number of effective coils, D = mean coil diameter and d = wire diameter. (7 Marks)

4. A leaf spring is made of plates 50 mm wide and 8 mm thick. The spring has a span of 700 mm. Determine the number of plates required to carry a central load of 45 kN. The maximum allowable stress in the plates is 200 MPa. What is the maximum deflection under this load? (7 Marks)

2008-2009

5. A cantilever type laminated spring (quarterelleptic) has a span of 0.5 meter. If each leaf be 8 mm thick and 72 mm wide, find the number of leaves so that the spring deflects 60 mm under an end load of 3kN. Determine maximum bending stress at this load. Also, determine the height from which this load may be allowed to fall so that maximum bending stress induced is 700 N/mm². Take $E = 2 \times 10^5$ N/mm²

(10 Marks)

COLUMNS AND STRUTS

2001-2002

1. From the first principles derive the expression for the critical buckling load for a column having one end fixed and one end hinged. (6½ Marks)

2. A straight steel bar, 1.5 m long and section 20 mm × 5 mm is compressed longitudinally until buckles. Using Euler's formula, estimate the maximum central deflection before the steel passes the yield point at 330 N/mm². Take $E = 200,000$ N/mm². (6½ Marks)

2002-2003

3. A slender column of length l is built in at its lower end A and laterally supported at its upper end. Find the first critical value of the compression load P. (6½ Marks)

4. Calculate the critical load of a strut which is made to a bar circular in section and 5 m long and which is pin jointed at both ends. The same bar when freely supported gives mid-span deflection of 10 mm with a load of 80 N at the centre. (6½ Marks)

2003-2004

5. A slender column of length l is built in at its lower end and free at upper end. Find the first critical value of the compressive load p. (6 Marks)

6. A hollow C.I. column whose outside diameter is 200 mm has a thickness of 20 mm. It is 4.5 m long and is fixed at both ends. Calculate the safe load of Rankine formula using a factor of safety of 4.

Take $\sigma_c = 550$ MPa, $a = \dfrac{1}{1600}$ (6 Marks)

2004-2005

7. In a column section, the length of the column is 40 times the length of each side of the square section. If both ends of the column are pinned and $E = 2 \times 10^4$ kN/cm², determine the critical stress set up in the column.

(6½ Marks)

8. How will you justify that Rankine's formula is applicable for all lengths of columns, ranging from short to long columns. (6½ Marks)

2005-2006

9. A rectangular masonary column has a cross-section 500 mm × 400 mm and is subjected to a vertical compressive load of 100 kN applied at point 'P' shown in Fig. 10 Determine the value of the maximum stress produced in the section. Is the section at any point subjected to tensile stresses?

(10 Marks)

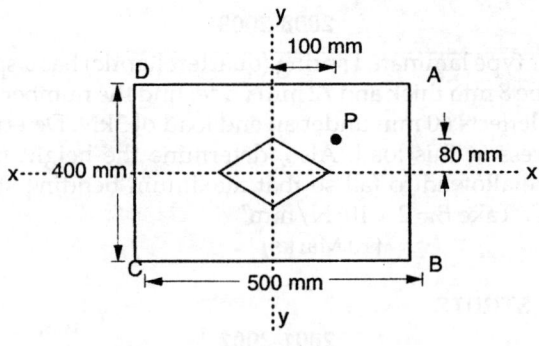

Fig. 10

2005-2006 Carry Over

10. Derive the equation to obtain buckling load for the column having one end hinged and other fixed. (7 Marks)

11. What are limitation of Euler's formula for the column? Explain with any one example. (6 Marks)

2006-2007

12. A mild steel hollow column has 100 mm external diameter and 60 mm internal diameter and 4 m length is used as a column. Determine the crippling load by Rankine's formula when both ends are hinged.

    Take $\sigma_c = 320 \text{ N/mm}^2$, Rankine's constant $a = \dfrac{1}{1600}$. (10 Marks)

13. Classing columns and struts with a short description of each classification. (5 Marks)

14. Write the limitation of Euler's formula for critical load. (5 Marks)

2007-2008

15. Explain middle quarter and middle third rules? What are the importance of these rules for concrete sections? (7 Marks)

16. State the assumptions made during the Euler's formula for a strut with pin jointed ends. Derive the Euler's crippling load for such a strut the general equations of bending and also the solution of the differential equation may be assumed. (7 Marks)

2008-2009

17. Explain middle third rule for rectangular sections. (10 Marks)

18. Derive an expression to obtain buckling load for the column which is neither too short nor too long. (10 Marks)

UNIT - IV

THIN CYLINDERS AND SPHERES

2001-2002

1. A mild steel cylinder has diameter to thickness ratio of 30. Find the internal pressure to which the cylinder should be subjected so that its volume is increased by 1/2000 of its original volume.

   Take $E = 200,000 \text{ N/mm}^2$. (6½ Marks)

2002-2003

2. A boiler drum consists of a cylindrical portions 2 m long, 1 m diameter and 25 mm thick, closed by hemispherical ends. In a hydraulic test to 10 N/mm², how much additional water will be pumped in after initial filling at atmospheric pressure?

Assume the circumferential strain at the junction of cylinder and hemisphere is same for both. For the drum material, E = 207000 N/mm².

μ = 0.3, For water K = 2100 N/mm². (6½ Marks)

2003-2004

3. A cylindrical shell 3 m long which is closed at the ends has an internal diameter of 1 m and a wall thickness of 15 mm. Calculate the circumferential and longitudinal stresses induced and also change in the dimensions of the shell, if it is subjected to an internal pressure of 1.5 MN/m². Take E = 200 GN/m² and μ = 0.3. (6 Marks)

2004-2005

4. Define thin cylinders. Derive an expression for circumferential stress and longitudinal stress for a thin shell subjected to an internal pressure.

(6½ Marks)

2005-2006

5. Derive the equations for circumferential stress and volumetric strain in a thin spherical shell under internal pressure. (10 Marks)

2005-2006 Carry Over

6. A cylindrical air drum is 2.25 m in diameter with plates 1.2 cm thick. The efficiencies of the longitudinal and circumferential joints are 0.75 and 0.40 respectively. If the tensile stresses in plating is to be limited to 120 MN/m², determine safe air pressure. (7 Marks)

7. A seamless spherical shell is of 8 m internal diameter and 4 mm thickness. It is filled with fluid under pressure until its volume increases by 50 CC. Determine the fluid pressure, taking E = 2 × 10⁵ N/mm² and v = 0.3. (7 Marks)

2006-2007

8. Prove that in case of a thin cylindrical shell, subjected to an internal fluid pressure, the volumetric strain is equal to twice the circumferential strain plus the longitudinal strain. (10 Marks)

2008-2009

9. A spherical tank, has a diameter of 20 meter and wall thickness 15 mm if the permissible stress in the material is 120 MPa determine the maximum pressure at which a gas can be stored in the tank. Determine the increase in diameter and volume of the tank due to gas pressure.

Take: E = 200 GPa and Poisson's ratio (μ) = 0.3 (10 Marks)

THICK CYLINDER

2001-2002

1. What is the difference between thin and thick cylinders? State the assumptions made in the analysis of stress in thick cylinders. Derive Lames' equations to find the stresses in thick cylinders. (6½ Marks)
2. The cylinder of a hydraulic ram is of 160 mm internal diameter. Find the thickness required to withstand an internal pressure of 60 N/mm². If the maximum tensile stress is limited to 90 N/mm², and the maximum shear stress to 80 N/mm². (6½ Marks)

2002-2003

3. The cylinder of a hydraulic ram is of 6 cm internal diameter. Find the thickness required to withstand an internal pressure of 40 N/mm², if the maximum tensile stress is limited to 60 N/mm² and the maximum shear stress to 50 N/mm². (6½ Marks)
4. Derive Lame's equations to find out the stresses in thick spherical shells. (6½ Marks)

2003-2004

5. The maximum stress permitted in a thick cylinder, radii 8 cm and 12 cm, is 20 N/mm², the external pressure is 6 N/mm², what internal pressure can be applied? Plot curves showing the variation of hoop and radial stresses through the material. (6½ Marks)

2004-2005

6. A thick spherical shell having internal radius of 75 mm is subjected to an internal pressure of 25 N/mm². If the maximum hoop stress 100 N/mm². Find the thickness of the shell. (6½ Marks)
7. What do you mean by Lame's equations? How will you derive these equations? (6½ Marks)
8. Explain the following: (6½ Marks)
   (i) What is compound cylinder? What is its advantage over a single cylinder?
   (ii) Shrinkage allowance
   (iii) State assumptions made in Lame's Theory.

2005-2006

9. A thick cylinder with closed ends has 100 mm internal radius and 150 mm external radius. It is subjected to an internal pressure of 60 MN/m² and external pressure of 30 MN/m². Determine the hoop and radial stresses at the inside and outside of the cylinder together with longitudinal stress. (10 Marks)
10. How thick and thin cylinder are classified? Derive the equation for Hoop stress and radial stress in thick cylinder? (10 Marks)

2005-2006 Carry Over

11. Derive the equation to obtain the radial and circumferential stresses in thick shell subjected to external and internal pressure both. (7 Marks)

12. A thick cylinder of 150 mm outside and 100 mm inside radius is subjected to an external pressure of 30 MN/m². Calculate the maximum shear stress in the material of the cylinder at inner radius. (7 Marks)

13. Calculate the thickness of metal necessary for a cylindrical shell of internal diameter 160 mm to withstand an internal pressure of 25 MN/m², if maximum permissible tensile stress is 125 MN/m². (7 Marks)

2006-2007

14. Derive an expression for maximum principal stress on thick cylindrical shell subjected to external pressure. (10 Marks)

15. A hollow cylinder of 45 cm internal diameter and 10cm thickness contains the fluid under pressure of 850 N/cm². Find the maximum and minimum hoop stress across the section. (10 Marks)

2007-2008

16. Derive the Lame equations for the hoop and radial stresses in a thick cylinder subjected to an internal and external pressure and show how these may be expressed in graphical form. (10 Marks)

2008-2009

17. Derive an expression to determine stresses in thick-walled cylinder subjected to internal pressure only. (10 Marks)

UNIT - V

CURVED BEAM

2005-2006

1. A steel ring has a rectangular cross-section, 75 mm in the radial direction and 45 mm perpendicular to the redial direction. If the mean radius of the ring is 150 mm and maximum tensile stress is limited to 180 MN/m² calculate the tensile load the ring can carry. (10 Marks)

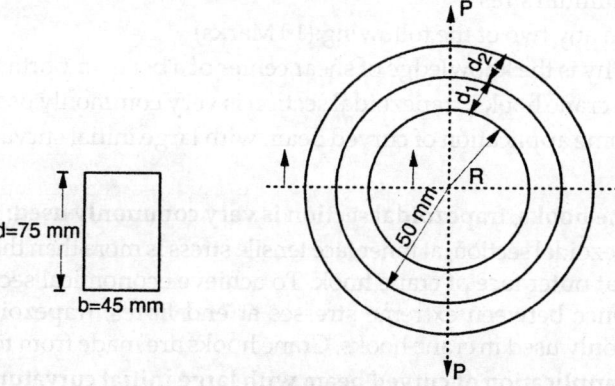

Fig. 11

2. A chain link (Fig. 12) is made of round steel of 15 mm diameter. If $R = 45$ mm, $L = 75$ mm and load applied is 1.5 kN. Determine the maximum compressive stress in the link and tensile stresses at the same section.

(10 Marks)

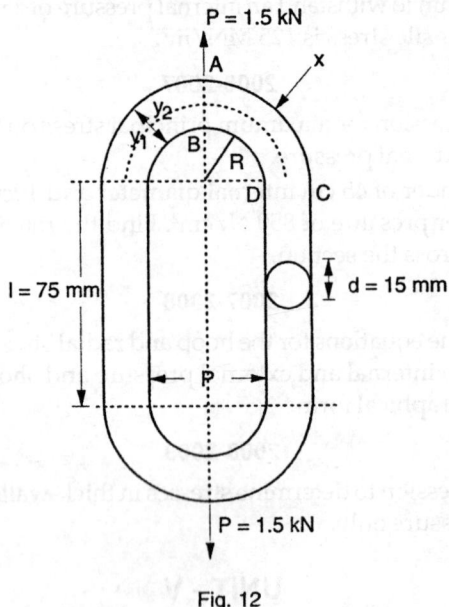

Fig. 12

2006-2007

3. A curved beam, rectangular in cross-section is subjected to pure pending with couple of + 40 kN - cm. The beam has width of 2 cm and depth of 4 cm and is curved in plane parallel to width. The mean radius of curvature is 5 cm. Find the position of the neutral axis, and the ratio of the maximum to the minimum stress.   (10 Marks)

4. Explain any two of the following:(10 Marks)
   (i)   Why is the knowledge of shear center of a beam important?
   (ii) In crane hooks, trapezoidal section is very commonly used.
   (iii) Some application of curved beam with large initial curvature.

SOLUTIONS

(ii) **In crane hooks, trapezoidal section is very commonly used:**

In trapezoidal section, at inner face tensile stress is more than the compressive stress at outer face of crane hook. To achieve economical section with less difference between extreme stresses at end fibres, trapezoidal section is commonly used in crane hooks. Crane hooks are made from forged steel.

(iii) **Some application of curved beam with large initial curvature:**

Rings, links and crane hooks are common engineering application of curved beam with large initial curvature.

2007-2008

5. Derive the equation to find the position of neutral axis for the following cross-sections of curved beam:

   (1) Rectangular section

   (2) Circular cross section (10 Marks)

6. Determine the numerical value of the ratio $\sigma_{max} / \sigma_{min}$ for the case of plane bending of a curved beam having 2.5×2.5 cm. Square cross-section if the radius of curvature of the centroidal axis is $R = 3.75$ cm. (10 Marks)

2008-2009

7. For curve bar of circular cross-section. Derive an expression to determine the distance of centroid from the neutral axis. (10 Marks)

UNSYMMETRICAL BENDING

2005-2006

1. A cantilever of length 1.2 m is of the cross-section as shown in Figure. It carries a vertical load of 10 kN at its outer end, the line of action being parallel with the longer leg and arranged to pass through the shear centre of the section (i.e. there is no twisting of the section). Working from first principles, find the stress setup in the section at points A, B and C given that the centroid is located as shown. Determine the angle of inclination of the N.A.

   $I_{xx} = 4 \times 10^{-6}$ m^4, $I_{yy} = 1.08 \times 10^{-6}$ m^4 (10 Marks)

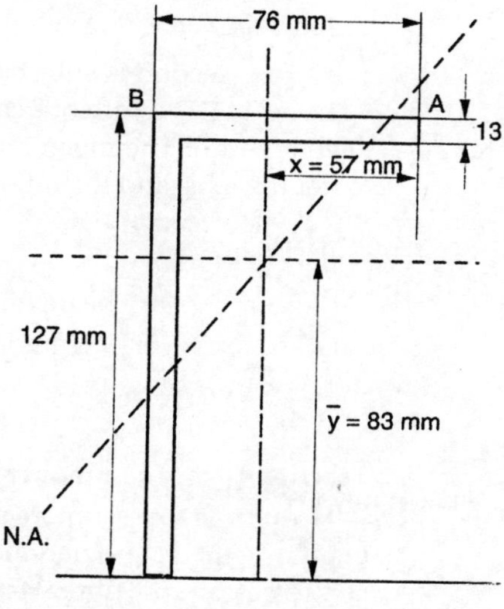

Fig. 13

2006-2007

2. What is shear center? Prove that the shear center for a thin-walled balanced z section coincides its centroid. (10 Marks)

3. A 6 cm × 4 cm × 0.6 cm unequal angle is placed with the longer vertical leg and is used as beam. It is subjected to a bending moment of 150 N-m acting in the vertical plane through the centroid of the section. Determine the maximum bending stress induced in the section.   **(10 Marks)**

2007-2008

4. What is shear center? Prove that the shear center for a thin-walled balanced z section coincides with its centroid.   **(10 Marks)**

— ❖❖ —

SOLVED UNIVERSITY QUESTIONS
2009-10
(Strength of Materials)

PAPER ID: 0429   **EME-302**

Q. 1(a) *At a point in a strained material, there are normal stresses of 30 N/mm², tension and 20 N/mm², compression on two planes at right angles to one another, together with shearing stresses of 15 N/mm² on the same planes. If the loading on the material is increased so that the stresses reach value of K times those given, find the maximum permissible value of K if the maximum direct stress in the material is not to exceed 80 N/mm², and maximum shear stress is not to exceed 50 N/mm².* **(10 Marks)**

SOLUTION Given

$\sigma_x = 30 \text{ N/mm}^2 \times K$

$\sigma_y = -20 \text{ N/mm}^2 \times K$

$\tau = 15 \text{ N/mm}^2 \times K$

$\sigma_{n1} \not> 80 \text{ N/mm}^2$

$\tau_{max} \not> 50 \text{ N/mm}^2$

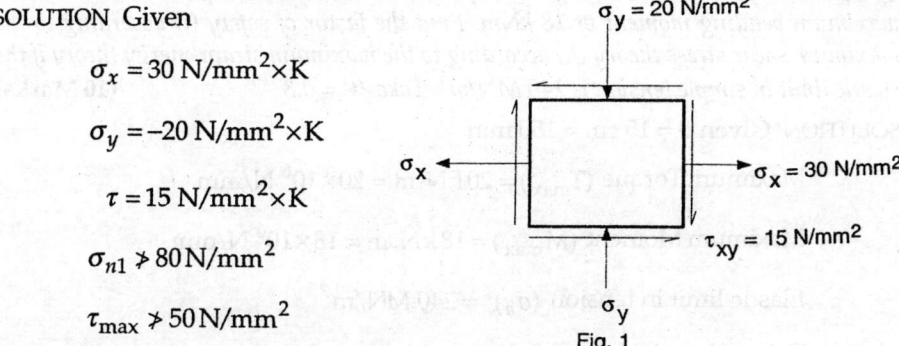

Fig. 1

Objective: To find the maximum permissible value of K

By Formula, we have

$$\sigma_{1,2} = \frac{\sigma_x + \sigma_y}{2} \pm \sqrt{\left(\frac{\sigma_x - \sigma_y}{2}\right)^2 + \tau_{xy}^2}$$

$$= \left[\frac{30 - 20}{2} \pm \sqrt{\left(\frac{30 - 20}{2}\right)^2 + (15)^2}\right] K$$

$$= (5 \pm \sqrt{(625 \times 225)}) K$$

$$= (5 \pm 29.15) K$$

$$= 34.15 \, K \text{ or } -24.15 \, K$$

So, $\sigma_{1(\text{maximum})} = 34.15 \text{ K}$

$$\sigma_{2\,(minimum)} = -24.15\,K$$

$$\therefore \qquad \tau_{max} = \left(\frac{\sigma_1 - \sigma_2}{2}\right)$$

$$= \left(\frac{34.15 + 24.15}{2}\right) = 9.15\,K$$

Given $\tau_{max} \not> 50\,N/mm^2$

So, $29.15\,K = 50$

$$\Rightarrow \qquad K = \left(\frac{50}{29.15}\right) = 1.71$$

Also, given $\tau_{max} \not> 80\,N/mm^2$

So, $34.15\,K = 80$

$$\Rightarrow \qquad K = \left(\frac{80}{34.15}\right) = 2.34$$

Hence, the maximum permissible value of K is 1.71. **Ans.**

Q. 1(b) *A shaft of 15 cm diameter is subjected to a maximum torque on 20 kNm and a maximum bending moment of 18 kNm. Find the factor of safety (i) according to the maximum shear stress theory (ii) according to the maximum strain energy theory if the elastic limit in simple tension is 240 MN/m². Take $\mu = 0.3$.* **(10 Marks)**

SOLUTION Given $d = 15\,cm = 150\,mm$

Maximum Torque $(T_{max}) = 20\,kN.m = 20 \times 10^6\,N/mm$

Maximum Moment $(M_{max}) = 18\,kN.m = 18 \times 10^6\,N/mm$

Elastic limit in tension $(\sigma_0)^* = 240\,MN/m^2$

Poisson's ratio $(v) = 0.3$

Objective: Factor of safety (fos)

Now fos according to Maximum Shear Stress theory

According to this theory failure of material will occur if τ_{max} in compound stress system = τ_{max} in simple stress system.

i.e. $\dfrac{\sigma_1 - \sigma_2}{2} = \dfrac{\sigma_0}{2}$

Now, we will compute τ_{max} (simple) and τ_{max} (compound)

By formula,

$$\tau = \frac{16\,T}{\pi d^3}$$

---

*We have denoted yield stress by σ_0

$$= \frac{16 \times 20 \times 10^3 \times 7}{22 \times 150 \times 150 \times 150} \, \text{N/mm}^2$$

$$= 30.168 \, \text{N/mm}^2$$

Bending Stress $(\sigma_b) = \left(\frac{M_{max}}{I}\right) \cdot y = \frac{18 \times 10^6}{\left(\dfrac{I}{y}\right)}$

$$= \frac{18 \times 10^6}{Z}$$

$$= \frac{18 \times 10^6}{\dfrac{\pi}{32}(150)^3} = 54.30 \, \text{N/mm}^2$$

Now, Principal Stresses, $\sigma_1, \sigma_2 = \dfrac{\sigma_b}{2} \pm \sqrt{\left(\dfrac{\sigma_b}{2}\right)^2 + \tau^2}$

$$= \frac{54.30}{2} \pm \sqrt{\left(\frac{54.30}{2}\right)^2 + (30.168)^2}$$

$$= 27.15 \pm 40.58$$

$$= 67.73 \text{ or } (-) \, 13.43 \, \text{N/mm}^2$$

Now, τ_{max} in Compound (or Complex) stress system

$$= \left(\frac{\sigma_1 - \sigma_2}{2}\right)$$

$$= \left(\frac{67.73 + 13.43}{2}\right) = 40.58 \, \text{N/mm}^2$$

Allowable stress $(\sigma_o) = \dfrac{\text{Stress at yield point}}{\text{fos}}$

$\therefore \qquad \sigma_o = \left(\dfrac{240}{\text{fos}}\right)$

Now, by Maximum Shear Stress theory

$$\frac{\sigma_1 - \sigma_2}{2} = \left(\frac{\sigma_o}{2}\right)$$

$$40.58 = \frac{240}{2 \times \text{fos}}$$

$$\Rightarrow \quad \text{fos} = \left(\frac{240}{2 \times 40.58}\right) = 2.95$$

$$\approx 3 \qquad\qquad\qquad \text{(fos is not taken in fraction)}$$

(ii) By Maximum Strain Energy Theory

$$\sigma_1^2 + \sigma_2^2 - 2\nu\,\sigma_1 \cdot \sigma_2 = \sigma_0^2$$

i.e. $\quad (67.76)^2 + (-13.43)^2 - 2 \times 0.3 \times 67.76 \times (-13.43) = \dfrac{(240)^2}{\text{fos}}$

$$\Rightarrow \quad 5317.\dot{\circ} = \frac{(240)^2}{\text{fos}}$$

$$\Rightarrow \quad \text{fos} = \frac{(240)^2}{5317.8} = 10.8$$

$$\therefore \quad \text{fos} = 11 \qquad \textbf{Ans.}$$

Q. 1(c) *Write short notes on any of the following:*   **(10 Marks)**
    (i) *Castigliano's Theorem*   (See Chapter 13)
    (ii) *Compatibility equations*   (See Chapter 3)
    (iii) *Three-dimensional stresses*   (See Chapter 3)

Q. 2(a) *A timber joist of 6 metre span has to carry a load of 15 kN/metre. Find the dimensions of the joist if the maximum permissible stress is limited to 8 N/mm². The depth of the joist has to be twice the width.*   **(10 Marks)**

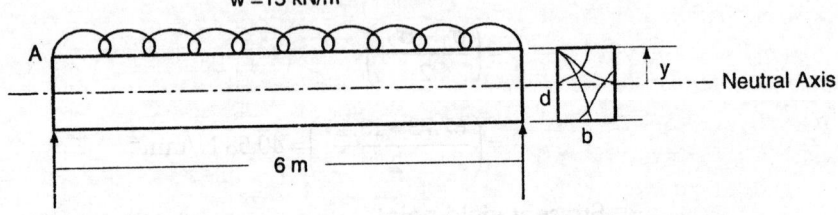

Fig. 2

SOLUTION   Given $\sigma_{\text{allowable}} = 8 \text{ N/mm}^2$

$$d = 2b$$

$$M_{\max} = \left[\frac{wl^2}{8}\right] = \frac{15 \times 10^3 \times 6}{8}$$

$$= 67{,}500 \text{ Nm}$$

$$= 67{,}500 \times 10^3 \text{ Nmm}$$

$$\text{MOI (I)} = \frac{bd^3}{12} = \frac{b \times (2b)^3}{12}$$

$$= \frac{8b^4}{12} = \frac{2b^4}{3}$$

Position of neutral axis $(\overline{y}) = \frac{d}{2} = \frac{2b}{2} = b$

Now, by bending formula,

$$\frac{M}{I} = \frac{\sigma}{y}$$

$$\frac{67,500 \times 10^3}{\dfrac{2b^4}{3}} = \frac{8}{b}$$

$$\frac{67,500 \times 10^3 \times 3}{2b^3} = 8$$

$$\Rightarrow \qquad b = \left(\frac{67,500 \times 10^3 \times 3}{16} \right)^{0.33}$$

$$\therefore \qquad b = 233 \text{ mm and } d = 2b = 466 \text{ mm} \qquad \textbf{Ans.}$$

Q. 2(b) *A beam, simply supported at ends A and B is loaded with two point loads of 60 kN and 50 kN at distance 1 metre and 3 metre respectively from end A. Determine the position and magnitude of maximum deflection. Take E = 2 × 10⁵ N/mm² and I = 8500 cm⁴.*
(10 Marks)

SOLUTION (See Page 10.37-10.39)

Q. 2(c) *Find the internal and external diameters required for a hollow shaft, which is to transmit 40 kW of power at 240 rev/minute. The shear stress is to be limited to 100 MN/m². Take outside diameter to be twice the inside diameter.*
(10 Marks)

SOLUTION Given: Power (P) = 40 kW = 40 × 10³ Watt

Speed (N) = 240 rpm

Shear stress (τ) = 100 MN/m²

$D = 2d$

Let di and do are internal and external diameter respectively

$$\text{Power (P)} = \frac{2\pi NT}{60}$$

$$\therefore \qquad T = \frac{P \times 60}{2\pi N}$$

$$= \frac{40 \times 10^3 \times 60 \times 7}{2 \times 22 \times 240} = 1590.90$$

$$\simeq 1591 \,\text{N.m}$$

$$= 1591 \times 10^3 \,\text{N mm}.$$

Using Torsion formula,

$$\frac{T}{J} = \frac{\tau}{R}$$

$$\frac{J}{R} = \frac{T}{\tau}$$

$$Z_p = \frac{1.592 \times 10^6}{100} = 1.592 \times 10^4$$

Now, $\quad \dfrac{\pi \left[D^4 - d^4 \right]}{16D} = 1.592 \times 10^4$

or, $\quad \dfrac{\pi \left[(2d)^4 - d^4 \right]}{16 \times 2d} = 1.592 \times 10^4$ $\qquad$ [Given $D = 2d$]

or, $\quad d^3 = 10807.6$

$\therefore \quad d = 22.109$ mm $\quad$ **Ans.**

and $\quad D = 2d = 2 \times 22.109 = 44.22$ mm $\quad$ **Ans.**

Q. 3(a) *A leaf spring has 12 plates each 50 mm and 5 mm thick, the longest plate being 600 mm long. The greatest bending stress is not to exceed 180 N/mm² and the central deflection is 15 mm. Estimate the magnitude of the greatest central load that can be applied to the spring. Take E = 0.206 × 10⁶ N/mm²* **(10 Marks)**

SOLUTION

Given, $n = 12, l = 600$ mm

$$b = 50 \text{ mm}$$

$$t = 5 \text{ mm}$$

Bending stress $\sigma_b \not> 180 \text{ N/mm}^2$

Deflection $(\delta) = 15$ mm

Central load $(W) = ?$

$$E = 0.206 \times 10^6 \text{ N/mm}^2$$

By formula,

$$\sigma_b = \frac{3}{2} \cdot \frac{Wl}{nbt^2}$$

$$180 = \frac{3}{2} \cdot \frac{W \times 600}{12 \times 50 \times (5)^2}$$

$$\therefore \qquad W = \left(\frac{180 \times 2 \times 12 \times 50 \times 25}{3 \times 600} \right) \text{Newton}$$

$$= 3000 \text{ Newton}$$

$$= 3 \text{ kN} \qquad \textbf{Ans.}$$

Q. 3(b) *Determine the section of a cast iron hollow cylindrical column 5 metre long with ends firmly built-in if it carries an axial load of 300 kN. The ratio of internal to external diameter is 3/4. Use factor of safety of 8. Take* $\sigma_c = 567 \, N/mm^2$ *and Rankine's constant* $a = 1/1600$.   **(10 Marks)**

SOLUTION

$$L = 5 \, m, \qquad \sigma_c = 567 \, N/mm2$$

$$P = 300 \, kN \qquad a = \frac{1}{1600}$$

$$\text{fos} = 8 \qquad \frac{d}{D} = \frac{3}{4} = 0.75$$

Objective: To find D and d.

Crippling load = Axial load × fos

$$= 300 \times 8 = 2400 \, kN$$

Area $\qquad A = \frac{\pi}{4}(D^2 - d^2)$

$$= \frac{\pi}{4}\{D^2 - (0.75D)^2\} = 0.3436 \, D^2$$

Radius of gyration $(K) = \sqrt{\dfrac{I}{A}}$

$$= \sqrt{\frac{\frac{\pi}{64}(D^4 - d^4)}{\frac{\pi}{4}(D^2 - d^2)}} = \sqrt{\frac{D^2 + d^2}{16}}$$

$$= \sqrt{\frac{D^2 + (0.75D)^2}{16}} = 0.3125 \, D$$

Now, since the ends of column are fixed i.e. it's both end are fixed.

Therefore, $\qquad l_e = \dfrac{l}{2} = \dfrac{5}{2}$

$$= 2.5 \, m = 2500 mm$$

Using Rankine formula,

$$P_{cr} = \frac{\sigma_c \cdot A}{1 + \alpha \left(\dfrac{l_e}{K}\right)^2}$$

$$2400 \times 10^3 = \frac{567 \times 0.3436 \, D^2}{1 + \dfrac{1}{1600}\left(\dfrac{2500}{0.3125 \, D}\right)^2}$$

$$194.84 \, D^4 - 2400 \times 10^3 D^2 - 9.6 \times 10^{10} = 0$$

$$\Rightarrow \qquad D^2 = 29194.6$$

$$\Rightarrow \qquad D = 170.86 \text{ mm}$$

So, $d = 0.75 \, D$

$$= 0.75 \times 170.86$$

Hence, computed value of diameter $(d) = 128.15$ mm.   **Ans.**

Q. 3(c) *From the first principles derive the expression for the critical buckling for a column having one end fixed and one end hinged.*   **(10 Marks)**

SOLUTION See Page No. 18.6 of the book.

Q. 4(a) *A cylindrical vessel 1.5 metre in diameter, 2 metre long and 1.5 cm thick is closed at both the ends by rigid plates and this cylinder is filled with water at atmospheric pressure. Find how much additional amount of water is required to be pumped so as to make the final pressure in the cylinder as 70 bar. Take E = 210 GN/m² and μ = 0.3 for the material of the cylinder. Bulk modulus of the water is 2.4 GN/m².*   **(10 Marks)**

SOLUTION Given $d = 1.5$ m $= 1500$ mm; $L = 2$ m $= 2000$ mm; $t = 1.5$ cm $= 15$ mm; $P = 70$ bar $= 0.7$ N/mm²; $E = 210$ GN/m² $= 210 \times 10^3$ N/mm².

Volumetric Strain $(\varepsilon_v) = \varepsilon_{v \, shell} + \varepsilon_{v \, fluid}$

$$= \frac{pd}{4tE}(5 - 4v) + \frac{p}{K}$$

$$= \frac{0.7 \times 1500}{4 \times 15 \times 210 \times 10^3}(5 - 4 \times 0.3) + \frac{0.7}{2.4 \times 10^3}$$

$$= 316.67 \times 10^{-6} + 2.917 \times 10^{-4}$$

$$= 6.083 \times 10^{-4}$$

$$d_v = \varepsilon_v \cdot V$$

$$= 6.083 \times 10^{-4} \times \frac{\pi}{4} \times 1500^2 \times 2000$$

$$= 215000 \text{ mm}^3 \qquad \textbf{Ans.}$$

Q. 4(b) *Calculate the thickness of metal necessary for a cylindrical shell of internal diameter of 80 mm to withstand an internal pressure of 25 N/mm^2, if the maximum permissible tensile stress is 125 N/mm^2.* **(10 Marks)**

SOLUTION Given $d = 80$ mm; $p_i = 25$ N/mm^2 and $p_o = 0$; $\sigma_{max} = \sigma_h = 125$ N/mm^2

Objective: To find the thickness of cylindrical shell.

By Lame's Equation,

$$\text{Hoop Stress } (\sigma_h) = \frac{B}{r^2} + A \text{ (Tensile)} \tag{I}$$

$$\text{Radial Stress } (\sigma_r) = \frac{B}{r^2} - A \text{ (Compressive)} \tag{II}$$

At $r_i = 40$ mm, $p_i = 25$ mPa

At r_o; $p_o = 0$

Substituting the value of p_i and p_o in eq. II

$$25 = \frac{B}{40^2} - A \tag{III}$$

$$0 = \frac{B}{r_o^2} - A \text{ hence, } A = \frac{B}{r_o^2} \tag{IV}$$

At $r_i = 40$ mm, $\sigma_h = 125$ N/mm^2

Hence, $\quad 125 = \dfrac{B}{40^2} + A \tag{V}$

Adding equation (III) and (IV), we get

$$150 = \frac{2B}{40^2}$$

$\Rightarrow \qquad B = 1,20,000$

Substituting value of B in equation (V), we get

$$125 = \frac{120000}{40^2} + A$$

$\Rightarrow \qquad A = 50$

From equation (IV)

$$A = \frac{B}{r_o^2}$$

$\Rightarrow \qquad 50 = \dfrac{120000}{r_o^2}$

$\Rightarrow \qquad r_o = 48.99 = 49$ mm

Hence, thickness of metal $(t) = r_o - r_i$

$$= 49 - 40 = 9 \text{ mm}$$

Q. 4(c) *Write short notes on any two of the following:*   **(10 Marks)**
  (i) *Lame's theory of thick cylinders.* (See Chapter thick cylinder)
  (ii) *Compound cylinder.* (See Chapter thick cylinder)
  (iii) *Radial, axial and circumferential stresses in thick cylinders.* (See Chapter thick
     cylinder)

Q. 5(a) *A curved bar of square section, 3 cm sides and mean radius of curvature 4.5 cm is
     initially unstressed. If a bending moment of 300 N-m is applied to the bar tending to
     straighten it, find the stresses at the inner and outer faces.*   **(10 Marks)**

SOLUTION Given $\bar{r}$ = mean radius of curvature

$$= 4.5 \text{ cm} = 45 \text{ mm}$$

$$r_i = \left(45 - \frac{h}{2}\right) = \left(45 - \frac{30}{2}\right)$$

$$= (45 - 15) = 30 \text{ mm}$$

$$r_i = (r_i + h)$$

$$= (30 + 30)$$

$$= 60 \text{ mm}$$

$$A = (30)^2 = 900 \text{ mm}^2$$

$$M = +300 \text{Nm} = 300 \times 10^3 \text{ Nmm}$$

Now, R_N = location of neutral axis radius

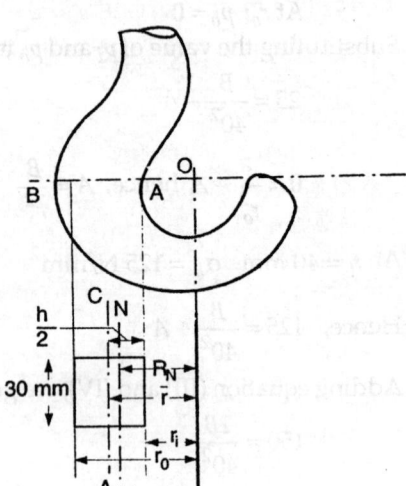

Fig. 3

$$= \frac{h}{\ln\left(\dfrac{r_o}{r_i}\right)} = \frac{30}{\ln\left(\dfrac{60}{30}\right)}$$

$$= \frac{30}{\ln(2)} = 43.28 \text{ mm}$$

$$e = (\bar{r} - R_N)$$

$$= (45 - 43.28) = 1.72 \text{ mm}$$

Stress at innermost faces $(\sigma_i) = \dfrac{M(R_N - r_i)}{A \cdot r_i \cdot e}$

$$= \frac{10^3 \times 300\,(43.28 - 30)}{900 \times 30 \times 1.72} \text{ N/mm}^2$$

$$= 85.78 \text{ N/mm}^2 \qquad \textbf{Ans.}$$

Stress at outermost faces $(\sigma_0) = \dfrac{M(R_N - r_o)}{A \cdot r_o \cdot e}$

$$= \frac{300 \times 10^3 \ (43.28 - 60)}{900 \times 60 \times 1.72} \ \text{N/mm}^2$$

$$= (-)\, 54.005 \ \text{N/mm}^2 \qquad \textbf{Ans.}$$

Q. 5(b) *A 60 mm × 40 mm × 6 mm unequal angle is placed with the longer leg vertical, and is used as a beam. It is subjected to a bending moment of 12 kN-cm acting in the vertical plane through the centroid of the section. Determine the maximum bending stress induced in the section.* **(See Unsymmetric Bending Chapter)** (10 Marks)

(N.B.: The formula of curved beam is based on the formula given by Winkler and Further Work by E.P. Popov—The Author of Mechanics of Solid, the prescribed text book is authentic in all Engineering colleges in India and Abroad, therefore reader(s) should not hesitate in applying these formulae for solving the problem for the curved beam).

Q. 5(c) *Write short notes on any two of the following:* (10 Marks)
  (i) *Centroidal Principal Axes.*
  (ii) *Compound cylinder.*
  (iii) *Radial, axial and circumferential stresses in thick cylinders.*

SOLUTION See the chapters on:
  (i) Unsymmetrical bending
  (ii) Curved Beam

— ❖❖ —

SOLVED UNIVERSITY QUESTIONS
(Strengh of Materials)
2010-11

PAPER ID: 0429   **Total Marks: 100**

Q. 1(a) *A two dimensional state of stress is given by:* $\sigma_{xx} = 10$ *MPs,* $\sigma_{yy} = 12.5$ *MPa. Determine the following, the plane is inclined at an angle of 30° from x-plane in anticlockwise direction.*

  (i) *Normal stress*   (ii) *Shear stress*

 (iii) *Resultant stress*   (iv) *Principal stresses at that point*

SOLUTION Given

$$\sigma_{xx} = \sigma_x = 10 \text{ MPa}$$

$$\sigma_{yy} = \sigma_y = 12.5 \text{ MPa}$$

$$\tau_{xy} = 2.5 \text{ MPa}$$

Since the plane is inclined at 30° with x-axis.

So, it (plane) is making 60° with y-axis.

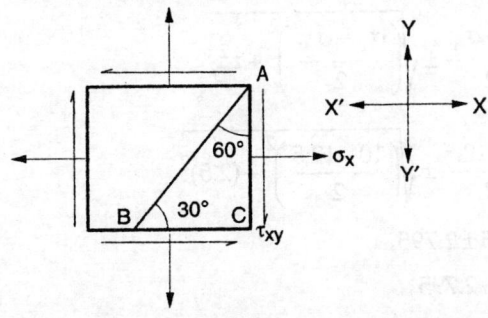

Fig. 1

[N.B.: This was done to match the formula given in this book in clause 2.3 where we have considered θ with the y-axis. Reader should always remember it. One can also use θ with x-axis, in that case other formula will be used as described in this book].

Normal stress on the inclined plane AB,

$$\sigma_\theta = \frac{\sigma_x + \sigma_y}{2} + \frac{\sigma_x - \sigma_y}{2} \cos\theta + \tau_{xy} \sin 2\theta$$

$$= \frac{10+12.5}{2} + \frac{10-12.5}{2}\cos 120° + 2.5 \sin 120°$$

$$= 11.25 + 0.625 + 2.165 = 14.04 \text{ N/mm}^2$$

Shear stress on the inclined plane AB

$$\tau_\theta = (-)\frac{\sigma_x - \sigma_y}{2}\sin 2\theta + \tau_{xy}\cos 2\theta$$

$$= (-)\frac{10-12.5}{2}\sin 120° + 2.5 \cos 120°$$

$$= 1.25 \sin 120° + 2.5 \cos 120°$$

$$= 1.25 \times 0.866 + 2.5 \times (-0.5)$$

$$= 1.0825 - 1.25$$

$$\therefore \qquad \tau_\theta = (-1)\,0.1675 \text{ N/mm}^2$$

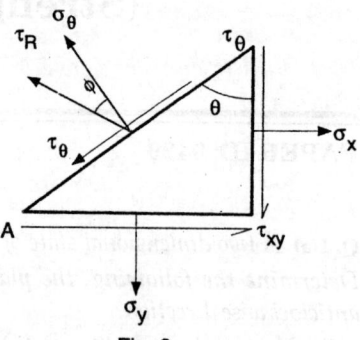

Fig. 2

Resultant stress on plane AB $(\sigma_R) = \sqrt{\sigma_\theta^2 + \tau_\theta^2}$

$$= \sqrt{(14.04)^2 + (0.1675)^2}$$

$$= 14.04 \text{ N/mm}^2$$

*Angle of obliquity, $\phi = \tan^{-1}\left[\dfrac{\tau_{xy}}{\sigma_\theta}\right]$

The principal stresses are given by following formula,

$$\sigma_{1,2} = \frac{\sigma_x + \sigma_y}{2} \pm \sqrt{\left(\frac{\sigma_x - \sigma_y}{2}\right)^2 + \tau_{xy}^2}$$

$$= \frac{10+12.5}{2} \pm \sqrt{\left(\frac{10-12.5}{2}\right)^2 + (2.5)^2}$$

$$= 11.25 \pm 2.795$$

$$\therefore \qquad \sigma_1 = 11.25 + 2.795$$

$$= 14.045 \text{ MPa} \qquad\qquad \text{(Max. or Major Principal Stress)}$$

$$\sigma_2 = 11.25 - 2.795$$

$$= 8.455 \text{ MPa} \qquad\qquad \text{(Min. or Minor Principal Stress)}$$

---

*Although ϕ i.e. angle of obliquity is not asked in the question, it is essential to compute it. ϕ is the inclination with the normal (σ_θ).
Here, ϕ comes to be very small.

Q. 1(b) *One end of a spring if fixed on horizontal plane with its axis in vertical direction. When it supports a mass of 10 kg, the spring is compressed by 2.0 cm. The maximum principal stress in the spring wire is 20 MPa and maximum shear stress is 10 MPa. Find the maximum value of the deflection and the stresses when the same mass is allowed to freely fall and strike the spring.*

SOLUTION Data insufficient.

Q. 1(c) *A bar of length 1.5 m, cross sectional area 20 cm² and mass 30 kg is hanging in vertical direction. A force of 200 N is applied at the free end of bar. Using Castigliano's Theorem, determine the elongation in the bar due to the force and self weight of the bar.*

SOLUTION

$$\text{Deflection } (\delta) = \left(\frac{\partial U}{\partial P} \right)$$

where U = Strain Energy

and P = Axial Load.

In this question weight of the bar is also taken into consideration.

Let us consider a small element dx at a distance from the free end. Let A be cross sectional and ρ is density of material of the bar and g = acceleration due to gravity. Then, axial force (P_x) due to self weight of the sample and the external force (P) $200\,N = \rho\,Axg + P$.

Now,   Strain Energy $(U) = \int_0^l \dfrac{P^2 x \cdot dx}{2AE}$

$$= \int_0^l \frac{(\rho A\,xg + P)^2\,dx}{2AE}$$

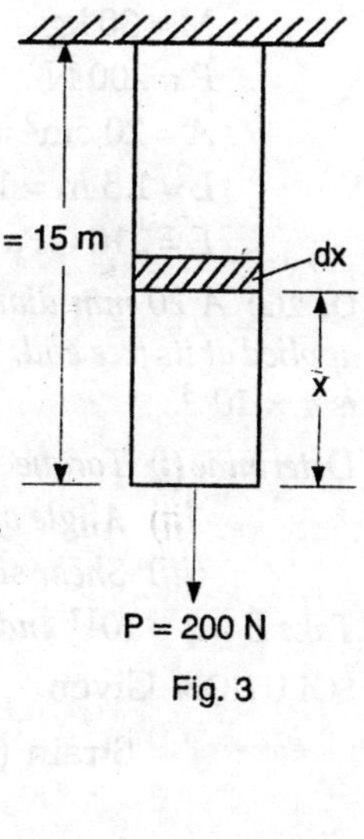

Now, by Castigliano's Theorem,

Deflection at a distance 'x' $(\delta) = \dfrac{\partial U}{\partial P}$

$$= \frac{\partial}{\partial P} \left(\frac{\rho Axg + P}{2AE} \right)^2 dx$$

$$= \frac{2\,(\rho Axg + P)}{2AE} \cdot dx$$

$\ell = 15\ m$

dx

x

$P = 200\ N$

Fig. 3

Hence for the entire length (i.e. $l = 1.5$ m)

$$\delta = \int_0^l 2 \left(\frac{\rho Axg + P}{2AE} \right) dx.$$

$$= \int_0^l \frac{2\rho Axg}{2AE}\,dx + \int_0^l \frac{2\rho dx}{2AE}$$

$$= \frac{2\rho Ag}{2AE} \int_0^l x\,dx + \frac{2\rho}{2AE} \int_0^l dx$$

$$= \frac{\rho Ag}{AE}\left[\frac{x^2}{2}\right]_0^l + \frac{P}{AE}[x]_0^l$$

$$= \frac{\rho Ag}{AE}\left[\frac{l^2}{2}\right] + \frac{P}{AE}[l]$$

$$= \frac{\dfrac{M}{V}\cdot A\cdot g\cdot l^2}{2AE} + \frac{P\cdot l}{AE}$$

$$= \frac{\dfrac{M}{V}\cdot (Al)\cdot gl}{2AE} + \frac{Pl}{AE}$$

$$= \frac{Mgl}{2AE} + \frac{Pl}{AE}$$

So, $$\delta = \frac{Mgl}{2AE} + \frac{P\cdot l}{A\cdot E}$$

Now, substitrute the value of M, g, l, A, E and P and get the result

$M = 30$ kg

$P = 200$ N

$A = 20$ cm$^2 = 20 \times 10^{-4}$ mm^2

$L = 1.5$ m $= 1.5 \times 10^3$ mm

$E = 210$ GPa (Assuming Steal)

Q. 2(a) *A 20 mm diameter shaft of length 500 mm is fixed at one end. A torque T is applied at its free end. The linear strain at the surface of shaft at an angle of 45° from axis is 4×10^{-3}.*

Determine (i) Torque

(ii) Angle of twist

(iii) Shear stress in the shaft.

Take $E = 2 \times 10^{11}$ and $G = 0.8 \times 10^{10}$

SOLUTION Given $d = 20$ mm $l = 500$ mm

Strain $(\phi) = 45° = 0.785$ $E = 2 \times 10^{11}$

$G = 0.8 \times 10^{10}$ $El = 4 \times 10^{-3}$

Objective: T, θ, τ

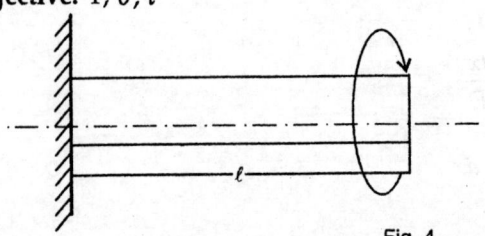
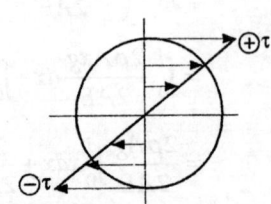

Fig. 4

We know that when torque (T) is applied to shaft, shear stress will be developed. In the upper layer $(+)\tau$ and lower layer $(-)\tau$ will develop and as a result the shaft will be twisted by angle ϕ.

If we recall relation between elastic constant then,

$$E = 2G(1+v)$$

$$2\times10^{11} = 2\times8\times10^{10}(1+v)$$

$\Rightarrow$ $v = 0.25$

Further,

$$\text{Linear Strain } (El) = \frac{\tau}{E} - v\left(-\frac{\tau}{E}\right)$$

$$= \frac{\tau}{E} + v\cdot\frac{\tau}{E}$$

$$4\times10^{-3} = \frac{\tau}{E}(1+v)$$

$$4\times10^{-3} = \frac{\tau}{2\times10^{11}}(1+0.25)$$

$\Rightarrow$ $\tau = 640\ \text{N/mm}^2$

Using Torsion formula,

$$\frac{T}{J} = \frac{\tau}{R}$$

$$T = \frac{J}{R}\times\tau = Z_p\times\tau$$

$$= \frac{\pi d^3}{16}\times\tau = \frac{\pi d^3}{16}\times640$$

$$= 1.005\times10^6\ \text{N.mm}\qquad \textbf{Ans.}$$

$$\text{Angle of Twist } (\theta) = \frac{\tau\cdot L}{R\cdot G} = \frac{640\times500}{10\times8\times10^{10}}$$

$$= 0.4\ \text{radian} = 0.4\times\frac{180}{\pi}$$

$$= 22.92°\qquad \textbf{Ans.}$$

Q. 2(b) *A fixed beam of length 2 m carries a concentrated load of 10 kN at its mid span. Determine the reaction and bending moment at the support and deflection at the mid span. Flexural stiffness of the beam is $2.0 \times 10\ Nm^2$.*

SOLUTION

By symmetry $R_A = R_B$ and $M_A = M_B$

$$R_A = R_B = \frac{W}{2} = \frac{10}{2} = 5 \text{ kN}$$

We know,

$$M_A = M_B = \frac{Wa^2b}{L^2}$$ [for shaft loaded at a distance a from left and b from right]

Now, putting $a = b = M_A = M_B = \dfrac{W \cdot a^3}{L^2}$

$$= \frac{W \cdot \left(\dfrac{L}{2}\right)^3}{L^2} = \frac{W \cdot L^3}{8L^2}$$

$$= \frac{W \cdot L}{8} = \frac{10 \times 2}{8}$$

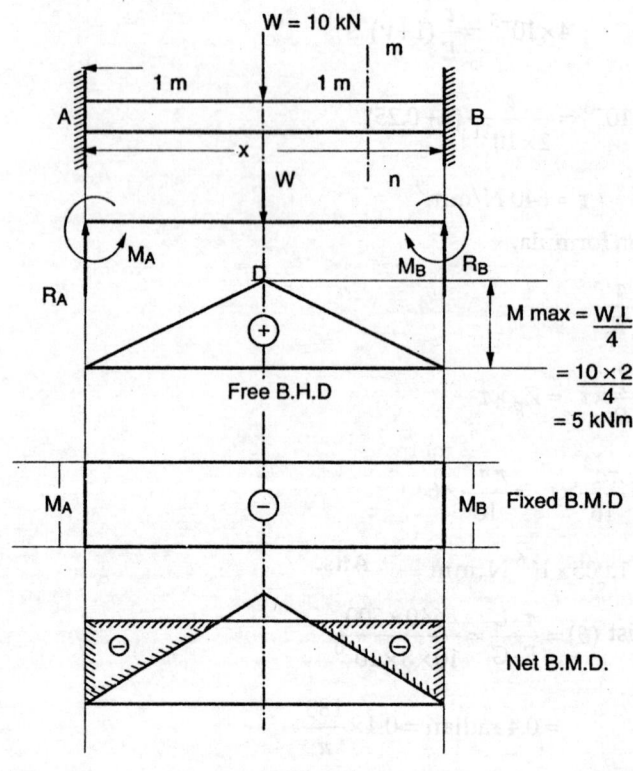

Fig. 5

$$\therefore \quad M_A = M_B = 2.5 \text{ kNM}$$

Consider an imaginary section MM at a distance x from left end

Then, by Macaulay's method,

$$M(x) = R_A \cdot x - M_A - W < x - 1 >$$

or, $EIy'' = 5x - 2.5 - 10 < x - 1 >$

Integrating both sides,

$$EIy' = \frac{5x^2}{2} - 2.5x - \frac{10}{2} < x - 1 >^2 + C_1$$

and $$EIy = \frac{5x^3}{6} - \frac{2.5x^2}{2} - \frac{5}{3} < x - 1 >^2 + C_1 x + C_2$$

BC are

at $x = 0, y = 0$ and $\dfrac{dy}{dx} = 0$

Therefore, $C_1 = C_2 = 0$

and $$y = \frac{1}{EI} \left[\frac{5x^3}{6} - \frac{2.5}{2} x^2 - \frac{5}{3} < x - 1 >^3 \right]$$

$A + x = 1m$ i.e. in the middle of beam

y at centre $= \dfrac{1}{EI} \left[\dfrac{5}{6} \times 1 - \dfrac{2.5}{2} \times 1 \right]$

$$= \frac{1}{EI} \left[\frac{5 - 7.5}{6} \right]$$

$$= -\left(\frac{2.5}{6} \right) \cdot \frac{1}{EI} \text{ metre}$$

$$= -0.416 \times \frac{1}{EI} \text{ metre}$$

$$= (-)\,0.416 \times \frac{1}{2 \times 10} \text{ metre}$$

$$= (-)\,0.0208 \text{ metre}$$

$$= (-)\,20.8 \text{ mm} \qquad \textbf{Ans.}$$

Q. 2(c) *A 100 mm × 150 mm wooden bar is to be symmetrically loaded with two equal forces P as shown in figure. Determine the position of loads and their magnitude when a bending stress of 10 MPa and shearing stress of 2.5 MPa are just reached. Neglect weight of the beam.*

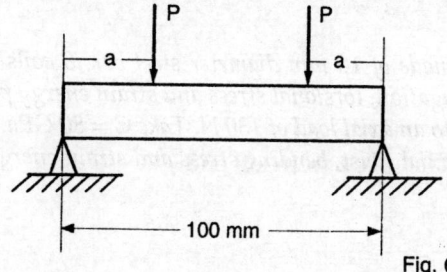

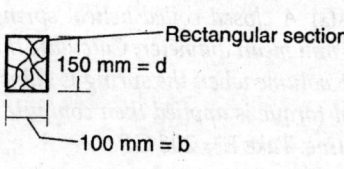

Fig. 6

SOLUTION

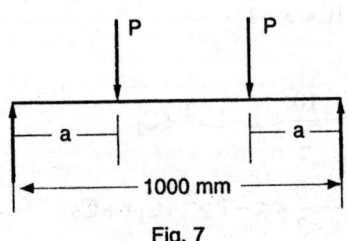

Fig. 7

Given: $b = 100$ mm, $d = 150$ mm
            $\sigma = 10$ MPa $\tau = 2.5$ MPa

Objective: To compute P

$$I = \frac{bd^3}{12} = \frac{100 \times 150^3}{12}$$

$$= 28.125 \times 10^6 \text{ mm}^4$$

Maximum shear stress $(\tau) = \dfrac{FAy}{bI}$

$$2.5 = \frac{P \times 100 \times 75 \times \dfrac{75}{2}}{100 \times 28.125 \times 10^6}$$

$\Rightarrow$ $P = 25000$ N $= 25$ kN   **Ans.**

Now, Position of load *i.e. a* is to be computed.

By Bending formula, $\dfrac{M}{I} = \dfrac{\sigma}{y}$

$$\frac{M}{28.125 \times 10^6} = \frac{10}{75}$$

$\Rightarrow$ $M = 3.75 \times 10^6$ N.mm

Maximum bending moment, $(M_{max}) = P \times a$

or, $3.75 \times 10^6 = 25 \times 10^4 \times a$

$\Rightarrow$ $a = 150$ mm   **Ans.**

Q. 3(a) *A closed coiled helical spring is made of 10 mm diameter steel bar, 8 coils of 150 mm mean diameter. Calculate the elongation, torsional stress and strain energy per unit volume when the spring is subjected to an axial load of 130 N. Take G = 80 GPa. If axial torque is applied then compute and axial twist, bending stress and strain energy/ volume. Take E = 208 GPa.*

SOLUTION

            Given, $d = 10$ mm, $n = 8$ mm

Mean diameter $D = 150$ mm

Modulus of rigidity $G = 80$ GPa

Axial Load $(W) = 130$ N

Objective: To compute τ and δ

<u>Case I:</u> **Spring subjected to an axial load.**

R = Mean radius $\dfrac{D}{2} = 75$ mm

Deflection $(\delta) = \dfrac{64\ WR^3 n}{Gd^4}$

$\quad = \dfrac{64 \times 100 \times 75^3 \times 8}{80 \times 10^3 \times 10^4} = 35.1$ mm $\qquad$ **Ans.**

Shear stress $(\tau) = \dfrac{16WR}{\pi d^3}$

$\quad = \dfrac{16 \times 130 \times 75}{\pi \times 10^3} = 49.66$ N/mm^2 $\qquad$ **Ans.**

Strain Energy per unit Volume $= \dfrac{\tau^2}{4G}$

$\quad = \dfrac{49.66^2}{4 \times 80 \times 10^3} = 7.705 \times 10^{-3}$ N/m^2 **Ans.**

<u>Case II:</u> **Spring Subjected to axial Torque**

$T = 9$ N·m $= 9 \times 10^3$ Nmm

$E = 200$ GPa $= 200 \times 10^3$ MPa

Axial twist $(\phi) = \dfrac{128TRn}{Ed^4}$

$\quad = \dfrac{128 \times 9 \times 10^3 \times 75 \times 8}{200 \times 10^3 \times 10^4}$

$\quad = 0.3456$ radian $\qquad$ **Ans.**

Bending stress $(\sigma) = \dfrac{32\ T}{\pi d^3}$

$\quad = \dfrac{32 \times 9 \times 10^3}{\pi \times 10^3} = 91.67$ MPa $\qquad$ **Ans.**

Q. 3(b) *A 5 m long column with fixed ends supports an axial load of 800 kN. The external diameter of the column is 240 mm. Determine the thickness of the column using Rankine Formula.*

Given that $a = \dfrac{1}{6400}$ *and working stress is 80 MPa.*

SOLUTION Given

$$L = 5m = 5000 \quad d = 240 \text{ mm}$$

$$a = \frac{1}{6400} \qquad \sigma = 80 \text{ MPa}$$

Objective: To calculate thickness 't'

Here, the effective length $(l_e) = \dfrac{l}{2}$

$$= \frac{5000}{2} = 2500 \text{ mm}$$

Area $A = \dfrac{\pi}{4}(D^2 - d^2)$

$$= \frac{\pi}{4}(240^2 - d^2)$$

Radius of gyration for hollow column,

$$K^2 = \frac{I}{A} = \frac{D^2 + d^2}{16}$$

By Rankine formula, $P_{cr} = \dfrac{\sigma_c . A}{1 + \alpha \left(\dfrac{l_e}{K}\right)^2}$

$$800 \times 10^3 = \frac{80 \times \dfrac{\pi}{4}(240^2 - d^2)}{1 + \dfrac{1}{6400}\left(\dfrac{2500 \times 16}{240^2 + d^2}\right)}$$

or, $\quad d^4 + 12.732 \times 10^3 d^2 - 2.385 \times 10^9 = 0$

$\Rightarrow \qquad d^2 = 42883.6$

$\Rightarrow \qquad d = 207 \text{ mm}$

Hence, thickness of column $(t) = \dfrac{D - d}{2} = \dfrac{240 - 207}{2} = 16.5 \text{ mm}$. **Ans.**

Q. 3(c) *Explain the term core of section with reference to short column. Derive an expression for finding out the core of a rectangular section.*
                                                                                    (10 Marks)

SOLUTION See chapter Combined Stress (Chp 8).

Q. 4(a) *A thin spherical vessel having diameter of 1.50 m is of uniform thickness. It is filled with water at a gauge pressure of 2 MPa. A relief valve attached to the vessel is opened and water is allowed to escape until the pressure falls to atmospherec. If the volume of water escaped is 4 litre, find the thickness of the plate of vessel. Bulk modulus of water is 2GPa and Young modulus of vessel material is 200 GPa and Poisson's ratio is 0.30.*

SOLUTION Given $d = 1.5$ m $= 1500$ mm; $p = 2$ MPa;

$dv =$ Volume escaped $= 4$ litre

$$= 4 \times 10^3 \text{ m}^3 = 4 \times 10^{-3} \times 10^9 \text{ mm}^3$$

$K = 2$ GPa $= 2 \times 10^3$ MFa

$v = 0.3$

Volume of the spherical shell (V) $= \dfrac{\pi}{6} d^3$

$$= \dfrac{\pi}{6} \times 1500^2 = 1.76 \times 10^9 \text{ mm}^3$$

Volumetric Strain for Compressible Fluid,

$$\varepsilon_v = \varepsilon_v \text{ (shell)} + \varepsilon_v \text{ (fluid)}$$

$$\dfrac{dV}{V} = \dfrac{3pd}{4tE}(1-v) + \dfrac{p}{K}$$

$$\dfrac{4 \times 10}{1.769 \times 10^9} = \dfrac{3 \times 2 \times 1500 \, (1-0.3)}{4 \times t \times 200 \times 10^3} + \dfrac{2}{2 \times 10^3}$$

$$2.261 \times 10^{-3} = \dfrac{0.007875}{t} + 1 \times 10^3$$

$\Rightarrow$ $\qquad\qquad\qquad\qquad t = 6.25$ mm $\qquad$ **Ans.**

Q. 4(b) *A thick cylinder of 160 mm internal and 240 mm external diameter is subjected to an external pressure 12 MPa. Determine the maximum internal pressure that can be applied if the maximum allowable normal stress is 36 MPa. Plot the variation of radial and hoop stresses.*

SOLUTION Given external diameter $(d_o) = 240$ mm

Internal diameter $(d_i) = 160$ mm

External pressure $(p_o) = 12$ mPa

Maximum allowable normal stresses $\sigma_h = 36$ MPa

Objective: $p_i = ?$

$r_i = 80$ mm; $r_o = 120$ mm

$\sigma_{h_i} =$ Hoop stress at inner face

$$\sigma_{h_i} = \dfrac{1}{r_o^2 - r_i^2}\left[p_i r_i^2 - p_o r_o^2 + r_o^2 \, (p_i - p_o) \right]$$

$$36 = \dfrac{1}{120^2 - 80^2}\left[p_i \times 80^2 - 12 \times 120^2 + 120^2 (p_i - 12) \right]$$

$$288 \times 10^3 = (80^2 + 120^2)\, p_i - 345.6 \times 10^3$$

$\Rightarrow$ $p_i = 30.46\, \text{MPa} \simeq 30.5\, \text{MPa} = $ radial stress at inner surface

This is the maximum internal pressure based on maximum allowable normal strain.

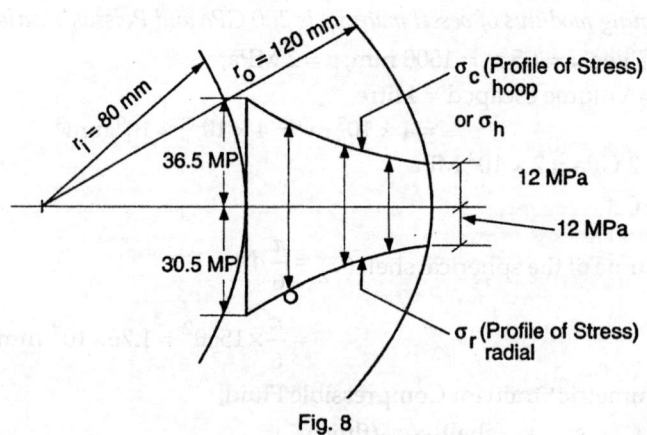

Fig. 8

Hoop stress at inner face $\sigma_{h_i} = \dfrac{1}{r_o^2 - r_i^2}\left[P_i r_i - p_o r_o^2 + (p_i - p_o)\, r_o^2\right]$

$$= \frac{1}{120^2 - 80^2}[30.5 \times 80^2 - 12 \times 120^2 + (30.5 - 12) \times 120^2]$$

$$= 36.1\, \text{MPa} \qquad \textbf{Ans.}$$

Hoop stress at out face $\sigma_{h_o} = \dfrac{1}{r_o^2 - r_i^2}\left[p_i r_i^2 - p_o r_i^2 - (p_i r_i^2 - p_o r_o^2)\right]$

$$= \frac{1}{r_o^2 - r_i^2}\left[p_o r_o^2 - p_i r_i^2 - (p_i - p_o)\right]$$

$$= \frac{1}{120^2 - 80^2}\left[\frac{12 \times 120^2 - 30.5 \times 80^2}{+80^2(30.5 - 12)}\right]$$

$$= \frac{1}{(120 + 80)\,(120 - 80)}\left[(12 \times 120)^2 - (30.5 \times 80^2) + (80^2 \times 18.5)\right]$$

$$= \frac{1}{200 \times 40}[96000]$$

$$= 12\, \text{MPa} \qquad \textbf{Ans.}$$

N.B. [To plot the exact graph the computation of radial stress and hoop stress at various inner radius and various outer radius is essential as is done in the Ex. 2 of thick cylinder. Here, not advised to do so as the same is not asked in question. However, rough sketch can be drawn showing the variation of stresses at inner and outer radius]

Check: Radial stress (σ_r) at inner surface

$$= \frac{1}{r_o^2 - r_i^2}\left\{(p_i - p_o)\, r_o^2 - (p_i r_i^2 - p_o r_o^2)\right\}$$

$$= \frac{1}{120^2 - 80^2}\left\{(30.5 - 12) \times 120^2 - (30.5 \times 80^2 - 12 \times 120^2)\right\}$$

$$= \frac{1}{200 \times 40}\left\{18.5 \times 120^2 - (30.5 \times 80^2 - 12 \times 120^2)\right\}$$

$$= \frac{1}{8000}\{244000\}$$

$= 30.5$ MPa $=$ Internal pressure. Hence OK.

Radial stress at outer surface

$$\sigma_{r_o} = \frac{1}{r_o^2 - r_i^2}\left\{p_o r_o^2 - p_i\, r_i^2 + (p_i - p_o r)\, r_i^2\right\}$$

$$= \frac{1}{120^2 - 80^2}\left\{12 \times 120^2 - 30.5 \times 80^2 + (30.5 - 12) \times 80^2\right\}$$

$$= \frac{1}{200 \times 40}[12 \times 14400 - 30.5 \times 6400 + 18.5 \times 6400]$$

$$= \frac{1}{8 \times 10^3}[96000]$$

$= 12$ MPa   **Ans.**

Q. 4(c) *Derive expressions for radial and hoop stresses in a thick cylinder with internal and external radii of a and b subjected to internal pressure p_1.*

SOLUTION See Chapter 17.

Q. 5(a) *A simply supported I section beam of span 2m carries a concentrated load of 4 kN at an angle of 20° from vertical as shown in figure. The load passes through CG of the section. Determine the maximum bending stress in the beam.*

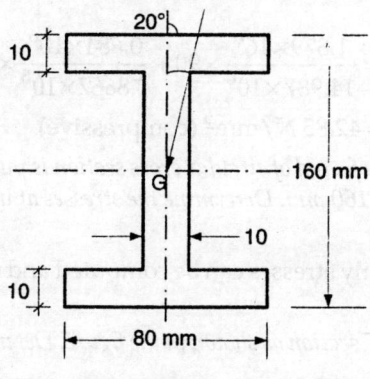

Fig. 9

SOLUTION Given $L = 2m$; $W = 4$ kN; $\theta = 20°$

Objective: To compute σ_{max}

$$M = +300 \text{Nm} = 300 \times 10^3 \text{ Nmm}$$

Now, R_N = location of neutral axis

$$I_{xx} = \frac{BD^3 - bd^3}{12} = \frac{80 \times 180^3 - 70 \times 160^3}{12}$$

$$= 14.987 \times 10^6 \text{ mm}^4$$

$$I_{yy} = \frac{10 \times 80^3}{12} + \frac{160 \times 10^3}{12} + \frac{10 \times 80^3}{12}$$

$$= 0.866 \times 10^6 \text{ mm}^4$$

Here, the symmetric axis are the principal axes

So, $I_{uu} = I_{xx} = 14.987 \times 10^6 \text{ mm}^4$

and, $I_{vv} = I_{yy} = 0.8667 \times 10^6 \text{ mm}^4$

Now, Maximum Bending Moment $M_X = \dfrac{W_X L}{4} = \dfrac{W \cos\theta \times L}{4}$

$$= \frac{4 \cos 20° \times 2}{4} = 1.879 \text{ kNm}$$

$$M_Y = \frac{W_Y \cdot L}{4} = \frac{W \sin\theta \times L}{4}$$

$$= \frac{4 \sin 20° \times 2}{4} = 0.684 \text{ kN.m}$$

Maximum Stress $(\sigma_A) = \dfrac{M_u}{I_u} \times y_A + \dfrac{M_v}{I_v} \times x_A$

$$= \frac{1.879 \times 16^6}{14.987 \times 10^6} \times 90 + \frac{0.684 \times 10^6}{0.8667 \times 10^6} \times 40$$

$$= 42.85 \text{ N/mm}^2 \text{ (compressive)} \quad \textbf{Ans.}$$

Q. 5(b) *A steel ring made of a rod of circular cross section is pulled by a force of 8 kN. The mean diameter of a ring is 160 mm. Determine the stresses at inside and outside the ring. Take E = 200 GPa.*

(N.B.: In this question only stresses can be computed and not increase in diameter due to insufficient data.

Q. 5(c) *An open ring has T section as shown in the figure. Determine the stresses in points P and Q.*

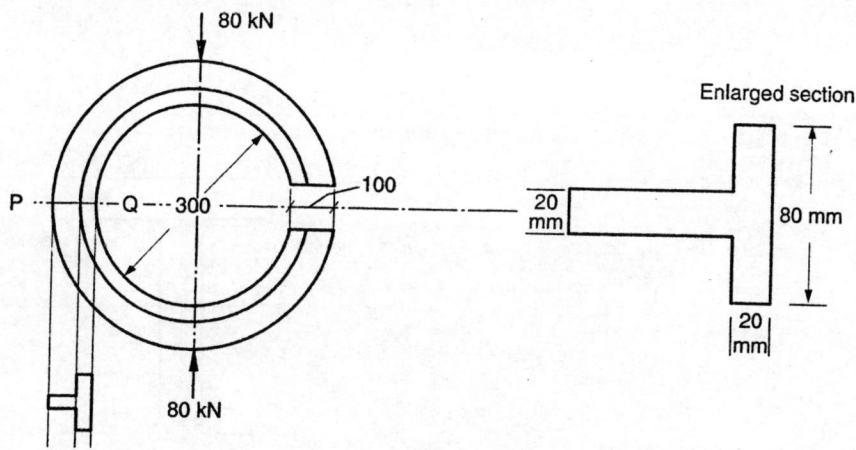

Fig. 11

[N.B.: Reader may choose any method to solve the problem and in each case answer will be same before decimal. A little difference in answer does not mean that solution is wrong. **Do not make approximation in computing eccentricity(e).**

Otherwise answer will deviate too much. Take $\pi = \dfrac{22}{7}$].

The problem is solved in Chapter 19, of this book.

— ❖❖ —

SOLVED UNIVERSITY QUESTIONS
(Semester-III) 2011-12
(Strength of Materials)

PAPER ID: 0429   **EME-302**

SECTION -A

Note: Attempt all questions. $2 \times 10 = 20$

Q. 1 *State Castigliano's first theorem.*

Q. 2 *Define principal plane and principal stress.*

Q. 3 *What do you mean by 'strength of a shaft'?*

Q. 4 *State Mohr's theorems for beams.*

Q. 5 *What are the limitations of Euler's formula?*

Q. 6 *Write short notes on wire winding of cylinders.*

Q. 7 *What are the various stresses induced in closed coil helical springs?*

Q. 8 *What are the assumptions made in Lame's equation?*

Q. 9 *Write down the expression for Winkler-Bach formula.*

Q. 10 *Why the shear centre is called the centre of twist?*

SOLUTION Q. 1 to 10 —See the corresponding chapters in this book.

SECTION -B

Note: Attempt any *three* questions. $10 \times 3 = 30$

Q. 1 *Derive an expression for major and minor principal stresses on an oblique plane when the body is subjected to direct stresses in two mutually perpendicular directions accompanied by a shear stress.*

Ans. See theory of compound stresses in this book.

Q. 2 *What is Macaulay's method? Where is it used? Find an expression for definition for a simply supported beam with an eccentric point load, using Macaulay's method.*

SOLUTION See theory in chapter Deflection of beam.

For expression of deflection for a simply supported beam with eccentric point load. See Example 1 Page 10.15.

Q. 3 *Find the expression for cripping load for a long column where one end of the column is fixed and other end is hinged.*

SOLUTION See theory of Column and Strut.

Q. 4 *What do you mean by a thick compound cylinder? How will you determine the hoop stresses in a thick compound cylinder?*

SOLUTION See theory of compound stress and mention Case - I, when there is no fluid and Case - II, when fluid is admitted.

Q. 5 *Derive an expression for neutral axis of circular cross section.*

SOLUTION See the chapter Curved Beam having Circular Section and prove

$$R_N = \frac{(\sqrt{r_i} + \sqrt{r_o})^2}{4} \quad \text{or} \quad R_N = \frac{d^2}{4(2\bar{r} - \sqrt{4\bar{r}^2 - d^2})}$$

SECTION -C

Note: Attempt *all* questions. $10 \times 5 = 50$

Q. 1 *At a certain point in a strained material, the intensities of stresses on two planes at right angles to each other are 20 N/mm² and 10 N/mm² both tensile. They are accompanied by a shear stress of magnitude 10 N/mm². Find graphically, the location of principal planes and evaluate the principal stresses.*

SOLUTION Given $\sigma_x = 20 \text{ N/mm}^2$

$$\sigma_y = 10 \text{ N/mm}^2$$

$$\tau_{xy} = 10 \text{ N/mm}^2$$

Objective: To find the location of principal planes and to compute principal stresses.

Steps for Solving Problem

1. Choose suitable scale so that the given problem can be accomodated in the examination sheet.
   Let $4 \text{ cm} = 10 \text{ N/mm}^2$

2. Make x and y axes with origin O.

3. Take σ_x and σ_y on the positive side i.e. R.H.S. and mark them. Similarly, scale of $\tau_{xy} = 4 \text{ cm}$ at A and B after drawing perpendicular at A and B.

or

$CD = R = 4.5 \text{ cm}$ on measuring

$$\sigma_{ave} = OC = \frac{\sigma_x + \sigma_y}{2}$$

$$= \frac{1}{2}(20 + 10) = 15 \text{ MPa}$$

$$R = \sqrt{CA^2 + AD^2}$$

$$CA = OA - OC$$

$$= 20 - 15 = 5 \text{ MPa}$$

Principal Stresses

$$\sigma_{max} = \sigma_1 = OA' = OC + CA'$$

$$= \sigma_{average} + \text{Radius of circle}$$

$$= 15 \text{ MPa} + 4.5 \text{ cm} \qquad \textbf{Ans.}$$

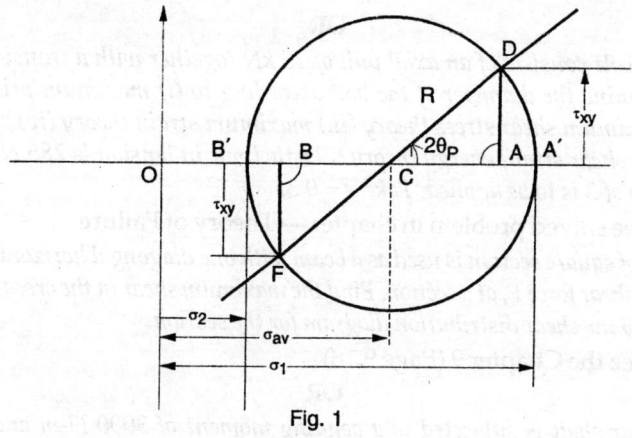

Fig. 1

$$= 15 \text{ MPa} + (4.5 \times 2.5) \text{ MPa}$$
$$= 15 \text{ MPa} + 11.25 \text{ MPa} = 26.25 \text{ MPa}$$

Similarly,

$$\sigma_{minimum} = \sigma_2 = OB' = OC - CB'$$

$$= \sigma_{average} - \text{Radius of circle}$$

$$= 15 \text{ MPa} - 4.5 \text{cm}$$

$$= 15 \text{ MPa} - (4.5 \times 2.5) \text{ MPa}$$

$$= 15 \text{ MPa} - 11.25 \text{ MPa} = 3.75 \text{ MPa} \quad \textbf{Ans.}$$

or

[Measure OA' and OB', which will give maximum and minimum principal stresses (after converting the scale) on measurement σ_1 = maximum principal stress = 26.25 MPa and σ_2 = minimum principal stress = 3.75 MPa.]

Principal Planes

$$\tan 2\theta p = \frac{DA}{CA} = \frac{10}{5} = 2$$

$$2\theta p = \tan^{-1}(2) = 63.43$$

$$\theta p = 31.71 \quad \textbf{Ans.}$$

Now, we can obtain the orientation for the principal plane as shown in figure.

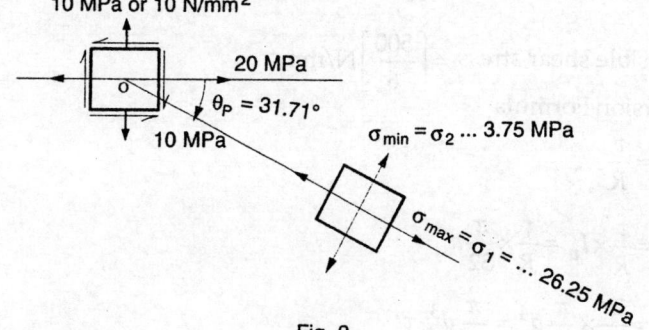

Fig. 2

OR

The load on a bolt consists of an axial pull of 15 kN together with a transverse shear of 7.5 kN. Determine the diameter of the bolt according to (i) maximum principal stress theory (ii) maximum shear stress theory (iii) maximum strain theory (iv) strain energy theory and (v) shear strain energy theory. Elastic limit in tension is 285 N/mm², and a factor of safety of 3 is to be applied. Take v = 0.3.

SOLUTION See solved problem in chapter — Theory of Failure.

Q. 2 *A beam of square section is used as a beam with one diagongal horizontal. The beam is subjected to shear force F, at a section. Find the maximum shear in the cross section of the beam and draw the shear distribution diagram for the section.*

SOLUTION See the Chapter 9 (Page 9.18)

OR

A solid circular shaft is subjected to a bending moment of 3000 N-m and a torque of 10000 N-m. The shaft is made of 45C8 steel having ultimate tensile stress of 700 MPa and a ultimate shear stress of 500 MPa. Assuming a factor of safety as 6, determine the diameter of shaft.

SOLUTION Given $M = 3000$ Nm

$\qquad T = 10,000$ N.m

$\qquad \sigma_{ultimate} = 700$ MPa $= 700$ N/mm²

$\qquad \tau_{ultimate} = 500$ MPa $= 500$ N/mm²

$\qquad$ fos $= 6$

$\qquad d = ?$

Here the shaft is subjected to combined loading.

i.e. $\qquad$ Bending Moment (M) and Torque (T)

So, equivalent torque $(T_e) = \sqrt{M^2 + T^2}$

$$= \sqrt{(3000)^2 + (10,000)^2} = \sqrt{9 \times 100} \times 100$$

$$= 10.44 \times 100 \text{ Nm} = 1044 \text{ metre}$$

$$= 1044 \times 10^3 \text{ Nmm}$$

Permissible tensile stress $= \dfrac{\sigma_{ultimate}}{fos} = \left[\dfrac{700}{6}\right]$ N/mm²

and, permissible shear stress $= \left[\dfrac{500}{6}\right]$ N/mm²

Now, by Torsion Formula

$$\frac{T_e}{I_p} = \frac{\tau}{R}$$

$\therefore \qquad T_e = \dfrac{\tau}{R} \times I_p = \dfrac{\tau}{R} \times \dfrac{\pi}{32} d^4$

$$= \frac{2\tau}{d} \times \frac{\pi}{32} d^4 = \frac{\pi}{16} d^3 \cdot \tau$$

$$T_e = \tau \cdot \frac{\pi}{16} d^3$$

$$1044 \times 10^3 = \frac{600}{6} \times \frac{\pi}{16} \times d^3 \qquad ...(\text{I})$$

$$\Rightarrow \qquad d = \left(\frac{1044 \times 10^3 \times 96 \times 7}{22 \times 500} \right)^{0.33}$$

$$\boxed{d = 38.50 \text{ mm}}$$

Further, from Bending formula $\dfrac{M_e}{I_p} = \dfrac{\sigma_t}{y}$

$$\frac{M_e}{\left(\dfrac{\pi d^4}{64}\right)} = \frac{700}{6} \times \frac{1}{\left(\dfrac{d}{2}\right)}$$

$$\frac{M_e \times 64}{\pi d^3} = \frac{700}{6} \times 2$$

or, $\qquad \dfrac{\pi d^3}{M_e \times 64} = \dfrac{6}{700 \times 2}$

$$\Rightarrow \qquad d^3 = \left(\frac{6 \times M_e \times 64}{\pi \times 1400} \right) \qquad ...(\text{II})$$

Now, $\quad M_e = \dfrac{M + \sqrt{M^2 + T^2}}{2} = \dfrac{3000 + \sqrt{(3000)^2 + (10,000)^2}}{2}$

$$= \frac{3000 + \sqrt{109} \times 100}{2} = \frac{3000 + 1044}{2}$$

$$= \frac{4044}{2} = 2022 \text{ Nm}$$

$$= 2022 \times 10^3 \text{ Nmm}$$

Substituting the value of M_e in eqn. II

$$d^3 = \left(\frac{6 \times 2022 \times 10^3 \times 64 \times 7}{22 \times 1400} \right)$$

$$\therefore \qquad d = \left(\frac{6 \times 2022 \times 10^3 \times 64 \times 7}{22 \times 1400} \right)^{0.33}$$

$$\boxed{d = 53.87 \text{ nm}}$$

Taking $d = 53.87$ mm being larger diameter.

This is computed value of shaft diameter.   **Ans.**

Q.3 *A hollow C.I. column whose outside diameter is 200 mm has a thickness of 20 mm. It is 4.5 m long and is fixed at both ends. Calculate the safe load by Rankine's formula using a factor of safety of 4. Calculate the slenderness ratio of Eular's and Rankine's critical loads. Take 550 N/mm, $\alpha = 1/1600$ in Rankine's formula and $E = 9.5 \times 10^4$ N/mm².*

SOLUTION See Column and Strut solved problem on Page 18.13.

OR

An opcn coiled helical spring, made out of 20 mm, diameter steel rod has 10 complete turns at a mean diameter of 150 mm, the angle of helix being 15°. An axial load of 400 N is applied. Compute (i) deflection under load and (ii) maximum intensities of direct and shear stresses, induced in the section of the wire. Take $G = 0.84 \times 10^5$ N/mm² and $E = 2 \times 10^5$ N/mm².

ŞOLUTION Given, opened coiled having helical angle $(\alpha) = 15°$

> Coil diameter $(D) = 150$ mm
> Number of turn $(n) = 20$ mm
> Axial load $(W) = 400$ N
> Wire diameter $(d) = 20$ mm
> $G = 0.84 \times 10^5$ N/mm²
> $E = 2 \times 10^5$ N/mm²

Objective: (i) To compute deflection (δ)

> (ii) To compute σ_b and τ_{max}

By formula of open coiled helical spring

$$\delta = \frac{64\,WR^3 n}{d^4 \cos \alpha}\left[\frac{\cos^2 \alpha}{G} + \frac{2\sin^2 \alpha}{E}\right]$$

$$= \frac{64 \times 400 \times (125)^3 \times 10}{(20)^4 \times \cos 15°}\left[\frac{(\cos 15°)^2}{0.84 \times 10^5} + \frac{2 \times (\sin 15°)^2}{2 \times 10^5}\right]$$

$$= \frac{64 \times 400 \times (125)^3 \times 10}{(20)^4 \times \cos 15° \times 10^5}\left[\frac{(0.966)^2}{0.84} + \frac{2 \times (0.258)^2}{2}\right]$$

$$= \frac{3234989.648 \times 1.177464}{10^5}\ mm$$

$$\boxed{\therefore\ \delta = 38.09\ mm}\qquad \textbf{Ans.}$$

Maximum Bending Stress:

$$\sigma_b = \frac{M}{I}\cdot y \ \text{ by Bending formula,}$$

$$= \frac{WR \sin \alpha}{\frac{\pi}{64} d^4} \times \frac{d}{2}$$

$$= \frac{32 \, WR \sin \alpha}{\pi d^3}$$

$$= \frac{32 \times 400 \times 125 \times 0.258 \times 7}{22 \times 8000}$$

$\therefore \qquad \sigma_b = 16.418 \, \text{N/mm}^2 \qquad$ **Ans.**

Maximum Shear Stress

$$\tau_{max} = \frac{16T}{\pi d^3}$$

$$= \frac{16 \times WR \cos \alpha}{\pi d^3}$$

$$= \frac{16 \times 400 \times 125 \times \cos 15^\circ \times 7}{22 \times (20)^3}$$

$$= \frac{16 \times 400 \times 125 \times 0.966 \times 7}{22 \times 8000}$$

$$= 30.73 \, \text{N/mm}^2 \qquad$$ **Ans.**

Q. 4 *In a cylindrical shell of 0.6 m diameter and 0.9 m long is subjected to an internal pressure 1.2 N/mm². Thickness of the cylinder wall is 15 mm. Determine longitudinal stresses, circumferential stress and maximum shear stresses induced and change in diameter, length and volume. Take E = 200 GPa and 1/m = 0.3.*

SOLUTION Given $d_i = 0.6$ m $\therefore r_i = 0.3$ m = 300 mm

$\qquad l = 0.9$ m

$\qquad p_i = 1.2 \, \text{N/mm}^2$

$\qquad t = 15$ mm

$\qquad E = 200$ GPa and $v = 0.3$

So, $\qquad d_o = (d_i + 2t) = 0.6 + 2 \times \dfrac{15}{1000}$

$\qquad\qquad = 0.6 + 0.030 = 0.630$ metre

$\qquad\qquad = 630$ mm

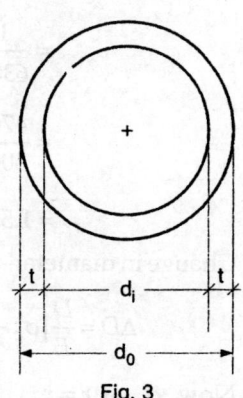

Fig. 3

Objective: To compute σ_l, σ_c, τ_{max}, ΔD, Δl, and ΔV

Longitudinal Stress $(\sigma_l) = \dfrac{p_i r_i^2 - p_o r_o^2}{r_o^2 - r_i^2}$

Here, $p_o = 0$

$$\therefore \qquad \sigma_l = \frac{p_i r_i^2}{r_o^2 - r_i^2}$$

$$= \frac{1.2 \times (300)^2}{(630)^2 - (300)^2} = 0.35 \text{ N/mm}^2 \qquad \textbf{Ans.}$$

Circumferential stress (σ_c) when the cylinder is subjected to only internal pressure (p_i).

$$\sigma_{c_{max}} = \frac{p_i r_i^2}{r_o^2 - r_i^2} \left(\frac{r_o^2}{r_i^2} + 1 \right)$$

$$= p_i \left(\frac{r_o^2 + r_i^2}{r_o^2 - r_i^2} \right) = 1.2 \left(\frac{630^2 + 300^2}{630^2 - 300^2} \right)$$

$$= \frac{1.2 \times 486900}{306900} = 1.904 \text{ N/mm}^2$$

Maximum shear stress, occurs at inner radius (r_i)

$$\therefore \qquad \tau_{max} = \frac{(p_i - p_o) r_o^2}{r_o^2 - r_i^2} \qquad\qquad\qquad \left[\tau_{max} = \frac{B}{r^2} \right]$$

But $p_o = 0$ as not given in question

Therefore, $\tau_{max} = \dfrac{p_i r_o^2}{r_o^2 - r_i^2}$

$$= \frac{1.2 \times 630}{630^2 - 300^2}$$

$$= \frac{476280}{306900}$$

$$= 1.55 \text{ N/mm}^2 \qquad \textbf{Ans.}$$

Change in diameter

$$\Delta D = \frac{D}{E} [\sigma_c - v \cdot \sigma_r - v \cdot \sigma_l]$$

Now, σ_r at $r = r_o$

σ_r is maximum when $r = r_o$

$$\therefore \qquad \sigma_r = \frac{B}{r^2} - A$$

$$= (-)\frac{p_o r_o^2}{(r_o^2 - r_i^2)}\left[\frac{r_i^2}{r^2} - 1\right]$$

At $r = r_o$, $\qquad \sigma_r = (-)\frac{p_o r_o^2}{(r_o^2 - r_i^2)}\left[\frac{r_i^2}{r_o^2} - 1\right]$

$$= (-)\frac{p_o \cdot (r_i^2 - r_o^2)}{r_o^2 - r_i^2}$$

$$= p_o \text{ (maximum}$$
$$= \text{atmospheric pressure}$$
$$= 1.044 \, \text{kgf/cm}^2$$

$$= 1.044 \times 0.981 \times 10^5 \, \text{N/m}^2$$

$$= \frac{1.044 \times 0.981 \times 10^5}{10^{-6}} \, \text{N/mm}^2 = 0.1024 \, \text{N/mm}^2$$

Take $\sigma_{r_i} = -p_i = (-)1.2 \, \text{N/mm}^2$ and $\sigma_{r_o} = -p_o = (-)0.1024 \, \text{N/mm}^2$

$\therefore \qquad \Delta D_i = \frac{2r_i}{E}\left[\sigma_{c_i} - v\sigma_{r_i} - v\sigma_l\right]$

$$\Delta D_o = \frac{2r_o}{E}\left[\sigma_{c_o} - v\sigma_{r_o} - v\sigma_l\right]$$

$\therefore \qquad \Delta D = [\Delta D_o - \Delta D_i]$

Similarly, $\Delta l = \frac{l}{E}\left[\sigma_l - v \cdot \sigma_r - v \cdot \sigma_c\right]$

Substituting the value of σ_l, σ_r and σ_c we can compute Δl (express in mm).

Since, σ_r is compressive, so $\sigma_r = (-)p_i$

N.B.: Remember $p_o < p_i$ otherwise cylinder will collapse.

OR

The external diameter of a steel color is 200 mm, and the internal diameter increases by 0.125 mm when shrunk on to a solid steel, shaft of 125 mm diameter. Find the reduction in diameter of the shaft, the radial pressure between the collar and the shaft and hoop stresses at the inner surface of the tube. Take E = 210 GPa and Poisson's ratio = 0.3.

SOLUTION Data insufficient.

Q.5 *A beam of T-section (flange 100 × 20, web 150 × 10) is 2.5 m in length and is simply supported at the ends. It carries a load of 3.2 kN inclined at 20° to the vertical and passing through the centroid of the section. Its E = 200 GPa. Calculate:*

(i) *Maximum tensile stress*

(ii) *Maximum compressive stress*

(iii) *Deflection due to load*

(iv) *Position of neutral axis.*

SOLUTION

First centroid of *T*-section is required.

So, $\bar{y} = \dfrac{100\times20\times10+150\times10\left(\dfrac{150}{2}+20\right)}{100\times20+150\times10} = 46.4$ mm

As, section is symmetrical about *Y*-axis therefore principal axis pass through the centroid *G* and are along *UU* and *VV* axes.

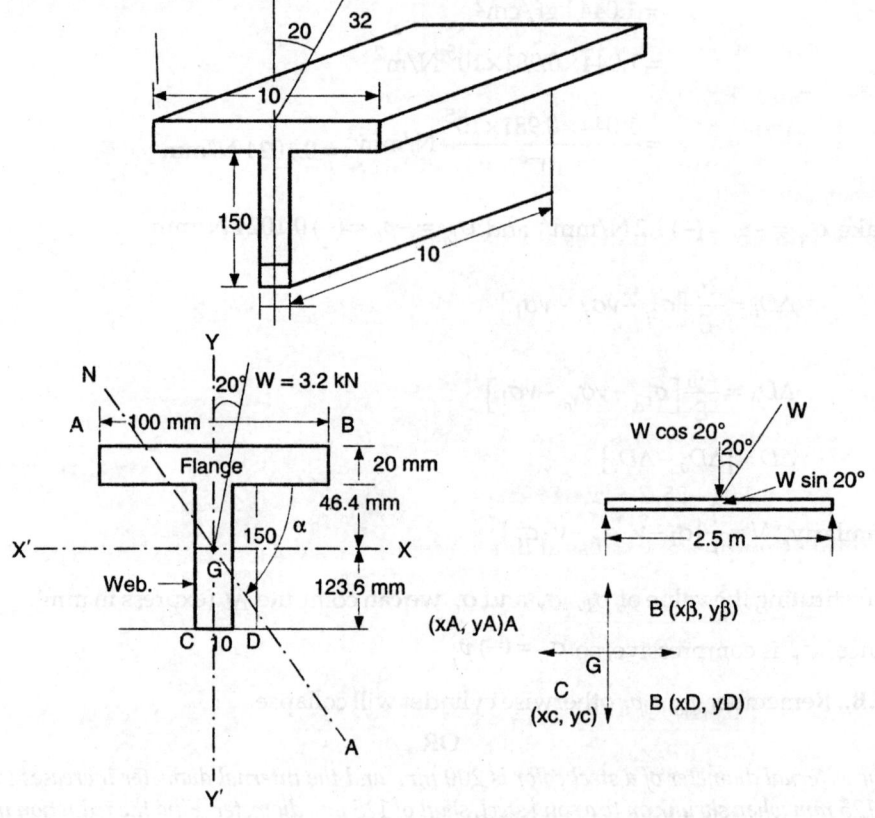

Fig. 4

$$I_{XX} = I_{UU} = \left[\frac{100\times20^3}{12}+100\times20\,(46.4-10)^2\right]$$

$$+\left[\frac{10\times150^3}{12}+150\times10\,(123.6-75)^2\right]$$

$$= [66666.67 + 2649920] + [2812500 + 3542940]$$

$$= 9.07 \times 10^6 \text{ mm}^4$$

$$M_X = M_U = \frac{(W \sin 20°) \times l}{4} \quad \left[M_{max} \text{ for simply supported beam} = \frac{Wl}{4} \right]$$

$$= \frac{3.2 \sin 20° \times 2.5}{4} = 0.684 \text{ kNM}$$

$$M_Y = M_V = \frac{W \cos 20° \times l}{4}$$

$$= \frac{3.2 \cos 20° \times 2.5}{4} = 1.879 \text{ kNM}$$

M_U will cause maximum compressive stress at B and D and maximum tensile stress at A and C.

M_V will cause maximum compressive stress at A and B and maximum tensile stress at C and D.

Now, Maximum Tensile stress at C:

$$\sigma_C = \frac{M_U \times Y_c}{I_{VV}} + \frac{M_V}{I_{uu}} \times x_c$$

$$= \left(\frac{0.684 \times 5 + 10^{-6}}{1.579 \times 10^{-6}} + \frac{1.879 \times 123.6 \times 10^{-6}}{9.07 \times 10^{-6}} \right) \text{MN/m}^2$$

$$= 2.04 + 25.6 = 27.64 \text{ MN/m}^2 \quad \textbf{Ans.}$$

Maximum Compressive stress at B:

$$\sigma_B = \frac{M_U \times (50 \times 10^{-3})}{I_{VV}} + \frac{M_V \times (46.4 \times 10^{-3})}{I_{uu}}$$

$$= \left(\frac{0.684 \times 50 + 10^{-3}}{1.679 \times 10^{-6}} \times 10^{-3} + \frac{1.879 \times 46.4 \times 10^{-3}}{9.07 \times 10^{-6}} \right)$$

$$= 20.37 + 9.61 = 29.98 \text{ MN/m}^2 \quad \textbf{Ans.}$$

Deflection (δ) due to inclined load

Now, $\delta_R = \sqrt{\delta x^2 + \delta y^2}$

$\delta x = \delta_{max} \cdot \sin \theta$

and $\delta y = \delta_{max} \cdot \cos \theta$

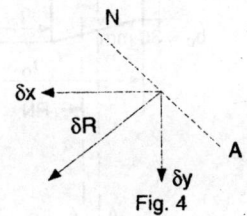

Fig. 4

For simply supported beam with load at centre x

$$\delta_{max} = \frac{Wl^3}{48\ EI}$$

$\therefore$

$$\delta_R = \sqrt{\left(\frac{Wl^3}{48\ EI_W}\right)^2 \cdot \sin^2\theta + \left(\frac{Wl^3}{48\ EI_V}\right)^2 \cdot \cos^2\theta}$$

$$= \frac{Wl^3}{48E}\sqrt{\frac{\sin^2\theta}{I_{VV}} + \frac{\cos^2\theta}{I_{UU}}}$$

$$= \frac{(3.2\times10^3)\times(2.5)}{48\times200\times10^9}\sqrt{\frac{\sin^2 20°}{1.679\times10^{-6}} + \frac{\cos^2 20°}{1.679\times10^{-6}}} = 1.20\ mm \qquad \textbf{Ans.}$$

Let α = Inclination of neutral axis with x-axis then we have,

$$\tan\alpha = \frac{I_x}{I_y}\tan\theta$$

$$= \frac{I_{UU}}{I_{VV}}\tan\theta = \frac{9.07\times10^{-6}}{1.679\times10^6}\tan 20°$$

$$= 1.95$$

Hence, $\sigma = 62.85°$ **Ans.**

OR

Determine the maximum stress in the frame of the 100 kN punch press as shown in the figure below.

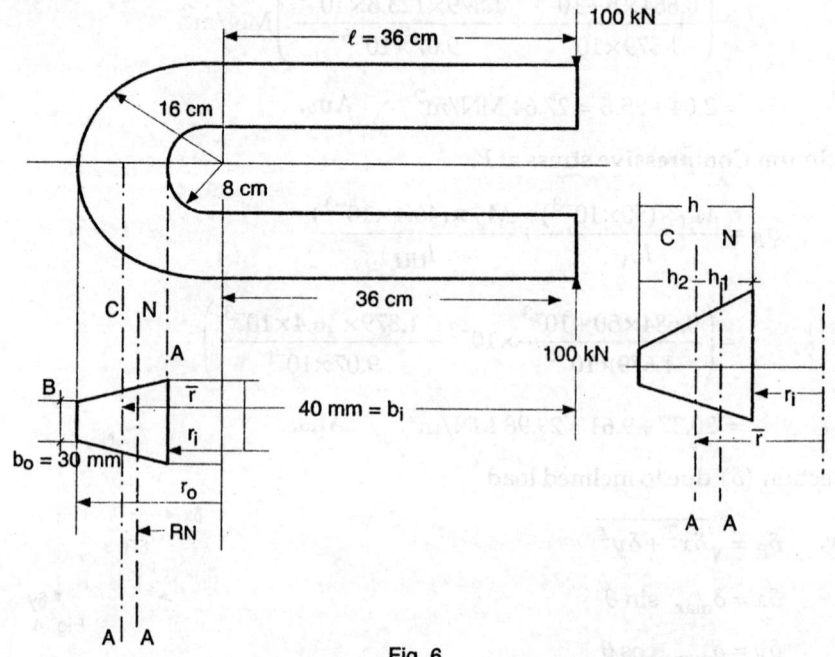

Fig. 6

SOLUTION

$$h = (r_o - r_i) = (16 - 8) = 8 \text{ cm} = 80 \text{ mm}$$

$$\bar{r} = (r_1 + h_1)$$

$$h_i = \frac{h}{3}\left(\frac{b_i + 2b_o}{b_i + b_o}\right) = \frac{80}{3}\left(\frac{40 + 2 \times 30}{40 + 30}\right)$$

$$= \frac{80}{3}\left(\frac{40 + 60}{70}\right) = \frac{80}{3} \times \frac{100}{70}$$

$$= \frac{800}{21} = 38.09 \text{ mm}$$

$$\bar{r} = (r_i + h_i)$$

$$= (80 + 38.09)$$

$$= 118.09 \text{ mm}$$

R_N for trapezoidal section

$$R_N = \frac{A}{(b_o - b_i) + \left(\dfrac{b_i r_o - b_o r_i}{h}\right)\ln\left(\dfrac{r_o}{r_i}\right)}$$

$$= \frac{\dfrac{1}{2} \times 80\,(40 + 30)}{(30 - 40) + \left(\dfrac{40 \times 160 - 30 \times 80}{80}\right)\ln\left(\dfrac{16}{8}\right)}$$

$$= \frac{40 \times 70}{-10 + \left(\dfrac{6400 - 2400}{80}\right)\ln 2}$$

$$= \frac{2800}{-10 + 50 \times 0.693}$$

$$= \frac{2800}{-10 + 34 \times 34.65}$$

$R_N = 113.59$ mm for trapezoidal section.

Now σ_A and σ_B can be computed as solved in curved beam chapter.

B.Tech (Sem. III)
Examination 2013-14
Strength of Materials and Machine Drawing-I
Section-A

Attempt *all* questions

1. (i) Define principal plane and principal stress.

  (ii) Explain complementary shear stress.

 (iii) Draw the Mohr's circle for pure shear.

 (iv) Define neutral axis.

  (v) What do you understand by section modulus?

 (vi) Explain point of contraflexure in a beam.

(vii) What do you understand by effective length of the column?

(viii) Explain torsional stiffness and torsional flexibility.

 (ix) Differentiate between thin cylinder and thick cylinder.

  (x) Define shear centre.

Section-B

Attempt *all* questions

1. Derive an expression for deformation of conical bar hung to a ceiling having diameter 'D' and height 'L', weight density of bar ρ and Young's modulus is E.

2. (a) Write the assumption for pure bending and also derive the bending equation.

   (b) Find the deflection of cantilever *l* at free end by area Moment Method.

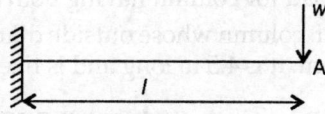

3. What are leaf springs ? Find maximum deflection and maximum bending stress in semielliptical type spring.

4. Write the assumptions for Lami's equation and also derive the expression for Lami's equation.

5. What do you understand by unsymmetrical bending? Prove that the sum of moment of inertia about any rectangular axis is constant.

Section-C

Attempt *all* questions

1. Show that if E is assumed correct, an error of 1% in the determination of G will involve an error of about 5% in the calculation of Poisson's ratio when its correct value is 0.25.

OR

A point in a strained material is subjected to a tensile stress 65 N/mm² and compressive stress of 45 N/mm², two mutually perpendicular planes and shear stress of 10 N/mm² are acting on these planes. Find the normal, tangential and resultant stresses on the plane inclined 30° with the plane of compressive stress.

2. Draw the shear force and bending moment diagram for the beam given below.

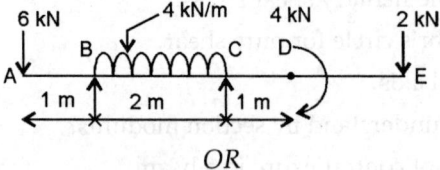

OR

Find deflection at point B and C of beam given below.
$E = 200$ GPa, $I = 19802.8$ cm⁴.

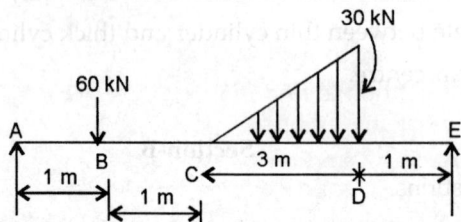

3. Deduce an expression for the extension of an open coiled helical spring carrying an axial load W. Take 'α' as the inclination of coils, d as the diameter of the wire and 'R' as mass radius of the coil. Find by what percentage the axial deflection of the coil is neglected for spring in which $\alpha = 25°$. Assume n and R remain constant.

    (i) Write the assumption for Euler's theory and derive an expression for critical load for column having both end fixed.

    (ii) A hollow C.I. column whose outside diameter is 200 mm has a thickness of 20 mm. It is 4.5 m long and is fixed at both end. Calculate the safe load of Rankine formula using FOS 4. $\sigma_c = 550$ MPa, $\alpha = \dfrac{1}{1600}$.

4. A boiler drum consists of a cylinder 2 m long, 1 m diameter and 25 mm thick closed by hemispherical ends. In a hydraulic test 10 N/mm², how much additional water will be pumped in after initial filling at atmospheric pressure ?

Assume the circumferential strain at junction of cylinder and hemisphere is same for both drum material.

$E = 207000 \text{ N/mm}^2, \mu = 0.3, \quad K = 2100 \text{ N/mm}^2.$

OR

A compound cylinder is to be made by shrinking one tube onto another so that the radial compressive stress at the junction is 28.5 N/mm². If the outside diameter is 26.5 cm and the bore 12.5 cm, calculate the allowance for shrinkage at common diameter which is 20 cm and $E = 2100000 \text{ N/mm}^2$.

5. Locate the shear centre with sketch for the section as shown below:

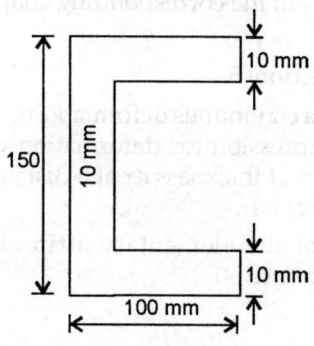

OR

Derive the equation to find the position of neutral axis for the following cross-section of curved beam:

(i)   Rectangular X-section

(ii) Circular X-section

Section-A

1. See answer (i) to (x) in the corresponding chapters of this book.

Section-B

1. Since conical bar is a continuous deformable body so to derive the expression for deformation we will take an element of thickness dx at a distance x from the top end of bar.

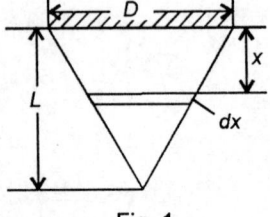

Fig. 1

Then the radius of the elementary strip at a distance x from the base is

$$= \left(\frac{L-x}{L}\right) \times \frac{D}{2}$$

Load on the elementary strip

$$\Delta P = \frac{1}{3}\pi\left[\left(\frac{L-x}{L}\right) \times \frac{D}{2}\right]^2 \cdot (L-x) \cdot \rho \cdot g$$

where ρ = density of the conical bar material

Area of elementary strip

$$\Delta A = \pi\left[\left(\frac{L-x}{L}\right) \cdot \frac{D}{2}\right]^2$$

Stress on the elementary strip $(\sigma) = \dfrac{\Delta p}{\Delta A}$

$$= \frac{1}{3}(L-x) \cdot \rho \cdot g$$

Extension of strip $= \left(\dfrac{\sigma}{E}\right) \cdot dx$

$$= \frac{1}{3E}(L-x) \cdot \rho \cdot g\, dx$$

Total extension of the conical bar $(\delta) = \dfrac{\rho g}{3E}\displaystyle\int_0^L (L-x)\,dx$

$$\therefore \qquad \delta = \frac{\rho g L^2}{6E} \qquad \textbf{Ans.}$$

2. (a) See chapter — Bending
    (b) See chapter — Deflection of beam
3. See chapter — Spring
4. See chapter — Thick cylinder
5. See chapter — Unsymmetrical bending

Section-C

1. Given E is correct; $v = 0.25$
    From the given condition
    $$E = 2G (1 + v) \qquad \qquad \text{...(I)}$$
    and $E' = 2 \times 1.01 \, G (1 + v')$ ...(II)
    As $E = E'$ (given)
    So, $1.01 (1 + v') = 1 + v$
    or, $1.01 + 1.01 \, v' = 1 + 0.25$
    or, $1.01 \, v' = 1.25 - 1.01$

    or, $v' = \dfrac{0.24}{1.01} = 0.2376$

    $\therefore$ % error $= \dfrac{v - v'}{v} \times 100 = \dfrac{0.25 - 0.2376}{0.25} \times 100$

          $= 4.96\% \simeq 5\%$ **proved**

    OR

    Given $\sigma_x = 65 \text{ N/mm}^2$
               $\sigma_y = -45 \text{ N/mm}^2$
               $\tau_{xy} = 10 \text{ N/mm}^2$
    To find $\sigma_{30°}$, $\tau_{30°}$ and $\sigma_{\text{resultant}}$

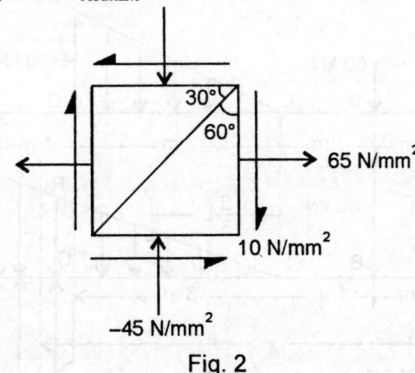

Fig. 2

Here $\theta = 60°$

So, $\sigma_{30°} = \dfrac{\sigma_x + \sigma_y}{2} + \dfrac{\sigma_x - \sigma_y}{2} \cos 2\theta + \tau \sin 2\theta$

$= \dfrac{65 - 45}{2} + \dfrac{65 + 45}{2} \cos 120° + 10 \sin 120°$

$= 10 + 55 \times \left(-\dfrac{1}{2}\right) + 10 \times \dfrac{\sqrt{3}}{2}$

$= 10 - 27.5 + 5\sqrt{3}$

$= 10 - 27.5 + 8.66$

$= -8.84 \text{ N/mm}^2$

$\tau_{30°} = \left(\dfrac{\sigma_x - \sigma_y}{2}\right) . \sin 2\theta + 10 \cos 120°$

$= -\dfrac{65 + 45}{2} \sin 120° + 10 \cos 120°$

$= -55 \sin 120° + 10 \cos 120°$

$= -55 \times \dfrac{\sqrt{3}}{2} - 10 \times \dfrac{1}{2}$

$= -27.5 \times 1.732 - 5 = -52.63 \text{ N/mm}^2$

$\sigma_{\text{resultant}} = \sqrt{(\sigma_{30°})^2 + (\tau_{30°})^2}$

$= \sqrt{(8.84)^2 + (-52.63)^2} = 53.36 \text{ N/mm}^2$

Fig. 3

Section-C

2. See chapter – Shearing Force and Bending Moment

OR

Find the deflection at point B and C

$E = 200 \text{ GPa}; \quad I = 19802.8 \text{ cm}^4$

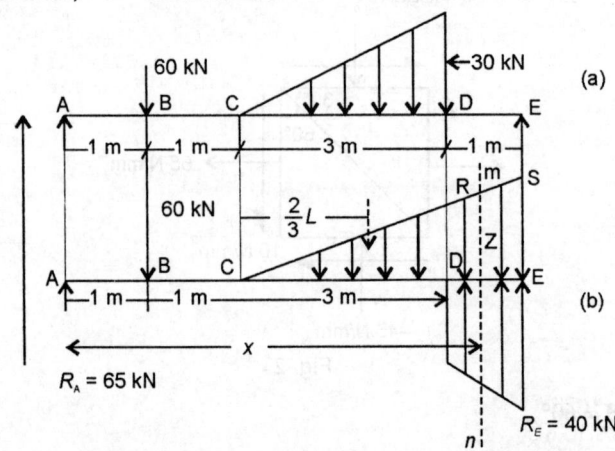

Fig. 4

Step 1 : Find reaction at support A and E first

Step 2 : Extend the triangular load up to right hand to apply Macaulay's method.

Step 3 : Take a section mn at a distance x from A

Step 4 : Find equation of $M(x)$ by applying Macaulay's method.

Step 5 : Find slope equation (y') by integrating equation of $M(x)$ with constant c_1.

Step 6 : Find deflection equation (y) by integrating equation of slope (y') with constant C_2.

Step 7 : The constants C_1 and C_2 can be found by applying boundary condition.

From Fig. 4(a)

$$R_A + R_B = 60 + \frac{1}{2} \times 3 \times \overset{15}{\cancel{30}} = 60 + 45$$

$$= 105 \text{ kN}$$

Taking moment about A

$$R_E \times 6 = 60 \times 1 + 60 + \frac{1}{2} \times 3 \times \overset{15}{\cancel{30}} \ (2+2)$$

$$= 60 + 180 = 240 \text{ kN}$$

$$R_E = 40 \text{ kN} \uparrow \ ; \ R_A = 65 \text{ kN} \uparrow$$

Corresponding to x, let Z be the rate of load which can be found from similar triangles CRD and CSE.

From similar triangles

$$\frac{Z}{30} = \frac{x-2}{3}$$

$$Z = \frac{30}{3} \langle x-2 \rangle$$

$$= 10 \ \langle x-2 \rangle$$

Now,

$$M(x) = R_A \cdot x - 60 \ \langle x-1 \rangle - \frac{1}{2} \ \langle x-2 \rangle \times z \times \frac{1}{3} \ \langle x-2 \rangle$$

$$+ \frac{30}{2} \ \langle x-5 \rangle \ \langle x-5 \rangle + \frac{1}{2} \ \langle x-5 \rangle \times 10 \ \langle x-5 \rangle \times \frac{1}{3} \ \langle x-5 \rangle$$

or, $$E \, Iy'' = 65x - 60 \ \langle x-1 \rangle - \frac{1}{2} \ \langle x-2 \rangle \times 10 \ \langle x-2 \rangle \times \frac{1}{3} \ \langle x-2 \rangle + 15 \ \langle x-5 \rangle^2$$

$$+ \frac{5}{3} \ \langle x-5 \rangle^3$$

or, $E\ Iy'' = 65x - 60 \langle x-1 \rangle - \dfrac{5}{3} \langle x-2 \rangle^3 + 15 \langle x-5 \rangle^2 + \dfrac{5}{3} \langle x-5 \rangle^3$

Integrating both sides

$E\ Iy' = 65\dfrac{x^2}{2} - 30 \langle x-1 \rangle^2 - \dfrac{5}{3\times4} \langle x-2 \rangle^4 + \dfrac{15}{3} \langle x-5 \rangle^3 + \dfrac{5}{3\times4} \langle x-5 \rangle^4 + C_1$

...(I)

Again integrating Eq. (I)

$E\ Iy = 32.5\dfrac{x^3}{3} - \dfrac{30}{3} \langle x-1 \rangle^3 - \dfrac{5}{3\times4\times5} \langle x-2 \rangle^5 + \dfrac{15}{3\times4} \langle x-5 \rangle^4$

$+ \dfrac{15}{3\times4} \langle x-5 \rangle^4 + \dfrac{5}{3\times4\times5} \langle x-5 \rangle^5 + C_1x + C_2$ ...(II)

B.C. are

At $x = 0$, $y = 0$ $C_2 = 0$

At $x = 6$, $y = 0$ [from Eq. (II)]

$0 = \dfrac{32.5}{3} \times 6^3 - 10 \times 5^3 - \dfrac{1}{12} \times 4^5 + \dfrac{5}{4} + \dfrac{1}{12} + C_1 \times 6$

$C_1 = -167.66$

Substituting the value of $C_1 = -167.66$ and $C_2 = 0$

In Eq. (II), we get the generalise equation of elastic curve of the beam

i.e. $y = \dfrac{1}{EI}\left[32.5\dfrac{x^3}{3} - 10 \langle x-1 \rangle^3 \dfrac{1}{12} \langle x-2 \rangle^5 + \dfrac{5}{4} \langle x-5 \rangle^4 \right.$

$\left. + \dfrac{1}{12} \langle x-5 \rangle^5 + x \times (-167.66) \right]$ ...(III)

Now to get deflection at B and C i.e. y_B and y_C, put $x = 1$ and $x = 2$ in turn in Eq. (III)

Now, for y_B put $x = 1$

$\therefore y_B = \dfrac{1}{EI}\left(\dfrac{32.5}{3} \times 1^3 - 167.66 \right)$

[neglecting negative value inside the bracket < >]

$= -\dfrac{156.63}{EI}$ similarly, putting $x = 2$, y_C can be obtained.

Now $y_C = \dfrac{1}{EI}\left[32.5 \times \dfrac{(2)^3}{3} - 10 + 2 \times (-167.66) \right]$

$= \dfrac{1}{EI}\left[32.5 \times \dfrac{8}{3} - 10 - 335.32 \right]$

$$= \frac{1}{EI}\left[86.66 \times - 10 - 335.32\right]$$

$$\therefore \qquad y_c = (-)\frac{258.66}{EI} \qquad\qquad\qquad \textbf{Ans.}$$

(neglecting (–) value inside the < >)

3. See theory on spring

OR

(i) See theory on Euler in chapter column and strut

(ii) See solved problem on column and strut

4. See solved problem on thin cylinder

OR

See the solved problem on compound cylinder (thick cylinder).

5. See the problems on shear centre in unsymmetrical bending.

OR

See the theory on curved beam for

(a) Rectangular section

(b) Circular section

To find the position of neutral axis *i.e.* R_N.

B. Tech.
(Sem III) (Odd Sem)
Theory Examination 2014-15
Mechanics of Solids

[Time : 3 hours]   [Total mark : 100]

1. Attempt any four questions: [4 × 5 = 20]

   (a) Prove that the maximum Shear Stress in the body is the half of the difference between maximum principal and minimum principal stresses.

   (b) Derive the expression for extension in the vertically suspended bar due to self weight.

   (c) Find the free end deflection in cantilever beam with uniformly distributed load by Macaulay's method.

   (d) A mild steel hollow cylinder has diameter to thickness ratio of 25. Find the internal pressure to which the cylinder should be subjected so that its volume is increased by 5×10^{-4} of its original volume. Take $E = 2 \times 10^5$ and $\mu = 0.3$.

   (e) Under what conditions unsymmetrical bending occurs in a beam. Also state the position of neutral axis.

   (f) Derive the expression of the value of constant (h^2) in curved beam for rectangular cross-section area beam.

2. Attempt any two questions :   [2 × 10 = 20]

   (a) At a point in a strained material, stresses are applied as shown in Fig. 1, find out the normal and shear stress on the oblique plane, principal stresses and principal strain.

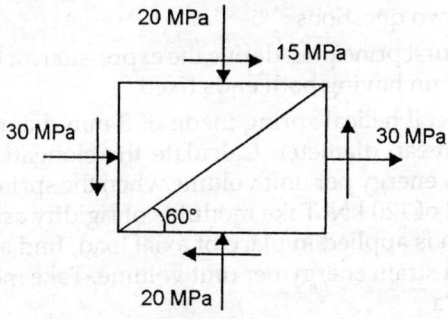

Fig. 1

   (b) The load on a bolt consists of an axial pull of 20 kN together with a transverse shear of 10 kN, calculate the diameter of bolt according to

   (1) Maximum total strain energy theory

   (2) Maximum shear strain energy theory (if $\mu = 0.3$)

   (Take elastic limit in tension 280 MPa and Factor of safety = 3)

(c) Write the assumptions for pure bending and also derive the equation for bending.

3. Attempt any two questions :

(a) Determine the deflection at the mid and slope at the end of the beam in terms of *EI* for a beam as shown in Fig. 2.

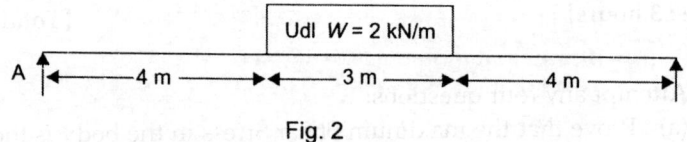

Fig. 2

(b) A solid steel shaft of 60 mm diameter is fixed rigidly and coaxially inside a bronze sleeve 90 mm external diameter. Calculate the angle of twist in a length of 2 m of the composite shaft due to action of a torque of 1 kN-m. Take G (steel) = 80 GPa, G (bronze) = 42 GPa.

(c) A shearing force of 180 kN acts over a T-section shown in Fig. 3. Draw the shear stress distribution curve (take $I = 1.134 \times 10^8$ mm^4).

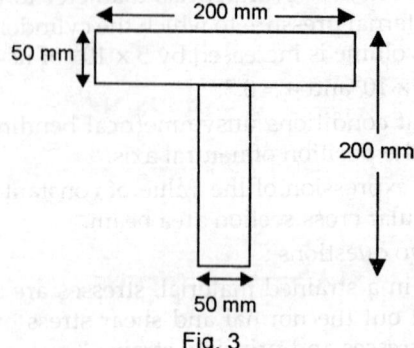

Fig. 3

4. Attempt any two questions :   [2 × 10 = 20]

(a) From the first principles, derive the expression for the critical buckling for a column having both ends fixed.

(b) A closed coil helical spring made of 8 mm diameter has 12 coils of 150 mm mean diameter. Calculate the elongation, torsional stress and strain energy per unit volume when the spring is subjected to an axial load of 120 kN. Take modulus of rigidity as 80 GPa. If a torque of 9 kN-m is applied in place of axial load, find axial twist, bending stress and strain energy per unit volume. Take modulus of elasticity as 200 GPa.

(c) A compound steel tube is composed of a tube 200 mm internal diameter and 300 thickness, shrunk on a tube of 200 mm external diameter and 25 mm thickness. The radial pressure of the junction is 12 N/mm^2. The composed tube is subjected to an internal fluid pressure of 80 N/mm^2. Find the variation of the hoop stress over the wall of the compound tube.

5. Attempt any two questions :   **[2 × 10 = 20]**

   (a) A crane hook having trapezoidal horizontal cross-section is 50 mm
        wide inside and 300 mm wide outside. Thickness of the section is
        60 mm. The crane hook carries a vertical load of 200 kN whose line
        of action is 50 mm from the inside edge of the section. The centre of
        curvature is 60 mm from the inside edge. Determine the maximum
        tensile and compressive stresses in the section.

   (b) If principal moments of inertia of section are I_{uu} and I_{vv} and X and Y
        axes inclined to an angle θ to U-V axis, then prove that

        $$I_{xx} + I_{yy} = I_{uu} + I_{vv}$$

   (c) A simply supported I-section beam of span 1.5 m carries a
        concentrated load of 8 kN at an angle of 20° from vertical as shown
        in Fig. 4. Load passes through the centroid of the section. Determine
        the maximum bending stress in the beam.

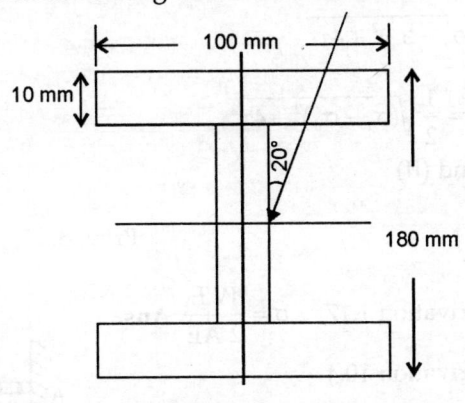

Fig. 4

1. (a) By formula, $\tau_{max} = \dfrac{1}{2}\sqrt{(\sigma_x - \sigma_y)^2 + 4\tau^2}$ ...(I)

Further by formula,

$$\sigma_{1,2} = \frac{\sigma_x + \sigma_y}{2} \pm \frac{1}{2}\sqrt{(\sigma_x - \sigma_y)^2 + 4\tau^2}$$

Hence,

$$\sigma_1 - \sigma_2 = \frac{1}{2}\left[(\sigma_x + \sigma_y) + \sqrt{(\sigma_x - \sigma_y)^2 + 4\tau^2} - (\sigma_x + \sigma_y) + \sqrt{(\sigma_x - \sigma_y)^2 + 4\tau^2}\right]$$

$$= 2 \times \frac{1}{2}\sqrt{(\sigma_x - \sigma_y)^2 + 4\tau^2}$$

$$\therefore \quad \left(\frac{\sigma_1 - \sigma_2}{2}\right) = \frac{1}{2}\sqrt{(\sigma_x - \sigma_y)^2 + 4\tau^2}$$ ...(II)

From Eqs. (I) and (II)

$$\tau_{max} = \left(\frac{\sigma_1 - \sigma_2}{2}\right)$$ **Proved.**

(b) See the derivation 1.17, $\sigma = \dfrac{W.L}{2\,AE}$ **Ans.**

(c) See the derivation 10.4

$$y_B = y_{max} = (-)\frac{wl^4}{8EI}$$ **Ans.**

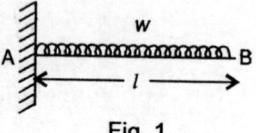

Fig. 1

(d) See the chapter thin cylinder.

(e) See theory of unsymmetrical bending 20.2, position of neutral axis 20.3.

(f) General formula for h^2 (constant) for any section of curved beam is

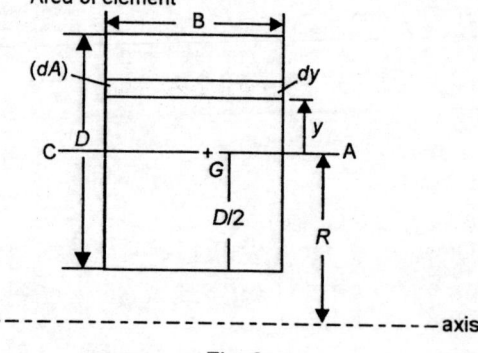

Fig. 2

$$h^2 = \frac{R^3}{A} \int \frac{dA}{R+y} - R^2$$

where R = Radius of curvature

y = Distance of the element (dA) from centroidal axis

dA = Area of element = $B.dy$

A = Area of the section = $B \times D$

Now, dA = area of element = $B.\,dy$

For rectangular section beam

$$h^2 = \frac{R^3}{B \times D} \int_{-\frac{D}{2}}^{+\frac{D}{2}} \frac{B.\,dy}{R+y} - R^2$$

$$= \frac{R^3}{D} [\log e\,(R+y)]_{-D/2}^{+D/2} - R^2$$

$$= \frac{R^3}{D} \left[\log e \left(\frac{R + \dfrac{D}{2}}{R - \dfrac{D}{2}} \right) \right] - R^2$$

$$= \frac{R^3}{D}.\log e \left(\frac{2R+D}{2R-D} \right) - R^2$$

2. (a) See the solved problem of this book in the corresponding chapter.

   N.B.: Principal strain in this problem cannot be worked out since ε_x, ε_y and γ_{xy} is not given.

   (b) See problem 15.4 solved in this book.

   (c) See the theory and derivation of bending in this book.

3. (a) Applying equilibrium condition

   $R_A + R_B = 2 \times 3 = 6$ kN

   Taking moment about B:

   $R_A \times 11 = 2 \times 3\,(1.5 + 4)$

   $\qquad\quad\;\; = 2 \times 3 \times 5.5$

   $\therefore \quad R_A = \dfrac{33.0}{11} = 3$ kN

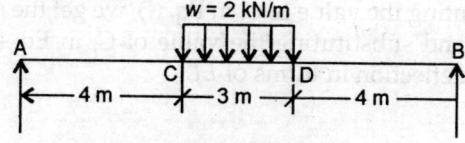

Fig. 3

Now the next step will be to extend the u.d.l up to extreme end B. Since we have extended u.d.l. extra so the same has to be subtracted by applying u.d.l. on the bottom of beam portion DB. Refer to Fig. 4.

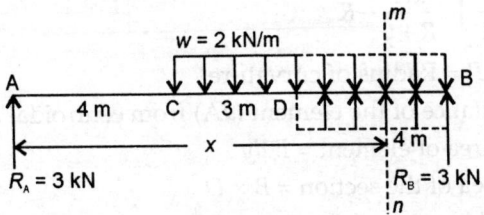

Fig. 4

Taking section mn at a distance x from A.

Applying Macaulay's method

$$M(x) = R_A \cdot x - \frac{2}{2}\langle x-4\rangle^2 + \frac{2}{2}\langle x-7\rangle^2$$

$$EI\,y'' = 3x - \langle x-4\rangle^2 + \langle x-7\rangle^2$$

Integrating both sides,

$$EI\,y' = \frac{3x^2}{2} - \frac{\langle x-4\rangle^3}{3} + \frac{\langle x-7\rangle^3}{3} + C_1 + \dots \qquad \dots\text{(I)}$$

Again integrating both sides

$$EI\,y = \frac{\cancel{3}x^3}{2\times\cancel{3}} - \frac{\langle x-4\rangle^4}{4\times3} + \frac{\langle x-7\rangle^4}{4\times3} + C_1 x + C_2 + \dots \qquad \dots\text{(II)}$$

B.C are at $x = 0, y = 0 \Rightarrow C_2 = 0$

at $x = 11, y = 0 \Rightarrow$ from Eq. (II)

$$0 = \frac{(11)^3}{2} - \frac{\langle 11-4\rangle^4}{12} + \frac{\langle 11-7\rangle^4}{12} + C_1 \times 11$$

$$C_1 = \frac{1}{11}\left[\frac{(7)^4}{12} - \frac{\langle 4\rangle^4}{12} + \frac{\langle 11\rangle^3}{2}\right]$$

$$= \frac{1}{11}\left[\frac{7^4 - 4^4 - 6\times11^3}{12}\right]$$

$$= \frac{1}{11}\times\left[\frac{49\times49 - 16\times16 - 121\times66}{12}\right] = (-)\,44.25$$

Now substituting the value of C_1 in Eq. (I), we get the equation of slope in terms of EI and substituting the value of C_1 in Eq. (II) we will get the equation of deflection in terms of EI.

Now

$$EIy = \frac{x^3}{2} - \frac{\langle x-4\rangle^4}{12} + \frac{\langle x-7\rangle^4}{12} - 44.25x$$

At middle of the beam deflection will be maximum

Middle of the beam = 4 + 1.5 = 5.5 m,

So at $x = 5.5$ m, we will get the maximum deflection

$$\therefore \quad EI\, y_{max} = \frac{5.5^3}{2} - \frac{(5.5-4)^4}{2} + 0 - 44.25 \times 5.5$$

$$\downarrow$$

(It is zero being negative)

$$= \frac{5.5^3}{2} - \frac{1.5^4}{2} - 243.375 = -162.71$$

$$\therefore \quad y_{max} = (-)\frac{1}{EI}162.71$$

Slope at A is θ_A, we put $x = 0$ in Eq. (I)

$$EI \cdot \theta_A = 0 + C_1$$

$$\therefore \qquad\qquad \theta_A = \frac{C_1}{EI}$$

$$= (-)\frac{44.25}{EI} \qquad \textbf{Ans.}$$

2. (b) $\left[\text{Hint: } \theta = \dfrac{T.l}{G_1 J_1 + G_2 J_2} \right]$

3. (c) See chapter—Shear stresses in beam – Solved problem.

4. (a) See chapter—Column and strut.

   (c) See chapter—Spring—Solved problem.

   (c) See chapter—Thick Cylinder—Problems on compound cylinder.

5. (a) See chapter—Curved beam—Trapezoidal section.

   (b) See chapter—Unsymmetrical bending, Product Moment of Inertia—Theory.

   (c) See the solved problem of Unsymmetrical Bending.